WITHDRAWN

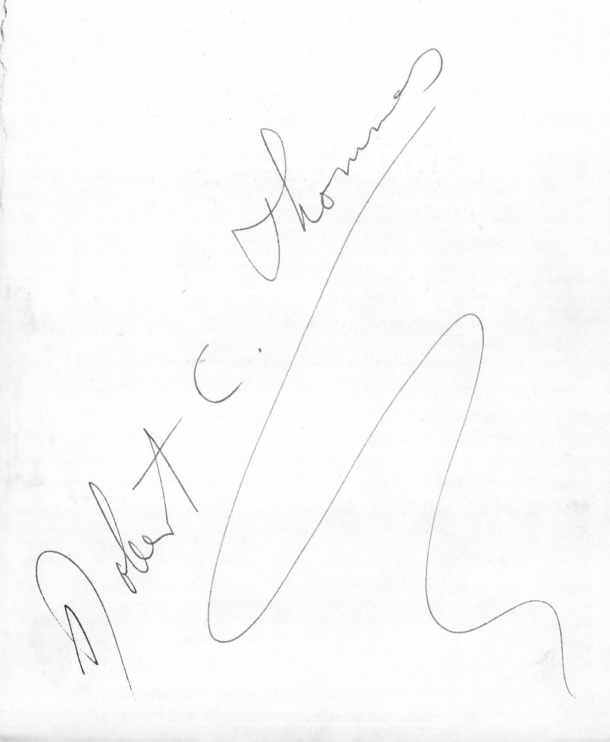

Essentials of CLINICAL ENDOCRINOLOGY

Essentials of CLINICAL ENDOCRINOLOGY

Norman G. Schneeberg, M.D.

*Clinical Professor of Medicine (Endocrinology and
Metabolism), Hahnemann Medical College and Hospital;
Head, Section of Endocrinology (Hahnemann), Philadelphia
General Hospital, Philadelphia, Pa.*

With 210 illustrations and 2 color plates

Saint Louis

The C. V. Mosby Company

1970

DEDICATION

To Helen, Susan, and Karen

Contributors

HARRY BANGHART, M.D.

Chief, Outpatient Service, Veterans Administration Hospital, Butler, Pa.

GORDON BENDERSKY, M.D.

Assistant Professor of Medicine, Hahnemann Medical College and Hospital, Philadelphia, Pa.

BERNARD A. ESKIN, M.S., M.D.

Clinical Assistant Professor of Obstetrics and Gynecology, Woman's Medical College of Pennsylvania; Chief, Endocrine Section, Division of Obstetrics and Gynecology, Albert Einstein Medical Center, Philadelphia, Pa.; Visiting Professor of Obstetrics and Gynecology, Rutgers Medical School, New Brunswick, N. J.

SUKHAMOY PAUL, M.D.

Resident in Endocrinology (1968 to 1969), Philadelphia General Hospital, Philadelphia, Pa.

RALPH A. SHAW, M.D., Ph.D.

Associate Professor of Medicine (Endocrinology and Metabolism), Hahnemann Medical College and Hospital, Philadelphia, Pa.

KEITH D. SMITH, M.D.

Associate Member, Division of Endocrinology and Reproduction, Research Laboratories; Adjunct, Section of Endocrinology and Metabolism, Albert Einstein Medical Center; Assistant Professor of Medicine, Temple University Medical Center, Philadelphia, Pa.

ANNA STEINBERGER, M.S., Ph.D.

Associate Member, Division of Endocrinology and Reproduction, Albert Einstein Medical Center, Philadelphia, Pa.

EMIL STEINBERGER, M.D.

Chairman, Division of Endocrinology and Reproduction, Research Laboratories; Attending Physician in Charge, Section of Endocrinology and Metabolism, Division of Medicine, Albert Einstein Medical Center; Associate Professor of Medicine, Temple University Medical Center, Philadelphia, Pa.

Preface

The increasing body of endocrine knowledge flows like a river, ever widening and becoming more voluminous as it progresses. The *Essentials of Clinical Endocrinology* strives to distill an aliquot of this knowledge to a presentable and digestible essence. It is designed for the student, the resident, and the practicing physician who are untutored in endocrine matters and who seek a didactic introduction or brief review of the subject. Clinical features are stressed, with particular emphasis on the practical aspects of therapy. No attempt is made to compete with the several available comprehensive endocrine texts; the book is not planned as a reference manual for endocrinologists or as a bibliographic repository. For the sake of brevity, references have been restricted to significant reviews and to literature either directly quoted or extremely pertinent. I make obeisance and sincere apologies to all of the omitted authors referred to as "et al." and to the numerous sources of information that must remain unacknowledged because of the exigencies of space. For the same reason several topics received short shrift and others, including endocrines and cancer, laboratory techniques, and several of the metabolic disorders of bone and of lipid metabolism, were completely omitted. At the time of the preparation of the chapters on the thyroid gland, the newly proposed nomenclature and classification (Werner, S. J.: J. Clin. Endocr. **29**:860, 1969) was not available.

It is a pleasure to acknowledge the advice and assistance of a number of colleagues and friends. Dr. Milton Tellum (deceased) and Dr. Alexander Nedwich of the Department of Pathology, Hahnemann Medical College, gave unstintingly of their time and expertise in the selection of gross and histologic specimens to be photographed and composed a pathologist's description of each. Dr. George Wohl, formerly Director of Radiology at the Philadelphia General Hospital, and Dr. Marvin Haskin of Hahnemann provided a number of the x-ray films. Dr. Lewis C. Mills and Dr. Allen Lewis read several chapters and gave advice and criticism. Dr. S. Leon Israel reviewed the chapter on female endocrinology, and Dr. Elliot Mancall read and criticized the chapter on neuroendocrinology. Dr. Sukhamoy Paul and Dr. Carlos Minnig, former residents in endocrinology of the Philadelphia General Hospital, were of great assistance. Mr. Joseph Poppel did most of the photography and Miss Marjory Stodgel made all the original drawings. The library staff of Hahnemann could always be depended on to find the unfindable. Mrs. Bernice Heller reviewed the final manuscript and made many necessary editorial corrections. All the rough and final copies were typed by Mrs. Ruth Davis. Apologies are due my co-authors, who so courteously masked their frustrations when their efforts were subjected to alterations and deletions.

Norman G. Schneeberg, M.D.

Contents

Color plates

Essentials of CLINICAL ENDOCRINOLOGY

Chapter 1

General principles of endocrinology

Endocrinology has been defined as "the study of the internal secretions." Claude Bernard first coined the term "internal secretions" in a lecture at the Collège de France in 1855. Until recent years, The Endocrine Society, an organization of American endocrinologists, was called "The Association for the Study of Internal Secretions." The word "hormone" (Greek *hormaō*, "I stir up") was suggested by W. B. Hardy and introduced by Bayliss and Starling. "Endocrine" literally means "to separate within" from Greek *endon*, "within," and *krinein*, "to separate."

The function of the endocrine system is to secrete intracellularly synthesized hormones into the circulation to be transported to nearby or distant sites of action. They serve as agents for the transfer of information from one set of cells to another for the good of the cell population as a whole. That they are effective in extraordinarily low concentration suggests that they function as stimulators, regulators, pacemakers, or catalysts of preexisting metabolic processes rather than as direct participants in biochemical reactions. They bear a close relationship to the more rapidly functioning regulator, the nervous system. Together these systems, endocrine and nervous, constitute a biologic communication network that serves to integrate the various physiologic functions of the organism, permitting and instituting alterations in its metabolism, behavior, and development to conform to external and internal environmental demands. A few hormones such as epinephrine and insulin act very rapidly, producing their effects in minutes, whereas most require a more prolonged interval to exert physiologic action.

The endocrine system consists of three components: (1) the endocrine cell that "sends" a specific chemical message to other cells, (2) the cell that "receives" the message, and (3) the environment through which this information is transported. In some instances the relationship is direct (first-order reaction), whereas in others the chemical message excites a second endocrine cell to transmit its chemical message to the final site of action, a tissue cell (second-order reaction). There is evidence to suggest that the chain of communication may be even more extensive (third-order reaction). Thus a hypothalamic neurosecretion may transmit its message to an anterior pituitary cell, which in turn secretes a trophic hormone. The latter stimulates the response of its target endocrine cell to secrete a hormone, which then attaches to a cellular receptor site and provokes an effect. Hormones may exert inhibitory rather than stimulatory effects (feedback control by target-cell secretion acting upon the anterior pituitary and/or hypothalamus) or may alter the physical and chemical state of a substance (TSH → thyroglobulin proteolysis). The action of one hormone may be altered or conditioned by another. For example, an excess of thyroid hormone increases the rate of adrenocortical hormone metabolism and may thus unmask adrenal insufficiency; it may increase the rate of insulin degradation and will thus be diabetogenic. An excess of insulin will trigger an outpouring of catecholamines from the adrenal medulla. Some hormones such as catecholamines, glucagon, and cortisol exhibit synergistic actions, whereas others such as GH or insulin and cortisol, and insulin versus cortisol or epinephrine show antagonistic actions. Hormones, after exerting their cellular effect, presumably are chemically transformed into metabolites by oxidation-reduction, conjugation, deiodination, or proteolysis. These reactions occur chiefly in the liver, to a lesser extent in the kidney, but also in other tissues and in the target cell. Metabolites have been viewed as inert by-products, but it is not inconceivable that they may exert some regulatory control upon hormone action.

The cell (end organ) receiving the chemical message may exhibit varying degrees of responsiveness to the hormonal signal. With extreme hormonal deprivation there is a state of hypersensitivity, whereas relative insensitivity may obtain if the cell has been flooded with the hormone. Specific hypersensitiveness is illustrated by the excessive hair follicle response to testosterone observed in dark-skinned females. Complete failure of end-organ response to parathyroid hormone occurs in pseudohypoparathyroidism and to vasopressin in nephrogenic diabetes insipidus. The sensitivity of certain target organs to the action of a specific hormone suggests that special receptor sites are present in tissue cells that may be likened to a key (the hormone) that fits certain locks (the target cell) and not others. Thus the characteristic biologic response is triggered in the sensitive tissue.

CHEMICAL NATURE OF HORMONES

1. *Steroids*—compounds derived from acetate and cholesterol having the basic cyclopentanoperhydrophenanthrene organic molecule
   a. *Adrenal cortex*—corticosteroids, aldosterone, androgens, estrogens, and progesterone
   b. *Testicle*—testosterone, estrogens
   c. *Ovary*—estrogens, progesterone
2. *Proteins* and *polypeptides* of varying size and complexity synthesized from amino acids; precise chemical configuration of only insulin, ACTH, and growth hormone known
   a. *Anterior pituitary*
      Large polypeptides—ACTH, GH, LTH, MSH
      Glycoproteins—protein + a carbohydrate group (TSH, FSH, LH)
   b. *Posterior pituitary*—octapeptides—vasopressin and oxytocin
   c. *Parathyroid*—parathyroid hormone
   d. *Thyroid*—thyroxine, triiodothyronine, thyrocalcitonin
3. *Low molecular weight amines*
   a. *Adrenal medulla* and *neurons (catecholamines)*—epinephrine and norepinephrine.

SYNTHESIS AND SECRETION OF HORMONES

For some endocrine tissues, particularly those secreting steroids, a great deal is known about the biosynthetic pathways, but little is known concerning the mechanisms of biosynthesis in many glands producing complex protein hormones. Most organs exhibit a basal level of secretion, show sporadic increases, and retain only small quantities of hormone, though the thyroid stores considerable pre-formed thyroxine. Secretion is not uniform but may display a circadian or diurnal rhythm (adrenocortical steroids), a cyclicity dependent on other events (estrogen, progesterone, and pituitary gonadotrophins), or dependence on a particular stimulus (insulin in response to elevation of blood sugar in the pancreatic artery). Certain hormones are released by stress (adrenocortical steroids and medullary catecholamines), by exposure of the organism to light stimulation (egg laying of hens), by coitus (ovulation of rabbits), or by suckling (lactation). Hormones may be stored in follicles in large quantities (thyroid) or in granules in small amounts (vasopressin, catecholamines).

TRANSPORT OF HORMONES

Blood, lymph, and extracellular fluids compose the transport phase, bearing hormones from the site of synthesis to sites of cellular action and ultimately to sites of metabolic inactivation and degradation. Plasma is not a passive diluent but provides specific proteins for binding and transport of circulating hormones. Bound hormone is biologically inactive and serves as a reservoir to liberate free hormone in minute quantities for diffusion into extracellular and intracellular phases.

MECHANISM OF HORMONE ACTION

The mechanism of hormonal action at the cellular or molecular level is unknown. Hormones constitute a chemical signal that stimulates a complex physiologic response. Obvious biologic effects of a hormone may be remote from its primary molecular action. Hormones may initiate a chain of events, only the last link being observable. The hormone secreted by a gland may require alteration before its biologic activity is established. Three-dimensional structural properties of a hormone may be fundamental to its physiologic activity. The interaction between hormone and tissue cell may involve specific groups on the hormone molecule with complementary groups on a cell macromolecule or "receptor." The receptor, or hormone-receptor combination, may initiate a series of secondary reactions giving rise to the characteristic response. Certain inklings as to the nature of the receptor have been forthcoming. One of the current theories of vasopressin action that may be applicable to other protein hormones is that the peptide SS group of vasopressin reacts with the SH group on a membrane receptor. The resulting disulfide bridge linking hormone and cellular membrane modifies the membrane, rendering it permeable to water (p. 21).

Four hypotheses have been offered to explain the action of hormones. None are mutually exclusive, and all may explain some fundamental characteristic of hormonal mechanisms.

The enzyme hypothesis

Since complex metabolic cellular reactions are basically enzymatic, it seems logical to account for hormone action, potent in such low concentrations, as one of enzyme control perhaps similar to the function of a catalyst. Hormones therefore alter, regulate, stimulate, or inhibit the rate and intensity of biochemical reactions by their control of enzymes. Biochemical reactions that are affected by hormones may nonetheless proceed, albeit at a much decelerated rate, even in the absence of the hormone. The completely thyroidectomized animal, for example, does not die in the absence of thyroid hormones but continues to exist at a subnormal metabolic rate. Hormones may alter or remove an enzyme inhibitor or stimulate an activator.

Cyclic 3′,5′-AMP (C-AMP) serves as such an activator or intermediary in a number of diverse hormonal reactions and has come to be recognized as a "second messenger" responsive to the hormone that is the first messenger. It is formed from its precursor ATP through the catalytic action of adenyl cyclase, an enzyme that is often located in cell membranes (Fig. 1-1). C-AMP is increased by several pituitary hormones (ACTH, TSH, LH, vasopressin) and by parathyroid hormone, catecholamines, and glucagon, whereas it is decreased by insulin. The cellular concentration of C-AMP rises or falls in response to the hormonal stimulus and sets off various appropriate physiologic responses within the cell, depending on the available mechanisms. For reviews, see Sutherland et al., 1968, and Butcher, 1968.

Enzymatic processes are dependent on

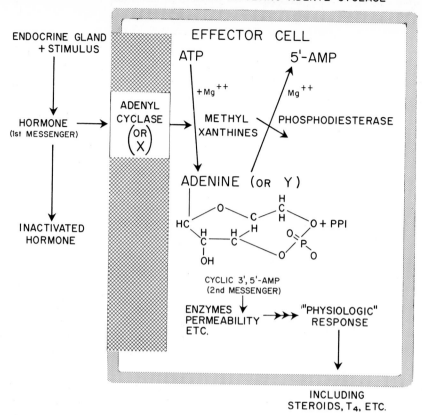

Fig. 1-1. Cyclic AMP, the "second messenger." (From Sutherland, E. W., et al.: Circulation **37**: 279, 1968, by permission of the American Heart Association, Inc.)

substrates, coenzymes, hydrogen ions, inorganic ions, the concentration and distribution of the enzyme, and certain intracellular structures such as mitochondria. Scores of enzyme systems have been shown to be affected or to interact with various hormones. However strongly the "enzyme hypothesis" may be defended, one must admit that the evidence in its favor remains far from being established. The strongest case has been made for a key role of C-AMP.

The cell-permeability hypothesis

Both insulin and ACTH exert clear-cut effects on *cellular* permeability, and attempts have been made to relate this phenomenon to subsequent intracellular enzymatic function (Hechter and Lester, 1960). The theory suggests that the primary action of hormones is on the cell membrane or on a specific receptor of the membrane and that subsequent metabolic transformations proceed thereafter without further hormonal influence. The reaction of hormonal sulfhydryl groups with cell-wall proteins, as previously discussed, may be implicated. The permeation of a substrate through the cell wall may constitute a signal that initiates subsequent reactions.

The "control of gene activity" hypothesis

The theory of control of gene activity is based on the observation that an insect steroid hormone called ecdysone is involved in the control of insect molting and metamorphosis (Karlson and Sekeris, 1966). Ecdysone has been shown to enter the cell nucleus and to produce "puffs" or other evidences of gene activation indicative of the synthesis of specific messenger ribonucleic acid (mRNA) from DNA. mRNA is then transferred from the nucleus to the cytoplasm and combines with ribosomes to produce "polysomes." Other hormones, particularly steroids as well as GH, ACTH, and thyroxine, have been shown to stimulate mRNA synthesis, but this stimulation may not be the primary reaction. The rat uterus shows an increase in blood flow within 30 seconds after administration of estrogen, but new RNA synthesis occurs 1 hour later and new protein synthesis 2 hours later. The same time lag is noted after corticosteroid injections when RNA synthesis occurs long after an increase in liver blood flow (van Overbeck, 1966).

The cytoskeleton (cytostructural) hypothesis

The electron microscope revolutionized our knowledge of the structure of the cell. The cell is now visualized as a complexity of structures all interconnected by a canal-like system penetrating the cytoplasm from cell surface to and including the nucleus. The structure, spatial relationships, macromolecular assemblages, electron interactions, and ionic constituents may be altered or reoriented by hormonal action. The hormone-receptor complex, formed at the cell surface, can thus spread through the subcellular structures, changing the molecular and electronic orientation of the cellular proteins. This thesis has been developed primarily by Hechter and his associates, who found that insulin significantly modified the structure of muscle (Hechter and Halkerston, 1964).

INACTIVATION, DEGRADATION, AND EXCRETION OF HORMONES

Hormones are inactivated by various mechanisms prior to excretion. In many instances the transformations facilitate excretion by rendering the hormone soluble in urine. The metabolic cycle of anterior pituitary hormones is in the main unknown, but there is evidence that they are metabolized or inactivated by their target organ (TSH by thyroid gland, etc.). The liver is the prime organ of degradation for many hormones; the kidney and other tissues may contribute. Thyroxine, for example, is deiodinated, deaminated, and conjugated primarily by the liver and to a certain extent by the kidney. Adrenal corticosteroids are reduced in the liver to water-soluble tetrahydro compounds, cortoles, and cortolones and are excreted as glucuronides and sulfate conjugates.

In addition to hormones secreted by recognized endocrine glands, a number of other humoral substances are secreted by various tissues into the circulation and have been the subject of controversy as to whether they should be labeled true hormones. These include gastrin, enterogastrone, secretin, cholecystokinin, and pancreozymin from the gastrointestinal tract; renin, angiotensin, and erythropoietin from the kidney; and relaxin from the placenta. Glomerulokinin is a hypothetical hormone that is thought to be responsible for the diurnal cycle of glomerular filtration rate. The prostaglandins are compounds of prostanoic acid found in human seminal plasma and other tissues that exhibit vasodepressor, smooth muscle-stimulating, and certain metabolic effects.

SOME IMPORTANT GENERAL CONSIDERATIONS RELATING TO THE DIAGNOSIS AND TREATMENT OF ENDOCRINE DISORDERS

1. Clear-cut endocrinopathies (myxedema, Addison's disease, hypopituitarism) have often been overlooked for years because of their relative rarity and the unfamiliarity of physicians with their manifestations. Psychoneurotic patients are often mistakenly thought to be suffering from an endocrine disorder and often unnecessarily receive protracted treatment with hormones. Pseudohypothyroidism is the most prevalent example.

2. Most endocrine disorders are fairly

clear-cut and not difficult to diagnose by those familiar with them. Borderline cases, however, do exist because evidence of deficiency may become noticeable only when a large part of a gland has been destroyed. Immediate diagnosis in most cases is not critical. A period of further observation will permit the disorder to flower to recognizable proportions. It is preferable, except in emergency situations, to make a definite diagnosis before instituting treatment, though therapeutic trials, if properly conducted, may be informative.

3. The patient suffering from an endocrine gland deficiency is quite sensitive to replacement therapy even in small doses. The response is almost invariably dramatic, leaves little doubt as to its efficacy, and is maintained. The neurasthenic patient responds equivocally and benefits are often temporary. In such instances the physician may find himself successively augmenting the dose of hormone replacement in a vain attempt to repeat the initial response.

4. There are a host of disorders commonly thought to be endocrine in origin by the uninitiated but usually found to be due to developmental defects, familial or genetic faults, or emotional disorders. These include mongolism, Laurence-Moon-Biedl syndrome, progeria, Werner's syndrome, etc. and are discussed in Chapter 25. Homosexuality, most cases of impotency, obesity, and alopecia totalis are not endocrine disorders.

REFERENCES

Baulieu, E. E.: A 1966 critical survey of steroid hormone metabolism. In Martini, L., Fraschini, F., and Motta, M., editors: International Congress on Hormonal Steroids, proceedings of the second congress, Milan, May 23-28, 1966, Amsterdam, 1967, Excerpta Medica Foundation, International congress ser. no. 133, p. 37.

*Butcher, R. W.: New Eng. J. Med. **279**:1378, 1968.

Haynes, R. C., Jr., et al.: Recent Progr. Hormone Res. **16**:121, 1960.

Hechter, O., and Halkerston, I. D. K.: On the action of mammalian hormones. In Pincus, G., Thimann, K. V., and Astwood, E. B., editors: The hormones, physiology, chemistry and applications, vol. 5, New York, 1964, Academic Press, Inc., p. 697.

Hechter, O., and Lester, G.: Recent Progr. Hormone Res. **16**:139, 1960.

Karlson, P., and Sekeris, C. E.: Recent Progr. Hormone Res. **22**:473, 1966.

Schwartz, I. L., and Hechter, O.: Amer. J. Med. **40**:765, 1966.

*Sutherland, E. W., et al.: Circulation **37**:279, 1968.

van Overbeck, J.: Science **152**:721, 1966.

*Significant reviews.

Chapter 2

Neuroendocrinology, the hypothalamus, and the pineal gland

The endocrine and nervous systems are closely allied, exerting reciprocal influences as they serve as regulators of bodily functions and of homeostatic mechanisms. Neuroendocrine control is centrally rather than peripherally maintained. The axis of this control is CNS → hypothalamus → anterior pituitary → target gland. Hypothalmic neurons possess nervous and secretory functions and elaborate humoral agents. Neural connections of the hypothalamus are complex and numerous, providing a rich network of neural circuits connecting ascending cord and bulbar tracts and descending tracts from the cortex and thalamus. Impulses reaching the hypothalamus are transferred via internuclear connections and discharged to autonomic and motor centers.

Fig. 2-1 is a simplified diagram of some of the neural connections and pathways carrying stimuli from higher cerebral centers (cortex, midbrain, rhinencephalon) to hypothalamic nuclei and the pituitary. Pathologic involvement of these tracts may cause disturbances of hypothalamic–anterior pituitary function. For example, bilateral fornix section in the monkey disrupts the diurnal variation of urinary corticoids, and lesions of the diencephalon and midbrain in the cat reduce the adrenal secretion of aldosterone and cortisol. Patients with localized pretectal-area or temporal-lobe disease exhibit abnormal patterns of corticotrophic regulation of the diurnal pattern of plasma corticoids. Bilateral amygdala destruction has been reputed to produce thyroid atrophy when performed early in life. Removal of portions of the hippocampus and amygdala produced hypersexuality and abnormal sexual behavior. Stimulation of the amygdala produced ovulation in the rabbit.

The three large afferent tracts are shown in Fig. 2-1. Important *efferent* pathways are the following:

1. Hypothalamic nuclei to midbrain in tegmentum vagus area and spinal cord (motor for cholinergic and adrenergic fibers of autonomic nervous system and for secretion of epinephrine by adrenal medulla)
2. Mammillothalamic tract—mammillary body to dorsomedial nucleus of thalamus and anterior nucleus; relays to mesopallium concerned with visceral and emotional feelings and to neocortex with maintenance of alert wakefulness
3. Hypothalamohypophysial system

HYPOTHALAMIC FUNCTIONS

1. Contributes to regulation of blood pressure, heart rate, body temperature, respiration, pilomotor function, sleep-waking, mood reactions, emotional tone (rage, fear), pupillary size
2. Contributes to regulation of gastrointestinal peristalsis (increase or decrease) and urinary bladder contraction; correlates visceral and olfactory impulses

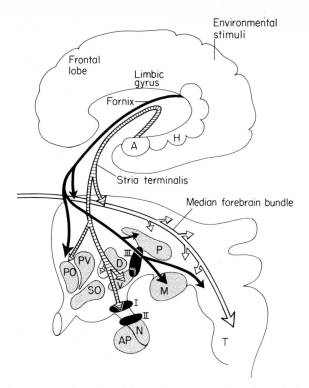

Fig. 2-1. Hypothalamus and main telencephalic connections. Hypothalamic lesions producing neuroendocrine syndromes, as described in text, are labeled **I, II,** and **III. A,** Amygdala; **AP,** anterior pituitary; **H,** hippocampus; **N,** neurohypophysis; **T,** tegmentum. *Hypothalamic nuclei:* **D,** Dorsomedial; **M,** mammillary; **P,** posterior; **PO,** preoptic; **PV,** paraventricular; **SO,** supraoptic; **V,** ventromedial. (Modified from Gloor, P.: Telencephalic influences upon the hypothalamus. In Fields, W. S., editor: Hypothalamic-hypophysial interrelationships, Springfield, Ill., 1956, Charles C Thomas, Publisher.)

3. Regulation of food intake—bilateral destruction of small area in extreme lateral portion of lateral hypothalamus in rats and cats leads to cessation of eating (feeding center); unilateral electrical stimulation provokes increased food intake; mechanism of hypothalamic effects on feeding unknown

4. Production of neurohormonal anterior pituitary–stimulating factors (releasors, releasing factors)

5. Production of neurohypophysial hormones (oxytocin, vasopressin)

ANATOMY OF HYPOTHALAMUS

The hypothalamus is a small structure (weight, about 4 grams) situated in the ventral diencephalon, divided by the third ventricle into right and left halves. Its bounds are indistinctly defined, and its anatomic relationships are extraordinarily complex. Dorsally lies the thalamus; ventrally the tuber cinereum and infundibulum; anteriorly the anterior commissure, lamina terminalis, and optic chiasm; and posteriorly the interpeduncular fossa. The hypothalamic nuclei are more or less distinct cellular conglomerations arranged in groups (Fig. 2-1). The supraoptic and paraventricular are the most easily identified in man. The paired supraoptic nuclei are over the lateral portion of the optic tract, and the paraventricular are contiguous to the third ventricle. The *median eminence* comprises the central portion of the tuber cinereum, is continuous with and forms the upper part of the infundibular stem and neurohypophysis, and forms the

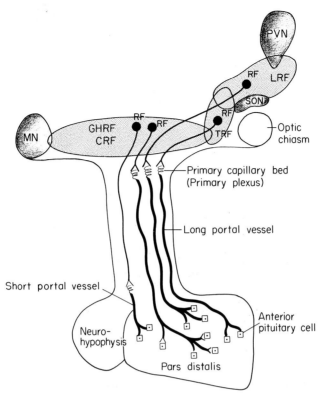

Fig. 2-2. Theoretical sites of origin of releasing factors (RF) and the hypothalamo–anterior pituitary portal circulation. **CRF,** Corticotrophin-releasing factor; **GHRF,** growth hormone-releasing factor; **LRF,** luteinizing hormone–releasing factor; **MN,** mammillary nucleus; **PVN,** paraventricular nucleus; **SON,** supraoptic nucleus; **TRF,** thyrotrophin-releasing factor. (Modified from Adams, J. H.: Brit. Med. J. **2:**1619, 1964; from Baker, B. L.: In Crosby, E. C., Humphrey, T., and Lauer, E. W.: Correlative anatomy of the nervous system, New York, 1962, The Macmillan Co.)

base of the hypothalamus and floor of the third ventricle.

HYPOPHYSIAL PORTAL CIRCULATION

The median eminence of the hypothalamus and the infundibular stem contain a rich capillary bed, or primary plexus, that is fed by branches of the superior hypophysial arteries. The primary plexus contains elaborate capillary tufts and spike formations (Fig. 2-2). Linking the hypothalamus and anterior pituitary is a collection of portal vessels that take origin in the primary plexus, form vascular trunks that traverse the hypophysial stalk in parallel fashion, and divide into a large sinusoidal capillary bed in the anterior

pituitary parenchyma. Long portal vessels traverse the anterior surface of the stalk, and short portal vessels originate in the lower infundibular stem below the diaphragma sellae (Fig. 2-2). The portal trunks are noncontractile (Worthington, 1960), but a variety of stimuli markedly alter the rate of blood flow by inducing dilatation or constriction of the arterioles of the primary plexus.

Stalk section leads to anterior pituitary insufficiency, provided vascular regeneration is prevented by placing a barrier between the cut ends of the stalk. The short portal vessels do not provide sufficient circulation to salvage more than a minimum of the adenohypophysis when the long portal vessels are completely severed. Electrical stimulation of the hypothalamus evokes an appropriate adenohypophysial response only if the stalk is intact. Similar stimulation directly to the adenohypophysis fails to elicit trophic hormone release, showing the dependence of its secretions on the hypothalamus. Pituitary tissue cultures exhibit increased production of ACTH, GH, and TSH when hypothalamic extracts are added. Vascular links between the pars distalis and the pars nervosa that may transmit neurohypophysial hormones to the anterior pituitary have been identified.

SECRETION OF HYPOTHALAMUS

The hypothalamus is a rich source of a number of pharmacologically active compounds including serotonin, histamine, sympathin (norepinephrine plus epinephrine), acetylcholine, gamma-aminobutyric acid, substance P (smooth-muscle activator), oxytocin, lysine and arginine vasopressin, alpha-MSH, and beta-MSH.

Releasing factors (RF)

In addition, neurohormones are elaborated by neuroendocrine cells in the median eminence and upper pituitary stalk. Their axons terminate in the region of convoluted vessels of a primary capillary bed (primary plexus) as illustrated in Fig. 2-2, from which the hypophysial portal vessels originate. The direction of blood flow proceeds from the hypothalamus to the pars distalis. The current chemotransmitter hypothesis visualizes these neurohormones being conveyed along the following pathway: axon → primary capillary bed → portal vessel → anterior pituitary cell. The neurohormones are called "releasing factors" (RF) because they stimulate the release of anterior pituitary trophic hormones. They may also regulate the biosynthesis of the trophic hormones and can maintain the morphology, differentiation, and function of pituitary grafts (Reichlin, 1966). RF's are named after the trophic hormone whose release they control. Currently RF's for ACTH (CRF), GH (GRF or SRF), TSH

(TRF), FSH (FRF or FSH-RF), LH (LRF or LHRF), and MSH (MRF or MSH-RF) have been identified, as well as inhibitors for MSH and prolactin in human and animal hypothalamic tissues. TRF, CRF, and LRF have been isolated from the portal circulation, and several RF preparations have been administered to humans, with evidence of the release of the appropriate pituitary trophic hormone.

The control of prolactin secretion is fundamentally different from that of other anterior pituitary hormones. Various influences that interfere with the production of ACTH, TSH, FSH, LH, and GH promote increased secretion of prolactin. The central nervous system exerts inhibitory control upon prolactin by means of a *prolactin-inhibiting factor* (PIF). It has been suggested, on the basis of experiments in rabbits, that a single hypothalamic factor may both inhibit prolactin release and stimulate LH secretion. In young animals a hypothalamic center has been identified with the release of FSH before puberty. Lesions in this area may delay the onset of puberty. The pineal body may also exert an inhibiting control upon sexual maturation.

Releasing factors respond to appropriate and various stimuli and may be inhibited by target organ hormones (that is, feedback control). One of the important regulators of RF release is the target organ hormone itself, which, having been elaborated under RF stimulation, may in turn inhibit RF secretion, thus comprising a feedback control or servomechanism analogous to the effect of room temperature on the thermostatic control of a heating system (Fig. 2-3). There is also evidence to suggest that feedback control, particularly with respect to the thyroid gland, may be exerted directly on the pituitary. CRF responds to stress and to vasopressin and is inhibited by cortisol. A short or "internal feedback" circuit has been proposed whereby anterior pituitary hormones themselves act upon hypothalamic neurons. An inverse relationship has been suggested between ACTH and TSH secretions; TRF

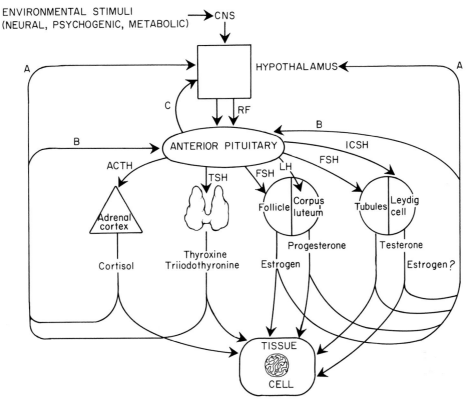

Fig. 2-3. Feedback control from target glands shown in **A** to the hypothalamus, **B** to the anterior pituitary, and **C** from anterior pituitary to hypothalamus. Only the adrenal cortex, thyroid, and gonads are shown to illustrate the relationship. **ACTH,** Adrenocorticotrophin; **FSH,** follicle-stimulating hormone; **ICSH,** interstitial cell–stimulating hormone; **LH,** luteinizing hormone; **RF** releasing factor; **TSH,** thyrotrophin.

stimulates the secretion of TSH and appears to inhibit ACTH, whereas inhibition of ACTH promotes greater amounts of TSH in response to TRF.

There are probably distinct locales of origin in separate hypothalamic regions for each RF (Fig. 2-2). Attempts to specifically localize these areas must be viewed as conjectural, particularly since this concept is challenged by investigators who believe that hypothalamic control is more diffuse. Adams et al., 1966, proposed that the individual portal vascular links from hypothalamus to anterior pituitary appeared to be strictly circumscribed, a finding that suggested that a particular RF might be transported by an individual portal vessel to a specific small group of anterior pituitary cells. It has been proposed (Mess et al., 1967) that some or all

RF secretions may arise outside the hypothalamus and be stored in the median eminence. By stimulation, destruction, and grafting experiments, various workers have tentatively, and with numerous reservations, assigned TRF to an area behind and above the optic chiasm in the rostral half of the hypothalamus, gonadotrophins (FRF, LRF) to an area extending from the TSH area posteriorly at the infundibulum to the mammillary nuclei, and both CRF and GRF to the middle and anterior regions of the median eminence between TRF and gonadotrophin-RF (Fig. 2-2).

The concept of a simple feedback system whereby the concentration of target organ hormone circulating through the hypothalamic centers regulates the elaboration of the releasing factors (Fig. 2-3) may be subject to various modifying factors that make the feedback mechanism more complex than was originally conceived. Gonadotrophin secretion, for example, is influenced not only by the concentration of circulating gonadal steroids but also by environmental stimuli. Copulation induces ovulation, and light may alter the estrus cycle of certain species. The complexity of neuroendocrine feedback influences is illustrated by experiments showing that manipulation of the hormone milieu of newborn animals may profoundly and permanently affect their subsequent biologic functioning. For example, thyroxine administration to the newborn rat permanently suppressed thyroid functioning (Bakke and Lawrence, 1966).

TRF, the first hypothalamic hormone to be identified chemically, is a simple compound consisting of three amino acids— glutamic acid, histidine, and proline (Burgus et al., 1969; Bøler, et al., 1969). A peptide that contains the amino acids of alpha-MSH plus alanine, threonine, and leucine, named alpha-1-CRF, has been separated from hypothalamic extracts rich in CRF activity. Beta-CRF, considered to be the true physiologic CRF, is an analogue of vasopressin and contains all the amino acids of lysine vasopressin, together with serine and histidine. Another compound isolated from hog pituitaries is designated alpha-2-CRF and bears similarities to alpha-MSH.

For reviews of RF, see Reichlin, 1963, 1966; Greep, 1963; and Guillemin, 1964.

HYPOTHALAMIC DISORDERS

The hypothalamus and its connecting pathways can be the site of a variety of pathologic states. Some may be due to specific space-taking lesions, whereas others cannot be defined pathologically but are presumed to be due to deranged neuroendocrine function.

Specific organic lesions involving hypothalamus or its afferent or efferent pathways

These disorders may be tumors or vascular (aneurysms, A-V communications), inflammatory, or degenerative lesions. Among 60 autopsied cases reported by Bauer, 1954, 4 were caused by craniopharyngiomas, 8 astrocytomas, 5 hyperplasias (congenital malformations), 4 infundibulomas, and 3 pinealomas. The remainder were represented by a variety of neoplastic lesions. Among the *inflammatory lesions* were 7 cases of encephalomeningitis or encephalitis, and among the *degenerative lesions* was 1 case each of tuberous sclerosis and arteriosclerotic degeneration. Aneurysms of the internal carotid artery may simulate a pituitary tumor. Internal hydrocephalus due to obstruction of the duct of Sylvius and tumors of the third ventricle may impinge upon or compress the hypothalamus.

Table 2-1. Hypothalamus-linked symptoms and signs; incidence and frequency of occurrence as first manifestation of hypothalamic disease (60 cases)*

Hypothalamus-linked symptoms and signs	*Number of cases*	*Number of cases appearing as first manifestations*
Sexual abnormalities		
Precocious puberty 24 }	43	21
Hypogonadism 19 }		
Diabetes insipidus	21	2
Psychic disturbances	21	7
Somnolence	18	6
Obesity	15	1
Thermodysregulation	13	4
Emaciation	11	2
Convulsions (automatic crises)	9	1
Disturbances of sphincteric control (urinary, rectal)	5	0
Bulimia	5	2
Anorexia	4	0
Dyshidrosis	4	0

*From Bauer, H. G.: Endocrine and other clinical manifestations of hypothalamic disease, J. Clin. Endocr. 14:13, 1954.

The resulting neuroendocrine syndromes cause varying combinations of endocrine and neurologic disorders suggesting adenohypophysial involvement, disordered antidiuretic hormone production, or more diffuse involvement of the afferent tracts.

The most common disturbances are precocious puberty or hypogonadism found in 24 and 19 of 60 cases, respectively (see Table 2-1 and Bauer, 1954).

Infundibular and pituitary stalk lesions

High lesions (at level of median eminence) (Fig. 2-1, *I*) involve all neurosecretory axons, may involve the nuclei, and may disrupt most pathways from hypothalamus to both anterior and posterior pituitary. There is loss of all or most RF's and vasopressin-oxytocin. The clinical picture combines adenohypophysial insufficiency and diabetes insipidus.

Low lesions (junction of pituitary stalk and pituitary) (Fig. 2-1, *II*) affect all hypophysial portal vessels except the short branches taking origin below the diaphragma sellae and, because the sole blood supply of the pars distalis is from the portal circulation, they may produce infarction of the adenohypophysis. The hypothalamus–posterior pituitary neural links are not as likely to be involved. Surgical stalk section will produce "low lesions." The clinical picture is that of more or less adenohypophysial insufficiency; the lower the section, the more profound the insufficiency. Diabetes insipidus will be absent or mild because the hypothalamic nuclei of ADH origin (p. 16) will release their secretions into the general circulation without being completely dependent on the stored ADH of the neurohypophysis.

Parainfundibular lesions

Lesions near the infundibulum, that is, parainfundibular (Fig. 2-1, *III*) (Rothballer, 1966), do not impinge upon the hypothalamic-hypophysial pathways, and the resulting clinical picture is less well defined. Precocious puberty is one of the more common syndromes seen in lesions behind the median eminence. Disturbances of feedback control, as demonstrated by abnormal responses to dexamethasone suppression or to the metyrapone test for endogenous ACTH secretion, may be demonstrated occasionally.

Intrahypothalamic lesions

Though the area of the hypothalamus is quite small ("the size of the terminal phalanx of a grown man's thumb"—Bauer, 1954), lesions within its substance produce syndromes of markedly varying patterns that defy attempts at classification. This variation is a consequence of the numerous functions under hypothalamic control. Lesions are rarely confined to a focus or to one nucleus. Any combination of disturbances of the known functions of the hypothalamus may occur. There may be loss of one or more RF's, producing partial or complete anterior pituitary hypofunction, of which hypogonadism is the most common expression. Loss of an inhibitor, such as prolactin-inhibiting factor, may result in galactorrhea, or loss of a hypothetical gonadotrophin inhibitor may result in precocious puberty. Obesity or cachexia, somnolence, diabetes insipidus, disturbance of sleep control, hypothermia, convulsions, rage, and expressions of loss of emotional control may occur alone or in various combinations.

Diffuse cerebral lesions

Cerebral lesions are not well defined, but various neurologic disturbances such as congenital brain disorders, temporal lobe lesions, epilepsy, and brain trauma have been described.

Nonspecific and presumed hypothalamic lesions

Patients presenting neuroendocrine syndromes in whom no organic lesion is demonstrable must be classified as "nonspecific" or of "presumed hypothalamic origin." Any of the disorders listed as "specific organic lesions" in which no organic pathology is demonstrable may be so classified. Thus adenohypophysial hypofunction, in which no intrasellar lesion is found at surgery or autopsy, may be of hypothalamic origin.

Laboratory studies of hypothalamic disease

There are no specific laboratory tests of hypothalamic function. Studies related to the diagnosis of diabetes insipidus will be discussed in Chapter 3. Loss of the normal diurnal pattern of plasma corticosteroid concentration is the most common abnormality. The second most frequently distorted response is the secretion of GH after insulin hypoglycemia. The availability of potent RF-extracts in the future should provide the best means of estimating hypothalamic insufficiency.

THE PINEAL GLAND

The pineal gland of fish and amphibians contains sensory cells that resemble retinal cone cells and can convert light waves into nervous impulses. It was theorized that this "third eye" became an ultimately calcified vestigial organ in mammals. Nonetheless, it was recognized for years that delayed or precocious puberty was not infrequently associated with a pineal tumor, though it was believed that its effects depended on pressure or irritation of the posterior hypothalamus or to alteration of cerebrospinal fluid pressure. Kitay, 1954, later described a correlation between delayed puberty, particularly in girls, and parenchymatous pineal tumors, whereas nonparenchymatous lesions that destroyed the pineal, such as gliomas or teratomas, appeared to correlate best with precocious puberty. Thus pineal hyperfunction produced delayed puberty, and pineal hypofunction caused precocious puberty, changes that could well be explained by a hypothetical pineal hormone that exerted an inhibitory influence on gonadal function.

In 1917 McCord and Allen found that bovine pineal extracts blanched frog skin, and in 1958 Lerner et al. isolated the active principle that contracted the pig-

ment granules in melanocytes and called it *melatonin*. The biosynthesis of this hormone and the description of many of its physiologic actions has been the work of Wurtman, Axelrod et al., 1969, who found that it depended on the methylation of serotonin and other indoles under the enzymatic control of hydroxyindole-O-methyl transferase (HIOMT), an enzyme found only in the pineal gland. The activity of HIOMT and the regulation of melatonin synthesis is controlled by environmental lighting. In experimental animals kept in a continuous-light environment, the pineal gland was small and contained little HIOMT and melatonin in contrast to animals kept in the dark, in whom HIOMT and melatonin synthesis was increased. Under normal conditions of alternating light and dark, there is a diurnal rhythm of melatonin production. Thus the pineal serves as a transducer for converting environmental lighting into an endocrine message. Exposure to constant light accelerates the induction of estrus and increases the fraction of time that the animal spends in estrus. Animals kept in darkness spend more time in diestrus, and their ovaries grow at a slower initial rate. Blind girls experience menarche at a younger age than their light-perceiving sisters. The pineal and brain have no direct neural connections. Light impulses are transmitted from the retina by an unknown route to the superior sympathetic cervical ganglia and thence via postganglionic fibers to the parenchymal cells of the pineal.

The physiologic role of the pineal and of melatonin and related hormones remains unknown. They appear to exert a significant effect on gonadal function, serve to antagonize melanocyte-stimulating hormone (MSH), and act on neurons of the central nervous system that utilize serotonin, the precursor of melatonin, and their neurotransmitter. They are probably the mechanism that transmits information about environmental light-dark cycles in the regulation of other neuroendocrine functions. For recent reviews, see Wurtman et al., 1969, and Relkin, 1966.

REFERENCES

Adams, J. H., et al.: Brit. Med. J. **2**:1619, 1964.

Adams, J. H., et al.: Neuroendocrinology **1**: 193, 1965-1966.

Bakke, J. L., and Lawrence, N.: J. Lab. Clin. Med. **67**:477, 1966.

Bauer, H. G.: J. Clin. Endocr. **14**:13, 1954.

Bøler, J., et al.: Biochem. Biophys. Res. Commun. **37**:705, 1969.

Burgus, R., et al.: C. R. Acad. Sci. (Paris), t. 268, **14**:2116, 1969.

Crosby, E. C., Humphrey, T., and Lauer, E. W.: Correlative anatomy of the nervous system, New York, 1962, The Macmillan Co., p. 314.

Gloor, P.: Telencephalic influences upon the hypothalamus. In Hypothalamic-hypophysial interrelationships, Springfield, Ill., 1956, Charles C Thomas, Publisher, p. 75.

*Greep, R. O.: Architecture of the final common pathway to the adenohypophysis, Fertil. Steril. **14**:163, 1963.

*Guillemin, R.: Hypothalamic factors releasing pituitary hormones, Record Progr. Hormone Res. **20**:89, 1964.

Kitay, J. I.: J. Clin. Endocr. **14**:622, 1954.

Lerner, A. B., et al.: J. Amer. Chem. Soc. **80**: 2587, 1958.

McCord, C. P., and Allen, F. P.: J. Exp. Zool. **23**:207, 1917.

Mess, B., et al.: The topography of the neurons synthesizing the hypothalamic releasing factors. In Martini, M., Fraschini, F., and Motta, M., editors: International Congress on Hormonal Steroids, proceedings of the second congress, Milan, May 23-28, 1966, Amsterdam, 1967, Excerpta Medica Foundation, International Congress ser. no. 132, p. 1004.

*Reichlin, S.: New Eng. J. Med. **269**:1182, 1246, 1296, 1963; **275**:600, 1966.

*Relkin, R.: New Eng. J. Med. **274**:944, 1966.

*Rothballer, A. B.: Bull. N. Y. Acad. Med. **42**: 257, 1966.

Scharrer, E., and Scharrer, B.: Neuroendocrinology, New York, 1963, Columbia University Press.

Worthington, W. C., Jr.: Endocrinology **66**:19, 1960.

*Wurtman, R. J., et al.: The pineal, New York, 1969, Academic Press, Inc.

*Significant reviews.

Chapter 3

The neurohypophysis (posterior pituitary gland) and diabetes insipidus

NEURAL PATHWAYS TO THE NEUROHYPOPHYSIS

The neurohypophysis originates as an invagination of the neural ectoderm in the floor of the third ventricle and is therefore a direct continuum of the nervous system. The *hypothalamo-neurohypophysial system* is composed of at least two paired hypothalamic nuclei, the *supraoptic* (S.O.) and paraventricular (P.V.), the *median eminence*, the *infundibular stem (pituitary stalk)*, and the *neurohypophysis (posterior pituitary, infundibular process, or pars neuralis*—Fig. 3-1). The nuclei are located in the anterior ventral hypothalamus, are sharply defined, richly vascularized, and composed of thousands of large, often bipolar, deeply staining cells. The S.O. nuclei are the larger and straddle the lateral portion of the optic chiasm. The P.V. nuclei are broad, flat, vertical plates that occupy a portion of the wall of the third ventricle. The *supraoptico-hypophysial tract* is made up of thousands of axons of these nuclei traversing the infundibular stem and terminating in the neurohypophysis as branches in close relationship to capillaries. A smaller tubero-hypophysial tract takes origin from small- to medium-sized, poorly staining cells in the tuber cinereum.

NEUROSECRETION

The highly specialized neurons of the S.O. and P.V. nuclei secrete small granules *(neurosecretory granules)* that are transported by axoplasmic flow along the axons of the hypothalamo-neurohypophysial tract and accumulate in bulbous axon terminals on the basement membranes of capillaries of the posterior pituitary (Fig. 3-1, *B*). Granules containing vasopressin (ADH) have been separated from those containing oxytocin (O), and it has been postulated that the two hormones originate from separate neurons situated in distinct hypothalamic areas and are released independently. ADH may originate principally in the S.O., and oxytocin may originate in the P.V. nuclei. The posterior pituitary is not an endocrine gland in the strict sense, therefore, but serves as a reservoir for the discharge of hormones into the systemic circulation under the stimulus of the hypothalamic nuclei. The final liberation of the hormone may be from an action potential arriving at the terminus of the neuron releasing a transmitter such as acetylcholine, which provokes the release of ADH and/or oxytocin.

The neurosecretory granules consist of oxytocin and ADH specifically bound to a protein carrier (neurophysine). This peptide-neurophysine complex is dissociated prior to release, and free hormone is secreted into the circulation. The granule is surrounded by a membrane, and the released hormones pass through the membrane, the cell wall, and the capillary endothelium, leaving an empty synaptic

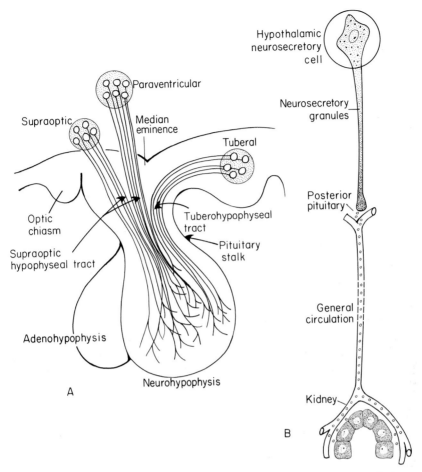

Fig. 3-1. Schematic diagram of the neurohypophysial tracts. **A,** Nuclei and fiber tracts. **B,** Diagram of a single neuron showing neurosecretory granules flowing down the axon fiber to be discharged into the circulation and thence to the renal tubule. (Modified from Scharrer, E.: Arch. Anat. Micr. Morph. Exp. **54:**359, 1965.)

vessel behind. The axon terminals are in proximity to the capillary basement membranes and are separated from the capillary lumen by a connective-tissue extracellular space, by the capillary basement membrane, and by the endothelium.

When the infundibular stalk is transected, granules accumulate proximal to and disappear distal to the section. A high section induces neuronal degeneration and permanent diabetes insipidus (D.I.), whereas a low transection or removal of the posterior pituitary gland does not. Water deprivation rapidly depletes the granular content of the entire neurohypo-

physial tract; rehydration promotes a reaccumulation of the neurosecretory granules.

HORMONAL RELEASE

Sachs and Haller, 1968, proposed that 10% to 20% of the total neurohypophysial ADH is in a "readily releasable" pool and that subsequent secretion takes place at a greatly reduced rate. There is no apparent control for the selective release of ADH and oxytocin. Both are frequently secreted simultaneously under the influence of a variety of stimuli, though certain physiologic changes favor a degree of selectivity (that is, hemorrhage—ADH predominates; suckling—oxytocin predominates). During late pregnancy and in the puerperium, the two hormones are released independently.

Osmotic receptors. Increased osmotic concentration of plasma produced by saline administration or water deprivation promotes ADH and oxytocin secretion and thus antidiuresis, uterine contractions, and milk ejection. Hypotonic saline inhibits ADH secretion and induces diuresis. An increase in the calcium content of neurohypophysial tissue promotes hormonal release. The osmoreceptors are probably located in the diencephalon and/or along the course of the internal carotid artery.

Volume receptors. Volume receptors are sensitive to changes in blood volume and to stretching-contracting of blood vessel walls, especially in the thoracic cavity (left atrium, intrapericardial pulmonary veins), and initiate, via the vagus nerves, afferent neural stimuli that may contribute to the regulation of hormone release. A decrease in carotid and perhaps aortic arterial pressure, a fall in cardiac output or extracellular or intrathoracic volume may stimulate a release of ADH, whereas the reverse of these changes inhibits ADH release. Osmotic pressure changes in the carotid blood may also be of importance. Massive hemorrhage is the most powerful stimulus to ADH release. Dehydration both increases osmotic blood concentration and reduces blood volume.

Other reflex stimuli. Suckling and parturition evoke oxytocin release, whereas stress has an inhibitory effect. The vagus nerve may exhibit both inhibiting and stimulating control of ADH secretion. Upright posture, emotional stress, or pain stimulate ADH, whereas supine position and occasionally emotional stress may inhibit ADH.

Drugs. Acetylcholine, nicotine, anesthetics, barbiturates, and morphine stimulate, whereas atropine, ethanol, diphenylhydantoin, and possibly epinephrine inhibit ADH release. The supraopticohypophysial neu-

ron may be cholinergic. Acetylcholine induces antidiuresis, and the anticholinesterase diisoprophyl fluorophosphate (DEP) initially causes antidiuresis and later D.I.

NEUROHYPOPHYSIAL HORMONES

The four known naturally occurring neurohypophysial hormone compounds are octapeptides with similar molecular structures differing only in the amino acids in the third and eighth positions (Fig. 3-2). There is a ring of five amino acids between the disulfide (S–S) bridge, which is critical for biologic activity. Reduction of the disulfide bond inactivates the hormone. Position eight is of prime importance. For example, substitution of arginine or lysine for leucine of oxytocin reduces oxytocic activity but enhances vasopressor and antidiuretic properties. The most potent ADH in man and dogs is *arginine vasopressin,* whereas in pigs *lysine vasopressin* is equally, if not more, potent. The physiologic action of lysine vasopressin, the source of most commercial vasopressin preparations, is very similar to that of the arginine compound. The structural formula for ox vasopressin is shown in Fig. 3-3.

Arginine vasotocin was synthesized by Katsoyannis and Du Vigneaud, 1958, before it was learned that arginine vasotocin was the naturally occurring ADH of most nonmammalian vertebrates. Other active peptide compounds found in various vertebrate species are isotocin, mesotocin, and glumitocin. A large number of synthetic analogues have been prepared. For a review of chemistry and structure, see Walter et al., 1967.

ADH and oxytocin are found in approximately equal quantities. The human fetal ADH/O ratio may be as high as 28, but it falls with advancing age and is 1 at full term (van Dyke, 1955).

CIRCULATING HORMONES

The circulating neurohypophysial hormones are confined to plasma and are minimally bound, if at all, to globulin frac-

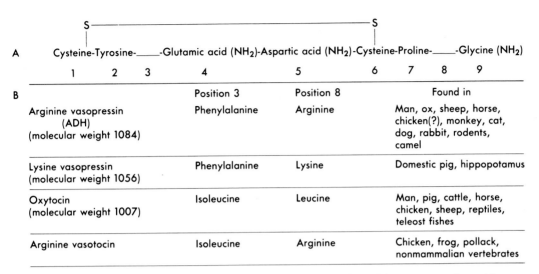

A, Basic molecular structure:

Cysteine-Tyrosine-_____-Glutamic acid (NH₂)-Aspartic acid (NH₂)-Cysteine-Proline-_____-Glycine (NH₂)

1   2   3   4   5   6   7   8   9

	Position 3	Position 8	Found in
Arginine vasopressin (ADH) (molecular weight 1084)	Phenylalanine	Arginine	Man, ox, sheep, horse, chicken(?), monkey, cat, dog, rabbit, rodents, camel
Lysine vasopressin (molecular weight 1056)	Phenylalanine	Lysine	Domestic pig, hippopotamus
Oxytocin (molecular weight 1007)	Isoleucine	Leucine	Man, pig, cattle, horse, chicken, sheep, reptiles, teleost fishes
Arginine vasotocin	Isoleucine	Arginine	Chicken, frog, pollack, nonmammalian vertebrates

Fig. 3-2. A, Basic molecular structure of the neurohypophysial hormones with positions 3 and 8 left blank. **B,** Changes in positions 3 and 8 that constitute the four known compounds. The listing of animals in which the compounds have been identified was taken partly from Sawyer. (From Sawyer, W. H.: Neurohypophyseal secretions and their origins. In Nalbandov, A. V., editor: Advances in neurology, Urbana, Ill., 1963, University of Illinois Press.)

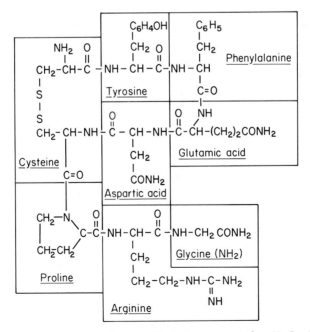

Fig. 3-3. Structure of ox vasopressin. (Modified from van Dyke, H. B.: Recent progress in hormone research XI, New York, 1955, Academic Press Inc.)

tions of serum proteins. Most of the activity in rat plasma is not ultrafiltrable, whereas in the dog approximately 70% appears to be free. The accuracy of published measurements of hormone concentrations in plasma has been questioned. Bioassay methods determine the ADH content of the unknown specimen by measuring the decrease in urine flow in the hydrated ethanol-anesthetized male rat after intravenous administration (Kleeman and Fichman, 1967). For a review of the bioassay of ADH, see Share, 1967. It has been estimated that there is only about 0.2 mU./100 ml. of blood (equivalent to about 0.3 mμg. of pure arginine vasopressin) during physiologic antidiuresis (van Dyke, 1955). The plasma level in unstressed hydrated subjects is approximately 1 to 2 mU./ml. (Kramar et al., 1966).

PHYSIOLOGIC EFFECTS OF NEUROHYPOPHYSIAL HORMONES

The major physiologic effects are on the following:

1. *Semipermeable membranes*—renal tubule, skin, and bladder of amphibians
2. *Contractile units*—myoepithelial cells surrounding mammary alveoli, smooth muscle of blood vessel or uterus

Because of almost identical molecular structures, oxytocin and ADH exhibit similarities in physiologic action. Though vasopressin is primarily an antidiuretic hormone, it exhibits oxytocic action, and oxytocin shares some antidiuretic effects. Table 3-1 lists their relative physiologic activities.

VASOPRESSIN (ADH)

Arginine vasopressin is the physiologic ADH. The ingestion of excess water dilutes the plasma Na and increases plasma volume; the osmoreceptor, sensitive to a 1% decrease in plasma osmolarity, inhibits the release of ADH. Water deprivation raises the plasma Na and contracts plasma volume. The osmoreceptor, sensitive to an increase of about 2% in plasma osmolarity, signals a release of ADH, the nephron retains water, and the plasma Na is restored to its previous concentration.

Kidney regulation of urine production

In 1951 Wirtz et al. suggested that the loop of Henle constituted a "countercurrent exchanger." A small osmotic gradient is established between the nephron loops and the interstitium, with the osmolarity of intraluminal water and interstitium increasing as Henle's loop is approached. In the thin descending limb (Fig. 3-4, *A*), Na and Cl are transferred from tubule to interstitium and carry large amounts of water (passive "obligatory" transfer). Intraluminal water increases in tonicity as it traverses the descending limb and becomes more dilute in the thicker distal limb (Fig. 3-4, *B*). Na is again transferred from lumen to interstitium, and in the

Table 3-1. Relative activities of neurohypophysial hormones*

Hormone	Rat antidiuretic	Rat vasopressor	Rat oxytocic	Rabbit milk ejector
Oxytocin	1	4	500	430
Lysine vasopressin	165	240	5	30
Arginine vasopressin	400	400	5	30
Arginine vasotocin	200	245	125	270

*Based on data from Sawyer, W. H.: Antidiuretic hormones and other antidiuretic agents. In DiPalma, J. R., editor: Drill's pharmacology in medicine, ed. 3, New York, 1965, with permission of McGraw-Hill Book Co.

absence of ADH, large volumes of hypotonic water are produced. The mechanism is shown in Fig. 3-4, *b* (Black, 1960). The numerals are units of concentration, and an active transfer of water is postulated from the upper to the lower limb of the loop. The concentration thus increases in the upper limb, being highest in the loop and decreasing in the lower limb; a small difference of only 1 unit is maintained across the dividing membrane. *ADH acts upon the epithelium of the distal tubule and collecting ducts to increase their permeability to water.* Urine therefore becomes increasingly concentrated in the collecting ducts, resulting in the production of urine hypertonic to plasma. When ADH is reduced or absent, as in D.I., the distal nephron becomes more impermeable to water, and the kidney excretes an abundant volume of hypotonic

urine. About 80% to 85% of the 120 ml./ min. of glomerular filtrate together with Na and Cl is iso-osmotically and passively absorbed, independent of ADH control in the proximal convoluted tubules, primarily under osmotic control. Distal tubular resorption (facultative) of most of the remaining 15% is an active process under ADH control. Despite the apparent impermeability of the distal nephron to water in the absence of ADH, some water resorption can occur despite ADH deprivation. Slower rates of water flow can produce some increase in water concentration. ADH also promotes osmotic transfer of water and active transport of Na through frog skin and urinary bladder and may reduce glomerular filtration by constricting the afferent arteriole in mammals. Under certain circumstances ADH may exhibit a dual effect; small doses may cause diuresis

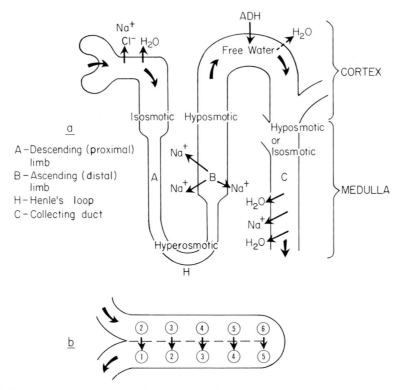

Fig. 3-4. Nephron, production of concentrated urine by the "countercurrent exchanger" hypothesis, and action on ADH. (**a** modified from Sawyer, W. H.: Antidiuretic hormones and other antidiuretic agents. In DiPalma, J. R., editor: Drill's pharmacology in medicine, ed. 3, New York, 1965, with permission of McGraw-Hill Book Co.; **b** from Black, D. A. K.: Recent advances in renal disease, Philadelphia, 1960, J. B. Lippincott Co.)

and larger doses, antidiuresis. For a review of water metabolism, ADH, and the kidney, see Kleeman and Fichman, 1967.

Corticosteroids tend to increase glomerular filtration (GFR) and may play a role in inhibiting ADH secretion and ADH inactivation by the liver. Aldosterone promotes increased tubular absorption of Na and its passively absorbed water. Its increased concentration promotes Na conservation, and its decreased concentration allows renal Na excretion. Thus the regulation of body water and extracellular osmotic pressure is a complex adjustment of multiple factors that together maintain a remarkable constancy of serum osmolarity in man. In a study by Dashe et al., 1963, the serum osmolar concentration of 25 subjects changed only 1 milliosmole/kg. of H_2O after $6\frac{1}{2}$ hours of water deprivation (285 ± 4.4 mOsm./kg. to 286 ± 5.5 mOsm./kg.). The greatest individual change was an increase of 6 mOsm./kg. or a decrease of 5 mOsm./kg.

Mechanism of ADH action

There are four hypotheses to explain the cellular action of ADH (Orloff and Handler, 1967).

The *hyaluronidase theory* supposes that ADH stimulates secretion of hyaluronidase into urine by the kidney, thus altering cellular permeability.

The *mechanical theory* visualizes binding of ADH to a receptor, thus mechanically producing cellular pores through which water flows. The disulfide bridge of vasopressin may play a role in binding the hormone to sulfhydryl groups of the renal tubular proteins.

The *series-barrier theory* supposes that in order to explain the paradox of ADH stimulation of Na, water, and urea movement without stimulation of permeability for other small related molecules, it was suggested that there were two cellular barriers in series, the one being vasopressin-insensitive of fixed permeability and the other vasopressin-sensitive. Thus vasopressin effected increased permeability in the porous barrier only, permitting passage of substances (Na, water, urea) not blocked at the outer barrier, whereas the diffusion of other molecules interdicted by the fixed permeability of the outer barrier was not altered by the hormone.

Cyclic 3′,5′-AMP (C-AMP) theory proposes that the concentration of C-AMP, produced by the action of adenyl cyclase on adenosine triphosphate (ATP), is regulated by ADH, and C-AMP is an intracellular mediator in the action of ADH. It is responsible for the augmentation in Na transport and osmotic water flow, which characterizes the physiologic response to ADH.

Vasopressor action of ADH

The first recognized property of neurohypophysial extracts was their ability to raise blood pressure by inducing peripheral vasoconstriction. It seems improbable that ADH serves any physiologic role in the regulation of blood pressure or cardiovascular function, though it appears to enhance vascular reactivity to catecholamines. The same is probably true for the vasodepressor response of birds (avian vasodepressor action) exhibited primarily by oxytocin and to a lesser extent by ADH. Cardiovascular effects of neurohypophysial hormones have been reviewed by Farrell et al., 1968. ADH may cause intestinal hyperperistalsis in large doses and may be a corticotrophin releaser.

OXYTOCIN

Oxytocin increases the frequency and intensity of uterine contractions and facilitates sperm migration by stimulating fallopian tubal contractions. It is secreted during labor and influences uterine motility, but the problem of whether it initiates or simply maintains labor has not been solved. Plasma levels of 50 mU./ml. during pregnancy and over 150 mU./ml. in the second stage of labor have been reported (Farrell et al., 1968). Oxytocin induces contraction of the myoepithelial cells that surround the alveoli and small ducts of the lactating breast and forces milk from the alveoli into the ducts (milk ejection).

Previously secreted milk stored within alveoli is made available for milking or suckling. It also possesses weak antidiuretic action. ADH demonstrates minimal oxytocic activity (Table 3-1) and may cause contraction of intestinal smooth muscle when administered in pharmacologic doses. A synthetic oxytocin is available for therapeutic induction and stimulation of labor and for postpartum uterine atony. It is supplied in ampules (1 ml. = 10 U.S.P. units, and 0.5 ml. = 5 U.S.P. units). A nasal spray containing synthetic oxytocin has been advocated in breast engorgement to promote milk ejection.

INACTIVATION AND EXCRETION

The half-life for circulating ADH in man is 8 to 20 minutes and for oxytocin in pregnant women 3 minutes. After vasopressin injection only about 5% to 15% appears in the urine. Both the *kidney* and to a lesser extent the *liver* rapidly inactivate neurohypophysial hormones probably by an enzymatic process (oxytocinases, vasopressinases) that involves reversible reduction of the disulfide bridge. Increased ADH-like material has been described in the plasma and urine of patients with hepatic cirrhosis and other edema states, but the suggestion that it causes or contributes to edema remains unproved. Other tissues, particularly mammary, probably possess these aminopeptidase enzymes and contribute to metabolic destruction and inactivation of neurohypophysial hormones.

DIABETES INSIPIDUS

Diabetes insipidus (D.I.) is a state of vasopressin (ADH) deficiency resulting in uncontrolled diuresis.

Pathophysiology

Bilateral destruction of the S.O. (and P.V.?) nuclei, or complete transection of the hypothalamo-neurohypophysial tracts, promotes retrograde degeneration of the axons and nuclei, interdicts the discharge of ADH into the circulation, and renders the distal renal nephron impermeable to water, resulting in uncontrolled diuresis of hypotonic urine. Incomplete lesions may produce only transient D.I. In the monkey, if only 15% of functional tissue remains intact, D.I. will not occur. It is probable, however, that ADH does not function on an all-or-none basis. Urine volume tends to vary inversely with the percentage of residual cells in the S.O. nuclei. Destruction of all or most of the *median eminence* seems critical. Following experimental transection of the hypothalamo-neurohypophysial tracts, a three-phased response has been described (Fisher et al., 1938).

1. *"Transient phase"*—initial polyuria, polydipsia lasting up to 10 to 11 days
2. *"Normal interphase"*—subsidence of diuresis for 2 to 11 days
3. *Permanent D.I.*

The interphase is due to the release of ADH from degenerating neurohypophysial tissue. If all damaged neurohypophysial tissue is removed, the interphase does not occur. Low stalk transection, or this plus total hypophysectomy, may cause little or no permanent D.I., because the important median eminence and the nuclei, with a large part of the axon, remain intact. High stalk section almost invariably results in D.I.

An intact adenohypophysis is critical for the maintenance of experimental D.I. Anterior pituitary insufficiency is associated with a reduction in glomerular filtration and tubular function and a diminution of urinary solutes (urea, NaCl). Polyuria is increased during corticosteroid or ACTH administration; somatotrophin (GH) exhibits synergistic action with these hormones. Thyroidectomy may occasionally ameliorate D.I., whereas thyroxine may promote the maintenance of diuresis.

Etiology

The following are causes of diabetes insipidus:
1. Idiopathic (primary)
2. Organic (secondary)
   a. *Tumor*—primary or metastatic lesion involving neurohypophysial tracts;

brain or intrasellar tumors (cranio-pharyngioma)

b. *Trauma*—basilar skull fracture, bullet wound, hemorrhage

c. *Infections*—encephalitis, meningitis, granulomatous (tuberculosis, sarcoidosis)

d. *Infiltrative lesions*—Hand-Schüller-Christian, xanthomatosis, leukemia, lymphoma, eosinophilic granuloma

e. *Vascular lesions*—aneurysms, A-V communications, hemorrhage

f. *Miscellaneous*—pellagra, Laurence-Moon-Biedl syndrome, tuberous sclerosis

Approximately one third of all cases are idiopathic (primary). Rarely these cases are congenital or familial (hereditary) and may be a sex-linked recessive characteristic or more often an autosomal dominant (Thomas, 1957). The few autopsied cases have shown a chronic degenerative process of the S.O. and P.V. nuclei, with marked nerve cell loss and gliosis. The remainder are caused by an organic lesion involving the hypothalamo-neurohypophysial system. The possibility that some cases are due in part to enhanced inactivation of ADH has been suggested, though the evidence favoring this concept is quite tenuous. Idiopathic familial (hereditary) D.I. is most prevalent in infancy, and cranio-pharyngioma is most prevalent in later childhood.

Clinical features

Incidence. Relatively rare.

Symptoms. The onset is usually acute, with *persistent, unremitting polyuria* and *polydipsia.* Enuresis occurs in children. The urinary output is increased (4 to 12 liters or more daily), and the specific gravity is reduced (less than 1.005). During periods of reduced food intake, the urine output may fall considerably. Variation in the severity of D.I. is caused by partial states of ADH deficiency or variations in solute load, depending on dietary differences. The urine volume can be less than 3,000 ml./day, and the urine osmo-larity can be near isotonicity in states of severe water or salt depletion or when adrenocortical or adenohypophysial insufficiency is present. *Water deprivation* does not diminish urine volume or increase osmolarity. If diuresis is prolonged, it leads to dehydration, weakness, restlessness, and eventually hypotension and collapse. Patients deprived of water may drink their own urine or any available fluid. When the chronology of symptoms can be ascertained, polyuria precedes polydipsia. A preference for cold water is common. Nocturia and disturbed sleep cause fatigue and irritability. Patients are usually able to prevent dehydration by frequent ingestion of fluid. If there is a disorder of the thirst mechanism engendered by drugs or central nervous system disease, dehydration occurs rapidly.

There may be symptoms of an organic lesion of the CNS (headache, visual disturbances) and/or of adenohypophysial insufficiency. It is important to be cognizant of the ameliorative effects of anterior pituitary, adrenocortical or thyroid insufficiency that may partially mask D.I. Substitution therapy in such instances will restore polyuria. The symptoms of surgically induced or traumatic D.I. follow the phases previously discussed (see discussion on pathophysiology, p. 23).

Signs. There are no physical signs of D.I. per se. Neurologic changes may be secondary to an organic lesion, and signs of anterior pituitary insufficiency may be due to interruption of the hypothalamo-hypophysial portal circulation or to intrasellar pathology. Other manifestations are a consequence of the underlying lesion. *Because of the frequency of secondary D.I., careful examination and prolonged observation are essential to ensure detection of an organic lesion in all apparent primary cases.*

Laboratory findings

The diagnosis of D.I. is unlikely if the specific gravity of a casual urine exceeds 1.015 or if water deprivation promotes increased urine concentration. Nevertheless, some patients, probably with partial or mild D.I., have concentrations to 1.010 or higher. The following four tests are the commonly employed diagnostic procedures. Subjects who have been receiving vasopressin or other therapy must withhold medication prior to testing to permit diuresis to be reestablished. Coffee, tea, and smoking are interdicted.

Vasopressin test. Pitressin, 100 mU./kg. I.V. or 0.3 U./kg. subcutaneously, is administered to a well-hydrated subject, and urine is collected in 15-minute samples for 2 hours; the urine flow in milliliters per minute and the specific gravity and/or osmolarity are measured. Marked antidiuresis and increased osmolarity occur in normal subjects and in D.I., but not in nephrogenic D.I. or in some cases of severe renal disease. In patients with psychogenic polydipsia and/or diabetes insipidus, there may be a poor response to vasopressin, presumably because of tubular resistance resulting from prolonged diuresis. If water drinking is controlled in the former or vasopressin therapy is instituted for about 2 weeks in the latter, the tubular response is restored.

Hypertonic saline. Hypertonic saline, by increasing the osmolarity of blood bathing the osmoreceptor centers, evokes a release of ADH (Carter and Robbins, 1947). Therapy is stopped to reestablish maximal diuresis, and fluids are withheld, but food is permitted. The subject is hydrated with water, 20 ml./kg. orally, for 1 hour. Some workers give an I.V. infusion of 5% dextrose in saline to ensure adequate urine flow. An indwelling catheter is desirable. Urine specimens are collected in 15-minute aliquots; urine flow of at least 5 ml./min. in two 15-minute control samples is essential. An I.V. infusion of hypertonic saline (2.5% to 3%) is started at a rate of 0.25 ml./kg./min. for 45 minutes. If no decrease in urine flow occurs during the infusion or in the first two postinfusion periods (15 minutes each), 0.1 unit of Pitressin is given I.V., and effect on urine

flow is observed for 30 to 60 minutes. Volume and specific gravity or osmolarity of each 15-minute urine specimen is measured. An antidiuretic response fails to occur in D.I. Response to Pitressin occurs in D.I. but not in nephrogenic D.I.

SOURCES OF ERROR

1. Hypertonic saline is a potent stimulus and may elicit a normal response in mild or partial D.I.

2. Normal subjects may fail to respond if the serum osmolarity is not raised above 300 mOsm./kg.

3. Adequate urine flow throughout the test is essential; a falling urine flow after the saline infusion may lead to a false assumption of an ADH response.

4. Patients with prolonged psychogenic polydipsia may fail to respond because the renal tubule has lost its sensitivity to ADH.

Nicotine test. Nicotine activates the S.O. nuclei to secrete ADH. The patient is made well hydrated, and a test dose of 0.5 mg. nicotine salicylate is injected I.V. in 3 to 5 minutes to determine the patient's sensitivity to the drug. The dose is then increased by 0.25 to 0.5 mg. every 30 minutes until an antidiuretic response or symptoms of CNS toxicity (vertigo, nausea, or vomiting) occur. The effective dose range is 0.5 to 3 mg. Cigarette smokers require the larger doses and may fail to respond. Significant antidiuresis fails to occur in most, but not all, cases of D.I.

Water deprivation test. Water deprivation raises the osmolarity of blood and stimulates the osmoreceptors to release ADH. The procedure of Eisenberg, 1965, is recommended:

1. Permit water during night.
2. 7 A.M.: Weigh patient nude at hourly intervals to end of test. Collect hourly specimens for volume, specific gravity, and, when indicated, osmolarity and creatinine. Draw blood at 7 A.M. for serum osmolarity and creatinine. Do not allow patient access to food or fluids; surreptitious drinking will invalidate the results.
3. If within 6 hours urine flow begins to fall to less than 50% of initial value, obtain blood specimens at midpoint of two consecutive urine collection periods. Determine

osmolarity and creatinine on both blood and urine, and compare with baseline value (7 to 8 A.M.). If decrease in urine flow is associated with weight loss (more than 3%), give patient amount of water equal to that lost from start of water deprivation. When urine flow has again increased, administer vasopressin 0.5 unit in 5% dextrose water I.V. over 1 hour. Collect urine hourly and weigh patient hourly for 4 more hours.

4. If there is no significant decrease in urine flow in 6 to 8 hours, obtain one blood specimen midway in an hourly urine collection for serum and urine osmolarity. Administer vasopressin and obtain urine hourly and weigh patient hourly for 4 more hours. Determine urine and serum osmolarity on the last one or two specimens.

Patients with D.I. will excrete large volumes of dilute urine until body weight has decreased 3% to 5%. With this degree of fluid loss, serum becomes hypertonic, and glomerular filtration rates will decrease 50% or more. This process may cause a fall in urine volume and an increase in urine osmolarity and be interpreted as a normal response to water deprivation. Patients with psychogenic polydipsia may have low serum osmolarity at the beginning of the test. Thus water deprivation may not elevate serum osmolarity sufficiently to stimulate the release of ADH. By measuring both serum and urine osmolarity, one can recognize the apparently normal response in the patient who fails to produce urine hypertonic to serum. Dashe et al., 1963, found a urine/serum osmolarity ratio of 1.9 or greater, whereas in D.I. the ratio was less than 1 in over half their patients and always less than 1.9. Though water deprivation may be unpleasant, the 6-hour test is usually well tolerated and is not associated with any serious complications.

A normal or partial response to nicotine and a failure to respond to hypertonic saline have been interpreted as indicating the presence of functioning neurosecretory tissue in the hypothalamus, but a selective failure of osmoreceptor function. In subjects with both anterior and posterior pituitary necrosis (as in some cases of Sheehan's syndrome), the normal reservoir of stored ADH may be deficient, with the production of a D.I.-like syndrome but with responsiveness to nicotine because the hypothalamic nuclei are more or less intact.

Differential diagnosis

Most of the disorders causing polyuria and polydipsia listed below can be recognized with little difficulty. The principal differential is between D.I., psychogenic polydipsia, and nephrogenic D.I.

1. Diabetes insipidus
2. Nephrogenic diabetes insipidus
3. Nephropathy with hypokalemia
4. Chronic renal disease (water-losing nephritis)
5. Psychogenic, hysterical, or compulsive water drinking
6. Diabetes mellitus
7. Renal disease (with or without potassium deficiency)
8. Hypercalcemia
9. Diuretic therapy
10. Disorder after large doses of corticosteroids and desoxycorticosterone acetate

Nephrogenic D.I. Nephrogenic D.I. (renal, vasopressin-resistant) is a rare hereditary disorder, transmitted as a sex-linked dominant gene attached to the X chromosome, with variable penetrance in the female heterozygous carriers (Schoen, 1960), characterized by its severity, high mortality rate, growth retardation, and mental deficiency. There is inability to respond to administered vasopressin, and assays for antidiuretic activity in the plasma of patients have been positive, implying that ADH production is normal. The disorder appears in male infants soon after birth, but female heterozygous carriers may rarely present mild symptoms. Schoen emphasizes the importance of attempting to identify the female carriers with renal concentration tests in view of the high mortality rate in their offspring. Treatment consists of maintaining an adequate supply of water to prevent dehydration and decreasing solute intake with special feeding formulas. Increased sweat electrolyte has been described in some infants, and clinical improvement has been observed with hydrochlorothiazide therapy. Renal resistance to ADH is also found in chronic renal disease and in hypokalemia.

Psychogenic polydipsia. In psychogenic polydipsia (primary polydipsia, compulsive or hysterical water drinking) (Table 3-2) the differential from D.I. may be difficult to judge in patients with long-standing symptoms, apparent emotional stability, and equivocal laboratory tests. A preference for ice water is typical of D.I. There should be little difficulty in recognizing true D.I. in patients who have had recent neurosurgical procedures or who show evidence of intracranial lesions. The administration of placebo injections may restore normal fluid balance in compulsive water drinkers. One difficulty in differentiating the two forms of polyuria is the tubular resistance to ADH that may appear in hysterical polydipsia and even in D.I.

Treatment

Vasopressin promotes antidiuresis, reduces thirst and polydipsia, and restores fluid balance. Other therapeutic measures, appropriate to the underlying cause, may be indicated in secondary D.I. (neurosurgical, irradiation, etc.), or associated adenohypophysial insufficiency. Available preparations are as follows.

Aqueous vasopressin (Pitressin, posterior pituitary extract). Aqueous vasopressin is an aqueous solution of vasopressin in 0.5 ml. (10 pressor units) and 1 ml. (20 pressor units) ampules. The initial dose should be small to avoid side effects. One to 5 units is injected subcutaneously or I.M. one or more times daily as required. Because the duration of action is brief (3 to 6 hours), the aqueous solution is not practical for long-term therapy. It may also be given intranasally by dropper or spray or on cotton pledgets. Abdominal or uterine cramps, hypertension, facial pallor, or even angina pectoris may be caused by overdosage.

Table 3-2. Diabetes insipidus versus psychogenic polydipsia—some aids to the differential diagnosis

	Diabetes insipidus	*Psychogenic polydipsia*
Incidence of females (Barlow and De Wardener, 1959)	41%	79%
Psychogenic factors	Varied	Commonly neurotic, hysterical
Onset	Acute	Vague, gradual
Primacy of polydipsia	No	Yes
Serum osmolarity	Normal or high	Low
Water deprivation effect on		
Serum osmolarity	Raises	None
Urine/serum ratio (Dashe et al., 1962)	Below 1.9	Greater than 1.9
Constancy of fluid intake	Constant	Varies considerably; spontaneous remission after months or years
Vasopressin therapy	Improvement	No improvement; may cause water intoxication
Placebo therapy	No response	Response may occur

Posterior pituitary powder U.S.P. This powder is available as ¾ grain (48 mg.) capsules and insufflated as snuff or by a special nasal insufflator in doses of 10 to 50 mg. one or more times daily. Duration of action is 3 to 8 hours. Some patients experience distressing nasal irritation.

Vasopressin tannate in oil (Pitressin tannate in oil). Vasopressin tannate is a suspension in peanut oil, 5 pressor units/ml., for I.M. injection. Duration of action is 24 to 72 hours. Patients can be controlled with 0.5 to 1 ml. daily, and some require only 0.3 to 1 ml. every other day or every third day. They are instructed to titrate their needs by withholding each dose until the onset of polyuria. Warm slightly and shake the ampules vigorously prior to injection.

Synthetic lysine-8 vasopressin. Synthetic lysine-8 vasopressin is not yet available in the United States. It has been used as a nasal spray (50 U./ml. in normal saline used every 4 hours) or by I.M. injection. The nasal spray may be used in combination with vasopressin tannate injections to effect a reduction in frequency of injections. Duration of effect is not precisely determined, but I.M. administration produces peak weight gain in 4 to 6 hours.

Synthetic 2-phenylalanine lysine vasopressin is also not available in the United States.

Side effects, precautions, and other measures

When side effects constitute a threat to the patient's life, small doses may be used or other measures (see below) may be employed. In mild cases of D.I. specific therapy may be omitted if the patient can stave off dehydration by maintaining a large fluid intake.

Pregnancy. Vasopressin is safe in therapeutic doses. Posterior pituitary powder is interdicted because of oxytocic activity.

Coronary heart disease. There is danger of angina, coronary insufficiency, or myocardial infarction with large doses.

Intestinal hyperperistalsis. Usually only with large doses does hyperperistalsis occur.

Allergic reactions. Allergic reactions are rare but they may occur.

Water intoxication. Water intoxication is rare, except after neurosurgery. Occasionally a patient with D.I. continues to consume excess fluids habitually.

After neurosurgery. The patient is usually unconscious after neurosurgery; careful monitoring of fluid balance is essential to prevent water intoxication. Aqueous vasopressin (short duration of action) is preferred until thirst mechanism is restored.

Solute load. In patients who are difficult to control with vasopressin, reduction of the solute load has an antidiuretic effect. Such a regimen consists of a low-protein low-salt average-carbohydrate intake and constitutes a useful ancillary measure in the rare patient who, because of distressing side effects, may have to reduce the dose of vasopressin.

Corticosteroids or thyroid hormones. Corticosteroids or thyroid hormones may increase diuresis in patients with D.I.

Other drugs

Chlorothiazides. The mild antidiuretic action of chlorothiazides may be of benefit in patients who suffer side effects or are difficult to control with vasopressin. They are of particular value in nephrogenic D.I. The mechanism may be, in part, due to an increase of Na and water reabsorption in the distal nephron as a result of the negative Na balance induced by the drug. Urine volume, free-water clearance, and osmolarity decrease. Maintenance of antidiuresis after drug withdrawal can be accomplished by drastic reduction of Na intake.

DOSE

Chlorothiazide, 0.25 Gm. four times a day or 0.5 Gm. thrice daily. Hydrochlorothiazide, 25 mg. four times daily or 50 mg. thrice daily.

PRECAUTIONS. Avoid hypokalemia.

Aminopyrine. Aminopyrine has mild antidiuretic properties. Danger of agranulo-cytosis has limited its usefulness.

Spironolactone. Spironolactone has been found to exert a potentiating or synergistic effect with the chlorothiazides.

Chlorpropamide. Chlorpropamide, the oral hypoglycemic agent, exerts an anti-diuretic effect similar to that of vasopressin and may become the treatment of choice in certain patients with D.I.

INAPPROPRIATE ADH SYNDROME

This unusual disorder is characterized by (1) asymptomatic dilutional hypo-natremia without hyperkalemia, (2) increased body water and body weight usually in the absence of edema, (3) hypertonic urine with increased Na content, and normal renal, cardiac, and adreno-cortical functions. ADH is secreted "inappropriately" because, under normal circumstances, hyponatremia and reduced plasma osmolarity inhibit ADH release. A similar syndrome can be reproduced by the injection of Pitressin tannate in oil into normally hydrated humans. The augmented plasma volume increases glomerular filtration rate, inhibits aldosterone secretion, induces some increase of renal Na, and ultimately causes hyponatremia. There may be a redistribution of Na from extracellular to intracellular sites.

Etiology

The syndrome, of unknown etiology, was first observed in patients having bronchio-genic carcinoma and later in central nervous system disorders (primary and metastatic brain tumors, cerebral vascular disease, encephalitis, that is, "cerebral hyponatre-mia"), but it has also been observed in a variety of unrelated conditions (pulmonary tuberculosis, pneumonia, acute porphyria, and myxedema—and possibly Addison's disease, anterior pituitary insufficiency, congestive heart failure, and liver cirrhosis). It has been presumed to be due to ADH secretion, and a number of investigators have reported high values in serum and urine extracts. The mechanism of ADH increase is unknown but has been attributed to (1) CNS lesions stimulating hypothalamic nuclei, (2) volume receptors in the mediastinum sending impulses transmitted by the vagi, (3) changes in osmoreceptor threshold, (4) production of a substance capable of stimulating the hypothalamus, (5) an ADH-like peptide produced by bronchiogenic tumor cells (ectopic ADH syndrome). Large amounts of antidiuretic material have been assayed in tumor tissue and urine extracts from patients with lung cancer.

Symptoms and signs

The syndrome is usually asymptomatic, but when the serum Na falls below 120 mEq./L., there may be weight gain, edema, irritability, confusion, anorexia, weakness, nausea, vomiting, and convulsions.

Laboratory findings

1. Low serum Na, normal serum K, normal or elevated plasma volume
2. High urine osmolarity and Na content, low serum osmolarity
3. Normal or low BUN, normal creatinine clearance, GFR, absence of proteinuria
4. Failure to raise serum Na even when large amounts of NaCl are administered
5. Normal plasma and urinary 17-OHCS and urinary aldosterone

Differential diagnosis

The differential diagnosis is mainly from other causes of hyponatremia.

Sodium depletion. There is dehydration, elevated hematocrit, and high normal or high BUN. The cause is usually obvious (diarrhea, vomiting, excessive drug-induced diuresis, adrenal insufficiency, diabetic acidosis, salt-losing nephritis).

Dilutional hyponatremia. There is increased plasma volume and usually edema (nephrosis, congestive heart failure, liver cirrhosis). In psychogenic polydipsia the urine specific gravity is low (1.000 to 1.004).

Treatment

Fluid restriction (to about 500 ml./day) contracts the plasma volume and raises the serum Na to normal. In instances of water intoxication accompanying the syndrome, hypertonic saline may be necessary to restore electrolyte and fluid equilibrium. Treatment of the underlying pathology when possible will cause prompt regression of the syndrome. For a review, see Bartter and Schwartz, 1967.

REFERENCES

Barlow, E. D., and DeWardener, H. E.: Quart. J. Med. **28**:235, 1959.
*Bartter, F. C., and Schwartz, W. B.: Amer. J. Med. **42**:790, 1967.
Black, D. A. K.: Normal function. In Milne, M. D., editor: Recent advances in renal disease, proceedings of a conference held in London, Philadelphia, 1960, J. B. Lippincott Co., pp. 3-10.
Carter, A. C., and Robbins, J.: J. Clin. Endocr. **7**:753, 1947.
Dashe, A. M., et al.: J.A.M.A. **185**:689, 1963.
Eisenberg, E.: Calif. Med. **102**:353, 1965.
*Farrell, G., et al.: Ann. Rev. Physiol. **30**:557, 1968.
*Fisher, C., et al.: Diabetes insipidus and the neurohormonal control of water balance: a contribution to the structure and function of the hypothalamico-hypophyseal system, Ann Arbor, Mich., 1938, Edward Brothers, Inc.

———
*Significant reviews.

Katsoyannis, P. G., and Du Vigneaud, V.: J. Biol. Chem. **233**:1352, 1958.
*Kleeman, C. R., and Fichman, M. P.: New Eng. J. Med. **277**:1300, 1967.
Kramar, J., et al.: Amer. J. Med. Sci. **252**:87, 1966.
Orloff, J. and Handler, J. S.: Amer. J. Med. **42**:757, 1967.
*Palay, S. L.: Fine structures of neurohypophysis. In Waelsch, H., editor: Ultrastructure and cellular chemistry of neural tissues, New York, 1957, Paul B. Hoeber, Inc., Medical Book Department of Harper & Bros., pp. 31-49.
Randall, R. V., et al.: Proc. Mayo Clin. **23**:299, 1959.
Sachs, H., and Haller, E. W.: Endocrinology **83**:251, 1968.
Sawyer, W. H.: Antidiuretic hormones and other antidiuretic agents. In DiPalma, J. R., editor: Drill's pharmacology in medicine, ed. 3, New York, 1965, McGraw-Hill Book Co., Fig. 43-4, p. 694.
*Sawyer, W. H.: Pharmacol. Rev. **13**:225, 1961.
Scharrer, E.: Arch. Anat. Micr. Morph. Exp. **54**:359, 1965.
Schoen, E. J.: Pediatrics **26**:808, 1960.
Schwartz, W. B., et al.: Amer. J. Med. **23**:529, 1957.
*Share, L.: Amer. J. Med. **42**:701, 1967.
*Thomas, W. C., Jr.: J. Clin. Endocr. **17**:565, 1957.
van Dyke, H. B., et al.: Recent Progr. Hormone Res. **11**:1, 1955.
*Walter, R., et al.: Amer. J. Med. **42**:653, 1967.
Wirz, H., et al.: Helv. Physiol. Pharmacol. Acta **9**:196, 1951.

Chapter 4

The anterior pituitary gland (adenohypophysis)

ANATOMY

The pituitary gland is an ovoid structure cradled in a fibrous depression of the sphenoid bone, the sella turcica (hypophysial fossa). It is roofed over by a connective fold of dura mater, the diaphragma sellae, and joined to the diencephalon and hypothalamus by the pituitary stalk, which pierces the diaphragma sellae. Somewhat less than three fourths of its bulk consists of the yellowish anterior lobe. The rich capillary network of the neurohypophysis produces a gray-red color. It weighs approximately 0.5 gram in the male and 0.6 gram in the female, is said to be heavier in the Negro, and becomes markedly enlarged during pregnancy (primiparas 820 mg., multiparas 954 mg.) (Friedgood, 1946, pp. 1 and 2). There is a decline in the weight of the pituitary with aging, so that by 70 years of age it is about 20% of its maximal weight. The three divisions of the anterior lobe are shown in Fig. 4-1. The *pars distalis* is the major portion; the small *pars intermedia* may be vestigial but is probably the source of MSH; the *pars tuberalis*, a region of unknown functional significance, forms a thin sheath investing the *pars infundibularis* of the neurohypophysis.

Circulation

The adenohypophysis receives no direct arterial blood but is fed almost exclusively by the hypophysial portal system and receives blood that has first traversed a capillary bed (Fig. 2-2). Sheehan and Stanfield, 1961, to the contrary, believe that there is a significant direct arterial supply. The hypophysial-portal circulation is described on p. 9. The arterial blood supply originates in the superior hypophysial arteries (from the internal carotids and posterior communicating arteries). The inferior hypophysial artery supplies the neurohypophysis. The venous drainage is composed of a number of large veins draining into the cavernous and intercavernous sinuses.

Anatomic relationships (Fig. 4-2)

There is considerable variation in the shape and depth of the normal *sella turcica*. The average dimensions are anteroposterior 10.6 mm. (8 to 13 mm.) and depth 8 mm. (5 to 9 mm.). The depth and shape determine, to a large extent, the direction of expansion of a pituitary tumor. In 5% to 7% of cases there is bridging of the sella usually between the anterior and posterior clinoids. Occasionally the posterior clinoids are congenitally absent. The paired *sphenoid sinuses* are located anterior to and below the sella but may occasionally fill a large portion of the sphenoid bone, and there may even be pneumatization of the dorsum sellae.

The *optic chiasm* is located anterior to and above the sella turcica, though in Schaeffer's studies (Friedgood, 1946, p.

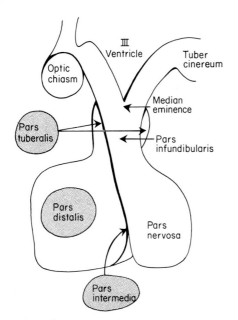

Fig. 4-1. The three divisions of the anterior pituitary lobe.

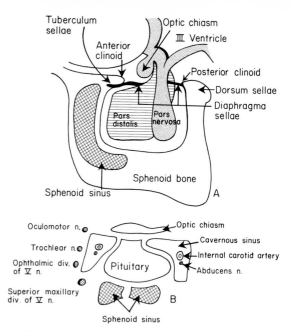

Fig. 4-2. Schematic lateral, **A,** and frontal, **B,** sections through the pituitary gland.

814) it was wholly or partly over the diaphragma sellae and hypophysis in 95% of cases. In 79% the pituitary was completely anterior and inferior to the chiasm and protruded somewhat laterally beyond the chiasm. The *cavernous sinuses* lie on either side of the sella turcica and contain the third, the fourth, the ophthalmic division of the fifth, and the sixth cranial nerves as well as the internal carotid artery. The oculomotor (third cranial) nerve passes forward through a lateral notch in the posterior clinoid process and may be compressed by an expanding pituitary tumor.

The posterior portion of the sella turcica is the *dorsum sellae* and the posterior clinoid process. This region may be thin walled and poorly calcified.

Embryology

The anterior lobe is derived from an ectodermal evagination of the roof of the fetal oral cavity (Rathke's pouch). The pars nervosa originates as an infundibular protrusion from the floor of the diencephalon of neural ectoderm that appears later,

forming the infundibular process behind Rathke's pouch. As Rathke's pouch invaginates further and lengthens, it loses its connection with the stomodeum and its tuberal portion surrounds the infundibular stalk. The neural invagination becomes more posterior and is pressed into and fuses with Rathke's pouch much as a small marble might be pressed into a larger sphere of putty. The pars intermedia is formed from the cells of Rathke's pouch in contact with the neural invagination that forms the pars nervosa.

A so-called *pharyngeal hypophysis* has been described as being located near the junction of the vomer and sphenoid and is derived from remnants of the oropituitary duct. It has been thought to exhibit physiologic activity occasionally. Craniopharyngioma is a suprasellar tumor derived from remnants of Rathke's pouch.

Cytology of the adenohypophysis

It would be desirable to adopt a functional classification so that cells secreting thyrotrophin would be called "thyrotrophic"; those secreting growth hormone

Table 4-1. Conventional classification and characteristics of adenohypophysial cells*

Cell type	Characteristics of cell granules and cells	Staining properties					Location in pars distalis	Proportions (%)		Hormone production
		Hematoxylin eosin	Periodic acid-Schiff–orange G (PAS)†	Acid hematein	Chromotrope aniline blue	Modified Mallory aniline blue		Male	Female	
Eosinophil (acidophil)	Dense granules Round cells with distinct cell boundaries	Pink	Schiff: negative Orange	Jet black	Red	Red	Posterolateral	36.8 (a)‡ 37.1 (b) 34.8 (c)	43.4 32.0 36.8	GH, LH LTH (prolactin) ACTH?
Basophil	Dense granules Large round or ovoid cells with distinct cell boundaries	Blue-purple	Schiff: intensely positive Red	Colorless (few fine black granules)	Blue	Blue	Peripheral, anterior, and inferior margins	16.9 (a) 12.3 (b) 21.0 (c)	7.0 13.8 20.4	ACTH TSH FSH
Chromophobe	Agranular Small cells with small nuclei and indistinct cytoplasm	0	0	0	0	0	Diffuse	52.2 (a) 38.0 (b) 22.8 (c)	49.6 39.6 23.6	ACTH? MSH? GH?
Amphophil	Large and small cells with vesicular nuclei and vague irregular cell boundaries; sparse round or polygonal cells *Hypertrophic variety contain giant nuclei*	Pale violet	Schiff: weakly positive Rose with rare pale orange granules	Gray	Mixed red and blue	Pale blue, occasional red	Central	10.0 (b) 19.7 (c) 2.1 (b) 1.4 (c)	12.7 17.8 1.8 1.4	TSH or many trophic hormones (b)

*Based on data from Burt and Velardo, 1954; Rasmussen, 1929, 1933; and Herlant, 1964.

†PAS for glycoproteins.

‡(a) Rasmussen, (b) Russfield, (c) Sommers.

(somatotrophin) would be "somatotrophic"; lactogenic hormone, "lactotrophic," etc. The International Committee for Nomenclature of the Adenohypophysis held its first meeting in Paris in 1963. The committee observed that a "functional nomenclature is preferable but not always possible since the cellular origin of some hormones is in doubt" (Purves, 1966). Histologic studies have been reevaluated in recent years by using the electron microscope, fluorescent-antibody techniques, radioautography, and differential centrifugation.

Three varieties of adenohypophysial cells—*acidophil, basophil,* and *chromophobe*—have been recognized by their tinctorial affinities for certain histologic stains. The chromophobe, being agranular, shows no affinity for the usual stains and was thought either to be converted into an acidophil or a basophil by the accumulation of specific granules or to represent the resting stage of these cells after discharge of granules. Table 4-1 illustrates this categorization and lists certain of their properties.

Attempts to assign specific hormonal loci to the acidophil and basophil as shown in Table 4-1 have been based on voluminous clinical and experimental evidence that will not be reviewed here, but in the light of more recent knowledge must be viewed as tenuous. Various investigators have devised their own classifications. Russfield, 1960, described the *amphophil* (Table 4-1), which she viewed as being more intimately correlated with trophic hormone content than with either the acidophil or the basophil. Golden, 1963, suggested that all cells are variants of a single cell type and that differences in granulation and staining characteristics are related to functional activity at the time of examination. Both Herlant, 1964, and Ezrin, 1958, 1963, offered their own modifications. That the chromophobe cell may be physiologically active is evidenced by the presence of chromophobe adenomas in some patients with acromegaly and in others after total adrenalectomy for Cushing's syndrome (Nelson's syndrome). Experimental pituitary tumors with adrenocorticotrophic, thyrotrophic, somatotrophic, and mammatrophic activity have resembled chromophobe adenomas. Cells that appear chromophobic by optical microscopy have been found to have fine peripheral granules when examined by electron microscopy.

An explanation for the observed regional cell localization of the various cells of the pars distalis (Table 4-1) has been sought by numerous investigators. Cells secreting ACTH, TSH, prolactin, and gonadotrophins are generally found in the median region, whereas the acidophil (STH-cell) is most commonly found laterally. Thus the most actively secreting cells are located centrally and the less active, peripherally. This situation may be induced by hypothalamic factors and is possibly related to the regional distribution of the hypophysial portal trunks. Anterior vessels appear to supply the central area of the pars distalis, dorsal or short-stalk portal vessels supply the lateral rostral areas, and neural-lobe portal vessels supply posterolateral and posterior areas, whereas deep median areas seem to be supplied by rostral neural portal vessels (or by the portal vessels from the lower infundibular stem).

For a review of the cytology of the adenohypophysis, see Purves, 1966.

HORMONES OF THE ADENOHYPOPHYSIS

The anterior pituitary gland elaborates seven trophic hormones, so named because their action is directed primarily upon specific target organs and their extra-target organ role is secondary or, in many instances, nonexistent. These hormones are the *thyrotrophic, adrenocorticotrophic, somatotrophic* (growth hormone), and *three* gonadotrophic hormones—*follicle-stimulating hormone, luteinizing hormone (interstitial cell–stimulating hormone* in the male), and *luteotrophic hormone* (identical with *prolactin* and *mammotrophin*). A seventh hormone, without a target gland, the *melanocyte-stimulating hormone*

(MSH, melanotrophin, intermedin) is believed to originate in the anterior pituitary but may be derived from the intermediate lobe. The parathyroids, adrenal medulla, islets of Langerhans, and to a large extent the zona glomerulosa of the adrenal cortex are independent of anterior pituitary control.

Thyrotrophin (thyroid-stimulating hormone—TSH)

Thyrotrophin regulates and stimulates all phases of thyroid activity. It may serve as an anatomic organizer of thyroid follicles, as shown by the reorganization of isolated thyroid cells into follicular structures when subjected to TSH. A deficiency causes thyroid atrophy ("pituitary" hypothyroidism). Highly purified extracts containing all the common amino acids except tryptophan (Friesen and Astwood, 1965), have been prepared from the pituitary gland of several species, but complete homogeneity has not yet been attained. TSH is a glycoprotein having a molecular weight of 28,000. Though it takes origin from cells of the pars distalis, substances exhibiting TSH characteristics have been detected in extracts from mammalian tuber cinereum, bovine median eminence, chorionic tissue, hydatidiform mole, choriocarcinoma, and testicular embryonal carcinoma.

Plasma TSH values are constant from day to day and throughout the day in an individual. The distribution volume of TSH is slightly larger than that of blood plasma and its half-life is 54 minutes in euthyroid subjects and 85 minutes in hypothyroid patients. The secretion rate in euthyroid subjects was calculated to be 110.1 μg./day (165.2 mU.) and 688.7 μg./day in hypothyroid patients (Odell et al., 1967).

The physiologic action of TSH depends apparently on both binding to the surface of thyroid follicle cells and penetration of their nuclei. The thyroidal iodide concentration, thyroglobulin iodination, synthesis of thyroid hormones, and secretion into the circulation are all augmented by TSH and

blighted by its absence. Thyroid metabolism is stimulated as reflected by an increase in glucose metabolism, O_2 consumption, DNA-RNA–protein synthesis, iodide metabolism, and phospholipid turnover. The rate of glucose oxidation is increased primarily via the hexose-monophosphate shunt. The binding of TSH to the surface of the follicle cell may activate adenyl cyclase and thus increase the conversion of ATP to cyclic AMP; the latter may serve as a mediator of TSH activity. When TSH is injected into animals, its thyroidal effect is rapidly apparent. Within minutes apical villi proliferate, pseudopods form, and colloid droplets appear in the apical cytoplasm. There is increased thyroid blood flow and hypertrophy and hyperplasia of the thyroid epithelium resembling hyperthyroidism.

TSH is inactivated by kidney, thymus, lymph nodes, liver, and the thyroid gland. A homeostatic feedback mechanism between TRF and/or TSH and the thyroid hormones serves to regulate TRF-TSH secretion. Thyroidectomy evokes a marked rise of circulating TSH, whereas the administration of TH inhibits TSH release and suppresses thyroid gland function. Various environmental stimuli (exposure to cold or heat) probably alter TSH secretion via the hypothalamic TRF. After the injection of ^{131}I-labeled–T_3 into experimental animals, ^{131}I-T_4 is found, and this metabolic conversion of T_3 to T_4 has been attributed to TSH. Other peptides such as alpha- and beta-MSH, ACTH, vasopressin, and synthetic peptides related to ACTH and alpha-MSH have TSH-like activity.

Bioassay of TSH

Histologic response of thyroid gland. The unknown serum is injected into a guinea pig or "stasis" tadpole, and the increase in cell height, colloid droplets, and/or change in percent of epithelium are measured. These methods are time consuming and laborious and have been supplanted by radioactive-isotope methods.

Radioactive-isotope methods. The most

popular radioactive-isotope method is the McKenzie method (1958), wherein the response of circulating ^{131}I to the unknown serum injected intravenously into mice, previously given radioactive iodine and pretreated with thyroxine to inhibit endogenous TSH, is measured. Normal values are 0.01 to 0.2 international milli-units/ml. of serum. Another method is the depletion of ^{131}I from the thyroid of chicks after TSH injection. An in vitro bioassay measures the release of ^{131}I-labeled iodine from guinea pig thyroid fragments, which is proportional to the concentration of TSH in the medium. The uptake of ^{32}P by the thyroid after TSH stimulation has also been used to assay TSH.

Radioimmunoassay method. The sensitivity of the radioimmunoassay method permits the detection of TSH and other anterior pituitary hormones in normal subjects. The mechanism is shown in Fig. 4-3, using growth hormone as an example. Antisera to TSH are prepared by injection into suitable animals, and the ability of unlabeled TSH (or "unknown plasma") to inhibit competitively the reaction of TSH-^{131}I with the antibody is measured

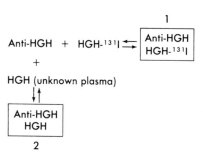

Fig. 4-3. Mechanism of the radioimmunoassay for human growth hormone (HGH). HGH is injected into rabbits and a HGH-antiserum is prepared (anti-HGH). To the unknown plasma, ^{131}I-labeled HGH (HGH-^{131}I) and the HGH-antiserum (anti-HGH) are added. The unknown plasma HGH and the HGH-^{131}I compete for binding anti-HGH. Thus labeled antigen (HGH-^{131}I) becomes displaced so that if the unknown HGH is high, a smaller amount of HGH-^{131}I will be bound, and if low, a larger fraction will be bound. Bound and free complexes are separated by chromatoelectrophoresis or by a double-antibody method (Morgan and Lazarow, 1962).

and correlated by comparison with known quantities of purified TSH. Free and antibody-bound TSH-^{131}I are separated by immunoprecipitation. Detection of plasma concentration of TSH as low as 1.5 mμg./ml. has been achieved. In euthyroid subjects, values range from 0 to 15 mμg./ml., and in primary hypothyroidism from 18 to 180 mμg./ml. In hyperthyroid patients no TSH was detected in 25 of 34 patients (Utiger, 1965).

Extrathyroidal actions of TSH

A number of physiologic actions of TSH have been described in the thyroidless animal, but there is as yet no proof that they constitute reactions to TSH alone because of impurities of the preparations used. The induction of increases of lipase and phosphorylase activity in adipose tissue is most suggestive of active extrathyroidal action.

Exophthalmos-producing substance (EPS) or factor (EPF)

Experimental exophthalmos has been produced in animals by the injection of anterior pituitary extracts and was attributed to their TSH content. Further studies, particularly by Dobyns and Steelman, 1953, showed that the exophthalmos-producing substance was probably not TSH but a closely associated distinct component of pituitary origin that could be separated from TSH and was thereafter called "exophthalmos-producing substance" or EPS. Though its role remains in doubt, it has been assayed in the serum of patients with severe exophthalmos and a correlation has been found between the severity of the exophthalmos and the assay titer. EPS has also been found in human, equine, bovine, and porcine pituitary extracts.

Adrenocorticotrophin (corticotrophin, ACTH)

ACTH is a straight-chain polypeptide containing 39 amino acids (Fig. 4-4) that was synthesized in 1963 (Schwyzer and Sieber, 1963). The complete structure of human ACTH has not yet been verified. A "precorticotrophin" activated by acid treatment of mammalian pituitary extracts may account for 80% of the total corticotrophic activity of the pituitary (Dasgupta et al., 1967). Though ACTH from various species either differs slightly in amino acid composition or in sequence, its biologic properties are similar. Species differences are expressed by changes in the 25 to 33 range of amino acid residues (Fig. 4-4). Full physiologic potency requires at least the first 24 amino acid residues of the 39 total, and complete potency by intravenous assay occurred with the 20–amino acid eicosapeptide (Friesen and Astwood, 1965).

Ciba has produced tetracosactide or Synacthen, consisting of the first 24 amino acids and exhibiting full trophic ACTH activity. It has been available in Europe. The structure and properties of MSH will be discussed later.

Bioassay of ACTH

1. Measurement of the depletion of ascorbic acid from the adrenal gland of a hypophysectomized rat (Sayers et al., 1948) can detect 0.25 mU. ACTH. Ascorbic acid can also be measured in the adrenal vein. The Sayers method has been modified by pretreatment of intact rats with cortisol to block endogenous ACTH,

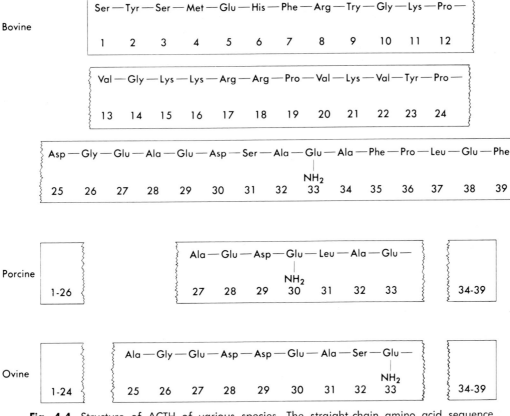

Fig. 4-4. Structure of ACTH of various species. The straight-chain amino acid sequence is fragmented for diagrammatic purposes. *Ala,* Alanine; *Arg,* arginine; *Asp,* aspartic acid; *Glu,* glutamic acid; *Glu-NH₂,* glutamine; *Gly,* glycine; *His,* histidine; *Leu,* leucine; *Lys,* lysine; *Met,* methionine; *Phe,* phenylalanine; *Pro,* proline; *Ser,* serine; *Try,* tryptophan, *Tyr,* tyrosine; *Val,* valine. (Adapted from Li, C. H.: Recent Progr. Hormone Res. **18:**2, 1962.)

thus eliminating the need for hypophysectomy.

2. Measurement of blood 17-hydroxycorticosteroids (17-OHCS) in the hypophysectomized dog (Nelson and Hume, 1955) can detect 0.5 to 1 mU. ACTH.

3. Similar to measurement 2 and more laborious but more sensitive is the fluorimetric measurement of corticosterone in the adrenal vein plasma of a hypophysectomized rat (Lipscomb and Nelson, 1959). This method can detect 0.03 to 0.06 mU. ACTH.

4. Radioimmunoassay—a method described by Yalow et al., 1964—detects 0.1 mU. ACTH.

Plasma ACTH is not detectable in anterior pituitary insufficiency and when suppressive doses of corticosteroids are administered. ACTH levels are elevated after adrenalectomy, in Addison's disease, in congenital adrenal hyperplasia, as a response to stress, and in Cushing's syndrome owing to bilateral adrenal hyperplasia or to some nonpituitary tumors producing an ACTH-like polypeptide. Cushing's disease with a functioning pituitary adenoma may be associated with very high levels.

Biosynthesis and secretion of ACTH

ACTH biosynthesis and/or secretion is under the control of, though not completely dependent on, a hypothalamic CRF. Cortisol, the most biologically active adrenocortical steroid, regulates the output of ACTH by an action either upon CRF, by direct action on the anterior pituitary, or possibly by both, that is, feedback control. Thus a fall of free plasma cortisol stimulates a CRF response, whereas an elevation inhibits its secretion. A circadian rhythm of ACTH secretion consisting of higher levels in the early morning gradually declining to lower levels in the afternoon coincides with a similar rhythmicity of adrenal 17-OHCS secretion and is dependent on the sleeping and waking cycle of the tested individual. Altering the sleep-wake schedule engenders a corresponding change in the diurnal pattern (Liddle, 1966). The rhythm of ACTH secretion is apparently not dependent on the stimulus of light, since blind individuals exhibit an identical pattern. It does not depend on cortisol feedback because the rhythm is maintained in Addison's disease.

The anterior pituitary contains small and relatively stable amounts of ACTH. Various workers have reported values of 0 to 30 I.U., 49 to 588 I.U., and 205 I.U. per gram of dried powder. Binding of ACTH in plasma to gamma globulin and beta-lipoprotein fractions has been described. Liddle, 1962, has shown that an infusion of only 4 U. of ACTH per hour evokes a maximal adrenal response. The half-life is from 1 minute up to 10 to 20 minutes and is the same in patients with Addison's disease and Cushing's syndrome as in normal subjects.

Stress

A variety of nonspecific stressful stimuli augment a basal level of activity of the CRF-corticotrophin-adrenocortical axis. The adrenal secretory rate is greatly accelerated, and there is a rapid rise of plasma corticosteroids that may reach four to five times the baseline value within 30 minutes (Fig. 4-5). This response is lacking in subjects with ACTH or adrenocortical insufficiency, and the inability of these patients to make the necessary metabolic adjustments to stressful stimuli (rise in blood pressure, increased gluconeogenesis and availability of glucose to tissues) can be fatal. The rise of plasma 17-OHCS may also be partly a consequence of a somewhat impaired peripheral degradation of cortisol, a situation that is particularly striking in liver disease. For example, an adrenalectomized dog on a constant dose of corticosteroid shows a rise of unconjugated 17-OHCS after trauma (Steenburg and Ganong, 1955). The stress may stem from physical trauma such as burns and fractures or from infections, drugs, hormones, toxins, anesthetics, surgical procedures, emotional stimuli, and

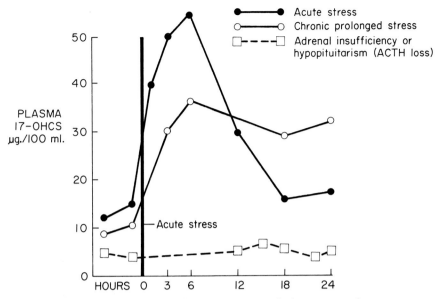

Fig. 4-5. Effect of nonspecific stress on the concentration of plasma cortisol.

various diseases. The stimuli they evoked converge upon the hypothalamus from the cerebral cortex, midbrain, and limbic system, and from peripheral nerves and the spinal cord, enter the complex connecting circuits of the hypothalamus and evoke a secretion of CRF. Both excitatory and inhibitory neural components, as well as circulating corticoid levels, contribute to the nature of the stress response. The response to stress permits the organism to adjust and to survive sudden emergencies or more chronic stressful situations (Selye's "alarm reaction").

Actions of ACTH

ACTH stimulates the zona fasciculata and reticularis of the adrenal cortex and promotes a rapid outpouring of adrenal corticosteroids (principally cortisol in humans, corticosterone in small animals) and androgenic steroids. It also exerts some control over the zona glomerulosa and the production of aldosterone, though the physiologic significance of this response is unsettled.

Mechanism of ACTH action (Hilf, 1965)

HAYNES-BERTHET THEORY. ACTH stimulates adrenocortical adenyl cyclase with the formation of cyclic adenosine-3′,5′-monophosphate (C-AMP), a phosphorylase activator. Active phosphorylase mediates the conversion of glycogen to glucose-1-phosphate → glucose-6-phosphate (G6P) via phosphoglucomutase. G6P can then be metabolized via the hexose monophosphate shunt with the production of TPNH. The latter supplies the cofactor for the energy required in steroidogenesis. Preparations of adrenal mitochondria to which C-AMP has been added stimulate the activity of an essential enzyme in adrenal steroidogenesis, 11β-hydroxylase. The critical biosynthetic reaction cholesterol → pregnenolone, which is currently viewed as the locus of ACTH action, has also been found to be the site of C-AMP activity.

PROTEIN SYNTHESIS. Protein synthesis has been suggested as a prerequisite for responsiveness of the adrenal cortex to ACTH and for steroidogenesis. ACTH may promote the formation of messenger RNA that acts at the adrenal microsome, resulting in the synthesis of a specific protein enzyme required for the elaboration of steroids. Current evidence, however, suggests that protein synthesis may not be necessary for the immediate response to

ACTH. It is possible that the Haynes-Berthet theory explains the regulation of the synthetic cycle and the protein hypothesis explains adrenal growth and continued response to ACTH stimulation.

Extra-adrenal effects of ACTH. Although most anterior pituitary trophic hormones depend on target gland response for physiologic action, unequivocal extra-adrenal actions of corticotrophin have been demonstrated (Lebovitz, 1965; Genuth and Lebovitz, 1965). A basal level of corticosteroid, however, appears to be necessary ("permissive action of corticosteroids"). In vitro experiments have shown a general increase in fat metabolism (increased oxygen consumption, glucose uptake and oxidation, triglyceride formation, and adenyl cyclase and phosphorylase activity). In vivo studies of carbohydrate metabolism have shown hypoglycemia, improved glucose utilization, and a rise in plasma insulin.

Melanophore-stimulating hormone (MSH)

The observations that hyperpigmentation is common in Addison's disease, that failure to promote pigmentation is characteristic of panhypopituitarism, and that pigmentation sometimes occurred when crude ACTH preparations were administered suggested that ACTH was the physiologic melanotrophic hormone. Later, a melanophore-stimulating hormone (MSH) was separated from ACTH, and it was found that ACTH had about one thirtieth the darkening activity of MSH on frog skin (Lerner and McGuire, 1964). It is currently believed that MSH, rather than ACTH, is responsible for pigmentation in endocrine disorders. Three MSH peptides have been identified in pituitary extracts, alpha-MSH and two beta-MSH's. The most potent, alpha-MSH, has been synthesized and is common to all species. The first 13 amino acid residues are identical in alpha-MSH and ACTH, though an acetyl group is attached to serine, the first amino acid of MSH. Both beta-MSH's contain 18 amino acids, though in humans 22 amino acids have been described. The exact site of MSH production is uncertain, but it is thought to originate in the intermediate lobe. An "MSH heptapeptide core" (met-glu-his-phe-arg-try-gly) is present in all preparations of ACTH and MSH and is probably responsible for the melanocyte-stimulating properties of ACTH (Li, 1961). Thus the hyperpigmentation of Addison's disease can be explained by the high levels of circulating ACTH.

Bioassay of MSH

MSH is often undetectable in normal individuals. (No international unit has been established.)

For *melanophore dispersion,* an unknown solution is injected into the dorsal lymph sac of a hypophysectomized frog, and the dispersion of melanophore in the web is measured under the microscope.

Isolated frog skin is incubated with unknown solution and darkening is measured.

Growth hormone (somatotrophin, STH, GH)

GH originates from the eosinophil cell of the adenohypophysis and is under the regulatory control of GRF. The human pituitary has a high concentration that exhibits little variation with age. Li, 1966, discovered that GH was a straight-chain polypeptide consisting of 188 amino acids. The molecular weight varies from 21,500 in humans to 47,800 in sheep. In contrast to other pituitary hormones, species specificity is an important property. Nonprimate GH is not effective in man or monkeys, whereas primate GH exhibits physiologic activity in both primates and man. Bovine and ovine preparations consist of branched polypeptides, whereas in man and primates there is a single polypeptide chain. All mammalian preparations appear to be active in the rat, although refractoriness to human and simian preparations occurs more rapidly than to bovine or whale. These species differences are summarized in Table 4-2. Li has hy-

Table 4-2. Biologic responses to growth hormones from various species*

Experimental animal	Pituitary growth hormone							
	Ox	Sheep	Man	Monkey	Pig	Whale	Horse	Fish
Man	–	–	+	+	–	?		
Monkey	–		+	+	–			
Sheep	+							
Goat	+							
Ox	+							
Rat	+	+	+	+	+	+	+	–
Mouse	+		+	+				
Guinea pig	–		–	–				
Dog	+		+	+	+			
Cat	+							
Tadpole	+							
Fish	+							
Molecular weight	45,000	47,800	21,500	25,400	41,600	39,900	—	—

*From Papkoff, H., and Li, C. H.: Hormone structure and biological activity; biochemical studies of three pituitary hormones, J. Chem. Ed. 43:41, 1966.

pothesized that there is an "active core" that is probably shared by all species. Trypsin digestion of bovine GH has yielded a substance with metabolic activity in humans. Enzymatic digestion of human GH to the extent of 40% NPN entailed no loss of biologic activity. For a review of the functional and immunologic specificity of GH, see Knobil and Hotchkiss, 1964.

Considerable controversy exists concerning the identity of GH and prolactin. Their separation into distinct chemical components has not yet been achieved, and as Li has suggested, the growth-promoting and prolactin activities of the adenohypophysis may be intrinsic properties of the same molecule. A polypeptide called "human placental lactogen" (HPL) or chorionic somatomammotropin has been isolated from the human placenta as early as the twelfth week of pregnancy in retroplacental as well as peripheral serum at term (Josimovich and MacLaren, 1962). It showed evidence of partial antigenic identity with human GH and has exhibited certain growth-promoting and prolactin-like activity. It is found in the plasma of pregnant women and disappears rapidly after delivery. For a review, see Grumbach et al., 1968.

Bioassay of GH

Tibia test. The tibia test is based on increased width of the proximal tibial epiphysial cartilage of hypophysectomized rats in response to GH administration. The test is relatively insensitive compared to newer methods.

Plasma-sulfation factor. The plasma-sulfation factor is a nondialyzable substance that stimulates the uptake of sulfate into mucopolysaccharides of hypophysectomized rat cartilage. The sulfation factor is not synonymous with GH. Its nature is obscure, but its presence in plasma appears to be dependent on circulating GH. The method lacks precision and reproducibility.

Radioimmunoassay. The methods of Glick et al., 1965, and Greenwood et al., 1964, are the most sensitive and specific.

The basis for the assay is similar to the original immunoassay for insulin described by Berson et al., 1956, as shown in Fig. 4-3. Greenwood et al. found normal adult male values of 3.2 mμg./ml.; acromegalics, 39.2 mμg./ml.; and children, 12 mμg./ml. Glick et al., 1965, were able to detect 0.25 mμg./ml. and found markedly elevated values in the umbilical veins of newborn and premature infants. Normal infants showed higher levels than adults. Values in children over 4 years of age were in the same range as adults, and there was no rise during periods of growth spurt in childhood or adolescence.

For a review of radioimmunoassays, see Selenkow et al., 1967.

Biosynthesis, secretion, and transport of GH

Circulating GH values fluctuate widely. Basal and ambulatory levels are higher in females than in males, and the GH-releasing mechanism is more sensitive in the female. Insulin hypoglycemia rapidly evokes a considerable rise, as does arginine, fasting, exercise, anesthesia, surgery, pyrogens, estrogens, vasopressin, and the inhibition of glucose utilization by the administration of 2-deoxyglucose. Feeding, glucose or corticosteroid administration, and severe malnutrition lower plasma GH values. The GH rise produced by pyrogens, major surgery, or I.V. amino acids is not affected by glucose administration. The rise induced by fasting and exercise does not occur in obese patients. The general concept is that GH responds to situations of carbohydrate deficit and that GH and glucose seem to bear a feedback relationship similar to that of other pituitary trophic secretions and their target organ hormone. A regulatory mechanism mediated by C-AMP stimulates the secretion of GH while blocking the release of insulin (Gagliardino and Martin, 1968). The half-life of circulating GH is approximately 23 minutes (Glick et al., 1965), but the metabolic effects observed after the injection of HGH into hypopituitary dwarfs may last 3 to 7 days.

Physiologic effects of GH

Investigations on the physiologic effects of GH were reported by Knobil and Hotchkiss, 1964; Raben, 1962; and Friesen and Astwood, 1965.

Protein metabolism. GH stimulates protein synthesis, producing an increase in protoplasm and positive nitrogen balance. There is enhanced intracellular incorporation of certain amino acids, fall in BUN and plasma amino acids, stimulation of the appearance of "sulfation factor" and of conversion of proline to hydroxyproline in collagen of hypophysectomized rat cartilage, increased incorporation of amino acids into cartilage, and cartilage growth.

Fat metabolism. GH mobilizes fat, inhibits lipogenesis, reduces carcass fat, raises plasma-free fatty acid (FFA), enhances the muscle uptake of FFA, lowers fat stores with the release of FFA from adipose tissue, increases liver fat, promotes ketosis, and lowers the respiratory quotient. Its protein anabolic action may depend on the availability of FFA.

Carbohydrate metabolism. GH was originally called "growth-diabetogenic hormone" because large doses of relatively crude extracts caused diabetes in intact dogs and cats, and smaller doses produced diabetes in partially depancreatized animals. The uptake of glucose by muscle and adipose tissue is retarded by GH. Long-term administration of human GH to pituitary dwarfs, however, has not produced glycosuria or hyperglycemia. GH in vitro stimulates the uptake, oxidation, and conversion to fatty acids of glucose and leucine by adipose tissue from hypophysectomized rats. It has been hypothesized that the anabolic action of GH may be mediated by insulin. Single injections of ^{14}C-labeled glucose to acromegalic subjects has revealed deviations similar to those found in diabetic subjects, namely, prolongation of the half-life, reduced fractional turnover rate, enlargement of the glucose pool size, and lowering of the oxidation rate of glucose to CO_2.

It has been suggested (Zierler and Rabinowitz, 1963) that an interplay of insulin and GH maintains metabolic homeostasis in the following manner: food ingestion → rise of blood glucose → insulin secretion → GH suppression → fall of FFA, promoting triglyceride synthesis; later a fall of blood glucose → secretion of GH → rise of FFA → protein synthesis. The sensitivity of man to injected insulin may be decreased by GH, but glucose tolerance is usually unchanged, though a slight decrease can occur. Hypophysectomized diabetic subjects maintained on insulin show an increased blood and urine sugar and ketosis when GH is injected. When intravenous GH is given to normal or diabetic individuals, a fall of blood sugar is observed in 20 to 30 minutes. An increase of urinary citrate has been a consistent finding after GH administration.

Mineral metabolism. GH causes retention of potassium, phosphate, sodium, and chloride, with expansion of extracellular fluid volume and an increase in aldosterone excretion. There is increased calciuria and intestinal absorption of calcium. In hypopituitary dwarfs, serum inorganic phosphorus and alkaline phosphatase rise.

Miscellaneous effects. There is augmentation of milk production in cows. GH is essential for full development of the lactating breast in the rat. In humans a renotrophic effect has been described, as evidenced by increased inulin and creatinine clearance, para-aminohippurate, and the Tm of para-aminohippurate.

Gonadotrophic hormones
Follicle-stimulating hormone (FSH)

FSH originates in the beta cell, a variety of basophil, of the anterior pituitary and is under the control of a hypothalamic releasing factor (FSH-RF, FRF). It is a glycoprotein containing 8% carbohydrate and has a molecular weight of about 30,000. Its physiologic action is described on p. 359. It is probable that FSH and LH are secreted more or less simultaneously in a certain ratio. The cyclic pattern of FSH secretion is an early follicular increase, a midcycle peak, and a luteal-phase decrease until the end of the menstrual cycle is reached. High values are found at the menopause and for some years thereafter. In the male, FSH causes growth of the seminiferous tubules and stimulates spermatogenesis; the secretion is not cyclical.

Bioassay of FSH. The bioassay for so-called urinary FSH is a misnomer because the gonadotrophic material of human urine is a mixture of FSH and LH, and the assay measures total human urinary gonadotrophins or "human pituitary" gonadotrophins (HPG).

UTERINE WEIGHT METHOD. Various modifications of the original Klinefelter et al., 1943, method by uterine weight are used. When gonadotrophins are injected into intact immature female mice, the ovaries are stimulated to secrete estrogen, and the latter induces hypertrophy of the uterus. Serial dilutions of extracts prepared from 24-hour urine collections are injected into immature female mice twice daily for 3 days. The gonadotrophin concentration is calculated by noting the most dilute specimen that induces a significant increase of uterine weight compared to controls. Results are reported in mouse units (M.U.), 1 M.U. being that amount of gonadotrophic hormone causing a 100% increase. Normal values usually range from 6 to 52 M.U./24 hours. Gonadotrophins are not detectable before puberty or in hypogonadotrophic hypogonadism.

OVARIAN WEIGHT AUGMENTATION REACTION. Urine extracts are injected into intact immature female rats and the ovaries are weighed. The weight is proportional to the concentration of urinary gonadotrophins.

RADIOIMMUNOASSAY. Current methods have been plagued by contamination of the FSH-antigens with LH; so reliability remains to be established. For a recent review of gonadotrophin bioassays and radioimmunoassays, see Albert, 1968.

Luteinizing hormone (LH, interstitial cell–stimulating hormone, ICSH)

LH is a glycoprotein that originates in the acidophil or possibly in a gamma cell of the anterior pituitary under the regulatory influence of a releasing factor (LRF). The chemical structure is unknown, but studies indicate that LH derived from sheep and human glands shows considerable differences in content of hexose, fucose, hexosamine, and sialic acid (Li, 1961). The amino acid composition is not dissimilar to ovine TSH. The molecular weight is 30,000 (sheep). The half-life of various preparations as determined by Parlow ranged from 17 minutes (rat LSH) to 294 minutes (chorionic gonadotrophin) (Friesen and Astwood, 1965). A small quantity of LH, together with FSH, induces ovulation and estrogen secretion. A midcycle rise in LH urinary excretion has been found by bioassay or immunoassay methods in women with ovulatory menstrual cycles. The physiologic actions of LH in the female are discussed in Chapter 14. In the male, LH is called ICSH because of its interstitial cell–stimulating properties. It promotes growth and maturation of the testicular Leydig cells and the secretion of testosterone.

Bioassay of LH (ICSH). Urinary extracts are injected into hypophysectomized male rats and the ventral prostate gland is weighed. One unit of ICSH equals the amount that induces a 100% increase. A more sensitive method measures the depletion of ascorbic acid in the ovaries of immature rats. Plasma radioimmunoassay determinations in females show an abrupt large peak at the midpoint of the menstrual cycle.

Chorionic gonadotrophin (CG)

CG is derived from the placental cytotrophoblast and is measured in pregnancy tests. It is produced in increasing quantities, reaching a maximum in the third month of gestation. High values are found in patients with chorionepithelioma and hydatidiform mole, and in men with testicular teratoma. It is a glycoprotein that physiologically, chemically, and immunologically resembles pituitary LH.

Luteotrophic hormone (LTH, prolactin, lactogenic hormone, mammotrophic hormone)

LTH of bovine and ovine origin is a single-chain polypeptide consisting of 211 amino acid residues, with a molecular weight of approximately 25,000. Thus far the only prolactin protein isolated from human pituitaries also exhibits marked GH activity, and all human GH preparations show some prolactin activity. Attempts to separate the two in human pituitary fractions have failed, though in other species complete separation has been accomplished. LTH maintains the function of the corpus luteum of experimental animals and stimulates the secretion of progesterone. It is apparently identical with prolactin, a lactogenic hormone that stimulates and maintains lactation. Increased amounts of prolactin, as well as ACTH and adrenocortical steroids, are secreted during parturition and serve to initiate lactation. Other hormones (GH, thyroxine, insulin, and parathyroid hormone) are necessary to elicit maximum milk production and milk ejection (oxytocin) but are not essential for milk secretion. In the rat the synergistic action of estrogens, progesterone, GH, and adrenal steroids, together with prolactin, is necessary to promote mammary ductal and alveolar proliferation and growth, but prolactin is clearly the major hormone involved. Ovarian hormones promote mammary growth mainly by stimulating the secretion of prolactin and possibly GH, by synergizing with these hormones, and by sensitizing the mammary gland to these hormones. Mechanisms of the function of the human breast may or may not be identical, since studies with purified extracts are lacking. Whether LTH plays a physiologic role in the human female is uncertain. For a review, see Meites and Nicoll, 1966.

Other physiologic activities similar to those of GH have been ascribed to prolactin. They include stimulation of protein synthesis, diabetogenic action, and calorigenic properties. In amphibians it induces migration to water (water-drive phenomenon) and in birds promotion of nesting behavior. Fish accustomed to salt water can adapt to the osmotic stress of fresh water because of their ability to secrete prolactin.

Bioassay of prolactin

PIGEON CROP SAC ASSAY OF RIDDLE. The unknown is injected I.M. into immature pigeons daily for 4 days. The crop sac weight is compared to an international standard. The sensitivity of the test is increased 100 to 10,000 times if a "local" crop sac test is used (Lyons, 1958). Using a single injection, local pigeon crop weight technique, and the Sulman method

for human whole blood extraction, Simkin and Goodart, 1960, reported the following results: no prolactin activity in 8 children, 6 normal young men, 7 normal young women in the first half of the menstrual cycle; definite prolactin activity in 13 lactating women and in 10 women in the second half of the menstrual cycle. Hypophysectomy in adult female rats and in one oophorectomized woman abolished prolactin activity of the blood. There is no standardized method to elicit prolactin secretion.

LABORATORY TESTS OF ANTERIOR PITUITARY FUNCTION

Most tests of anterior pituitary function depend on an evaluation of target gland activity (Fig. 4-6). Quantitative measurement of circulating pituitary hormones is still in the experimental stage, and the techniques remain too complex for the average laboratory. The most critical test would be the augmentation of circulating

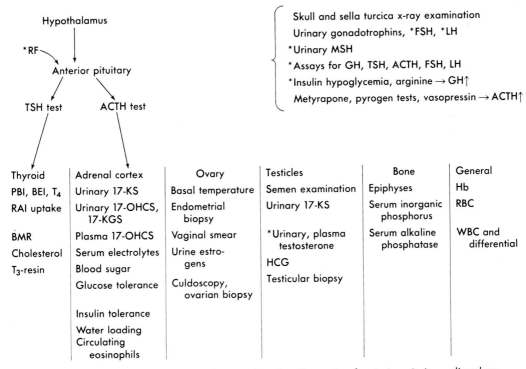

Fig. 4-6. Survey of laboratory studies used in the diagnosis of anterior pituitary disorders. Tests not generally available are marked by an asterisk.

blood levels of pituitary hormones in response to the injection of an appropriate hypothalamic releasing factor (RF). For example, Bernard-Weil et al., 1967, infused a corticotrophin–RF preparation (fraction H of Garilhe) in 14 subjects and found a significant rise of plasma corticosteroids.

Direct anterior pituitary tests

Urinary gonadotrophins. Persistent absence is evidence of pituitary gonadotrophic failure, although this also occurs in primary thyroid myxedema. Sedatives, tranquilizers and analgesics may interfere with gonadotrophin release. Loss of gonadotrophins and probably GH are usually the first laboratory evidence of hypopituitarism. The results of a single determination may be misleading, and at least two or preferably several 24-hour urine specimens should be tested. Since selective failure of pituitary trophic hormones is not uncommon, the presence or absence of the gonadotrophins does not necessarily reflect the condition of the entire gland.

X-ray examination of skull and sella turcica. A significant enlargement of the sella turcica is accepted as prima facie evidence of a pituitary tumor, though other mechanisms are possible. Examination of the ocular fundi and mapping of the visual fields may be an ancillary aid. Radiologic examination of the skull may reveal the typical changes of acromegaly, or cerebral or intrasellar calcifications.

Assays for TSH, GH, ACTH, and MSH

The assay methods for TSH, GH, ACTH, and MSH have been discussed previously. The TSH and GH determinations are available commercially, but the cost is high.

Provocative tests

Measures to provoke secretion of a pituitary hormone are used as gauges of endogenous hormone reserves.

ACTH by metyrapone. The test for

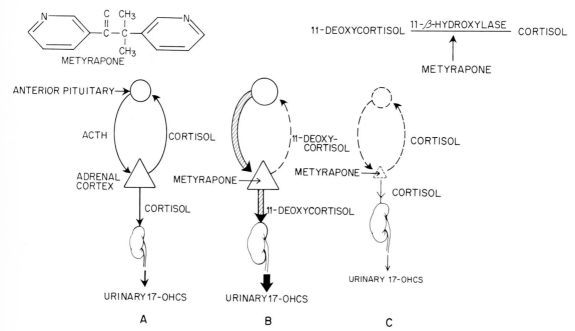

Fig. 4-7. Metyrapone test. **A,** Normal anterior pituitary-adrenocortical feedback control. **B,** Metyrapone blocks cortisol production, resulting in excessive release of pituitary ACTH. **C,** Failure to respond in pituitary insufficiency. Site of action of metyrapone in biosynthesis of cortisol is shown at top right. Chemical formula of metyrapone at top left.

ACTH provides an indirect estimate of pituitary ACTH reserves (Liddle, 1962) (Fig. 4-7). Metyrapone (methopyrapone, 2-methyl-1,2-di-3-pyridyl-1-propanone, Metopirone, SU-4885) blocks the adrenocortical synthesis of cortisol by selectively inhibiting 11β-hydroxylase, one of the essential adrenal biosynthetic enzymes. Plasma cortisol is therefore markedly reduced, and its precursor, 11-deoxycortisol, quantitatively replaces it. Since the latter is a weak inhibitor of pituitary ACTH, the loss of cortisol evokes an outpouring of ACTH that can only result in a further rise of plasma and urinary 11-deoxycortisol and urinary tetrahydro-11-deoxycortisol. The usual chromogenic method of measuring urinary 17-OHCS or 17-KGS does not distinguish between urine cortisol and its metabolites and deoxycortisol and metabolites, so that increased urinary deoxycortisol causes a substantial increase of the urinary 17-OHCS in normal subjects. The elevated urinary values for deoxycortisol may be measured directly.

ORAL TEST. The dosage for the oral test is 500 to 750 mg. orally every 4 hours for 6 doses (after food or milk to prevent transient vertigo); 24-hour urines are collected the day before, the day of metyrapone administration, and the day after for determination of 17-OHCS and/or 17-KGS. The latter determination is the more sensitive, since the rise of 17-KGS has been found to be double that of the Porter-Silber chromogens.

INTRAVENOUS TEST. The dosage for the I.V. test is 30 mg. of metyrapone ditartrate/kg. body weight in 1,000 ml. normal saline solution infused I.V. for 4 hours. Urine is collected for the preceding 24 hours and the 24 hours of the day of the test. Urinary 17-OHCS and 17-KGS are determined. A modification entails measurement of plasma levels of 11-deoxycortisol before and after the infusion.

In patients with normal pituitary ACTH reserves, the urinary 17-OHCS increases by two to three times or more. Failure to respond indicates deficient ACTH reserves

and/or adrenocortical hypofunction, and the responsiveness of the adrenals must be ascertained by performing an ACTH test. Chlorpromazine and related drugs, as well as corticosteroids, ACTH, and estrogens, interfere with the response. Whether attempts to quantitate the responses that are less than normal and to ascribe varying degrees of hypothalamic and/or pituitary failure (that is, limited pituitary reserve) are justified is not established. The metyrapone test depends on many variables, such as the completeness of absorption when the oral test is used, the degree of interference with 11β-hydroxylase, and the plasma reduction of cortisol, and at best can provide only a rough estimate of pituitary-ACTH secretion. Though untoward effects are rare, Addisonian crisis and fatalities in adults have been reported.

ACTH by pyrogen test. A pyrogen such as lipid-polysaccharide-polypeptide complex (endotoxin) derived from *Salmonella abortus equi* is injected I.V. in a dose of 0.25 μg. Plasma cortisol is measured before the infusion and 30, 60, 120, 180, and 240 minutes after the infusion. The pyrogen stimulates ACTH secretion and causes an abrupt rise in plasma cortisol at 120 minutes, whereas in hypopituitarism there is no response.

ACTH by vasopressin. With vasopressin, there is a clear-cut prompt rise in plasma cortisol, presumably by evoking a CRF $\rightarrow$ ACTH response or by mimicking the action of CRF. Ten units of synthetic lysine-vasopressin is given I.M., and plasma cortisol is measured at 0, 30, 60, and 120 minutes. Smaller doses may be necessary in patients sensitive to the stimulation of intestinal motility, and the test is contraindicated in cardiovascular disorders and particularly in coronary heart disease. Acute hypertension and asthmatic episodes have occurred. Failure to respond to vasopressin and/or metyrapone has been interpreted as indicative of an anterior pituitary lesion, whereas failure to respond to the pyrogen or other stressors may point to the hypothalamus-CRF mechanism. The site of action of vasopressin remains doubtful, however, but many workers believe it causes a release of CRF.

ACTH by insulin. When 0.1 unit of insulin per kilogram of body weight is injected I.V., a prompt increase of plasma 17-OHCS occurs, similar to that evoked by vasopressin, and is an index of endogenous ACTH reserves.

GH. Because GH values in some normal subjects may be undetectable, measures to provoke an increased blood concentration are necessary to assess GH reserves. The most commonly employed agent is insulin in an I.V. dose of 0.1 U./kg. There is a normal increase of plasma GH exceeding 5 mμg./ml., or a threefold to fiftyfold rise of plasma GH, at 30 to 60 minutes in response to a significant decrease of blood sugar. Intravenous arginine (30 grams) provokes a tenfold rise in the male. A pyrogen, Piromen, in an I.V. dose of 0.5 μg./kg., also induces a considerable GH response. Elevated plasma GH levels fall in normal subjects during a glucose tolerance test but fail to change in most patients with acromegaly.

TSH. Attempts to devise a measure of TSH reserve, similar in principle to the metyrapone test for ACTH, with the use of antithyroid drugs could not be confirmed (Schneeberg and Kansal, 1966).

Indirect estimates of GH

The *serum inorganic phosphorus concentration* serves as a rough indirect estimate of circulating GH being elevated (above 4.5 mg./100 ml.) in active acromegaly and gigantism and in growing children. Unfortunately, in juvenile hypopituitarism low values are not consistently found. The maximum fall of serum inorganic phosphorus to insulin-induced hypoglycemia is greatly reduced in acromegaly. *Serum alkaline phosphatase* measurements are also of limited diagnostic value. *Delayed epiphysial maturation* and *dental development* are characteristic of juvenile hypopituitarism.

Miscellaneous

Mild anemia, particularly evident in males, and a relative lymphocytosis and eosinophilia may be found in anterior pituitary insufficiency. The BMR is usually reduced. When insulin is injected I.V. (0.1 U./kg. in the provocative tests for ACTH and GH, blood sugars are also measured at 0, 20, 30, 45, 60, 90, and 120 minutes (insulin tolerance test). In normal subjects the blood sugar falls less than 50% and returns to the baseline value within 90 to 120 minutes. In hypopituitarism (and in adrenocortical insufficiency) the fall is greater and the blood sugar fails to return to the baseline value (hypoglycemia unresponsiveness). In fact, serious hypoglycemia can occur, and one employs a smaller dose of insulin (0.044 U./kg.) when the diagnosis seems likely. Low fasting blood sugar values and a flat oral glucose tolerance curve are common in hypopituitarism. A prolonged glucose tolerance test (6 hours) can provoke hypoglycemia. There is an impaired ability to excrete a water load.

Suppression tests

The ability of a target gland secretion to inhibit or block the effects of its appropriate pituitary trophic hormone is called a "suppression test" and is utilized as an aid in the diagnosis of target organ disorders. Thus in Cushing's syndrome, because of adrenocortical hyperplasia, a specific dose of a corticosteroid fails to inhibit ACTH, and in hyperthyroidism the exhibition of thyroid hormone fails to block TSH. These failures will be discussed in later chapters.

Tests of target organ function

The tests of target organ function are listed in Fig. 4-6 and will be discussed in subsequent chapters dealing with the various target glands. Target organ function is reduced when the particular trophic hormone of that gland is deficient, but the target gland usually retains its capacity to respond to trophic hormone stimulation.

This capacity forms the basis for the ACTH, TSH, and HCG tests.

ACTH stimulation test. When ACTH is administered to a normal individual, adrenocortical steroidogenesis and secretion are markedly augmented. Maximal adrenocortical stimulation is induced when plasma ACTH values are approximately 5 mU./100 ml. (Liddle, 1962). In hypopituitarism the adrenal cortex is relatively dormant and inactive but is responsive to exogenous ACTH stimulation, whereas in primary adrenal insufficiency (Addison's disease) the adrenal cortex is either totally destroyed or too attenuated to respond. At times in pituitary insufficiency adrenocortical response is attained only after repeated ACTH stimulation with priming doses. A great variety of procedures have been devised. Most of them consist of intravenous infusions of an aqueous preparation of a lyophilized ACTH powder, and measurement of the response of plasma and/or urinary 17-OHCS. The availability of depot preparations of ACTH now permits prolonged adrenal stimulation by intramuscular injections comparable to that obtained with intravenous infusions. Since there is no standardized procedure, one must select the most suitable technique and acquire experience in its use. The I.M. ACTH-gel test is performed as follows: (1) Baseline 24-hour urine specimens are collected for 2 days, and two daily fasting venous blood samples are obtained; (2) ACTH-gel 40 U. are given I.M. every 12 hours for 4 days; (3) on the last 2 days 24-hour urine specimens are collected, and fasting blood samples are obtained. The 17-OHCS concentration is measured on all blood and urine samples. Typical results are shown in Fig. 4-8. If it is inconvenient to give 40 U. every 12 hours, similar results may be obtained by giving 80 U. once daily. The 4-day test is necessary to ensure maximal

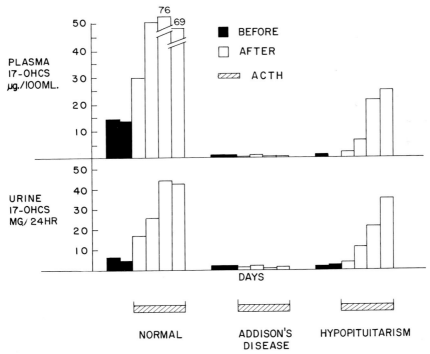

Fig. 4-8. ACTH (Thorn) stimulation tests showing contrasting results obtained in patients with primary adrenal insufficiency (Addison's disease) and secondary adrenal insufficiency (hypopituitarism).

stimulation. If 17-OHCS values can be obtained quickly, the test may be terminated whenever a significant urine and/or plasma increase is noted. If results are equivocal with the I.M. test, an I.V. test should be done, using a 4- to 8-hour infusion of 25 to 50 U.

Anaphylactic reactions to ACTH are rare. With the I.V. technique, the reaction is apt to be more profound, but the infusion can be quickly terminated. With I.M. injections, reactions are not as likely to be fatal. Patients with probable or known adrenocortical insufficiency should be protected by a small dose of synthetic corticosteroid preparation before and throughout the test (dexamethasone 0.5 mg. or triamcinolone 4 mg. every 12 hours). Synthetic β^{1-24}-corticotropin, at present not commercially available, is less antigenic and is useful as a potent ACTH compound in patients who are sensitive to or who have acquired resistance to ACTH.

Thyrotrophin (TSH) test. TSH induces a substantial increase of RAIU and of serum PBI and T_4 in normal subjects and in patients with hypopituitarism. In myxedema there is no thyroid tissue to respond and these indices remain unchanged. Taunton, 1965, compared the numerous techniques for performing the test and concluded that 5 units of TSH given I.M. daily for 3 days produced maximal thyroid stimulation (mean final ^{131}I value is $41\pm16\%$ in euthyroid subjects and $32\pm10\%$ in hypopituitarism). Occasional hypopituitary subjects will require priming with multiple doses to obtain a response (Fig. 4-9), and rarely no response occurs. That such refractoriness is possible is shown by one report that in 15 of 95 cases only a small mass of dense scar tissue was found in the thyroid region (Sheehan and Summers, 1949). The phenomenon of low thyroid reserve will be discussed in Chapter 9. Suppression of thyroid function with thyroid hormone treatment, even when prolonged, will not interfere with the TSH test, though prior iodine will inhibit ^{131}I uptake, and only the PBI response persists. Toxic reactions to TSH are uncommon. They include transient thyroiditis,

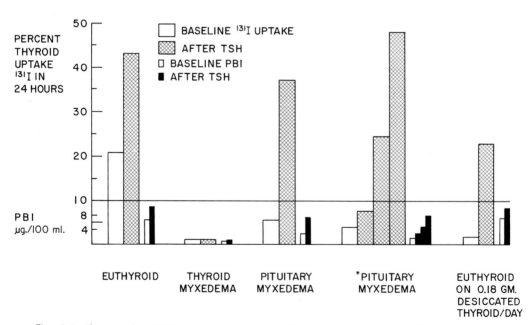

Fig. 4-9. Thyrotrophin (TSH) test in myxedema. The asterisk is an example of a case of pituitary myxedema that failed to respond after a single injection of TSH but did respond after subsequent injections.

fever, nausea, vomiting, headache, urticaria, tachycardia, and cardiac arrhythmias. In patients with anterior pituitary insufficiency, TSH may induce sufficient thyroid hormone secretion to rapidly raise body metabolism and provoke adrenocortical insufficiency. For a review of the TSH test, see Burke, 1968.

Human chorionic gonadotrophin (HCG) test. Testicular functional response to HCG serves to differentiate primary testicular failure from failure secondary to hypopituitarism. Various techniques have been described. The author gives 1,000 I.U. HCG I.M. daily for 5 to 10 days, and a baseline 24-hour urinary 17-KS is compared to the 24-hour urine specimen collected on the fifth day. Injections are continued beyond day 5 until the 17-KS value is reported. A rise of 50% to 100% above the baseline is found in hypogonadotrophic hypogonadism. If the rise is equivocal, HCG injections are continued and a second urine is collected on day 10. Determination of urine and/or plasma testosterone is a further refinement of the test.

REFERENCES

Albert, A.: J. Clin. Endocr. **28:**1683, 1968.

Bernard-Weil, E., et al.: Evaluation of hypothalamo-pituitary-adrenal function by the vasopressin (or C:R:F) test. In Martini, L., Franchini, F., and Motta, M., editors: International Congress on Hormonal Steroids, proceedings of the second congress, Milan, May 23-28, 1966, Amsterdam, 1967, Excerpta Medica Foundation, International Congress Ser. no. 132, p. 1149.

Berson, S. A., et al.: J. Clin. Invest. **35:**170, 1956.

°Burke, G.: Ann. Intern. Med. **69:**1127, 1968.

Burt, A. S., and Verlardo, J. T.: J. Clin. Endocr. **14:**979, 1954.

Dasgupta, P. R., et al.: Acta Endocr. **55:**31, 1967.

Dobyns, B. M., and Steelman, S. L.: Endocrinology **52:**705, 1953.

Ezrin, C., et al.: J. Clin. Endocr. **18:**917, 1958.

Ezrin, C., et al.: Histology of the human pituitary in relation to Thyrotropic secretion. In Werner, S. C., editor: Thyrotropin, Springfield, Ill., 1963, Charles C Thomas, Publisher, p. 129.

Friedgood, H. B.: Endocrine function of the hypophysis, New York, 1946, Oxford University Press, Inc.

°Friesen, H., and Astwood, E. B.: New Eng. J. Med. **272:**126, 1272, 1328, 1965.

Gagliardino, J. J., and Martin, J. M.: Acta Endocr. **59:**390, 1968.

Genuth, S., and Lebovitz, H. E.: Endocrinology **76:**1093, 1965.

°Glick, S. M., et al.: Recent Progr. Hormone Res. **21:**241, 1965.

Golden, A.: Cytologic reflections of altered human adenohypophyseal function. In Werner, S. C., editor: Thyrotropin, Springfield, Ill., 1963, Charles C Thomas, Publisher, p. 138.

Greenwood, F. C., et al.: Brit. Med. J. **1:**25, 1964.

Grumbach, M. M., et al.: Ann. N. Y. Acad. Sci. **148:**501, 1968.

°Herlant, M.: Int. Rev. Cytol. **17:**299, 1964.

°Hilf, R.: New Eng. J. Med. **273:**798, 1965.

Josimovich, J. B., and Maclaren, J. A.: Endocrinology **71:**209, 1962.

Klinefelter, H. F., Jr., et al.: J. Clin. Endocr. **3:**529, 1943.

°Knobil, E., and Hotchkiss, J.: Ann. Rev. Physiol. **26:**47, 1964.

Lebovitz, H. E.: Effects of anterior pituitary trophic hormones on extra-target organs. In Taylor, S., editor: Proceedings of the Second International Congress on Endocrinology, 1964, Amsterdam, 1965, Excerpta Medica Foundation, International Congress Ser. no. 83, p. 1239.

Lerner, A. B., and McGuire, J. S.: New Eng. J. Med. **270:**539, 1964.

Li, C. H.: Postgrad. Med. **29:**13, 1961.

°Li, C. H.: Recent Progr. Hormone Res. **18:**1, 1962.

Li, C. H., et al.: J. Amer. Chem. Soc. **43:**41, 1966.

°Liddle, G. W., et al.: Recent Progr. Hormone Res. **18:**125, 1962.

Liddle, G. W.: Arch. Intern. Med. **117:**739, 1966.

Lipscomb, H., and Nelson, D. H.: Fed. Proc. **18:**95, 1959.

McKenzie, J. M.: Endocrinology **63:**372, 1958.

°McKenzie, J. M.: Physiol. Rev. **48:**252, 1968.

°Meites, J., and Nicoll, C. S.: Ann. Rev. Physiol. **28:**57, 1966.

Morgan, C. R., and Lazarow, A.: Proc. Soc. Exp. Biol. Med. **110:**29, 1962.

Nelson, D. H., and Hume, D. M.: Endocrinology **57:**184, 1955.

Odell, W. D., et al.: J. Clin. Invest. **46:**953, 1967.

Papkoff, H., and Li, C. H.: J. Chem. Educ. **43:**41, 1966.

°Significant reviews.

*Purves, H. D.: Cytology of the adenohypophysis. In Harris, G. W., and Donovan, B. T., editors: The pituitary gland, vol. 1, Berkeley, Calif., 1966, University of California Press, p. 147.

*Raben, M. S.: New Eng. J. Med. **266**:31, 82, 1962.

Rasmussen, A. T.: Amer. J. Path. **5**:263, 1929; **9**:459, 1933.

Russfield, A. G.: Cancer **13**:790, 1960.

Sayers, M. A., et al.: Endocrinology **42**:379, 1948.

Schneeberg, N. G., and Kansal, P. C.: J. Clin. Endocr. **26**:579, 1966.

Schwyzer, R., and Sieber, P.: Nature **199**:172, 1963.

*Selenkow, H. A., et al.: Radiol. Clin. N. Amer. **5**:317, 1967.

Sheehan, H. L., and Stanfield, J. P.: Acta Endocr. **37**:479, 1961.

Sheehan, H. L., and Summers, V. K.: Quart. J. Med. **18**:319, 1949.

Simkin, B., and Goodart, D.: J. Clin. Endocr. **20**:1095, 1960.

Sommers, S. C.: Lab. Invest. **8**:588, 1959.

Steenburg, R. W., and Ganong, W. F.: Surgery **38**:92, 1955.

Taunton, O. D., et al.: J. Clin. Endocr. **25**:266, 1965.

Utiger, R. D.: J. Clin. Invest. **44**:1277, 1965.

Yalow, R. S., et al.: J. Clin. Endocr. **24**:1219, 1964.

Zierler, K., and Rabinowitz, D.: Medicine **42**:385, 1963.

Chapter 5

Diseases of the anterior pituitary gland

ANTERIOR PITUITARY INSUFFICIENCY (SIMMONDS' DISEASE, SHEEHAN'S SYNDROME)

Physiology

Hypophysectomy leads to atrophy of the target organs (thyroid, adrenal cortex, ovary, or testicle—Fig. 5-1). To produce panhypopituitarism in dogs, one must remove 97% to 99% of the anterior lobe. When 75% to 95% is removed, there is partial hypopituitarism (gonadal or gonadal and thyroidal insufficiency); less than 75% removal is associated with no detectable endocrine abnormality. In man approximately 90% to 95% of the pituitary must be destroyed in order to produce clear-cut evidence of pituitary insufficiency.

Effects on carbohydrate metabolism

The fasting blood sugar is normal or somewhat lowered; hypoglycemia is uncommon, in part owing to diminished insulin production. Glucose tolerance tests may be normal or show various patterns (flat, delayed rise and fall, or terminal hypoglycemia). There is insulin hypersensitivity and a delayed restitution of the blood sugar when insulin is administered intravenously (insulin hypoglycemia unresponsiveness). However, when smaller doses of insulin (0.05 to 0.033 U./kg. body weight) are infused into a well-nourished hypophysectomized human, the insulin tolerance curve is comparable to the curve in intact subjects using 0.1 U./kg. body weight. The administration of HGH restores the normal response to insulin and tends to increase the low circulating insulin levels. In diabetic patients hypophysectomy markedly reduces or may abolish the need for insulin, probably owing chiefly to the loss of GH.

Visceral and skeletal effects

In long-standing panhypopituitarism there is reduction in size of the heart, liver, kidneys, and other visceral organs, but there are no histologic abnormalities. There is decreased cardiac output and oxygen consumption associated with microcardia. The reduction of kidney size results in a decrease in glomerular filtration rate, renal plasma, and blood flow. Gastric acid and volume of secretion are reduced. The bones are smaller than normal, and mild osteoporosis may occur. The muscles are small because of a reduction in the size and number of fibers.

Hematologic effects

Moderate normocytic anemia is frequently present. The total white cell count is generally normal, but there is a tendency to slightly elevated or high normal lymphocytes and eosinophils in patients with adrenocortical insufficiency. Platelet counts are normal. The bone marrow is either normal or shows various nonspecific changes.

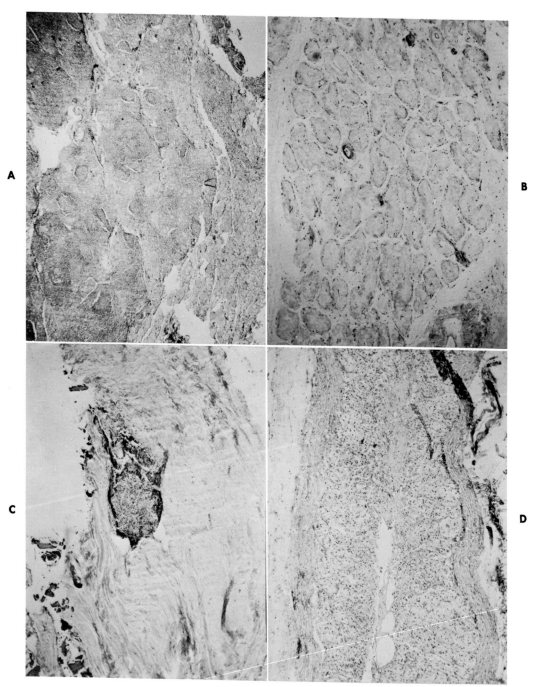

Fig. 5-1. Panhypopituitarism. The sella turcica contained no recognizable pituitary tissue but was occupied by a cyst. **A,** Atrophic thyroid gland infiltrated with lymphocytes. **B,** Atrophied testis with "shadow tubules" devoid of germinal epithelium or Sertoli cells. Leydig cells are absent. **C,** Cyst wall contained a remnant of partially hyalinized adenohypophysis. **D,** Adrenal gland. The zona glomerulosa occupies most of the cortex.

Causes

The lesions that can cause anterior lobe hypopituitarism are listed below in approximate order of frequency:

Sheehan's syndrome—postpartum necrosis

Benign tumor—chromophobe adenoma, eosinophilic adenoma, mixed chromophobe-eosinophilic adenoma, craniopharyngioma

Nonspecific necrosis and fibrosis

Granulomas—sarcoidosis, histiocytosis

Infections—tuberculosis, lues, mycoses, moniliasis, bacterial infections

Lipoidoses (Hand-Schüller-Christian disease)

Vascular lesions—intracranial aneurysms, cavernous sinus thrombosis, temporal arteritis, internal carotid aneurysm

Hypothalamic (with normal pituitary)—tumor, infection, granuloma, histiocytosis, idiopathic

Metastatic neoplasm, brain tumor

Pituitary carcinoma

Functional lesions—due to malnutrition, anorexia nervosa?

Iatrogenic lesions—hypophysectomy, target organ hormone withdrawal, drugs (busulfan)

Hemachromatosis

Traumatic lesions—basilar skull fracture, hemorrhage, avulsion of stalk

The commonest lesion is postpartum ischemic necrosis (Sheehan's syndrome), which comprises at least 75% of the cases in women. In men a pituitary tumor is the principal lesion. Sarcoidosis has recently been reported as a cause of giant-cell granulomas of the anterior pituitary. Trauma of the skull with basilar fracture, hemorrhage, or avulsion of the pituitary stalk can lead to destruction of the pituitary. However, only 9 documented examples have been reported (Klachko et al., 1968). Of particular interest are those rare cases of hypopituitarism with an intact pituitary gland. Escamilla and Lisser, 1942, in their review of Simmonds' disease, listed 14 examples. Gross pathology of the hypothalamus has only rarely been found, but physiologic failure with loss of RF's can be postulated. So-called functional or physiologic hypopituitarism can be the result of prolonged malnutrition. Cases of unitrophic deficiency of a pituitary hormone may be caused by loss of the appropriate RF.

Clinical picture

Sheehan's syndrome may be more common than is generally believed. Sheehan's estimate was 2 severe and 7 moderately severe cases per 10,000 people. We discovered 4 previously unrecognized cases among 35 survivors of postpartum hemorrhage and/or shock (Schneeberg et al., 1960). Pituitary insufficiency is almost twice as prevalent in females as in males.

Past medical history. A history of previous postpartum complications (hemorrhage, shock, infection, morbidity) may first alert the clinician to the diagnosis. Sheehan's syndrome, however, has occasionally followed an apparently normal pregnancy. Pituitary necrosis can occur in diabetes mellitus and after severe infections. Plaut, 1952, found fibrotic pituitary lesions 13 times among 149 unselected autopsies of adult males.

Because *Sheehan's syndrome* is the commonest cause of pituitary insufficiency, the description of its particular features will dominate the ensuing discussion.

Pathogenesis of Sheehan's syndrome. Postpartum hemorrhage and shock leads to arteriospasm of the vascular supply of the anterior pituitary and stalk. The portal blood flow is impeded, favoring portal thrombosis and thrombosis of the sinusoids and small capillaries of the pars distalis (Sheehan and Stanfield, 1961). Infarction, necrosis, and fibrotic repair ensue. Beernink and McKay, 1962, attribute these changes to disseminated intravascular coagulation. Pituitary necrosis has been found after eclampsia, premature separation of the placenta, infected abortion, premature rupture of the membranes with chorioamnionitis, amniotic fluid embolization, placenta praevia, and afibrinogenemia.

Clinical picture of Sheehan's syndrome. The typical syndrome is characterized by failure of lactation in the puerperium, amenorrhea, loss of axillary and pubic hair, genital and breast atrophy, superinvolution of the uterus, sterility, and various degrees of hypothyroidism and/or adrenocortical insufficiency. Patients with advanced cases may appear prematurely senile because of weight loss, pale wrinkled skin, and apathetic personality. Less severe examples may include isolated or various combinations of deficiencies of anterior pituitary trophic hormones. The disorder may be manifest shortly after the puerperium (failure of lactation) and becomes progressively worse after an interval of months or may not manifest itself for years. The clinical picture may vary considerably and may include a spectrum from an extremely mild or latent form to the typical syndrome described above. It may be unmasked only when some stressful situation precipitates an adrenocortical crisis, hypoglycemia, or coma.

Symptoms and signs. The symptoms and signs of anterior pituitary insufficiency, (with particular emphasis on Sheehan's syndrome), or panhypopituitarism,* that is, total loss of trophic hormones, are outlined below:

Symptoms
  Amenorrhea, infertility (female)
  Failing libido, impotence (male)
  Postpartum failure to lactate
  Weakness, fatigue, loss of sense of well-being
  Anorexia, weight loss (mild)
  Cold intolerance, lack of perspiration, dry skin
  Psychic—personality and mood changes, apathy, intellectual impairment
  Gastrointestinal—nausea, vomiting, vague indigestion, flatulence, pain
  Coma, convulsions, restlessness, delirium.
  Neurologic (usually secondary to brain tumor) —visual disturbances, headache
  Hypoglycemia
Signs
  Asthenia, lassitude, weakness
  Dull expression, apathy
  Skin dry, inelastic, pale, wrinkled, atrophic, lacks pigment
  Loss of axillary and pubic hair
  Decrease of beard (male)
  Breasts atrophic (female)
  Atrophy of mons, labia, vagina, uterus
  Premature senility
  Blood pressure low, postural hypotension, pulse slow, small heart
  Body temperature subnormal
  Myxedema occasionally present

*Many authors reserve the diagnosis of panhypopituitarism for combined anterior hypopituitarism and diabetes insipidus.

Less than total deficiency, that is, partial hypopituitarism, is more common. The mild form, frequently seen early in patients with pituitary tumors, involves gonadotrophin and probably GH loss with little or no TSH or ACTH deficiency. Selective (unitrophic) hypogonadotrophism may occur without apparent cause, may be an inherited tendency, and may be associated with anosmia (Kallman's syndrome, 1944), syndactyly, color blindness, and mental deficiency, with the Laurence-Moon-Biedl syndrome, with Friedreich's ataxia, or in association with Addisonian adrenocortical insufficiency. If the onset is before puberty, there is sexual infantilism. The exact frequency of occurrence of the combined loss of gonadotrophin-TSH or gonadotrophin-ACTH is not known, though the former is the more prevalent.

An *isolated* (unitrophic, monotrophic) *deficiency of a trophic anterior pituitary hormone* is rare. Apparent, selective trophic hormone failure may represent an early stage of more severe hypopituitarism and may later progress to loss of other trophic hormones. A deficiency of one pituitary hormone may mask the features of a more diffuse loss of function. Approximately 10 patients with isolated loss of ACTH have been reported. Solitary absence of TSH has been described in 10 patients, of GH in 3 patients,* and of gonadotrophin in some 250 patients. The last has not been further differentiated as to loss of FSH, LH, or both, and such diagnostic precision is not generally available at the present time. The diagnosis of an isolated deficiency depends on (1) clinical and laboratory evidence of end-organ hypofunction of a single gland or end organ, (2) increase of end-organ hormone secretion when stimulated by the trophic hormone (that is, response to TSH, ACTH, gonadotrophins, or growth hormone), and (3) when possible, demonstration of the loss of a single anterior pituitary hormone by plasma radioimmunoassay. One can

*Considerably more have been described since this writing.

only speculate as to the cause of unitrophic anterior pituitary insufficiency. A significant reduction of pituitary acidophils was described in a dwarfed female (Hewer, 1944), and a reduction of basophils was reported in a patient with selective loss of ACTH (Perkoff et al., 1960). Hypothalamic deficiencies with selective loss of a single RF are possible but unproved. Circulatory impairment of specific trunks of the hypophysial portal circulation affecting selected areas of the pars distalis is another hypothetical explanation. For a review see Odell, 1966.

HYPOGONADOTROPHISM. Loss of sexual function is an early, almost constant, and sometimes isolated feature of hypopituitarism.

Female. Oligomenorrhea or scanty menses progresses to amenorrhea. Vasomotor flushes do not occur. There is loss of libido. The mons veneris shrinks because of loss of fat, and pubic hair disappears or does not regrow if shaved. The vagina is atrophic, the mucosa thins, and vaginal smears lack the estrogen effect. The labia and uterus atrophy. The breasts, nipples, and areolae become smaller; erectile function is lost; and glandular tissue cannot be palpated. Feminine body contours regress somewhat because of loss of subcutaneous fat. Pallor is attributed to mild anemia, reduced cutaneous circulation, and hypopigmentation. Sterility is characteristic, but subsequent pregnancy has been reported and has been thought to promote clinical improvement in some patients by causing pituitary hyperplasia, whereas in others pregnancy has been followed by death.

Male. There is loss of libido and sexual potency. Semen volume falls eventually to zero, and there is oligospermia and/or aspermia. The testes atrophy and soften, and the penis and prostate shrink. Pubic hair thins, assumes a female pattern, and may eventually disappear completely. The beard thins, and shaving becomes infrequent or unnecessary (Fig. 5-2). Once secondary sex characters are well established, however, their regression is slow and often

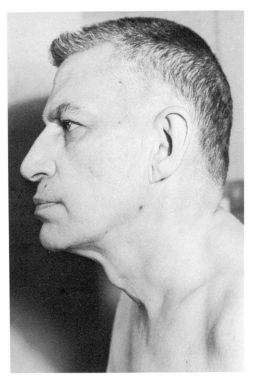

Fig. 5-2. Beardless facies of a 56-year-old male with a chromophobe adenoma of the pituitary and panhypopituitarism. Some features of acromegaly are evident. Axillary and pubic hair scant, libido absent, total sexual impotence.

incomplete. Thus some males with mild hypopituitarism may retain a modicum of sexual function for months and sometimes for years. Voice changes are rare unless the disorder is initiated during puberty or early adolescence. The pallid skin is smooth but may show the wrinkles and rhagades so characteristic of eunuchoid males.

HYPOTHYROTROPHISM. Pituitary hypothyroidism from a deficiency of TSH results in atrophy of the thyroid (Fig. 5-1, A). Occasionally there is myxedema that is indistinguishable from primary thyroid myxedema, but the clinical manifestations are not generally as profound. Normal robustness and sense of well-being give way to lethargy, asthenia, weakness, and fatigue. Part of this change can be attributed to associated adrenocortical insufficiency. The patient soon eschews physical activity and may become a chronic invalid. There are cold intolerance, anorexia, constipation, loss of muscle tone, myxedema tendon reflexes, paresthesias, myalgias, and arthralgias. Intellectual impairment, personality changes, and apathy ensue. The axillae are dry and lack the characteristic sweat odor of a healthy adult. The differential diagnosis of pituitary from primary thyroid myxedema is outlined in Table 5-1. The differential diagnosis is often difficult because primary thyroid myxedema leads to diminished function of other endocrine glands. Thus hypogonadism is common

in classic myxedema but is usually not as severe as in pituitary insufficiency. Adrenocortical insufficiency is demonstrable by laboratory studies rather than by clinical signs. Isolated thyrotrophin deficiency with complete preservation of other pituitary trophic functions may occur rarely and can be diagnosed by using the TSH test, and/or by measuring the plasma TSH concentration, and by demonstrating the preservation of other trophic hormones.

HYPOCORTICOTROPHISM. Adrenocortical insufficiency because of loss of ACTH differs from classic Addison's disease. There is

Table 5-1. Some laboratory and clinical findings of value in differential diagnosis of myxedema of pituitary or thyroid origin

	Pituitary hypothyroidism	*Primary thyroid hypothyroidism*
Response of PBI and radioiodine uptake to TSH	Marked (may require "priming" with several daily injections)	None
24-hour thyroidal radioiodine uptake	Low (occasionally up to 20%)	Usually 5% or below
Serum cholesterol	Usually normal or slightly elevated	Elevated (over 300 mg.)
Heart size by x-ray examination	Small	Large
Other signs of hypopituitarism	Yes (except in isolated TSH deficiency)	No
Loss of genital function	Profound	None or mild to moderate
Tolerance to administration of thyroid hormone	Poor; may cause severe side effects, adrenal crisis	Good
Blood pressure	Very low	Low normal, normal, or high
Urinary 17-OHCS	Very low	Low or low normal
Urinary 17-KS	Very low	Low or low normal
Metyrapone test	Abnormal	Diminished (or normal if dose of metyrapone is increased and administered for longer time)
Thyroid autoimmue antibodies	Absent	Often present
Plasma TSH	Absent	Usually very high

usually no hyperpigmentation, and electrolyte disturbances are less common. The zona glomerulosa remains intact after hypophysectomy in lower animals and may remain so in man (Fig. 5-1, *D*), though after long-standing hypopituitarism, aldosterone secretion is reduced, and responses to sodium restriction and surgical stress are also deficient. *Hypoglycemia* and *hypoglycemia unresponsiveness* occur as a consequence not only of ACTH but also of GH deficiency. The sudden termination of a glucose infusion in a hypopituitary patient can result in severe hypoglycemia and may be fatal. Hypopituitarism complicating *diabetes mellitus* causes an apparent improvement in carbohydrate tolerance, with diminished requirements for insulin and the occurrence of hypoglycemic episodes. These events have been called the "Houssay phenomenon in man" and refer to the amelioration of experimental pancreatic diabetes in animals by hypophysectomy, to their exquisite sensitivity to the hypoglycemic effects of insulin, and to the production of severe hypoglycemia after brief fasting (Houssay and Biasotti, 1930). Isolated loss of ACTH is discussed on p. 235.

HYPOSOMATOTROPHISM. Growth hormone deficiency in adults may be manifest only by hypoglycemia. The syndrome of pituitary dwarfism will be considered separately.

Laboratory findings

Urinary gonadotrophins. Urinary gonadotrophins are not detectable in most cases and normally are not found in children.

Bioassays or radioimmunoassays. TSH, ACTH, and MSH are undetectable in assays.

Immunoassay of GH. Since normal plasma GH levels may often be below the sensitivity of the immunoassay, single estimations may be of no diagnostic value, and therefore measures to evoke a rise of endogenous GH must be employed (p. 48). In one series of 25 patients (Rabkin and Frantz, 1966), all showed a diminished plasma GH response to insulin. GH was therefore presumed to be deficient in 100% of those patients, whereas gonadotrophin loss was found in 88%, ACTH in 56%, and TSH in 52%. Hypothyroid patients usually respond poorly. The administration of HGH causes a considerable retention of nitrogen in hypopituitarism.

Thyroid tests. There is responsiveness to TSH, though priming with more than one dose may be required (Fig. 4-9). The PBI, BEI, or T_4 is diminished (PBI 2 to 3.5 μg./100 ml.) but not so profoundly as in primary thyroid myxedema (PBI usually less than 2 μg./100 ml.). The BMR tends to be moderately lowered (about -15% to -20%), and the cholesterol, normal or slightly elevated. In cachectic patients, particularly if anemic, hypocholesterolemia occurs. Several cases of unexplained hyperlipemia with lactescent serum have been described. For a more complete discussion, see Chapter 6.

Adrenocortical tests. If ACTH is deficient, tests of adrenocortical function will reveal various degrees of hypoadrenocorticism. Plasma and urinary 17-OHCS are lowered but will be increased by ACTH stimulation. The *metyrapone* test (p. 46) will be abnormal in most patients. Some patients, with apparent deficiency of ACTH as gauged by metyrapone, have subsequently shown a normal corticosteroid response to pyrogens, insulin, or surgery, so that this test either may be a more sensitive index of endogenous ACTH reserves or may give false negative results. The presence of endogenous ACTH can also be assessed by measuring the plasma 17-OHCS response to vasopressin. The effects of pituitary insufficiency on tests of carbohydrate metabolism have been discussed (p. 48). All tests involving the use of glucose and insulin require 2 to 3 days of preparation, with an adequate carbohydrate intake, preferably 200 to 300 grams/day, or else false positive results may occur in patients who are malnourished but who may have normal pituitary-adrenal function. The water-loading test (Chapter 12) shows delayed excretion that becomes normal after ACTH or corticosteroid therapy; in Addison's disease (primary adrenocortical failure) cortisol therapy will restore normal water excretion, whereas ACTH will not. Serum electrolytes are frequently normal, but there may be hyponatremia. The serum potassium is normal, in comparison with Addison's disease, in which the potassium is often elevated. For a more complete discussion see Chapter 12.

Gonadal studies. There is a castrate type of vaginal smear and endometrial biopsy, low urinary estrogens, and ovarian atrophy revealed by culdoscopy. In the male there is oligospermia or aspermia, low or zero semen volume with low fructose content, low urinary 17-KS, and low plasma and urinary testosterone. Testicular biopsy shows atrophy of tubules, oligospermia, and a deficiency or absence of Leydig cells. A positive response to human chorionic gonadotrophin (HCG) injection (rise of urinary 17-KS and blood or urine testosterone) will serve to differentiate primary testicular failure from that secondary to hypopituitarism (p. 51).

X-ray studies. The presence of a pituitary or suprasellar tumor will heighten the physician's suspicion of hypopituitarism. Lateral sella turcica area measurements are often diminished in Sheehan's syndrome.

Differential diagnosis

Panhypopituitarism is usually not overlooked, but lesser degrees of pituitary insufficiency may resemble hypothyroidism,

Table 5-2. Differential diagnosis of anterior pituitary insufficiency from anorexia nervosa

	Anterior pituitary insufficiency	Anorexia nervosa
Sex	Female/male, 2:1	Female almost exclusively
Age	10 to 65 years	15 to 40 years; rare after 40
Onset	Gradual	Sometimes abrupt
Anorexia	Mild reduction of appetite	Profound; severe aversion to food; self-induced vomiting; hiding or discarding food
Emotional status	Asthenia; mental torpor	Disturbed, hysterical, alert
Weight loss	Slight or none	Emaciated
Physical activity	Reduced	Active out of proportion to emaciation
Axillary and pubic hair	Reduced markedly or absent	Preserved; may be slight loss
Genital atrophy	Severe	Little or none
Breasts	Marked atrophy	Atrophy due to weight loss; often very little true atrophy
Pallor	Definite, often severe	Little or none
Laboratory tests for pituitary function	Profoundly reduced	No change or mild reduction
Response to hormone replacement therapy	Clear-cut improvement	Equivocal or no response

adrenocortical insufficiency, eunuchoidism, obscure anemia, liver cirrhosis, chronic asthenic states, malignancy, chronic malnutrition, or senility. The differential diagnosis of long-standing anorexia nervosa from hypopituitarism may be difficult (Table 5-2). Many cases designated as "Simmonds' cachexia" prior to the advent of modern laboratory techniques were undoubtedly cases of anorexia nervosa. Chronic malnutrition may result in functional hypopituitarism so that the differential diagnosis may require a long period of observation. A rare cause of diagnostic confusion is *multiple target organ failure (pluriglandular insufficiency)*, which may simulate panhypopituitarism. There is hypogonadism, hypoadrenocorticism, and hypothyroidism without loss of gonadotrophic, corticotrophic, or thyrotrophic hormones, and failure to respond to the administration of these pituitary trophic hormones.

Treatment

The therapeutic regimen depends on an assessment of the hormonal deficiencies. Ideally, replacement therapy with the missing trophic hormones should restore and maintain target organ function. Except for ACTH and TSH, however, potent anterior pituitary extracts are not available for general use. Present-day therapy consists of the replacement of the missing target organ secretion. Prolonged use of ACTH and/or TSH is not practical because of expense, the need for parenteral administration, the danger of foreign protein reactions, and the eventual production of antibodies. Potent GH preparations are available for experimental use only. Long-term depot-ACTH therapy has been used successfully in a number of patients without untoward effects. In addition to replacement of hormonal deficiencies, other therapeutic measures may be necessary. Associated diseases may require treatment (tuberculosis, sarcoidosis). If a pituitary tumor is the responsible agent, radiotherapy or surgery may be necessary. Occa-

sionally diabetes insipidus coexists and must be controlled.

Corticosteroids. In panhypopituitarism, therapy with cortisol should precede the administration of thyroid hormone. The dosage is 20 to 40 mg. daily (p. 232). Mineralocorticoids are necessary only where electrolyte deficiencies have been demonstrated or possibly during severe stress. For details see p. 231. An *identification disk*,* or dog tag, stating the diagnosis and the need for corticosteroids should be worn. The patient and his family should understand the possible lethal effects of stress and the need for augmentation of dosage.

Thyroid hormone. For hypothyrotrophism, replacement with thyroid hormone is necessary. Sensitivity to the metabolic stimulus of thyroid hormone occurs in some patients, and therapy may rarely precipitate severe adrenocortical insufficiency. For this reason small initial doses (8 to 15 mg. daily) are used, with gradual increases and pretreatment with hydrocortisone. For details see p. 166.

Sex hormone therapy. Most patients with hypopituitarism lack gonadotrophic hormones and require replacement therapy.

FEMALE. In women from approximately 14 to 45 years of age, cyclic therapy with an estrogen or an estrogen-progesterone preparation to cause withdrawal bleeding is desirable. Ovulation has been induced by using as a source of FSH human gonadotrophin prepared from postmenopausal urines (Pergonal) or from human pituitary glands followed by human chorionic gonadotrophin, a rich source of LH. The only rationale for gonadotrophin therapy would be infertility. After age 45 one may prescribe a smaller dose of estrogen so as to prevent vaginal bleeding. Androgen therapy is rarely if ever indicated in a female. For details of treatment see Chapter 20.

MALE. Most men with hypopituitarism require therapy to restore libido, sexual

---

*Medic-Alert, Turlock, Calif.

potency, muscle tone, and physical vigor. In cases of long-standing hypogonadotrophic hypogonadism, full restoration of virility is only rarely attained. Fertility in these patients will not be restored until a potent FSH preparation is available, though spermatogenesis has been stimulated with human menopausal gonadotrophins (HMG). A long-acting depot testosterone is given by injection every 3 or 4 weeks. Oral tablets of methyltestosterone or fluoxymesterone may be used, to be either swallowed or employed as buccal tablets. Testosterone pellets may be implanted subcutaneously. For details concerning the therapy of male hypogonadism, see Chapter 21.

Prognosis. The immediate mortality for panhypopituitarism, particularly where there is severe hypoglycemia or coma, is high. Pituitary coma and pituitary apoplexy are lethal complications. The prognosis for long survival is good in cooperative, carefully supervised patients receiving adequate replacement therapy.

Diabetes insipidus with anterior pituitary insufficiency

Rarely diabetes insipidus (D.I.) complicates adenohypophysial insufficiency and may remain latent until replacement therapy restores diuresis. The lesion may lie in the hypothalamus astride the neurohypophysial tracts or may be secondary to posterior lobe destruction or necrosis in Sheehan's syndrome or intrasellar tumor. Septic emboli or embolic abscesses of the neurohypophysis have been described. D.I. is common after hypophysectomy. Laboratory studies for D.I. had best be postponed until the associated anterior lobe deficiencies have been treated so as to avoid any possible untoward effects of vasopressin or nicotine administration in a patient with adrenocortical insufficiency.

Hypopituitary coma

Coma may occur at any time but is usually a complication of long-standing hypopituitarism. It is frequently precipi-tated by stress and is manifested by increasing apathy, drowsiness, stupor, and finally deep coma. The diagnosis depends on recognition of stigmas of anterior pituitary insufficiency associated with severe hypotension, weak or almost imperceptible pulse, hypothermia, and cold dry skin. There may be hypoglycemia, hyponatremia, and hypochloremia. Acute adrenocortical insufficiency secondary to hypocorticotrophism is usually heralded by nausea and vomiting and leads to dehydration, fever, and vascular collapse. In some patients there is bradycardia and profound hypothermia, a state that Sheehan has compared to hibernation. The treatment is almost identical to that for Addisonian crisis (p. 233). After recovery from coma, one can proceed with substitution therapy as previously outlined.

Prepuberal anterior pituitary insufficiency (pituitary dwarfism, infantilism)

Etiology. The cause of most cases is obscure, and only a few have been autopsied. There can be congenital absence of the pituitary gland. Some may be due to deranged hypothalamic function, with loss of neurosecretory cells causing a deficiency of growth hormone–releasing factor (GRF) and other RF's. Craniopharyngioma, lipoid disorders (Hand-Schüller-Christian), or other space-taking lesions may impinge upon the median eminence and suprasellar area, interfering with the hypophysial portal circulation, or may extend into the sella turcica. Diabetes insipidus is common with space-taking or infiltrative suprasellar lesions. A biologically inactive GH was the apparent cause of a familial form of dwarfism reported by Laron et al., 1966. Gilford, 1903, described normally proportioned dwarfs (ateliotic) with or without sexual development. McKusick reported two families of sexually matured ateliotic dwarfs having the disorder because of an isolated GH deficiency inherited as an autosomal recessive trait (Rimoin et al., 1966).

Incidence. Only 6.7% of the 442 cases

of stunted growth reported by Martin and Wilkins, 1958, were attributed to hypopituitarism or hypothalamic involvement, and these authors considered pituitary deficiency to be the "least common cause of dwarfism."

Clinical manifestations. Growth failure may become evident in early infancy or in later childhood. Size at birth may be normal or subnormal. Growth does not cease but is greatly decelerated, and stature may be similar to that of children 3 or more years younger than the patient. Dental development is retarded, with pro-

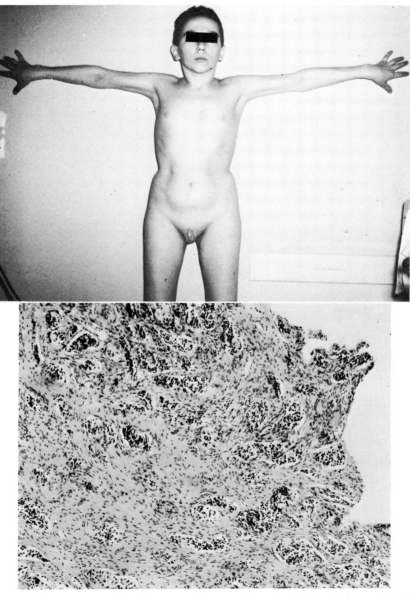

Fig. 5-3. Panhypopituitary dwarfism in a 33-year-old male. Height 53 in., weight 74 lb. Note boyish appearance, hairless body, and sexual infantilism. The testicular biopsy shows undeveloped tubules, architectural disorganization, interstitial fibrosis, and absence of Leydig cells.

longed retention of deciduous teeth. General health may not be impaired unless other pituitary hormones are deficient. There may or may not be various degrees of hypothyroidism and adrenocortical insufficiency. If there is hypogonadotrophism, sexual maturation will not occur at the time of puberty (infantilism). Occasionally hypoglycemic attacks may be prominent. There is no mental impairment.

Isolated GH deficiency has been rarely detected, but Grumbach's group (Goodman et al., 1968) studied 35 patients with growth deficiency by radioimmunoassay and found that 16 satisfied the criteria for this diagnosis. Hypoglycemia was a feature in 56%. They tended to have round doll-like facies with a normal head circumference, a pudgy appearance with height more retarded than weight, bone age less retarded than height age, and delayed puberty with initiation or acceleration of pubertal development during HGH therapy.

Physical examination. Growth retardation is usually severe, unless the disorder commences in late childhood. Skeletal proportions are normal. An immature childlike appearance persists into adulthood, and there is sexual infantilism with absence of axillary and pubic hair and small immature genitalia (Figs. 5-3 and 5-4). Dwarfs can mature sexually when there are gonadotrophic hormones and responsive gonads.

Laboratory studies. The program of laboratory study is similar to that for the adult. However, prior to 10 to 12 years of age one does not expect to detect urinary gonadotrophins in the normal child. In pituitary dwarfs with ACTH deficiency, values of 17-OHCS and/or 17-KS are lower than one would expect for the age of the individual being studied. Normal urinary 17-OHCS in childhood is approximately 3.1 ± 1.1 mg./M.^{2} body surface (Wilkins, 1965). If GH assays are available, the response to insulin hypoglycemia, arginine or a pyrogen is measured (p. 48). When these are not available, one can obtain a rough index of GH by measuring the serum inorganic phos-

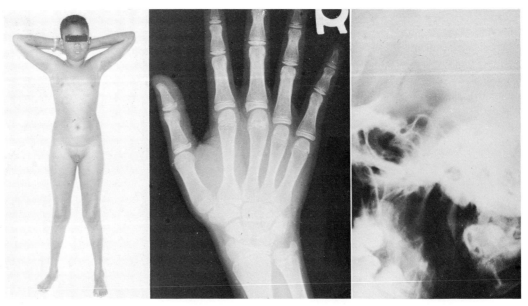

Fig. 5-4. Pituitary dwarfism in male Negro. Note sexual infantilism, good nutrition. Epiphyses of phalanges, radius, and ulna are unfused at age 21. The sella turcica is very small.

phate and alkaline phosphatase. Low values are characteristic of hypopituitarism. Hypercholesterolemia is common. X-ray examination of the epiphyses for retarded skeletal maturation is of great aid, though not specific. Skull films may reveal a hypoplastic sella turcica (Fig. 5-4) in idiopathic cases. This hypoplasia was found in 56.8% of 44 hypopituitary dwarfs in a study by Fisher and Di Chiro, 1964. An enlarged sella suggests a tumor, a craniopharyngioma, or other space-taking intracranial lesion. Silverman, 1957, and Riach, 1966, have published normal standards for the dimensions of the sella turcica in children.

Differential diagnosis of dwarfism. Precision in the diagnosis of dwarfism will undoubtedly improve with the availability of newer diagnostic tools but remains quite difficult, and often dwarfs must be observed into late adolescence before the cause becomes clear.

NUTRITIONAL DWARFISM. Caloric deficiency, even in the face of adequate protein intake, can result in growth impairment. The subcaloric intake detours protein from anabolic functions to satisfy energy requirements. Chronic infections (tuberculosis), celiac disease and diarrheas, cystic fibrosis of the pancreas, emotional disturbances with anorexia, or poverty can lead to nutritional deficiencies. Severe emotional disturbances associated with bizarre habits of eating and drinking may present features of hypopituitarism with short stature. When nutrition is improved, the growth rate is accelerated. Ultimate adult stature was not impaired in a study of 30 undernourished girls (Dreizen et al., 1967). The girls sustained a longer growth time that permitted them to eventually make up the deficit. Nutritional deficiencies may be viewed as examples of *functional hypopituitarism.*

DELAYED PUBERTY (CONSTITUTIONAL RETARDED GROWTH). Delayed puberty may frequently be mistaken for mild hypopituitarism. The differential diagnosis is discussed on p. 421.

PRIMORDIAL DWARFISM (MINIATURE ADULTS). An inherited congenital defect commencing during embryonic life may be the cause of primordial dwarfism. Various unknown factors may cause intrauterine growth retardation. Well-known examples are Tom Thumb, a circus dwarf of almost 100 years ago, and tribes of aboriginal pygmies. The disorder may also be inherited sporadically in families. Skeletal growth is usually seriously retarded but may exhibit gradations of growth stunting. Sexual maturation usually occurs and is not ordinarily delayed, and fertility may be unimpaired. These dwarfs are sometimes characterized by nanocephaly, and by craniofacial disproportions with a broad flat face, receding chin, and sunken nasal bridge. Bone age may be normal or slightly retarded, or may exhibit a mosaic pattern of varying degrees of maturation. Though the usual endocrine studies are normal, some patients so labeled in the past may prove to be examples of monotrophic GH deficiency. Rimoin et al., 1967, reported that African pygmies exhibited a normal GH rise after insulin-hypoglycemia or arginine infusion.

CRETINISM. Cretins are usually so easy to recognize that, except in early infancy, the differential from hypopituitary dwarfism is not difficult. Physical characteristics are outlined on p. 172. Epiphyses show the characteristic dysgenesis described by Wilkins, skeletal proportions are infantile, features of myxedema predominate, I.Q. is low, and the laboratory findings, particularly the response to TSH, are diagnostic.

GONADAL DYSGENESIS (OR GONADAL APLASIA). Gonadal dysgenesis (p. 372), a relatively common genetic disorder, is often confused with hypopituitary dwarfism because of sexual infantilism, amenorrhea, short stature, slight delay in bone age, and some reduction of urinary 17-KS. When the stigmas of Turner's syndrome are present (webbed neck, low hairline, increased carrying angle of the elbow, shield chest with widely spaced nipples, aortic coarctation), the diagnosis is obvious.

Height is rarely as seriously impaired and the delay of bone age is minimal. The karyotype is XO. There are characteristic x-ray findings in this syndrome not seen in hypopituitarism. Elevated levels of plasma GH have been reported, in contrast to the absence of measurable levels in pituitary dwarfs.

ACHONDROPLASTIC DWARFS (CHONDRODYS-TROPHY). The striking disproportion between the short arms and legs and the relatively normal trunk makes this condition rarely if ever mistaken for pituitary dwarfism. There is no endocrine disorder, and laboratory studies are normal.

MISCELLANEOUS CAUSES OF DWARFISM. A number of metabolic disorders (diabetes mellitus, disorders of calcium metabolism), chronic renal or hepatic disease, asthma, anemias with chronic anoxemia, and congenital or chronic cardiac diseases

can lead to impaired growth, and their presence should be ruled out before one embarks on any extensive endocrine survey. A host of osteodystrophies and congenital disorders are associated with short stature (Pott's disease of the spine, Hurler's syndrome, Laurence-Moon-Biedl syndrome, Seckel's bird-headed dwarfs, mongolism, dwarfism with microcephaly, Ellis–van Creveld syndrome, leprechaunism). Sexual precocity leads to early epiphysial closure.

Treatment of pituitary dwarfism. Human growth hormone (HGH) preparations are available only for investigational use under the control of the National Pituitary Agency. The first report of a collaborative study was made by Henneman, 1968. Forty-six of 50 patients showed clear-cut stimulation of growth. The average growth rate before treatment was 0.25 cm./month

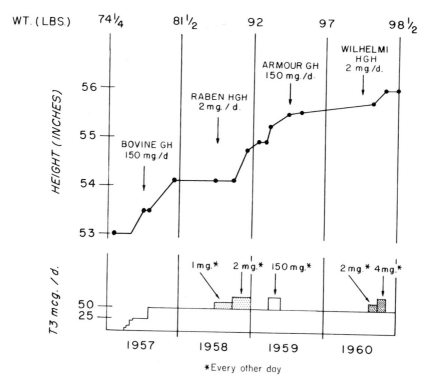

Fig. 5-5. Effect of HGH on the growth rate of the patient shown in Fig. 5-3. His height had been stationary for the previous 10 years. The bovine preparation was not effective; growth during 1957 was from the administration of triiodothyronine (T_3). The Raben preparation given in 1958 was the most effective. The asterisk means GH dose.

and during initial treatment with HGH, 0.65 cm./month. The usual doses given by most workers have been 2 to 4 mg. I.M. thrice weekly, though 2.5 to 5 mg. in one weekly injection has been effective. Some patients respond during prolonged treatment, whereas others become resistant after several months. Antibodies to HGH have been demonstrated, but their presence does not always correlate with therapy resistance.

Other measures to stimulate growth are less effective. Thyroid hormone in the hypothyrotrophic dwarf will induce some response (Fig. 5-5), and testosterone or other anabolic steroids will cause epiphysial maturation so that the growth spurt is prematurely curtailed by epiphysial closure. Panhypopituitary dwarfs will, of course, require substitution therapy with cortisol, and thyroid and gonadal hormones, as previously outlined.

PITUITARY TUMORS

Anterior pituitary tumors are classified according to the cell of origin as chromophobic, acidophilic, or basophilic adenomas. The last are rarely large enough to cause neurologic changes and will be discussed in Chapter 14 (Cushing's syndrome). Most are benign, but rarely they show rapid progression and malignant characteristics. "Invasive pituitary adenomas" are those which spread to areas contiguous to the hypophysis, and "pituitary carcinomas" spread to distant sites.

Structural effects (Schurr, 1966). The expansion of a pituitary tumor is conditioned by the size and shape of the sella turcica and the structure of the diaphragma sellae. The normal pituitary occupies only 50% of the volume of the sella turcica, so that a small tumor has room for considerable silent expansion. The posterior clinoids and the dorsum sellae are particularly vulnerable to pressure effects and are displaced posteriorly and subsequently eroded, decalcified, and finally destroyed by an expanding tumor. The floor of the sella turcica may be eroded,

and the tumor may rarely penetrate the sphenoidal sinus and protrude into the nasopharynx. The anterior clinoids are more resistant to tumor pressure. Invasive and malignant tumors may penetrate the cavernous sinus and produce abducens palsy or involvement of the trigeminal nerve, with severe facial pain. Tumors that break through the diaphragma sellae and penetrate the suprasellar region will compress and distort the optic chiasm or expand upward and backward to invade the hypothalamus and third ventricle.

Clinical manifestations. The signs and symptoms of a pituitary tumor may be (1) *endocrine*, because of interference with hypothalamic-hypophysial function and/or (2) *neurologic*, because of impingement upon neighboring structures and/or invasion of the third ventricle with obstruction of cerebrospinal fluid circulation. The endocrine manifestations differ somewhat in chromophobe adenomas and acromegaly and will be discussed separately.

Laboratory findings. Endocrine studies seek to reveal GH activity in acromegaly or evidences of hypopituitarism (p. 45) in acromegaly and chromophobe adenomas. Examination of the retina and mapping of visual fields are useful to investigate encroachment upon the optic tracts and chiasm.

Radiologic studies. Skull x-ray studies may show enlargement of the sella turcica or erosion or destruction of its floor, invasion of the sphenoid sinuses, distortion or destruction of the clinoid processes, or intrasellar or suprasellar calcifications. A balloon-shaped sella is found predominantly with an eosinophilic adenoma, whereas the sella tends to be more enlarged and cup shaped with a chromophobe adenoma. Chromophobe adenomas tend to cause more marked destruction of the dorsum sellae and more asymmetry of the sella. Rarely significant sellar enlargement may be caused by other brain tumors, intracranial aneurysms, pregnancy, myxedema, increased intracranial pressure, and the "empty sella" syndrome. A decision as to whether or not the sella is enlarged may be impossible when its diameters or total area is at the upper limit of normal. Serial x-ray films may be helpful in arriving at a diagnosis. Precision is increased by estimations of the *volume* of the sella turcica (Fig. 5-6). Air encephalography can demonstrate the extent of extrasellar spread. Carotid angiography may reveal lateral displacement of the cavernous segment of the internal carotid artery and elevation of the first part of the anterior cerebral artery. Arteriograms will also reveal in or near the sella an aneurysm that may be confused with a pituitary tumor. The term "empty sella" was coined to describe instances in which the pituitary gland appeared to be absent and the diaphragma sellae was incomplete. The pituitary gland is compressed to a narrow rim on the floor of the sella. The sella is remodeled and often enlarged sufficiently to mimic an intrasellar tumor. Sheehan also used the term empty sella to describe cases of severe postpartum necrosis of the adenohypophysis with extensive atrophy.

Chromophobe adenoma

Seventy percent to 90% of pituitary tumors are chromophobe adenomas; they are the commonest cause of enlargement of the sella turcica and produce a greater expansion of the pituitary fossa than other tumors. They are the most likely cause of pituitary insufficiency in adult males but are rare in children.

Pathology. Chromophobe adenomas consist of relatively agranular polygonal cells negative to PAS stain, though occasionally fine PAS-positive granules are seen.

Symptoms and signs. Duration is from a few days to many years. There is often a long delay in arriving at the diagnosis.

Onset. In the beginning the disease may be rapid, or slow and insidious.

Visual effects. Blurred vision and reduced visual acuity occur in one half to two thirds of all cases. The first physician consulted is usually an ophthalmologist. Visual field defects are common and are usually bitemporal hemianopia or temporal-field cuts. Papilledema usually indicates extension into the third ventricle. Sudden amblyopia is a symptom of probable hemorrhage in a pituitary tumor (pituitary apoplexy).

Headaches. Headaches are common and often severe, respond poorly to analgesics, and are often frontal or unilateral. Their occasional subsidence with the onset of visual disturbances has been attributed to rupture of the tumor through the diaphragma sellae.

Hypopituitarism. The expanding tumor

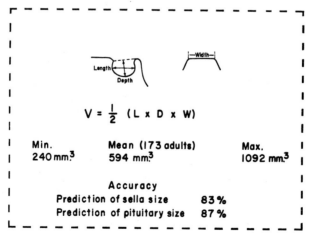

$$V = \frac{1}{2} (L \times D \times W)$$

Min.	Mean (173 adults)	Max.
240 mm.³	594 mm.³	1092 mm.³

Accuracy
Prediction of sella size   83%
Prediction of pituitary size   87%

Fig. 5-6. Volume of the sella turcica as calculated by Di Chiro and Nelson. (From Di Chiro, G., and Nelson, K. B.: Amer. J. Roentgenol. **87**:989, 1962.)

gradually encroaches upon normal anterior pituitary tissue. The earliest disturbances are loss of GH and hypogonadism, but with progression the picture of panhypopituitarism gradually emerges. Galactorrhea, usually evident only by milking the breast, is not rare; it may be due to interference with the secretion of prolactin-inhibiting factor.

Cranial nerve involvement (other than optic nerve). Nerve involvement is uncommon and is usually a sign of lateral spread into the cavernous sinus. There may be persistent diplopia because of oculomotor palsy, trigeminal involvement with facial pain, facial nerve palsy, involvement of the abducens nerve, and disturbances of olfaction and hearing.

Diabetes insipidus. D.I. is unusual but may occur when the supraopticohypophysial tracts are involved.

There is increasing evidence that some tumors labeled chromophobe adenoma may elaborate hormones. In certain cases of acromegaly in which hypophysectomy has been performed, a histologic diagnosis of chromophobe adenoma or mixed acidophil-chromophil has been made. A similar finding has been reported in a number of patients with Cushing's syndrome stemming from bilateral adrenocortical hyperplasia in whom, after adrenalectomy, visual defects and hyperpigmentation caused by excessive pituitary ACTH and MSH (Nelson's syndrome) developed.

Treatment of chromophobe adenomas. When a tumor is suspected but there is evidence neither of optic nerve or other neurologic involvement nor of endocrine disturbance, therapy is withheld and the patient is observed for evidence of progression. Eye grounds, visual fields, and skull films are repeated at regular intervals. Small tumors that are not growing rapidly can be controlled by supervoltage rotational radiotherapy. The average dose is 3,500 to 4,000 R in 3 to 4 weeks; rotational therapy tends to prevent brain damage, skin reactions, and permanent depilation. The response is slower than that achieved by surgery, and a histologic diagnosis is lacking. About 20% of chromophobe tumors are cystic and respond poorly. Operative decompression or hypophysectomy is reserved for patients having larger or rapidly expanding tumors whose vision is threatened and in whom previous radiotherapy has been unsuccessful. Complete removal of the tumor is rarely accomplished. The operative mortality varies from 0% to 10% but is considerably greater in patients with large tumors. It is advisable to support the patient with corticosteroids during and after surgery even when specific evidence of adrenocortical insufficiency is lacking and probably even if a normal metyrapone test is obtained. Vasopressin may be required if diabetes insipidus occurs.

Postoperative radiotherapy is favored by many surgeons, in the hope of avoiding recurrences. Some experts contend that even tumors causing visual impairment can be initially treated by radiotherapy, whereas other experts always favor a surgical approach. Late sarcomatous degeneration has been attributed to radiation. Recurrences may occur years later, and prolonged follow-up is recommended. Visual improvement is achieved after surgery in 55% to 75% of reported cases.

Pituitary apoplexy. Sudden hemorrhage into a tumor or area of infarction is a surgical emergency. There is acute loss of vision, fever, hypotension, mental deterioration, extraocular palsies, and even signs of a subarachnoid hemorrhage.

For reviews of three large series of chromophobe adenomas, see Fürst, 1966, Chang and Pool, 1967, and Elkington and McKissock, 1967.

Acromegaly

Acromegaly is a disorder caused by the hypersecretion of GH usually from an adenoma of the anterior pituitary in an adult.

Pathophysiology

Pituitary gland. The eosinophilic tumor is usually solid but may be cystic or show areas of hemorrhage, and it is ordinarily not large. Malignancy is rare. Occasionally there is eosinophilic cell hyperplasia rather than a tumor. In Ezrin's series (Gordon et al., 1962) the pathology in 29 cases was as follows: 18 mixed eosinophilic-chromophobic adenomas, 4 relatively pure eosinophilic, 2 chromophobic adenomas composed of "gamma" cells, 3 malignant adenomas of which 1 was eosinophilic, and 1 case of multiple adenomas. In addition to excessive GH secretion, there may be irritative hypersecretion of other pituitary hormones. Galactorrhea may be due to prolactin excess and adrenocortical enlargement and nodule formation because of excess ACTH. During stage I (hyperpituitarism) increased gonadal activity may occur but has not been proved to be caused by hypergonadotrophism. Goiter formation has been ascribed to excess TSH. The evidence, however, favors the role of excess GH alone accounting for all or most of the above changes.

Thyroid gland. The thyroid gland is frequently enlarged and may be nodular or contain adenomas. Hyperthyroidism may occur but is unusual. If hypopituitarism occurs, the thyroid atrophies. The *parathyroids* too may exhibit hypertrophy and may rarely become hyperactive. The thymus may persist and be enlarged.

Adrenal glands. The cortex is hypertrophied, and cortical nodules (or adenomas?) are common. Adrenocortical function is frequently normal but may be increased (elevated cortisol secretion rate and 17-KS hyperresponsiveness to ACTH) or reduced from pituitary insufficiency.

Carbohydrate metabolism. Plasma insulin is hyperresponsive to glucose, tolbutamide, and arginine. There is decreased sensitivity to insulin with insulin tolerance tests and frequently a diabetic glucose tolerance curve.

Ovary and testicle. Few data are available to substantiate a hypothesized early hypertrophy and hyperfunction. Gonadal atrophy is common because of hypogonadotrophism.

Visceral organs. Generalized marked splanchnomegaly occurs, though enlargement of the liver is most common. The heart and kidneys may be greatly enlarged. There is elevated glomerular filtration rate, renal plasma flow, and proximal tubular functions.

Bone. See the discussion on x-ray changes, p. 74.

Connective tissue. Generalized increase noted throughout ligaments, fascia, tendons, articular capsules, synoviae, peribronchiolar tissues, pancreas, heart, liver, and skin.

Multiple endocrine adenomatosis. Functioning tumors of other endocrine tissues, particularly the islets of Langerhans and the parathyroids, may coexist with acromegaly. It is frequently a hereditary disorder and may be associated with peptic ulceration of the upper gastrointestinal tract (Zollinger-Ellison syndrome).

Clinical features

Stages. To understand the various clinical phenomena of acromegaly, one must visualize the progression of the disease in stages as follows.

State I—Hyperpituitarism. Enlarging tumor actively secretes GH and perhaps other anterior pituitary trophic hormones.

Stage II—Plateau stage. When excessive secretory activity gradually subsides and progression of the disorder decelerates or ceases, the plateau stage is reached.

Stage III—Anterior pituitary insufficiency. When the tumor interferes with the elaboration of GH and other pituitary hormones, there is anterior pituitary insufficiency (Fig. 5-7).

These stages are outlined to serve as a guide and not to imply either the existence of hard-and-fast categories or of inevitable progression. A patient may display evidences of active GH secretion combined with signs of pituitary insufficiency. Bailey and Cushing described a transient mild form they called "fugitive acromegaly." Often even in florid acromegaly, the disease reaches a plateau, and progression

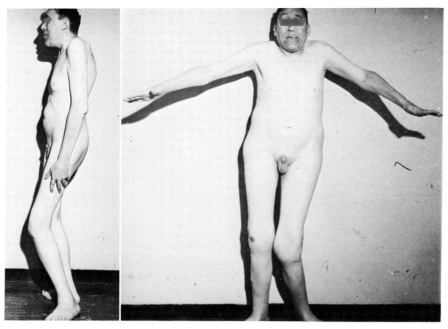

Fig. 5-7. Acromegalic gigantism in a 47-year-old male with panhypopituitarism. Intrasellar tumor operated on at age 13 years. Note acromegalic features, sexual infantilism, absence of body hair, severe degenerative arthritis of knees with subluxation and destruction of left knee joint.

ceases. It is not clear whether this is due to a spontaneous cessation of hypersecretion of GH, necrosis of the tumor (autohypophysectomy), or loss of end-organ response.

The clinical picture, described below, will therefore represent a composite pattern.

Onset. Usually the onset is slow and insidious. The patient may be scarcely aware of physical alterations for some time. In retrospect, the disorder is present 10 or more years before the diagnosis is made.

Sex. Males and females are equally affected.

Symptoms. The patient or his family notice the coarsening of facial features and the enlarged hands and feet. Disturbances of vision or persistent headaches usually constitute the first symptom. Early in the disease (stage I) there may be hyperhidrosis and increased physical strength, energy, libido, sexual energy, and potency. Later there is loss of strength, fatigue, loss

of the sense of well-being, and beginning hypogonadism. Muscle atrophy occasionally occurs. The complaints that can be ascribed to pituitary insufficiency (see list on p. 56) often develop, particularly in long-standing cases. *Headaches* are severe, persistent, generalized, or bitemporal. The *disturbance of vision* is usually slow and progressive but may occasionally be abrupt in onset. It is the most serious disturbance of acromegaly and classically consists of *bitemporal hemianopia* but may, however, cause various field defects affecting color vision initially. Temporary or even permanent symptomatic remissions may occur. Cushing described uncinate gyrus seizures preceded by olfactory and gustatory aurae because of interpeduncular extension of the hypophysial growth. The carpal tunnel syndrome, with acroparesthesias and pain affecting the thumb and middle three fingers, may occur and is due to the soft tissue and cartilaginous-bony thickening compressing the median nerve in the carpal tunnel. Muscle aches and pains and

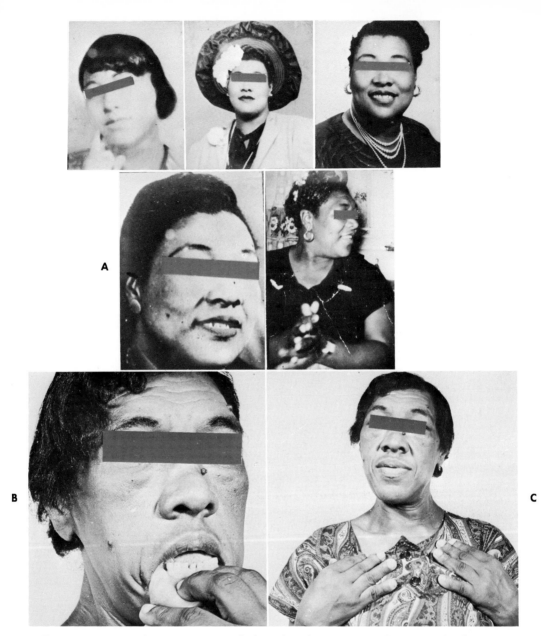

Fig. 5-8. Acromegaly. **A,** Five views before the obvious onset of acromegalic features. **B,** Note increased interdental spaces, coarsened features, nevi, and comedones. **C,** Note large nose, thick lips, prognathism, and large hands with thick bulbous fingers.

painful stiff extremities, joints, and spine are common.

Signs. There is overgrowth of the acral parts, coarsened features (Fig. 5-8), and large spadelike hands and feet (Fig. 5-9). The mandible usually is elongated and protrudes (prognathism or "lantern jaw"), causing dental malocclusion. There may be an impediment of speech because of tongue hypertrophy. The thyroid gland may be enlarged and nodular. The skin and soft tissues are coarse and thickened, and normal skin folds are accentuated, especially over the scalp and forehead,

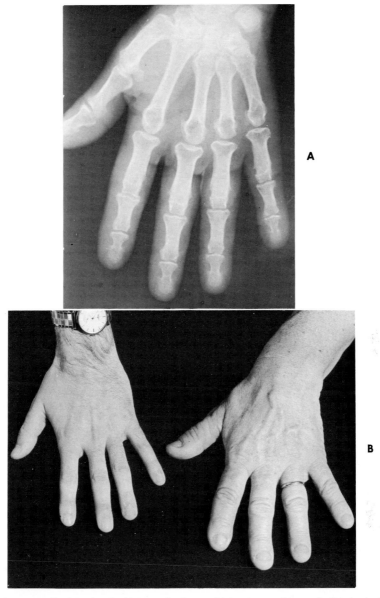

Fig. 5-9. Acromegalic hands. **A,** Note soft tissue thickening, tufting of distal phalanges, thickened phalangeal shafts, enlarged medial sesamoid bone, and periarticular spurs. **B,** An acromegalic hand on the right contrasted to normal male adult hand of comparable age.

producing corrugations. The skin may be oily and moist with comedones and acne because of hypertrophy and hyperplasia of sebaceous and sweat glands, but if hypopituitarism appears, the skin becomes dry. Acanthosis nigricans, a rare skin disorder, has been reported. Papillomas, nevi, and lipomas are common. There may be hypertrichosis in males, and hirsutism and occasionally even signs of virilism in women, associated with elevated urinary 17-KS. The furrows and folds of the knuckles are enlarged, and the fingers become bulbous or sausage shaped, chiefly because of soft-tissue thickening (Fig. 5-9). Joint enlargement resembles degenerative arthritis and may be the site of intra-articular effusions, subluxations, and deformity (Fig. 5-7). The interphalangeal and metacarpophalangeal joints of the hands and the knee joints are often painful and swollen. Rather than joint stiffness, there is excessive mobility because of a lax capsule. Hypertension is frequent and may be severe. There may be cardiac hypertrophy and even congestive failure. The cardiac muscle shows hypertrophy and fragmentation of muscle fibers, diffuse fibrous hyperplasia separating individual fibers, and atherosclerosis. Acromegalic cardiomyopathy is a serious complication found in approximately 10% of patients. Hepatic photoscans show the liver to be enlarged approximately one and one-half times normal, but this enlargement can only occasionally be detected by palpation (Preisig et al., 1966). An augmented excretory capacity for sulfobromophthalein was also observed. Galactorrhea is not unusual and may be discovered only by milking the breast. Symptoms and signs of hypopituitarism may be present (p. 56).

Laboratory findings

Plasma growth hormone (GH). Most untreated patients have plasma GH values above the normal of approximately 3 mμg./ml. The expected decrease of plasma GH provoked by *glucose* administration does not occur, but the rise that is normally evoked by *insulin* hypoglycemia may or may not obtain. The hoped-for association of high GH levels with clinical evidence of activity has not always been found.

Plasma sulfation factor, an index of serum GH (p. 41), is elevated in acromegaly.

Serum inorganic phosphorus (SIP). SIP is frequently elevated (that is, above 4.5 mg./100 ml.) and decreases after successful therapy. It has been used as an index of activity, but its accuracy is questionable. Elevation of the SIP also occurs in uremia, male hypogonadism, and hypoparathyroidism and is physiologic before the comple-

tion of puberty. During an augmented insulin tolerance test (0.3 U./kg. I.V.) in 14 acromegalic subjects, Massara et al., 1966, found a higher fasting level and a conspicuously smaller maximum fall of the SIP than was found in normal subjects. The serum alkaline phosphatase is frequently elevated.

Blood sugar. Elevated postprandial blood sugars and impaired glucose tolerance, the latter found in about 25% of cases, have been used as indices of activity but are too inconsistently abnormal to be reliable. Clinical diabetes is found in 10% to 20% of acromegalic patients, and the recession of documented diabetes is usually a reliable sign of reduced GH activity or even of the onset of pituitary insufficiency. The diabetic state may be latent, mild, or severe and may show insulin insensitivity.

Basal metabolic rate. The BMR is frequently high. Hyperthyroidism is unusual, and the PBI, RAIU, and other indices of thyroid function are normal, though the thyroxine-binding proteins may be altered. The hypermetabolism is extrathyroidal in origin.

"Forearm metabolism." In active acromegaly Rabinowitz and Zierler, 1963, found elevated-forearm O_2 consumption, net inward potassium movement, and a threefold enhanced release of free fatty acid (FFA) from adipose tissue. Intra-arterial insulin provoked decreased glucose and potassium movement into the forearm, but retention of the insulin effect on FFA movement.

Urinary hydroxyproline. Urinary hydroxyproline is inconstantly increased.

Urinary calcium. Urinary calcium is frequently elevated.

X-ray changes

Skull (Fig. 5-10). The sella turcica is enlarged in approximately 80% of cases and tends to be balloon shaped. The calvarium is thickened, the skull circumference is increased, and there may be hyperostosis frontalis interna in women. The

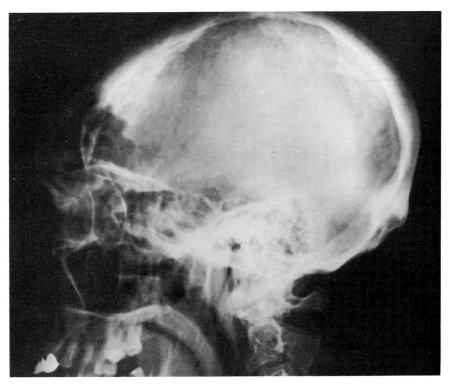

Fig. 5-10. Skull in acromegaly. Note thickened calvarium with hyperostosis, enlarged frontal and maxillary sinuses, and pneumatized mastoids. The sella turcica has been disorganized by previous hypophysectomy.

scalp is thicker than normal, and the ear cartilages may be calcified and ossified.

Paranasal sinuses. The frontal sinuses are often greatly enlarged, particularly in males, with bossing of the superciliary ridges, and the maxillaries are similarly hypertrophied.

Mastoids. Hyperpneumatization occurs in the mastoids.

Mandible. The mandible is enlarged and lengthened (prognathism). The mandibular angle is increased.

Vertebrae. The bodies of the vertebrae are elongated and widened because of periosteal proliferation of bone along the anterior and lateral surfaces. Hypertrophic spurs may be greater than expected for the age of the patient. There is often increased thickness of the intervertebral disks. Thoracic kyphosis occurs when the vertebrae are severely involved. Lumbar vertebrae show concave posterior borders.

Ribs. The ribs are enlarged and elongated, causing a large thorax with increased sagittal and coronal thoracic diameters. The lower sternum may be elevated. The costochondral junctions show a fusiform widening.

Hands and feet. The most constant finding is *thickening of the soft tissues of the fingers and toes.* Such thickening is most prominent at the proximal interphalangeal joints of the fingers. Tufting of the terminal phalanges is another pathognomonic finding but may occasionally be seen in normal subjects. The phalangeal, metacarpal, and metatarsal shafts may be thickened, whereas the shaft of the proximal phalanges of the feet tends to be narrowed. The bony articular surfaces of the joints of the hands and feet are separated widely, suggesting increased cartilaginous thickness. The medial *sesamoid bone* at the metacarpophalangeal joint of the first digit is enlarged. The *sesamoid index* is determined by measuring the greatest diameter in millimeters and multiplying by the greatest perpendicular diameter. In 100 control subjects (Kleinberg et al., 1966) the mean for both sexes was 20 (12 to 29), and among the 20 acromegalics the mean for men was 40 (30 to 63) and women 33 (31 to 35). Increased *heel-pad thickness* was described by Steinbach and Russell, 1964. In 103 normals the mean was 17.8 mm. (13 to 21 mm.), and in 29 acromegalics the mean was 25.6 mm. (17 to 34 mm.). However, 40% of Negroes and 9% of white individuals were found to have a heel-pad thickness of more than 21 mm. (Puckette and Seymour, 1967). A significant increase in skin thickness, demonstrated by a roentgenographic method, has been described (Sheppard and Meema, 1967).

Joints. Spurring is common, but joint narrowing as in degenerative arthritis is rare.

Pelvis. Beaking of the superior portion of the pelvic bones adjacent to the symphysis is seen. In women there is often flaring of the iliac bones and thinning of the pubic rami.

For a review of skeletal changes see Steinbach, 1959.

Differential diagnosis

The diagnosis may be difficult in early or very mild and transient cases. Certain coarse-featured large-boned individuals may resemble acromegalics, but the physiognomy remains unchanged throughout their adult lives. Examination of photographs from a family album may be useful. Patients with *myxedema, leontiasis ossea,* or *Paget's disease* may exhibit some superficial resemblances. *Pachydermoperiostosis* (idiopathic hypertrophic osteoarthropathy) is an uncommon familial disorder that usually affects young males and produces digital clubbing and certain facial and skeletal features that resemble acromegaly. It has been called "familial acromegaly" in older literature. Facial coarsening and slight enlargement of the hands and feet are sometimes found in normal pregnancy but subside after delivery.

Therapy

Judgment concerning the need for treatment depends on the activity or quiescence of the disease ("hot" or "cold"?) and whether the lesion compromises vision or is invading nearby structures. The following are some useful criteria of activity:

1. Progressive increase in clinical manifestations (further growth of hands, feet, acral parts, mandible)
2. An enlarging sella turcica and/or the appearance of thinning or erosion of the floor or destruction of the clinoid processes
3. Development or persistence of headaches
4. Progressive impairment of vision
5. Developing signs of hypopituitarism
6. Hypothalamic symptoms (diabetes insipidus)
7. Appearance of diabetes mellitus, or worsening of established diabetes
8. Serum inorganic phosphorus and urinary hydroxyproline elevation
9. Plasma GH elevation and abnormal response to glucose and to insulin
10. Active endochondral bone formation found upon biopsy of the costochondral junction (Sullivan et al., 1963) (normally not found in adults over 30 years of age or in quiescent acromegaly)

When the disease is inactive, therapy may be withheld and the patient is observed at intervals thereafter, with serial repetition of x-ray examinations and appropriate laboratory studies. Some authorities, however, stress the importance of treatment of all cases, even when they are apparently inactive.

Pituitary x-ray irradiation. Irradiation has been the favored treatment in patients who show slow progression and no mandatory reasons for immediate neurosurgery. The eosinophilic adenoma is more radiosensitive than the chromophobic tumor.

Conventional radiotherapy frequently appears to arrest the progression of acromegaly, but recurrences are not uncommon. Elevated plasma GH levels generally have not been reduced. More favorable results and restoration of normal GH concentrations have been achieved with heavy-particle, alpha, and proton radiation (Lawrence et al., 1963). Cobalt and rotational beam therapy avoids permanent depilation, radiation necrosis, and optic nerve damage. Local surgical implantation of radioactive materials (yttrium 90, gold 198) and the use of stereotactic cryohypophysectomy are promising newer modalities.

Surgery. Sudden or rapidly developing amblyopia because of pituitary apoplexy is a surgical emergency. Progressive visual impairment or signs of increased intracranial pressure are indications for surgical decompression and/or hypophysectomy, though visual difficulties per se are not accepted by all authorities as a contraindication to radiotherapy. Complete removal of the tumor cannot always be accomplished. Corticosteroids and vasopressin may be required (see discussion on chromophobe adenoma, p. 69). Surgery may be necessary if a trial of radiation is unsuccessful. An initial surgical approach in all cases has been advocated by some authorities who point to the unpredictable and often partial regressions achieved by radiation and its failure to reduce plasma GH values. Surgical decompression combined with local implantation of radioactive isotopes has been tried with considerable success. Postoperative x-ray irradiation is practiced by many neurosurgeons.

Complications of surgery include transient, or occasionally permanent, diabetes insipidus, cerebrospinal rhinorrhea (which may be brief or permanent), brain, optic nerve, or other cranial nerve damage, meningitis, osteomyelitis, and convulsive seizures. Permanent panhypopituitarism is a not infrequent sequela. An operative mortality of 0% to 10% must be expected and

is usually caused by hemorrhage or cerebral edema.

Estrogens. The possibility of suppressing GH hypersecretion by estrogen administration was suggested by the observation that the eosinophils of the anterior pituitary of experimental animals were depleted by large doses of stilbestrol and that the elevated SIP frequently was lowered by estrogen therapy. Clinical results, however, have been disappointing and unpredictable.

Replacement therapy for hypopituitarism is frequently required as the disorder progresses (see p. 61).

Prognosis. The outlook for duration of life and preservation of vision depends on multiple factors. The onset of hypopituitarism and/or diabetes insipidus complicates the prognosis. There are no adequate long-term statistics to judge the effects of radiation or surgical treatment. Conventional radiotherapy has usually been only partially successful, and recurrences are common. Heavy-particle, cobalt, and implantation radiation have had only a limited trial. The best long-term results seem to be achieved by hypophysectomy. Vision usually improves after successful treatment, and soft tissue thickening regresses, but the connective tissue hyperplasia and skeletal hypertrophy persist. Distortion of the physiognomy and enlargement of the acral parts tend to recede slowly, but the typical features of acromegaly often persist.

Gigantism

Gigantism occurs when GH hypersecretion arising from an eosinophilic pituitary adenoma originates before puberty. The disorder is rare and affects males predominantly.

Clinical features. Rapid growth may commence at any age but tends to appear late in childhood and early puberty. One of the most celebrated giants was the Alton boy. Excessively rapid growth began in infancy, and by age 9 years he was 6 feet tall; at 12 years his height was 7 feet, and at 18, 8 feet 3 inches (Behrens and Barr, 1932). The Trinity College skeleton is 8 feet 6 inches tall.

The epiphyses remain open, and growth may continue into early adulthood. Acromegalic features, at first not evident, begin to appear during adolescence. Secondary sex characters are often delayed in appearance and may never be fully mature (Fig. 5-7). Eunuchoidism is common. The shoulders are narrow, the trunk, arms, and legs are long, and the hands and feet are enormous. An unusual association of gigantism with "fractional hypopituitarism" (hypogonadism, hypothyroidism, and hypoadrenocorticism) and a normal sella turcica as revealed by x-ray examination has been described (Goldman et al., 1963).

Laboratory findings. Laboratory results are similar to those of acromegaly.

Differential diagnosis. Extraordinarily tall, large-boned, normal individuals may be mistaken for true giants. They usually have tall forebears, are often of North European or Scandinavian stock, are symmetrically proportioned, and show none of the stigmas of gigantism (that is, acromegaloid features, enlarged sella turcica, eunuchoidism, and characteristic changes in x-ray and laboratory findings). Rapid growth is observed in hyperthyroidism, various forms of precocious puberty, Klinefelter's syndrome, and eunuchoid states, but none of these resemble gigantism.

Therapy. The method of treatment is similar to that for acromegaly.

Craniopharyngioma

Craniopharyngiomas (craniopharyngeal duct tumors, Rathke pouch tumors, adamantinomas, suprasellar cysts) are tumors derived from remnants of the craniopharyngeal duct (Rathke's pouch). They are usually suprasellar in close relationship to the optic chiasm but may be found below the diaphragma sellae. The optic nerve tracts and chiasm are compressed and stretched or may even be incorporated into the tumor mass, and there may be compression or invasion of the third ventricle. Most or all of the tumor may lie within the sella turcica compressing or invading the pituitary gland.

Pathology. The tumors are oval or spherical, may be small and solid or large and cystic, and contain yellowish or reddish brown "motor-oil" fluid, cholesterol crystals, and grumous material (Love and Marshall, 1950). They tend to adhere firmly to surrounding neural tissue. The histology may resemble adamantinomas, but most consist of nests or whorls of squamous epithelium in a connective tissue stroma. They are benign.

Clinical features. Craniopharyngiomas are most prevalent in the first two decades. However, in Love and Marshall's series of 56 males and 44 females, 47% were 20 years of age or older. *Symptoms* and *signs* are caused by pituitary compression or invasion, involvement of the optic chiasm and nerves, and hypothalamic and/or third ventricle involvement. The neurologic phenomena (headache, vomiting, drowsiness, and other signs of increased intracranial pressure and visual loss) are the most common initial complaints. Hydrocephalus may result from invasion of the third ventricle. Compression or invasion of the hypothalamus may cause somnolence, diabetes insipidus, obesity, and interference with the passage of hypothalamic releasing factors to the anterior pituitary, resulting in hypopituitarism, dwarfism, and sexual infantilism. Froehlich in 1901 described a 14-year-old boy with a hypothalamic tumor, which may have been a craniopharyngioma, who showed short stature, sexual infantilism, obesity, and diabetes insipidus. Drowsiness, stupor, personality changes, vertigo, convulsive seizures, and uncinate fits may occasionally be prominent features.

X-ray findings. Suprasellar lesions may produce x-ray signs of increased intracranial pressure (that is, separation of cranial sutures) and usually depression of the clinoids, erosion of the dorsum sellae, and compression of the sella. There may be signs of an intrasellar tumor, however, with expansion of the sella turcica, widening of the outlet, and erosion or destruction of the clinoids. Areas of *calcification* are seen in over 50% of cases. Air encephalograms, ventriculograms, and arteriography may be useful in localizing the lesions.

Laboratory findings are principally related to adenohypophysial insufficiency and diabetes insipidus.

Differential diagnosis. Craniopharyngioma must be suspected when visual loss, signs of increased intracranial pressure, diabetes insipidus, and anterior pituitary insufficiency are combined with x-ray evidence of a suprasellar calcified mass. The differentiation from a pituitary adenoma is often difficult, but the latter is rarely calcified and usually produces a more uniform symmetrical expansion of the sella turcica. Brain tumors, optic nerve gliomas, and internal hydrocephalus may be mistaken for craniopharyngioma. Craniopharyngiomas are often misdiagnosed in adults because they have mistakenly been thought to be confined to children.

Treatment. Complete surgical extirpation has been possible in only a small percent of cases because of their proximity and adherence to vital brain structures. When the optic chiasm, hypothalamus, or third ventricle is involved, extirpation may endanger life or seriously damage these structures. In some instances a cyst may be aspirated and the collapsed capsule partially removed. If the third ventricle is obstructed, ventriculocisternostomy may induce a prolonged remission. Postoperative supervoltage x-ray irradiation may be beneficial. Measures to control diabetes insipidus and endocrine substitution therapy for hypopituitarism are employed as required. The prognosis is poor. Only 5 of 104 patients in Love and Marshall's series survived 10 years. However, Holmes et al., 1968, described 8 children who not only survived removal of the tumor but showed normal or superior rates of statural growth after operation.

REFERENCES

Beernink, F. J., and McKay, D. G.: Amer. J. Obstet. Gynec. 84:318, 1962.

Behrens, L. H., and Barr, D. P.: Endocrinology 16:120, 1932.

*Chang, C. H., and Pool, L.: Radiology 89:1005, 1967.

Di Chiro, G., and Nelson, K. B.: Amer. J. Roentgen. 87:989, 1962.

Dreizen, S., et al.: J. Pediat. 70:256, 1967.

*Elkington, S. G., and McKissock, W.: Brit. Med. J. 1:263, 1967.

*Escamilla, R. F., and Lisser, H.: J. Clin. Endocr. 2:65, 1942.

Fisher, R. L., and Di Chiro, G.: Amer. J. Roentgen. 91:996, 1964.

*Fürst, E.: Acta Med. Scand. 180:suppl. 452:1, 1966.

Gilford, H.: Practitioner 70:797, 1903.

Goldman, J. K., et al.: Amer. J. Med. 34:407, 1963.

Goodman, H. G., et al.: New Eng. J. Med. 278:57, 1968.

Gordon, D. A., et al.: Canad. Med. Ass. J. 87:1106, 1962.

*Henneman, P. H.: J.A.M.A. 205:828, 1968.

Hewer, R. F.: J. Endocr. 3:397, 1944.

Holmes, L. B., et al.: New Eng. J. Med. 279:559, 1968.

Houssay, B. A., and Biasotti, A.: Rev. Soc. Argent. Biol. 6:251, 1930.

Kallman, F. J., et al.: Amer. J. Ment. Defic. 48:203, 1944.

Klachko, D. M., et al.: J. Clin. Endocr. 28:1768, 1968.

Kleinberg, D. L., et al.: Ann. Intern. Med. 64:1075, 1966.

Laron, Z., et al.: Israel J. Med. Sci. 2:152, 1966.

Lawrence, J. H., et al.: J.A.M.A. 186:156, 1963.

Love, J. G., and Marshall, T. M.: Surg. Gynec. Obstet. 90:591, 1950.

Martin, M. M., and Wilkins, L.: J. Clin. Endocr. 18:679, 1958.

Massara, F., et al.: J. Endocr. 34:13, 1966.

*Odell, W. D.: J.A.M.A. 197:1006, 1966.

Perkoff, G. T., et al.: J. Clin. Endocr. 20:1269, 1960.

Plaut, A.: Amer. J. Path. 28:883, 1952.

Preisig, R., et al.: J. Clin. Invest. 45:1379, 1966.

Puckette, S. E., Jr., and Seymour, E. Q.: Radiology 88:982, 1967.

Rabinowitz, D., and Zierler, K. L.: Bull. Johns Hopkins Hosp. 113:211, 1963.

Rabkin, M. T., and Frantz, A. G.: Ann. Intern. Med. 64:1197, 1966.

Riach, I. C. F.: Brit. J. Radiol. 39:824, 1966.

Rimoin, D. L., et al.: Science 152:1635, 1966.

*Significant reviews.

Rimoin, D. L., et al.: Lancet **2:**523, 1967.

Schneeberg, N. G., et al.: J.A.M.A. **172:**20, 1960.

*Schurr, P. H.: Pituitary tumours in man, In Harris, G. W., and Donovan, B. T., editors: The pituitary gland, vol. 2, Anterior pituitary, Berkeley, 1966, University of California Press, p. 498.

Sheehan, H. L., and Stanfield, J. P.: Acta Endocr. **37:**479, 1961.

Sheppard, P. H., and Meema, H. E.: Ann. Intern. Med. **66:**531, 1967.

Silverman, F. N.: Amer. J. Roentgen. **78:**451, 1957.

*Steinbach, H. L., et al.: Radiology **72:**535, 1959.

Steinbach, H. L., and Russell, W.: Radiology **82:**418, 1964.

Sullivan, C. R., et al.: Proc. Mayo Clin. **38:**81, 1963.

Wilkins, L.: The diagnosis and treatment of endocrine disorders in childhood and adolescence, ed. 3, Springfield, Ill., 1965, Charles C Thomas, Publisher, pp. 66-67.

Chapter 6

The thyroid gland

ANATOMY

The thyroid gland is H or butterfly shaped with the wings as lateral lobes and the body as the isthmus. The isthmus is a thin ribbonlike band that crosses the trachea at the level of the second ring and connects the lower thirds of the lateral lobes. A pyramidal lobe, which varies greatly in size and is found in 25% of individuals, springs ordinarily from the left half of the isthmus and extends toward or to the hyoid bone. Accessory thyroid tissue is occasionally found at the base of the tongue (lingual thyroid) or in the neck. The gland is light reddish brown in adults, and its consistency resembles firm rubber. Its surface is smooth, somewhat lobulated, and well encapsulated. The adult weight is 20 to 35 grams, and it is larger in women than in men.

Blood supply

The arterial supply is from the left and right superior thyroid arteries (from the common carotid) and the inferior thyroid arteries (from the subclavians). An inconstant thyroidea ima (lowest thyroid) artery arises from the innominate artery. The vascular supply is extraordinarily rich, being twice as much blood per gram of tissue as that of the kidneys. Branches of the major arteries radiate in a network over the surface of the gland, penetrate the capsule, and extend inward along connective tissue septa. The two lateral thyroid lobes are subdivided into *structural lobes*, which are themselves further subdivided into *lobules*. Each lobule consists of 20 to 40 follicles bound by a fine connective tissue sheath and supplied by a small *lobular artery*, which feeds into the intricate capillary plexus that envelops each follicle (Johnson, 1955) (Fig. 6-1). Marked capillary proliferation occurs in experimental hyperplasia of the thyroid gland. There is a rich lymphatic network (Fig. 11-2) that forms large cisternae or bursulae in the interfollicular spaces interconnected by smaller lymph channels (Wissig, 1964).

Nerve supply

There is an autonomic nerve supply. Sympathetic innervation is from plexuses arising from cervical sympathetic ganglia and feeding along arterial trunks to enter the thyroid. The *parasympathetic innervation* arises from the vagus (ganglion nodosum) and passes to the thyroid through the superior and recurrent laryngeal nerves. The autonomic nerves exert control over thyroid blood flow and may thus make an important contribution to its physiologic activity.

Thyroid gland relationships

Important contiguous structures are of particular interest to the surgeon. The four *parathyroid glands* may be inadvertently removed during thyroidectomy,

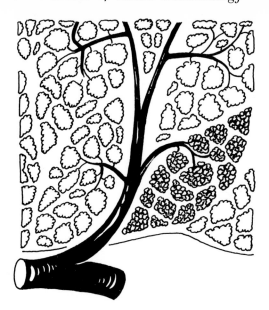

Fig. 6-1. Blood supply of the thyroid gland. A branch from a large surface vessel passes between structural lobes. Branches from the interlobar vessel enters the structural lobes and further subdivides to supply the thyroid lobules. (From Johnson, N.: Brit. J. Surg. **42:**587, 1955.)

particularly when they are within the thyroid capsule or even embedded in thyroid parenchyma. The *recurrent laryngeal nerves,* branches of the vagi, are found behind the lateral lobes in the tracheo-esophageal groove, but their course is inconstant.

EMBRYOLOGY

The thyroid gland arises from a midline collection of endodermal cells in the floor of the primitive pharynx that can be identified near the end of the first month of fetal life at the 3.5 to 4 mm. stage. From this primordium a hollow diverticulum appears that enlarges, forms a spherical vesicle, and remains attached to the pharyngeal floor by a narrow stalk. It begins to assume a bilobal or inverted Y shape, loses its lumen, and after further growth forms an isthmus connecting the two lateral lobes. Caudal migration, in part assisted by descent of the heart and septum transversum, elongates the stalk to form the

thyroglossal duct, which originates at the base of the tongue. The duct eventually is attenuated and disintegrates, though the cranial portion attached to the base of the tongue at the foramen cecum may persist for a time as a *lingual duct* that eventually disappears. A persistent portion of the distal duct becomes the *pyramidal lobe* (or process). The hyoid bone develops dorsal to the duct. Occasionally thyroid nodules are found behind the hyoid, attached to it, or rarely in the substance of the bone.

Thyroid follicles devoid of colloid appear at the latter part of the tenth week (58 mm.) and accumulate RAI and form colloid by the twelfth to fourteenth week (100 mm.). The formation of follicles in the developing thyroid may be influenced by TSH from the fetal hypophysis. The fourth pharyngeal pouches give rise to the ultimobranchial (postbranchial) bodies. Thyroid cysts and lateral aberrant thyroid tissue may arise from ultimobranchial remnants.

MICROSCOPIC STRUCTURE

The functional units of the thyroid gland are the follicles. They are spherical structures measuring 200 to 300 μ that rest on a thin delicate basement membrane and are supported by a narrow connective tissue interstitium richly endowed with vascular, lymphatic, and neural networks. The follicle is lined by a single layer of cuboidal epithelial cells that are specially adapted to accumulate iodide from the circulation and to synthesize and deliver thyroid hormone (TH) into the circulation. The lateral borders of the epithelial cells are in direct contact, the apices border the colloid, and the bases rest on a basement membrane that is in close apposition to the endothelium of the capillary plexus. The mean acinar-cell height tends to be proportional to the activity of the gland. Cells other than follicular epithelium have been described ("parafollicular," "C-cells") in the thyroid connective tissue that may be the source of thyrocalcitonin. The follicular lumen is filled

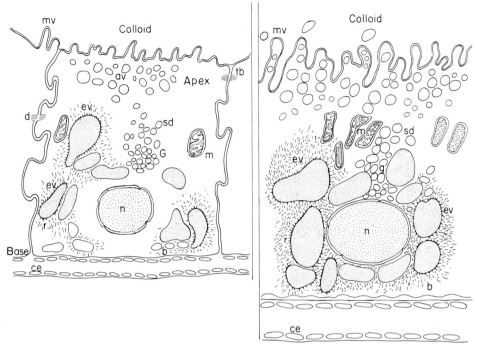

Fig. 6-2. Fine structure of the thyroid cell. Normal cell on the left and stimulated or hyperthyroid cell on the right. **av,** Apical vessels; **b,** basal plasma membrane; **ce,** capillary endothelium; **d,** dermosome; **ev,** ergastoplasmic vesicles; **G,** Golgi apparatus; **m,** mitrochondrion; **mv,** microvillus; **n,** nucleus; **r,** ribosomes attached to **ev** or free in cytoplasm; **sd,** secretory droplets; **tb,** terminal bar. The stimulated cell on the right is larger and shows intense proliferation of microvilli (many containing droplets). All other subcellular structures are enlarged and increased in number. The nucleus almost doubles in volume. Note gaps or fenestrations in capillary endothelium. The stimulated cell shows elongation of endothelial cells and invaginations of the basal plasma membrane, which can extend toward the nucleus. (Adapted from text and photographs in Wissig, 1964, and Nadler, 1964.)

with colloid that contains stored TH. A proteolytic enzyme whose activity parallels thyroid secretory function (protease) probably contributes to the hydrolysis of thyroglobulin in colloid and/or thyroid vesicles.

Knowledge of the detailed fine histologic structure of the thyroid has been reviewed by Wissig, 1964, Heimann, 1966, and others and is depicted schematically in Fig. 6-2. The *functional significance* of the subcellular structures of the thyroid has been the subject of intensive investigation. Nadler, 1965, has advanced the following hypothesis. The uniodinated protein moiety is synthesized by ribosomes and enters the ergastoplasmic vesicles. The Golgi ap-

paratus may be an important structure in colloid biosynthesis and may add the carbohydrate moiety. The release of the protein from these vesicles to the cell surface and to the follicular colloid "might be visualized like a bubble of soap coming up to the surface of the water where it explodes leaving a soap film. In a similar manner, the membrane of an apical vesicle reaching the cell surface would fuse with the plasma membrane of the cell and break up to release its content to the colloid."[*] All cells deliver thyroglobulin

[*]From Nadler, N. J.: In Cassano, C., and Andreoli, M., editors: Current topics in thyroid research, New York, 1965, Academic Press, Inc.

to the colloid at the same rate. Small follicles would therefore show a more rapid turnover rate than would large follicles. Iodination of thyroglobulin occurs either in the follicular colloid or at the cell-colloid interface, and, in all likelihood, the iodination process concentrates in the periphery of the lumen quite close to the apical surface of the follicular cell.

MECHANISM OF THYROID HORMONE SECRETION

The follicular lumen is filled with a thin clear refractile fluid called *colloid*. It contains thyroglobulin, a compact protein with a sedimentation constant of 19S and a molecular weight of approximately 670,000. Its molecular structure is still not completely known. It contains thyroxine (T_4) and triiodothyronine (T_3) in peptide linkage and thus is a reservoir of stored thyroid hormones. The mechanism of hormone secretion remains hypothetical. Deiss and Peake, 1968, have summarized the process as follows: Colloid droplets engulfed from the lumen by apical villi enter the cell by pinocytosis. Lysosomes, intracellular granular particles containing hydrolytic enzymes, migrate from the cell base toward the apex and fuse with the colloid droplets. Lysis of thyroglobulin occurs, and T_4 and T_3 are released and enter a capillary at the base of the cell. Glutathione (GSH) may play a role in the cleavage of the disulfide bridges in thyroglobulin. Some intact thyroglobulin enters the lymph and venous channels draining the thyroid gland. For a review see Seljelid and Nakken, 1969.

THYROID HORMONES
Chemistry (Fig. 6-3)

L-*Thyroxine (T₄) and* L-*triiodothyronine (T₃)* are the biologically active circulating thyroid hormones. They are composed of two ether-linked benzene rings with a hydroxyl at position 4' on the outer ring and an alanine side chain at position 1 on the inner ring. As shown in Fig. 6-3, loss of an iodine at position 5' produces T_3, an

extremely active compound, whereas loss of iodine at position 5 produces inert "reverse-T_3." T_3 has about five times the metabolic potency of T_4 and acts much more rapidly but more transiently. T_3 is bound less to plasma proteins and is more readily diffusible. In the chicken, T_4 is not protein bound and exhibits properties similar to T_3.

Other thyroxine analogues are shown in Fig. 6-3. The pyruvic and acetic acid compounds are metabolic products of T_4 and T_3, but there is doubt that any of the analogues found in tissues of experimental animals exert any physiologic activity. When T_4 has been incubated with kidney slices or homogenates, *tetrac* has been· found and *triac* has been formed from T_3 in rat kidney and muscle. Both compounds have shown some metabolic activity when given to hypothyroid humans. *Triprop* and *tetraprop* are more potent stimulators of tadpole metamorphosis than are T_3 or T_4, but, in general, no analogue has exhibited metabolic activity approaching that of T_4 and T_3.

Substitution of other halogens for the iodine atoms all but abolishes activity. For a review see Barker, 1964.

The *stereochemical* requirements for biologic activity have been reviewed by Jorgensen, 1964. The benzene rings are inclined at an angle of approximately 120 degrees and rotate about the ether linkage (Fig. 6-3). Jorgensen believes that the outer ring interacts with a thyroid hormone "functional receptor" and is responsible for biologic activity, and the inner ring, together with the ether-linking oxygen and the alanine side chain, attaches to a "binder receptor" at the site of hormone action.

Biosynthesis of thyroid hormones

The present concept of the biosynthesis of T_4 and T_3 is shown diagrammatically in Figs. 6-4 and 6-5. Plasma iodine (I^-) is derived from iodide ingested in food and drink, with perhaps a small fraction absorbed by the lungs and skin. The kid-

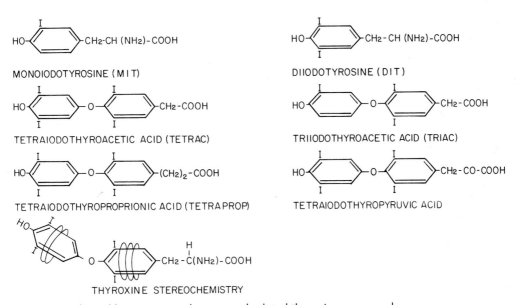

Fig. 6-3. Thyroid hormones, analogues, and related thyronine compounds.

ney and thyroid compete for the iodide, and a small amount is lost in the urine. Thyroid synthesis of T_4 and T_3 involves four phases. The fifth phase is that of secretion.

Iodide concentration (the iodide "trap"). The trapping of iodide from the low con-centration of perfusing arterial blood is accomplished by establishing a concentration gradient that can promote a ratio of thyroid iodide to serum iodide (the T/S ratio) of 20:1 or more in the normal resting gland. The trap is stimulated by TSH, is Na^+, K^+, and Mg^{++} dependent, is

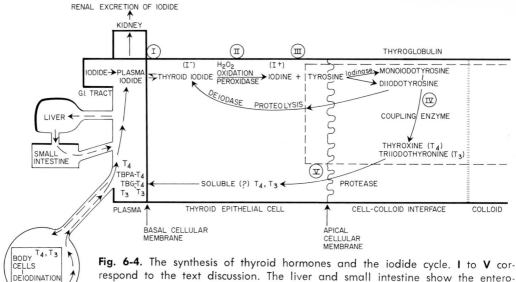

Fig. 6-4. The synthesis of thyroid hormones and the iodide cycle. **I** to **V** correspond to the text discussion. The liver and small intestine show the enterohepatic cycle. **TBG,** Thyroxine-binding globulin; **TBPA,** thyroxine-binding prealbumin.

slowed by hypophysectomy and anoxia, and is blocked by thiocyanate, perchlorate, digitalis glucosides, iodide, and other anions. That a concentration gradient exists seems certain, since the thyroid cell is approximately 50 mv. negative to colloid and extracellular fluid. Passive diffusion of iodide ions, possibly through membrane "pores," does occur but is probably negligible unless plasma levels are high. Iodide may combine reversibly with a carrier in the cell membrane and then pass irreversibly into an area of high I⁻ concentration. The energy required for trapping is supplied by high energy phosphate bonds. That the precise trapping site is unknown may be inferred by the knowledge that isolated thyroid cells free of colloid can concentrate ^{131}I and synthesize iodoproteins. Iodide trapping also occurs in the salivary glands, stomach, mammary glands, choroid plexus, and ciliary body of the eye but does not lead to iodothyronine synthesis and is not affected by TSH. The mammary glands quite actively form iodotyrosines and considerable PB^{131}I.

It has been suggested that there are two iodide compartments in the thyroid cell.

One, designated "first iodide pool," consists of readily dissociated and exchangeable iodide recently trapped from perfusing blood and quickly washed out by potassium perchlorate ($KClO_4$) or thiocyanate ($KSCN$). The "second iodide pool" is derived from the deiodination of iodotyrosines, is much larger than the first pool, turns over at a slower rate, does not exchange readily with plasma iodide, and is not released by $KClO_4$ or $KSCN$.

Liberation of iodine from iodide. Intracellular iodide [I⁻] is converted into a reactive form [I⁺] by hydrogen peroxide [H_2O_2] as the oxidizing agent and peroxidase as the catalyst, as shown in Fig. 6-4, *I* and *II*. The mechanism of the generating systems that produce H_2O_2 in the thyroid gland is unknown. Klebanoff et al., 1962, believe that peroxidase may catalyze both the generation of H_2O_2 and the oxidation of iodide as follows:

$$DPNH + H^+ + O_2 \xrightarrow{\text{peroxidase}} DPN^+ \; H_2O_2$$

$$H_2O_2 + 2I^- + 2H^+ \xrightarrow{\text{peroxidase}} 2\text{"Oxidized I"} + 2H_2O$$

Hydrogen peroxide may be produced by

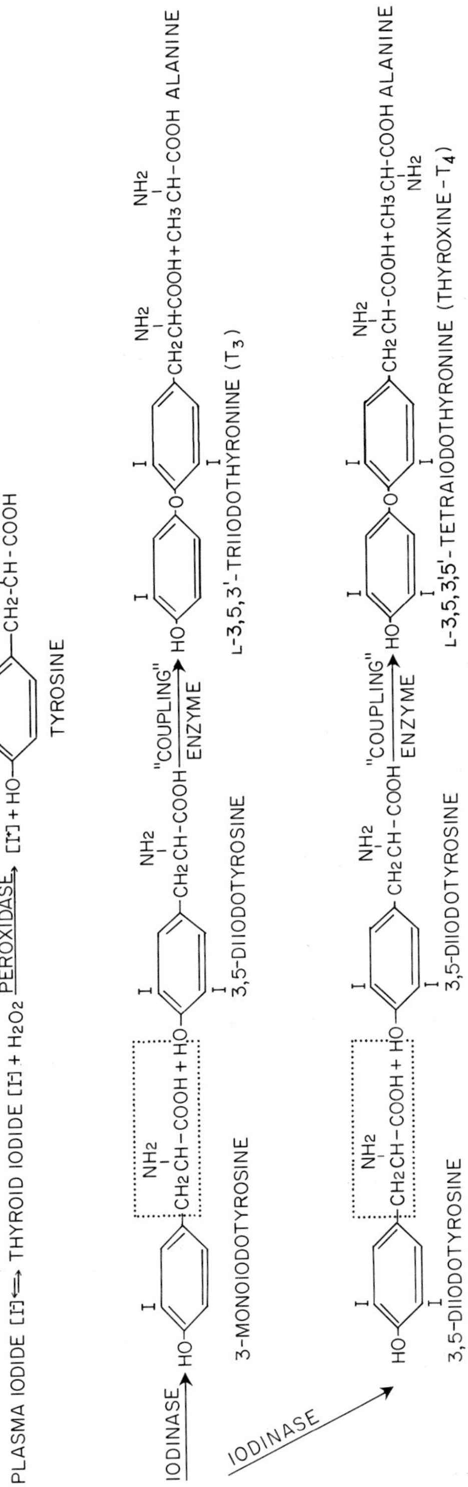

Fig. 6-5. Biosynthesis of thyroid hormones.

flavin-linked enzymes, since flavin adenine dinucleotide is a thyroid constituent.

Iodination of tyrosine (organification). "Active" iodine [I⁺] is instantaneously bound to tyrosine so that free iodide cannot be demonstrated unless a blocking agent such as thiourea is used. Within seconds after ^{131}I administration to an experimental animal, tyrosine-^{131}I can be detected. This reaction may be regulated by an enzyme called tyrosine iodinase, though the evidence for its role is tenuous. It is stimulated by triphosphopyridine nucleotide and flavin nucleotide and is inhibited by an antihydrogen peroxide enzyme, catalase. The oxidizing enzyme, peroxidase, and the iodinating enzyme, tyrozine iodinase, may be an iodinating complex originating in microsomal or membranous elements of the cell. The mitochondria may be the site of H_2O_2 production. Iodination occurs on peptide-linked tyrosine within the matrix of the thyroglobulin molecule. Whether mono-iodotyrosine (MIT) is a necessary precursor for the formation of diiodotyrosine (DIT) or whether both are formed simultaneously is an unsettled question, though the evidence favors the former. Tyrosine iodination is inhibited by antithyroid drugs of the thiourylene series by interfering with the iodination reaction directly and/or by blocking the oxidation (peroxidase) of iodide [I⁻] to the reactive state [I⁺]. The anions thiocyanate and perchlorate block the accumulation of iodide by the thyroid cell and also, in high concentration, inhibit organic binding.

Synthesis of T_4 and T_3 (coupling). T_4 and T_3 are formed by the coupling of iodinated tyrosines under the regulation of a hypothetical "coupling enzyme." The synthetic steps may occur as shown in Fig. 6-5, with MIT and DIT coupling to form T_3 and with two DIT molecules coupling to form T_4. There may be other pathways such as the deiodination of T_4 to T_3 or the iodination of T_3 to T_4, but there is little evidence to support the concept that either compound is the precursor of the other.

Secretion. The thyroid gland can store large amounts of available hormone adequate to supply tissue needs for several weeks and can therefore adjust to large variations in iodide intake. The mechanism of thyroglobulin hydrolysis has been discussed (p. 84). T_4, T_3, and some iodide are released from peptide-linkage within thyroglobulin and enter the circulation, but only under abnormal conditions are intact circulating iodotyrosines found.

Thyroid follicles vary considerably in size and are structurally and functionally heterogeneous. Smaller follicles show a more rapid ^{131}I turnover than do large follicles. Recently formed organic iodine is secreted preferentially before older organic iodine and thus the thyroid handles iodine in a "last come, first served" manner.

Deiodination of iodotyrosines

Proteolysis of thyroglobulin also yields iodotyrosines, which are deiodinated by deiodinase and their iodide reutilized to synthesize T_4 and T_3. This iodide, designated "second pool iodide," is much larger than trapped or "first pool iodide" and is largely retained, though a small amount may leak into the circulation. The concept of compartmentalization of iodides is challenged by workers who visualize a homogeneous situation where there is a single pool of iodide.

Extrathyroidal thyroxine formation

Young, thyroidectomized, experimental animals can be restored to a euthyroid state and resume normal growth and maturation when iodide is given in large amounts. Numerous similar observations have suggested that either T_4 is formed in the absence of the thyroid gland or iodide itself has thyroidlike properties. The question remains unsettled, but Taurog and Evans, 1967, have presented direct evidence of T_4 formation in iodide-injected thyroidectomized rats.

Regulation of thyroid hormone formation

TSH. *Pituitary thyrotrophin (TSH),* discussed on p. 35, is the major regulator of thyroid hormone synthesis.

Iodide. Thyroid activity varies inversely with the concentration of thyroidal iodide. Organic binding of iodide is markedly inhibited at a critical level of plasma inorganic iodide (20 to 35 μg. in rats, 6 to 12 μg./100 ml. in man). Tyrosine iodination and coupling are reduced, and the MIT/DIT ratio is increased. The inhibition usually is overcome when the iodide concentration recedes below the critical level and synthesis is renewed. This self-regulatory iodide-controlled phenomenon has come to be known as the Wolff-Chaikoff effect (Wolff and Chaikoff, 1948). It is an acute phenomenon; "escape" or adaptation to the inhibitory effects of large doses of iodide usually occurs within 48 hours, though the thyroid loses some of its ability to concentrate iodide (Braverman and Ingbar, 1963). Iodide deficiency stimulates thyroid function as shown by increased RAIU, T/S, and MIT/DIT ratios and iodide clearance. The regulation of thyroid function by iodide is independent of TSH, but the effects of TSH appear to be potentiated by thyroidal iodide depletion.

For a discussion of the synthesis of

Table 6-1. Antithyroid compounds*

Classification	Compound	Mechanism of action
Monovalent ions	Perchlorate Thiocyanate Chlorite, hypochlorite Iodate, periodate Nitrate	Block accumulation of iodide by thyroid† (competitive inhibition) Discharge of unbound iodide from thyroid Thiocyanate depresses organic binding of iodine (in large doses)
Thiourylenes (thiocarbamides)	Thiourea Thiouracil Propylthiouracil Methylthiouracil Methimazole	Inhibit oxidation of iodide (peroxidase reaction) Inhibit other biosynthetic intrathyroidal steps (coupling, iodination of tyrosine, formation of DIT) Propylthiouracil increases renal clearance of iodide, reduces peripheral degradation of T_4 and T_3
Aniline and amino-heterocyclic compounds	Para-aminosalicylates Para-aminobenzoates Sulfonamides Sulphonylureas Amphenone-B	Similar to thiocarbamides (with certain differences)
Miscellaneous compounds	Dinitrophenol, resorcinol, cobalt, phenylbutazone, iodides, sodium chloride	Various
Naturally occurring goitrogens (human and cattle feed)	Thiocyanates Progoitrin and goitrin	Block accumulation of iodide by thyroid gland

*Based on data from Greer et al., 1964.
†Can be overcome by increasing the dose of iodide.

thyroid hormones, see DeGroot, 1965, Wolff, 1964, and Rosenberg and Bastomsky, 1965.

Antithyroid agents

Goitrogenic compounds (Table 6-1) inhibit thyroid hormone (TH) synthesis, depress the circulating level of TH, and thus induce excessive TSH release, with resultant compensatory thyroid hyperplasia. Prolonged administration, particularly in large doses, may completely inhibit TH synthesis. Hypothyroidism ensues once pre-formed stores of hormone have been utilized. In experimental animals inhibition of peripheral activity has been demonstrated. For example, propylthiouracil retards the disappearance rate of serum $PB^{131}I$. Pharmacologic studies of the thiourylenes have been confined mainly to thiouracil. Antithyroid compounds are excreted in breast milk and are transported to the fetus via the placenta. In Fig. 6-6 the contrasting effects of two types of antithyroid compounds are illustrated. For a review of antithyroid drugs see Greer, 1964.

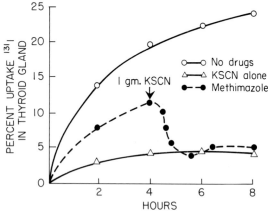

Fig. 6-6. Contrasting effects of a thiocarbamide (methimazole) and a monovalent anion (thiocyanate, KSCN) on thyroidal accumulation of radioiodine. KSCN prevents the thyroidal uptake of ^{131}I. Methimazole does not block uptake but does prevent organic binding; the free, unbound ^{131}I is then washed out of the gland by KSCN.

Circulating thyroid hormone (hormone transport)

The circulating TH concentration remains remarkably constant under normal conditions. The half-life of T_4 is 6.5 days, and that of T_3 1.3 to 2.6 days. This rate may be accounted for by differences in protein binding, rate of deiodination, and metabolic degradation. T_4 is the major circulating component; only very small amounts of T_3 are detectable. Nonetheless, a considerable contribution to the total biologic activity of TH is made by T_3. A given serum concentration of T_3 will be metabolically equivalent to roughly $5 \times 2\frac{1}{2} \times 2$, or 25 times the concentration of T_4 (Wiener, 1968). Almost all (99%) of the circulating T_4 is reversibly bound to carrier proteins. The mechanism of the binding is not clear but appears to result from forces of electrostatic attraction. T_3 is more loosely bound to protein, and a larger proportion remains unbound and is readily diffusible.

Thyroxine-binding plasma proteins (TBP)

Thyroxine-binding globulin. TBG is an alpha-globulin whose electrophoretic mobility is situated between alpha-1-globulin and alpha-2-globulin. It is present in human serum in an approximate concentration of 10 to 20 mg./L. and is believed to be a trace alpha-glycoprotein with a molecular weight of 40,000 to 45,000. It is the major carrier for circulating TH, occurs only in mammals, and exhibits a greater binding capacity in females than in males. A fall in binding capacity has been reported with increasing sexual maturation in males. TBG binds T_3 about 25% to 35% as firmly as T_4 and is only one third saturated under normal conditions. Complete saturation can occur when hormone levels rise as in hyperthyroidism, or where the concentration of TBG is reduced.

Thyroxine-binding prealbumin. TBPA (Ingbar, 1958) migrates anodal to albumin by electrophoresis. Its binding properties are similar to those of TBG, but it binds T_4 exclusively. It has a low carbohydrate content in contrast to TBG and a molecular weight of 61,000. Oppenheimer and Bernstein, 1965, studied a highly purified TBPA that contained no carbohydrate, had a molecular weight of 73,000, and had an average concentration in serum of 34 mg./100 ml. TBPA is the thyroid-binding protein in cerebrospinal fluid.

Thyroxine-binding albumin. Serum albumin transports little hormone under ordinary conditions but is capable of binding T_4 and T_3 if the capacity of TBG and TBPA is exceeded. Its binding affinity, however, is less than that of TBG or TBPA. The PBI remains normal in hypoalbuminemic states. If normal serum is enriched with minute amounts of labeled T_4, TBG binds $57\pm6.7\%$, TBPA $32\pm5\%$, and albumin $10.6\pm1\%$ (Oppenheimer et al., 1963).

Other protein carriers probably play a minor role. Binding is diminished by deiodination, the loss of an aromatic ring, loss of the OH^- group on the outer ring, or alterations in the alanine side chain.

Free circulating thyroxine

The proportion of nonprotein-bound ("free") TH constitutes less than 0.05% of the total. The protein-bound fraction is physiologically inert, whereas the free fraction readily diffuses into the extracellular space, penetrates cell membranes, and is responsible for thyroid-induced metabolic activity. The protein-bound fraction probably serves both as a reservoir and as a buffer to aid in the regulation of the concentration of free hormone. Thus the PBI and free hormone circulate in simple reversible equilibrium.

$$TBP{\cdot}T_4 \leftrightarrows T_4 + TBP$$

or

$$K = \frac{(T_4)(TBP)}{TBP{\cdot}T_4}$$

Table 6-2. Alterations in free thyroxine and thyroxine proteins in various clinical states*†

	Normal	Pregnancy	Hypothyroid	Hyperthyroid	Nonthyroid illness
PBI	N	↑	↓	↑	N or slightly ↓
Free T_4	N	Slightly ↓	↓	↑	N or slightly ↑
Maximal binding capacity — TBG	N	↑	Slightly ↑	N	N
Maximal binding capacity — TBPA	N	Slightly ↓	N	↓	↓

TBG binding elevated:	Myxedema, pregnancy, estrogens, contraceptive pill, acute porphyria (females), severe liver disease, perphenazine (Trilafon), genetic, familial
TBG binding decreased:	Androgens, diphenylhydantoin, corticosteroids Nephrosis Acidosis (respiratory or metabolic) Severe hypoproteinemia (occasional)
TBPA decreased:	Hyperthyroidism Nonthyroid illness, trauma, stress (surgery) Dinitrophenol, salicylates

*Based on data from Ingbar, S. H., and Freinkel, N., 1960; Oppenheimer et al., 1963, 1965.

†N = normal, ↑ = increased, ↓ = decreased. Changes reflect binding capacity and not necessarily total concentration.

TBP·T_4 is protein-bound thyroxine, T_4 is free thyroxine, TBP is total thyroxine-binding protein, and K is the dissociation constant at equilibrium. The buffering action of protein binding is illustrated by the marked alterations in PBI, and thus in thyroxine-binding proteins, that may occur without disturbing the euthyroid status of the subject (Table 6-2). The normal TSH-thyroid axis constitutes a homeostatic regulator that continually tends to maintain a constant level of free T_4. In pregnancy and during estrogen administration, TBG is increased. This change tends to increase binding → lower free T_4 → increase pituitary TSH secretion → increase thyroid secretion → restore free T_4. Free T_4 concentration is therefore not significantly altered, though in pregnancy the values tend to be slightly diminished.

In hyperthyroidism both free and bound hormone rise, though TBG remains unchanged and TBPA is decreased. The TSH-thyroid axis does not serve as a regulator, and hypersecretion is constantly maintained. Free T_4 tends to rise disproportionately to the bound fraction. Alterations of the concentration of free T_4 in various states are shown in Table 6-2 and are consistent with the thesis that it most accurately reflects the functional state of the thyroid gland. In a variety of nonthyroid heterogeneous illnesses, the maximal binding capacity and the absolute concentration of TBPA are reduced. The reduction noted after surgery has been attributed to a marked diminution in the synthesis of TBPA, a protein with a half-life of 1.9 days as compared to serum albumin with a half-life of 12.7 days (Oppenheimer and Bernstein, 1965). In febrile states T_4 may be displaced from the binding proteins, resulting in a somewhat elevated level of free T_4, though less than obtains in hyperthyroidism. Binding of T_4 to albumin may be affected by several anions. Diphenylhydantoin exhibits competitive inhibition of binding to TBG, and salicylates inhibit binding to TBPA (Hollander et al., 1967).

Distribution of thyroid hormones

Free circulating T_4 and T_3 are probably in reversible equilibrium with intracellular T_4 and T_3, though some hormone appears to be irreversibly bound. Studies of the tissue distribution of ^{131}I- and ^{14}C-labeled T_4 and T_3 show that T_3 is concentrated more rapidly. The liver concentrates and metabolizes thyroid hormones most actively, but skeletal muscle, by virtue of its bulk, accounts for most of the extravascular hormone. Little or none is concentrated by brain, spleen, and gonad. The hormones are found in the soluble cytoplasmic fraction of tissue cells. Tata, 1965, found in rat and rabbit muscle a "cellular thyroxine-binding protein" (C-TBP) that exhibited less thyroxine-binding capacity than did serum. C-TBP may regulate the availability of free thyroid hormones for metabolic processes.

Metabolism of thyroid hormones (degradation, excretion)

The liver is the principal site of thyroid hormone metabolism; kidney and skeletal muscle make important contributions. In liver disease the clearance of thyroid hormone may be retarded. Calvalieri and Searle, 1965, found that almost the entire plasma T_4 pool (126 μg. of T_4 iodine) enters and leaves the liver hourly. They visualize the liver as a reservoir, perhaps to buffer against sudden changes in the circulating level of hormone. There are three major metabolic disposal routes that may operate alone or in various combinations (Fig. 6-7).

Deiodination

Deiodinating enzymes (dehalogenases) have been found in many tissues. In skeletal muscle, deiodination is the only available metabolic transformation. The salivary glands can deiodinate TH, and the salivary iodide can be reabsorbed in the gastrointestinal tract, thus functioning as an "iodine cycle." Thyroxine dehalogenase is activated by flavins and ferrous ions and acts upon T_4 much more readily than upon

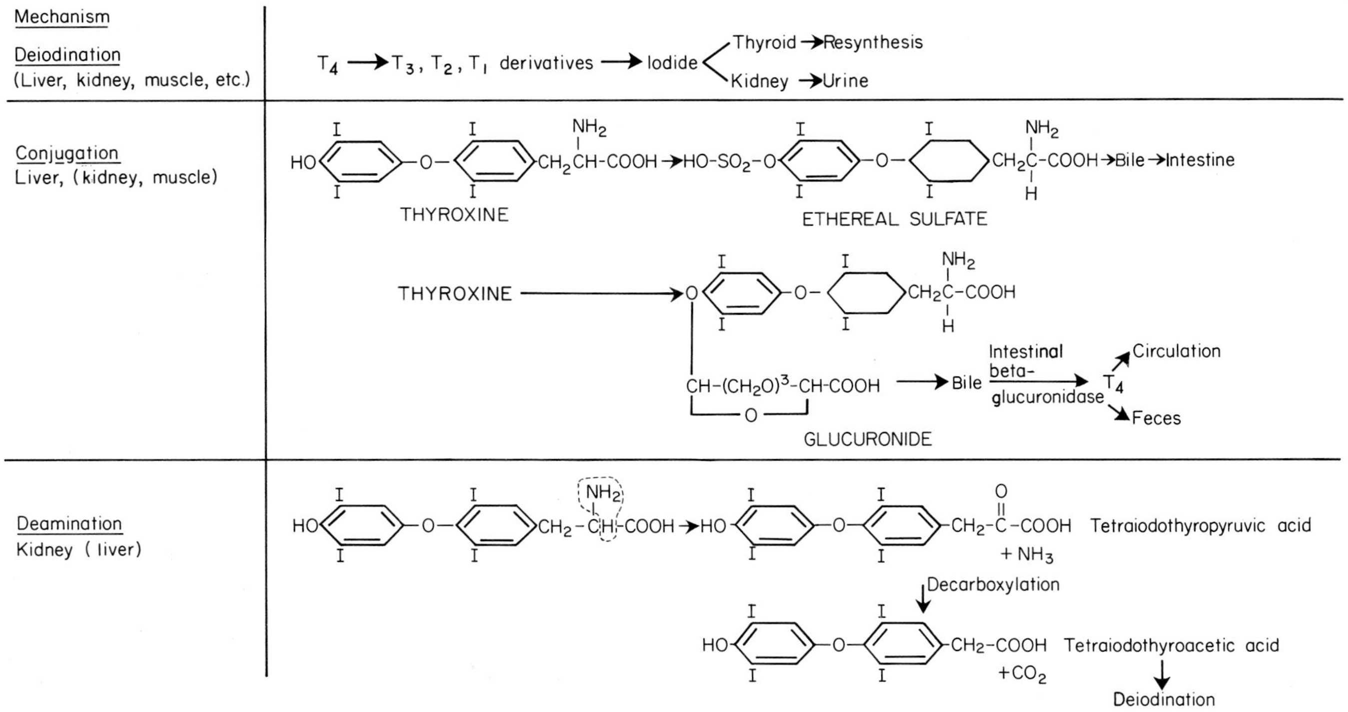

Fig. 6-7. The three major metabolic disposal routes for thyroid hormones. T_4, Thyroxine; T_3, triiodothyronine; T_2, diiodothyronine; T_1, monoiodothyronine.

T_3. Deiodination feeds iodide into the body iodide pool, from which the kidney may excrete it in urine and the thyroid may reutilize it for hormonal synthesis.

Conjugation

The glucuronidation of T_4 by the liver is one of the principal pathways of degradation and aids in the regulation of circulating hormone concentration. T_3 tends to conjugate preferentially with sulfates. The resulting glucuronides and ethereal sulfates (Fig. 6-7) are excreted in the bile and undergo intestinal hydrolysis (β-glucuronidase). Most of the freed hormone, or its derivatives, is reabsorbed into the circulation, and only a small portion is excreted in the feces. The liver-biliary excretion and reabsorption have been called the "enterohepatic cycle." The kidney and other tissues conjugate thyroid hormones to a lesser extent.

Deamination and decarboxylation

Deamination is the principal renal mechanism but is probably the least important pathway in the overall metabolic degradation of T_4 and T_3. The oxidative alteration of the alanine side chain produces the pyruvic acid analogue, and its decarboxylation produces the acetic acid analogue (Fig. 6-3). The loss of the iodine at the 5 position increases their potency, and it had been formerly suspected that these compounds, particularly in the triiodo form, were the metabolically active thyroid hormones at the cellular level. They are probably further deiodinated.

Physiologic action of thyroid hormones

Thyroid hormones (TH), the most important metabolic regulators of the body economy, have widespread effects on organ, cellular, subcellular, and enzymatic processes. Although TH's are apparently not essential for life, little is known about the effects of absolute deprivation, because there is the possibility of extrathyroidal sources of even minute quantities in the totally thyroidless organism. Thyroidectomized animals on a very low iodine intake show extreme debility. The administration of iodides to hypothyroid animals restores a eumetabolic state and an almost normal rate of growth and maturation.

METABOLIC EFFECTS
Calorigenesis and metabolic rate

In the absence of the thyroid gland, the BMR falls to about -40% to -50%. TH has no effect on the BMR of poikilotherms but is essential for metamorphosis of larval forms. Its action on O_2 consumption of isolated tissues is confined to liver, kidney, diaphragm, pancreas, heart, developing brain, and salivary gland, and it has little or no action upon lung, adult brain, spleen, gonads, thymus, lymph node, or skin. The mechanism of these differences in response is unknown, though the unresponsive tissue may lack a deiodinating enzyme necessary for TH activity. That T_4 appears to act mainly upon tissues in which protein and/or lipid metabolism are primary and carbohydrate metabolism is negligible suggests that its action may be upon some process that indirectly leads to increased O_2 consumption, and this may well be its primary action on protein biosynthesis (Sokoloff, 1967).

Temperature regulation

TH's are essential for thermoregulation and may be necessary for survival. Exposure to cold activates the TSH $\rightarrow$ TH system and permits normal function and growth of the organism at an environmental temperature that would be lethal to a hypothyroid animal. Humans with myxedema frequently have subnormal body temperatures, and in myxedema coma, striking falls in body temperature have been recorded.

Protein metabolism

In physiologic concentration TH is anabolic, whereas in large doses it induces catabolism, weight loss, and negative nitrogen balance, as well as increased lipid breakdown. The *catabolic* effect is not directly attributable to TH but is probably mediated by growth (GH) and corticosteroid hormones in response to a demand for carbohydrate. The *anabolic* effect is based on a direct stimulus of protein synthesis. The growth-promoting properties of GH administered to a hypophysectomized animal are considerably enhanced by the addition of TH. The rate of tissue protein synthesis is decreased in myxedema and is restored to normal after TH therapy. Very small doses of T_4 can maintain growth in thyroidectomized rats without showing an increase in O_2 consumption. Thus the primary action of TH is on protein synthesis rather than on O_2 consumption (Sokoloff, 1967).

Carbohydrate metabolism

The diabetogenic properties of TH have been known since Houssay first produced permanent diabetes by the administration of thyroid extract to partially depancreatized dogs (metathyroid diabetes). Abnormal glucose tolerance curves are commonly found in hyperthyroidism and are ascribed to rapid intestinal absorption from enhanced hexose phosphorylation, to elevated FFA concentrations, or to an inhibition of insulin release associated with increased sympathetic tone or responsiveness. Liver glycogen is depleted and synthesis is reduced in hyperthyroidism, but whether this is a specific effect or secondary to negative caloric balance and an increased demand for carbohydrate in extrahepatic tissues is not clear. Liver glycogen depletion is not overcome by the accelerated gluconeogenesis from protein induced by TH because the turnover rate of liver glycogen $\rightarrow$ glucose is likewise enhanced, and a tendency to a "starvation diabetes" is promoted. Muscle glycogen is similarly diminished after large doses of T_4, but smaller doses increase synthesis in vivo and in vitro. It has been assumed that the peripheral cellular uptake and utilization of glucose are increased by T_4 administration, but more recent work using constant intravenous infusions of glucose has failed to confirm this concept. The insulin content of the pancreas is reduced by T_4, and the rate of insulin degradation is accelerated in hyperthyroidism.

Lipid metabolism

Serum cholesterol, cholesterol ester, phospholipids, and total lipids are elevated in hypothyroidism. T_4 accelerates cholesterol synthesis, but the hypocholesterolemia characteristic of thyrotoxicosis is ascribed to even more greatly augmented cholesterol degradation and biliary excretion. In hypothyroidism the rate of synthesis is slowed, but the degradation-excretion rate is disproportionately slower, and the net effect is a raised level of serum cholesterol. That these effects may not be related to O_2 consumption is suggested both by the failure of dinitrophenol to alter serum cholesterol and the cholesteropenic action of D-thyroxine and other analogues at doses that have no effect on the BMR. However, the BMR measurement may be too gross to reflect small changes in cellular oxidation. The hypocholesterolemia and hypolipidemia of thyrotoxicosis may perhaps be primarily the result of weight loss and negative caloric balance rather than a specific effect of TH, since the serum cholesterol may be within normal limits in well-nourished hyperthyroid patients. Accelerated lipolysis, elevated values of basal plasma nonesterified fatty acids (NEFA) and often profound depletion of body fat are characteristic of severe hyperthyroidism.

Vitamin metabolism

Vitamin requirements are increased in thyrotoxicosis, and some of the symptoms have been ascribed to specific deficiencies. The evidence depends mainly on animal experiments, and there are only sparse data derived from investigating vitamin deficiencies in human thyroid disease.

Vitamin A. Carotenemia occurs in myxedema because the hepatic conversions of provitamin A (carotene) to vitamin A requires TH. In hyperthyroidism vitamin A deficiency may occur because of increased requirements, coupled with an increased rate of destruction. Attempts to demonstrate an antithyroidal effect of vitamin A have not been fruitful.

Vitamin B. The B-complex functions as cofactors in enzyme systems, and the increased cellular enzyme metabolism of hyperthyroidism increases the requirements for all the B vitamins. The blood and liver *thiamine* concentration is decreased, whereas urinary, stool, and sweat thiamine is increased. *Pyridoxine* and *pantothenic acid* deficiencies have been described in hyperthyroidism but are of doubtful clinical significance. *Vitamin B_{12}* is decreased in blood, tissue, and mitochondria of thyrotoxic rats, whereas in humans B_{12} deficiency has been described in myxedema. However, in human myxedema, achlorhydria may be the responsible agent. The liver deglycogenation of experimental hyperthyroidism can be prevented by the administration of B vitamins.

Vitamin C. Deficiencies in vitamin C have been reported in hyperthyroidism, but no specific relationship to thyroid disease, other than that caused by general malnutrition, has been described. Experimental thyrotoxic creatinuria has been ameliorated by ascorbic acid administration.

Vitamin D and calcium. There is an increased turnover of Ca, exchangeable-Ca pool, urinary Ca and phosphorus, fecal Ca, and occasionally x-ray–visible osteoporosis in human thyrotoxicosis. Hypercalcemia with a normal or slightly decreased phosphorus and increased alkaline phosphatase can occur. The mechanism is not clear but may be from a combined effect of increasing bone resorption and reducing intestinal absorption of Ca from a relative vitamin D deficiency. The parathyroid glands are normal. Vitamin D and supplemental Ca are required to combat this negative Ca balance. The effects of thyrocalcitonin will be discussed in Chapter 17.

Phosphates (Hoch, 1962)

Excess TH causes negative phosphate balance, decrease in liver and muscle ATP, and an increased breakdown of phosphocreatine. "Uncoupling" of oxidative phosphorylation has been shown in numerous studies both in vivo and in vitro. The rate of ^{32}P incorporation in liver, kidney, and muscle is diminished in thyrotoxic rats, and the turnover rate in the bones of thyrotoxic humans is increased.

Magnesium

Plasma magnesium (Mg) is low, the urinary excretion is increased, but the total and cellular exchangeable Mg is normal in hyperthyroidism. In hypothyroid patients, plasma Mg is elevated, the urinary excretion is decreased, fecal secretion is increased, and exchangeable Mg is reduced. Mg balance is positive in hyperthyroidism and usually negative in hypothyroidism. A defect in Mg transport in thyroid deficiency is probable. Ionic thyroidal transport of iodide is closely related to membrane ATPase activity, which is Mg^{++} dependent.

Systemic effects

Metamorphosis, development, and growth. Metamorphosis of tadpoles to frogs is dependent on an adequate TH milieu, though high concentrations of inorganic iodide are similarly active. Triac, tetrac, triprop, and tetraprop are more active than T_4 and T_3. Thyroidless tadpoles acquire giant proportions, and thyroid administration thereafter produces giant frogs. Mammalian fetal dependence on TH is demonstrated by the cretin. Brain, bone, and dental development is particularly vulnerable. Growth may be stimulated by TH and, in fact, a temporary acceleration of growth has been observed in juvenile hyperthyroidism. The dependence of the growth-stimulating properties of TH on growth hormone has been previously alluded to.

Nervous system. Lack of TH is associated with EEG abnormalities and elevated spinal fluid protein. Diminished cerebral blood flow and brain uptake of O_2 have been reported by some workers and denied by others. The same controversy exists concerning changes in cerebral functions in hyperthyroidism, some finding it augmented and others finding no alteration. TH does not affect the O_2 consumption of adult brain tissue studied in vitro. The mode of action of TH on the nervous system has been attributed to alterations in enzymes (particularly cholinesterase, succinic dehydrogenase), electrolyte changes, O_2 uptake, glucose metabolism, decreased availability of ATP, uncoupling, and decreased acetylcholine production.

Cardiovascular system. T_4 produces increased heart weight with a disproportionate increase of the right as compared to the left heart, an increased catecholamine uptake and myocardial concentration of norepinephrine in some but not all species of animals. The atria show higher concentrations than the ventricles. T_4 tends to inhibit enzymes necessary for catecholamine degradation. Reserpine almost completely depletes norepinephrine from the myocardium (Goodkind, 1966) and other tissues and may thus ameliorate some of the effects of severe thyrotoxicosis and thyroid storm.

Muscle function. Creatinemia and creatinuria are characteristic in hyperthyroidism and are possibly due to a fundamental disorder of creatine phosphate metabolism. ATP is the main source of the energy of muscle contraction. Actomyosin is an active Mg^{++}-dependent ATPase. Uncoupling of oxidative phosphorylation may be the fundamental cause of thyrotoxic myopathy. Muscle biopsies of hyperthyroid patients frequently show granular degeneration of fibers, with loss of striations, edema, and cellular infiltration, particularly with lymphocytes. Satoyoshi et al., 1963, found intracellular water, potassium, creatine, creatine phosphate, ATP, and creatine phosphokinase reduced in muscle tissue removed from hyperthyroid subjects as compared to controls. The administration of KCl, 3 Gm./day for 3 days, reduced serum creatine and creatinuria. In hypothyroidism, muscles contract slowly and the deep tendon reflexes show a characteristic delayed relaxation time (the "hung-up reflex" in myxedema).

Gastrointestinal function. Hyperthyroxinemia increases smooth muscle tone of the gastrointestinal tract and causes an acceleration of gastric emptying, hyperperistalsis with rapid transit time, and an increased frequency of stools. There may be a decreased volume of saliva and gastric hypoacidity or anacidity. The rate of intestinal absorption that is governed by phosphorylation mechanisms is increased in hyperthyroidism and reduced in hypothyroidism.

Liver function. Impaired liver function has been described in 40% to 90% of cases of hyperthyroidism in older reports. The deglycogenated liver cell of hyperthyroidism was thought to be susceptible to various toxins, of which T_4 was the most important. Hepatic pathology was undoubtedly more prevalent 25 to 40 years ago when the diagnosis was delayed and there was considerable weight loss, negative nitrogen balance, malnutrition, and vitamin deficiencies. One recent study (Dooner et al., 1967), however, did confirm the existence of histologic and functional evidence of liver damage.

Blood. Accelerated erythropoiesis, shortened red cell survival, accelerated disappearance of plasma Fe, and increased erythrocyte Fe utilization have been found in hyperthyroidism. Anemia occurs in hypothyroidism and has been explained as a physiologic adaptation to reduced tissue oxygen requirements. Although white cell counts are usually normal in hyperthyroidism, a mild leukopenia and a relative lymphocytosis are not uncommon. A specific elevation of antihemolytic factor (factor VIII) in hyperthyroidism and subnormal levels of a variety of coagulation factors have been reported.

Fluid and electrolytes. Effective renal blood flow and glomerular filtration seem to depend on adequate TH. The administration of TH to experimental animals increases renal function, as measured by enhanced O_2 consumption, creatinine clearance, and renal tubular function (Tm glucose, PAH, Diodrast). Impaired water excretion, found in myxedema, may be due to reduced glomerular filtration, low corticosteroid production, or inappropriate secretion of antidiuretic hormone with hyponatremia. The accumulation of water and salt-laden myxedema tissue is promptly reversed by thyroid therapy. Although subjects with hypothyroidism excrete a salt load normally, the total exchangeable and extracellular sodium stores are ordinarily high.

Mechanism of action of thyroid hormone

Attempts to define the fundamental mechanism of TH action have been frustrated by the complexity of the problem. In vitro observations may not mirror in vivo realities. In view of the long latent period of action, the search for a single function or locus of action may mask the possibility that TH sets off a chain reaction that, once accelerated, proceeds without TH intervention. The role of TH in supporting growth, metamorphosis, reproduction, and other functions is apparently not directly dependent on calorigenic and oxidative stimulation. Tata, 1965, suggests that the fundamental role of thyroid hormones may lie in their stimulation of protein synthetic capacity by subcellular components.

TH enhances the permeability of mitochondrial membranes and, by permitting cell water to enter, causes swelling of mitochondria and increased fragility. Because of the central role of mitochondria in energy transformations and liberation, this TH-induced change may be the fundamental action of the hormone. The labile high-energy phosphate bonds of ATP, derived principally from the oxidation of constituents of the Krebs cycle and fatty acids, provide the chemical energy for intracellular metabolism. The phenomenon of carrying energy or acting as a "carrier" has been called "coupling," and ATP is a "coupling agent." Agents that cause dissociation of oxidation reductions from energy production "uncouple" oxidative phosphorylation. Thus oxidation may proceed at a greater rate and phosphorylation at a lesser rate, so that less ATP is available for cellular function. Numerous investigators have shown that thyroxine, albeit in unphysiologically large doses, can produce uncoupling in mitochondria, and Luft et al., 1962, found "uncoupling in the mitochondria of skeletal muscle in 2 of 5 patients with hyperthyroidism." Peter, 1968, using a new technique for isolating skeletal-muscle mitochondria, found no evidence of uncoupling in patients with muscle weakness and thyrotoxicosis but suggested that the 1.7-fold average increase in the amount of mitochondrial protein per gram of muscle might account for the hypermetabolism of thyrotoxicosis. Hoch, 1962, has advanced the hypothesis that thyrotoxicosis may be a disease of mitochondria with uncoupling the basic defect. One of the initial effects of TH on cellular functions in vivo is to increase the capacity of the mitochondrial electron-transport system.

THE THYROID RELATIONSHIP WITH OTHER ENDOCRINE GLANDS

The thyroid-pituitary relationship has been discussed in Chapter 4. TH acts upon the metabolism of endocrine cells as it does upon all other body cells, so that the absence of TH causes a general decrease of endocrine functions.

Adrenal cortex. Corticosteroids and ACTH tend to inhibit thyroid function either by increasing the renal clearance of iodide or by inhibiting pituitary TSH. Thyroidal RAI accumulation and serum T_4 are usually, but not invariably, reduced. Excess TH, as in hyperthyroidism, shortens the half-life of plasma 17-OHCS, increases the excretion particularly of biologically inactive 11-ketonic metabolites of cortisone and thus the secretion of ACTH, and causes an increase in cortisol production. In thyroid crisis the adrenal insufficiency that sometimes occurs is caused by a dissolution of the homeostatic adjustment and by an augmented disappearance rate of circulating cortisol. The secretory rate of aldosterone is also increased.

Adrenal medulla. Many of the manifestations of thyrotoxicosis have been ascribed to sensitization of certain tissues to the effects of the catecholamines (p. 131). The thyroid-adrenal medullary relationships are complex, and their interactions are at present not clearly understood. Much of the experimental work is conflicting.

Gonads. A normal thyroid hormone milieu is essential for pituitary LH release, ovulatory menstruation, fertility, and fetal survival. Excess TH may retard appearance of the menarche, inhibit estrus in animals, and promote infertility and death of the fetus. In human myxedema anovulatory menstrual disorders characterized by excessive bleeding are common, whereas in hyperthyroidism hypomenorrhea, usually ovulatory, obtains. There has been a great deal of contradictory evidence concerning the effect of thyroxine on testicular function, some workers reporting stimulation and others inhibition.

For a review of thyroid physiology see Werner and Nauman, 1968.

THE THYROID GLAND AND PREGNANCY

There is an estrogen-induced rise of TBG early in pregnancy. The resultant increased binding of T_4 decreases the T_4 turnover rate and lowers the circulating level of free T_4. Pituitary TSH increases, promotes thyroid hyperplasia, enhances biosynthesis, and all but completely restores the level of free T_4, which remains slightly diminished so that the normal physiology of pregnancy is characterized by minimal thyroid hyperplasia. Thus a new level of thyroid function is established in which the serum T_4 concentration is increased, but its turnover rate is reduced so that total daily T_4 utilization remains unchanged. The pituitary-thyroid axis is more difficult to suppress during pregnancy than in the nonpregnant state. Chorionic tissue may elaborate a TSH-like material. Stimulation of the TSH-thyroid axis may be further enhanced by the increased urinary iodide found during pregnancy. The PBI rises from nonpregnant levels of 4 to 8 μg. to 6 to 12 μg./100 ml., and the BEI increases from a range of 3.2 to 6.4 μg. to 5.5 to 10.5 μg./100 ml. In molar pregnancy even higher levels have been found, and the RAIU, conversion ratio, and secretion rate are higher than in normal pregnancy. An increased incidence of complications of pregnancy, such as spontaneous abortion, prematurity, congenital malformations, and developmental retardation of the infant, is associated with a failure of this rise of the PBI and BEI. However, Man et al., 1968, reported an apparently innocuous but substantial decrease of the BEI in young pregnant women during weight gain, edema, or an acute respiratory infection. The level of PBI or BEI may be misleading because the concentration of free hormone circulating in the fetus undoubtedly determines its metabolic health. The thyroidal accumulation of RAI is increased and the T_3 RBC or resin uptake is reduced.

Since maternal TSH does not penetrate the placental barrier, the fetal thyroid must apparently depend on its own pituitary TSH, though the placenta may make some contribution. The fetal thyroid begins to accumulate RAI by the twelfth to fourteenth week and to synthesize hormone by the nineteenth to twenty-second week. There is evidence to suggest that the fetal TSH-thyroid feedback axis is established at least by the fifth month. The movement of T_4 and T_3 across the placental barrier is minimal, and at term the equilibration of hormone between mother and fetus is quite slow, though probably considerably faster for T_3 than T_4. Maternal hormone binding to serum proteins is stronger than fetal binding so that the normal hormonal gradient appears to be fetal→maternal. This may be the result of the transfer of placental estradiol principally to the maternal side. Estimates of placental clearance of maternal T_4 suggest that the amount reaching the fetal circulation almost equals the fetal requirements and that a placenta with a minimal reduction of transport rate can result in an inadequate supply to the fetus. About one third of athyreotic infants are born with some degree of hypothyroidism, as shown by retarded bone maturation. For reviews, see Herbst and Selenkow, 1965, and Werner, 1967.

LABORATORY TESTS OF THYROID FUNCTION

No test can substitute for the considered opinion of the sophisticated physician. Multiple testing is justified only in the most difficult diagnostic problem and even then should be selected with discrimination to provide maximum information with a minimum of inconvenience and expense to the patient. In attempting to interpret thyroid tests, the physician must be cognizant of the following:

1. There is no direct measure of thyroid function and no single ideal test. Each study usually mirrors one aspect of thyroid physiology.

2. Thyroid disorders are not all-or-none phenomena. One must expect, therefore, borderline values and inconsistencies.

3. The thyroid gland is an integral part of the total body physiology and can be affected by stress, infection, malnutrition, pregnancy, other endocrine disorders, and severe emotional disturbances.

4. Drugs, especially those containing iodide, are ubiquitous and profoundly alter many, but not all, studies.

A classification of thyroid tests is shown in Table 6-3. Those listed under the heading "Target organ" measure the impact of the thyroid hormones upon tissues and have been supplanted to a large extent by more specific tests utilizing radioactive iodine (RAI) or those that measure circulating blood levels of hormone.

Protein-bound iodine

Protein-bound iodine (PBI, serum-precipitable iodine) is probably the most frequently utilized test of thyroid function. Since there is no significant diurnal variation and food ingestion does not alter the value, blood specimens can be drawn in the physician's office regardless of the time of day. The PBI is not affected

Table 6-3. Classification of laboratory tests of thyroid function

Thyroid gland	*Circulating blood*	*Target organ*
Radioiodine	PBI	BMR
Accumulation (uptake)	BEI	Cholesterol
TSH and suppression tests	Serum thyroxine	Circulation time
Urinary excretion	By column chromatography	Galactose tolerance
Thiocyanate washout test	By competitive protein-bind-	Creatinuria
Scintigram	ing analysis	Creatine tolerance
Radioautogram	TSH effect on PBI and/or BEI	Alkaline phosphatase
Thyroid clearance	PB¹³¹I	Serum inorganic phosphorus
RAI turnover rate	Conversion ratio	ECG
RAI urinary excretion	"Free" thyroxine	Bone age (by x-ray)
Thyroid biopsy (needle, open)	Free thyroxine index	Salivary excretion RAI
	TBG index	
	T_3 resin or RBC test	
	Autoimmune antibodies	

by storing serum for days or even weeks at room temperature. Hemolysis introduces a dilutional error.

Method of determination

The partition of serum iodide is shown in Fig. 6-8. The serum proteins containing organic iodide are precipitated, washed to remove the inorganic iodide, and ashed in a muffle furnace. The iodide in the ash is then determined by measuring its catalytic effect on the reduction of yellow ceric ion by arsenious acid. The degree of decolorization is proportional to the iodide content.

It is obvious that the PBI is not necessarily synonymous with biologically active circulating hormone but is merely a measure of circulating organically bound iodide. Fortunately in 90% to 95% of cases it correlates well with the serum T_4 and is therefore a reasonably accurate index of thyroid activity.

Normal values

The normal range is 3.5 to 8 μg./100 ml. However, the overlap of normal and hyperthyroid patients is considerable in the 7 to 8 μg. range. *Infants* show elevated values during the first 12 weeks of postnatal

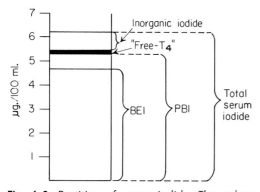

Fig. 6-8. Partition of serum iodide. The values are averages for euthyroid subjects. Serum T_4 ("by column") is equivalent to the BEI. PBI minus BEI equals nonhormonal biologically inactive PBI and consists of other iodinated amino acids, small amounts of iodotyrosines, other inert iodothyronines, and iodohistidines.

life, probably because of maternal or placental estrogens. The rise in pregnancy has been discussed (p. 99).

Elevated PBI because of nonthyroid factors

Iodides. A myriad of pharmaceutical products may contain sufficient iodide to precipitate with the plasma proteins and cause a spurious PBI elevation. Space does not permit a complete listing.

INORGANIC IODIDES. Inorganic iodides occur in saturated KI, Lugol's solution, compound tincture of iodine, cough mixtures, vitamin preparations, suntan lotions, gargles, Special K cereal, and some cod-liver oil preparations. Most vitamin preparations contain 0.1 mg. or less of iodide per capsule and, unless large amounts are ingested, will rarely in themselves raise the PBI but may be important by adding to other sources of iodide. The stable iodine content of ^{131}I is not sufficient to vitiate the PBI, but therapeutic doses of ^{131}I may institute the thyroidal secretion of nonthyroxine, iodinated proteins (thyroglobulin, iodotyrosine, iodohistidines) that enter the circulation and raise the PBI. Both iodized table salt and a seafood diet contain too little iodine to affect the PBI. If less than 200 mg. of iodine is ingested (corresponding to 4 minims of saturated solution of KI or 20 minims of Lugol's solution), the PBI determination will not be significantly affected (Friend, 1960). Most laboratories routinely check the inorganic iodide before measuring the PBI and eliminate specimens with a factitious elevation. Most inorganic iodides are eliminated in 3 to 5 days, though heavy dosage may require several weeks.

ORGANIC IODIDES. Organic iodides occur in all x-ray dyes, iodinated penicillin, Floraquin, Vioform, and Diodoquin. These iodides become bound to serum proteins, are not washed away in the determination of the PBI, and must be either metabolized before releasing the iodide for excretion or excreted unchanged or partially altered.

1. *Short-lived compounds* (3 to 10 days)—most of the contrast media used in pyelograms (Diodrast, Telepaque)
2. *Intermediate compounds*—Gallbladder (6 to 12 weeks), idopanoic acid, Priodax, Cholegrafin
3. *Long-term compounds*—may contaminate the PBI for many months or years (Lipiodol, Pantopaque, Teridax); barium sulfate contains less than 1 mg. iodide per examination and will not alter the PBI

Hormones

THYROID HORMONES. Thyroglobulin, desiccated thyroid, L-thyroxine sodium, and D-thyroxine sodium will raise the PBI of euthyroid subjects. In physiologic dosage, exogenous hormone supplants endogenous sources and there is no net effect on the PBI. Danowski et al., 1952, found that 1 grain of U.S.P. desiccated thyroid (Parke, Davis) administered daily to euthyroid subjects for 12 weeks had no effect on the PBI; 3 grains caused no rise in 7 of 9 subjects, but 6 grains consistently raised the PBI. Within a few days following cessation of thyroid therapy, the PBI decreased somewhat below control values, suggesting that endogenous hormone secretion had been suppressed by inhibition of pituitary TSH. The different quantitative effects of various thyroid hormones on the PBI will be discussed in Chapter 9. T_3 lowers the PBI by suppressing TSH. Since the doses used are small and the binding to serum proteins is minimal, its administration causes no net addition to the PBI. D-Thyroxine causes the greatest increase of the PBI.

ESTROGENS. Estrogens elevate the TBG and thus the PBI. *Oral contraceptive compounds* that contain estrogens raise the PBI within 3 to 7 days, and the elevation can persist for as long as 2 months after medication is stopped.

Nonhormonal iodoprotein. Nonhormonal iodoprotein may be secreted by the thyroid gland in chronic thyroiditis, after RAI therapy, in thyroid carcinoma, and in some forms of goiter, especially goitrous cretinism.

Decreased PBI because of nonthyroid factors

Hormonal factors. Anterior pituitary hypofunction with loss of TSH causes pituitary hypothyroidism. The PBI may be reduced in patients treated with large doses of corticosteroids, T_3, or androgens.

Antithyroid drugs. The compounds propylthiouracil, mercaptoimidazole, mercazoles, perchlorate, thiocyanate, para-aminosalicylic acid, para-aminobenzoic acid, resorcinol, cobalt, Butazolidin, and sulfonamides reduce thyroid function by various mechanisms and may lower the PBI. When certain foods (rutabaga, cabbage, turnip) possessing antithyroid properties are eaten in large amounts, and usually to the exclusion of other foodstuffs, the PBI may fall.

Other drugs. Salicylates and diphenylhydantoin (Dilantin) displace T_4 from TBG and lower the PBI. Mercurial diuretics lower the PBI for 24 to 48 hours after injection by forming an insoluble mercuric iodate in the test tube only when the PBI is determined by distillation techniques. Fluorides, amphenone, and chrysotherapy have been associated with a low PBI.

Nephrosis and liver cirrhosis. Nephrosis and liver cirrhosis may occasionally be associated with a low PBI because of an alteration or reduction of TBP or loss of PBI in the urine.

Butanol-extractable iodine (BEI)

The BEI is a more precise measure of T_4-iodine and does not include either the nonhormonal fraction of the PBI or the inorganic iodide (Fig. 6-8). Under certain conditions (chronic thyroiditis, Hashimoto's thyroiditis, thyroid carcinoma, goitrous cretinism, and after RAI therapy) the PBI is either increased or at variance with the true level of circulating hormone, and the BEI is more informative. The PBI/BEI ratio is normally 5:4 (that is, a 20% difference), but in the above-listed disorders the ratio is increased.

Method of determination

Serum is extracted with *n*-butanol, the extract is treated with an alkaline agent and evaporated, and the PBI is determined in the dried extract.

Normal values

Normal values are 3.2 to 6.4 μg./100 ml. and are 0 to 1.3 μg. (mean 0.6 μg.) lower than the PBI. The BEI is usually above 6.5 μg. in hyperthyroidism and below 3.1 μg./100 ml. in hypothyroidism, and there is less overlap with normal subjects than with the PBI. The BEI is subject to the same extrathyroidal influences as the PBI, except that it is not affected by inorganic iodides or nonthyroxine iodinated proteins but is increased by organic iodides.

Serum thyroxine (T_4) by column chromatography

T_4 can be separated from inorganic and organic iodides or iodotyrosyls by passage of the patient's serum through an ion-exchange resin column, subsequent elution from the column with acetic acid or other appropriate solvent and determination of the T_4-iodine by the usual method for the PBI. Values obtained are similar to the BEI (normal = 3.2 to 6.4 μg./100 ml.). The method eliminates contamination by iodides, including radiographic dyes, and is available at reasonable cost. Plastic columns containing an ion-exchange resin are commercially available. *The method has supplanted the PBI in many laboratories.*

Serum T_4 by competitive protein-binding analysis

T_4 is separated by ethanol extraction and then measured according to its effect on the passage of a standard tracer-T_4 and plasma solution through an anion-exchange resin in the test tube (Murphy et al., 1966). The method is not affected by iodide or mercury contamination but is lowered by Dilantin and T_3 and elevated by estrogens and pregnancy. A simplified modification uses a [131]I- or ^{125}I-resin sponge that is available commercially.* Normal values are 4 to 11 μg./100 ml., with a mean of 6.36 μg. for males and 6.60 μg. for females. Values below 3.6 μg. are found in hypothyroidism and above 9.8 μg. in hyperthyroidism, with a minimal overlap with euthyroid subjects. The method is gaining in popularity, especially because 5% to 8% of PBI determinations are invalidated by iodide contamination. A method for measuring serum T_3 has been described (Nauman et al., 1967).

Serum-free thyroxine

Serum-free thyroxine (free T_4) has not been sufficiently standardized to be recommended for routine use. It may be of value where the PBI, BEI, or T_4 fails to correlate with the clinical status of the patient, but the test is invalidated by iodide contamination and is affected by major alterations of TBP. Sterling and Brenner, 1966, described a simplified dialysis method that yielded the results shown below.

*Tetrasorb-125, Abbott Laboratories, North Chicago, Ill.

	Free T_4 (%)	Free T_4 iodine (mμg./100 ml.)	Free T_4 concentration (moles/L.)
Normal	0.046 ± 0.005	2.76 ± 0.50	5.4×10^{-11}
Hyperthyroidism	0.104 ± 0.026	13.08 ± 3.42	25.7×10^{-11}
Hypothyroidism	0.028 ± 0.008	0.38 ± 0.08	0.8×10^{-11}
Pregnancy	0.026 ± 0.004	2.35 ± 0.7	4.6×10^{-11}
Euthyroid "sick"	0.088 ± 0.036	4.76 ± 2.62	9.4×10^{-11}

The free T_4 iodine value (free $T_4\% \times$ PBI) showed much greater deviations from the normal in thyroid disorders. In pregnancy the PBI was elevated, but the free $T_4\%$ was low, yielding a free T_4 iodine in the low normal range. The Murphy-Pattee technique can also be applied to the determination of free T_4 as well as T_4 and TBG. The free T_4 value may not always accurately reflect thyroid function particularly in states of altered capacity of cells to accumulate T_4, such as in hepatic cirrhosis.

Thyroxine-binding globulin (TBG)

TBG is determined electrophoretically by measuring its capacity to bind ^{131}I-labeled T_4. The determination may serve to explain certain marked discrepancies in the serum PBI, BEI, or T_3-^{131}I–resin test but is rarely required in clinical diagnosis. Factors altering TBG are outlined in Table 6-2.

Studies using radioactive iodine (RAI)

Radioactive iodine uptake (RAIU)

The avidity with which the thyroid gland extracts iodide from the total body-iodide pool can be measured by labeling the pool with an isotope of iodine (usually ^{131}I) and measuring the percent of the tracer dose present in the thyroid gland at designated intervals of time. In hyperthyroidism the gland collects more ^{131}I and does so more rapidly, whereas in hypothyroidism it collects less. In most instances the collection rate and the quantity collected mirrors the thyrometabolic state of the patient, but the RAIU test does not necessarily reflect hormonal production and release. The kidney and thyroid compete for the circulating ^{131}I; the thyroid uptake is inversely proportional to the renal excretion.

Standard method. Carrier-free sodium iodide (^{131}I) is given by mouth after an overnight fast. The "tracer dose" ranges from 1 to 25 microcuries (μCi.), and even amounts of ^{131}I as little as 0.1 to 0.2 μCi. have been used with sufficient accuracy for clinical purposes. An identical dose is set aside to be used as a standard. Readings are made over the neck with a special counter (usually a sensitive scintillation crystal probe). Counts per unit of time are converted into percent of uptake by comparing the counts over the thyroid with the counts over a phantom thyroid containing the aliquot of ^{131}I that was set aside as a standard. A background reading and a thigh count are subtracted from the thyroid and phantom counts and appropriate corrections are made for the rate of decay of the ^{131}I.

Readings are usually done 24 hours after the administration of ^{131}I, both for convenience and because the uptake reaches a plateau at this time. Readings at 2, 4, or 6 hours are valuable in the diagnosis of hyperthyroidism; when a high early value is obtained, the 24-hour reading may be omitted. In severe hyperthyroidism the conversion and excretion of iodine may be so rapid that at 24 hours the amount of ^{131}I retained in the thyroid may be less than in the first 12 to 18 hours and may even fall within the euthyroid range. There are a number of reports attesting to the accuracy of measurements of thyroidal ^{131}I accumulation from 10 to 60 minutes after the tracer dose.

The *neck-thigh ratio* involves the simultaneous measurement of the uptake over the neck and thigh 2 hours after a tracer dose of ^{131}I and is an index of thyroidal accumulation. It has the following advantages over the standard RAIU test: (1) it is a simple ratio of counts so that no phantom is required; (2) the dose is small and need not be accurately measured, (3) it can be performed rapidly with a minimum chance of error by an unskilled technician, and (4) it has a high correlation with the thyroid clearance rate. The method is less accurate than the standard RAIU in the diagnosis of hypothyroidism.

Normal values. The normal values vary in different laboratories, in different sections of the country, and in different parts of the world. They tend to be higher in areas where the iodide content of food and water is low. No sharp line can be drawn between euthyroid subjects and patients with thyroid disease. Establishing a wide range of normal values will inevitably include more hyperthyroid and hypothyroid patients, whereas a narrow range will fail to include many euthyroid subjects. The *normal* 24-hour range varies from a low of 10% to 15% to a high of 40% to 50% (mean, 21% to 24%). In recent years there has been a trend toward lower normal values that may be related to iodides in the flour used in making bread. Values for hyperthyroid patients are usually over 50% (mean, 60% to 64%) and for hypothyroid subjects, less than 10%. Normal 2-hour uptakes are less than 15%.

Repetition of test. Tests repeated within 1 to 3 days show an error of ±3%; within 14 days, ±10%; beyond 14 days the differences in repeat tests may be greater than ±10%.

Factors causing a "false" high RAIU in euthyroid patients

1. A contracted total body-iodide pool because of iodide deficiency increases the avidity of the thyroid for iodide. This may be due to dietary deficiency as in endemic goiter or to a block in organification of thyroid accumulation produced by an antithyroid drug leading to a rebound rise of RAIU when the compound is withdrawn. Patients studied in an area of endemic goiter had a mean RAIU of 59%, and over half the patients had values above 58%.

2. Thyroid hyperplasia in a euthyroid patient may be seen in hyperplastic goiter, occasionally in Hashimoto's thyroiditis and in pregnancy.

3. Certain types of goitrous cretins have high uptake but fail to organify.

4. The increased uptake often found in renal failure is generally not large enough to be of clinical significance.

Factors causing a "false" lowering of RAIU in euthyroid patients. In general, most factors that induce spurious eleva-

tions of the PBI (that is, elevation of the plasma inorganic iodide, PII) will enlarge the total body-iodide pool and cause a reduction of RAIU. However, all PBI elevations do not change the pool content, and in some instances discordant effects will be observed. For example, most organic iodides raise the PBI and lower the RAIU. Teridax, however, causes an extraordinary elevation of the PBI but is without effect on the RAIU. When less than 1.5 mg. of stable carrier iodide is added to ^{131}I in patients with endemic goiter, there is no appreciable effect on the RAIU. The RAIU of euthyroid nongoitrous subjects is only slightly affected by 2 mg. or less of stable iodide. For a review of factors that alter the RAIU, see Grayson, 1960.

Several other isotopes of ^{127}I have been used in diagnostic tests. ^{132}I has a half-life of 2.3 hours as compared to 8 days for ^{131}I, a factor that reduces the radiation exposure to approximately a hundredth of that of ^{131}I and permits its freer use in repeated testing and when RAI studies are required in children and pregnant women. The background error caused by repeated testing is also reduced. ^{125}I has a half-life of 57 to 60 days and has a long chemical shelf life and low radiation dose to the patient. It has been used primarily for thyroid scans and provides greater contrast than does ^{131}I. ^{124}I, with a half-life of 4.2 days, has a greater time range and may prove useful in therapy.

Radioiodine-labeled triiodothyronine erythrocyte or resin test (ET$_3$ test, T$_3$ test)

When ^{131}I-labeled T$_3$ (T$_3$-^{131}I) is added to blood, plasma, or serum containing erythrocytes (or a resin), the thyroxine-binding proteins (TBP) will bind T$_3$-^{131}I, depending on their capacity or degree of previous hormonal saturation. The unbound T$_3$-^{131}I will be free for binding to the erythrocyte or resin. The various factors that affect the T$_3$ test are shown in Fig. 6-9. If TBP is saturated with excessive thyroid hormone as in hyperthyroidism, the capacity to bind added T_3-^{131}I will be reduced, and more will be bound to the red blood cell or resin (Fig. 6-9, *A*). If TBP is unsaturated because of a deficiency of thyroid hormone as in hypothyroidism, there will be unoccupied binding sites for the added T_3-^{131}I, and less will be free to be picked up by the RBC or resin (Fig. 6-9, *B*). If TBP is increased (as in pregnancy or with estrogen administration), it will present more binding sites, and the RBC or resin uptake will mimic hypothyroidism (Fig. 6-9, *D*). If binding is interfered with and T_4 is displaced or if there is a low binding capacity, the resin uptake will be increased (Fig. 6-9, *C* and *E*). Thus the T_3 test is not only an index of thyroid function but also an indirect measure of the binding capacity of TBP,

that is, the quantity of T_3-^{131}I bound to the RBC or resin is directly proportional to the saturation of TBP.

Method. T_3-^{131}I is added to blood and incubated for 2 hours. The red cells are separated and washed, and the T_3-^{131}I content is counted and calculated as a percent of the total T_3-^{131}I added. A hematocrit correction must be made. Most laboratories now use serum and substitute a resin for the RBC. A recent innovation is to designate the results obtained in a large pooled serum as 1.0, or 100%, and compare the patient's serum to the pool. This method insures uniformity and more comparable results from different laboratories. The "thyro-binding index" involves labeling the resin with T_3-^{131}I and determining the amount of the label leaving the resin and

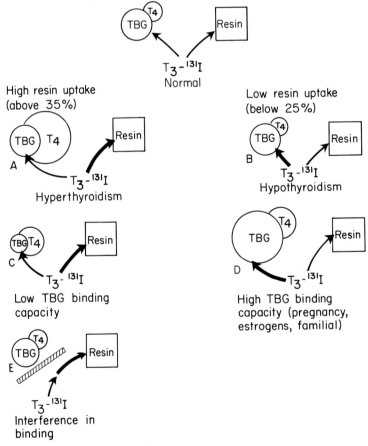

Fig. 6-9. T_3-resin test and factors that may influence the results. See text for explanation.

entering the plasma. The results thus become a reciprocal of the more usual techniques. The resin test is simpler in that frozen serum can be stored for later determinations, the hematocrit correction is unnecessary, and the effect of RBC abnormalities is eliminated.

Normal values. Accepted normal values are as follows:

Red blood cell test: 10% to 17% in males, 10% to 19% in females

Resin test: 23% to 35%

Pooled serum method: 0.82 to 1.3 (82% to 130%)

Thyro-binding index:

Euthyroid 1.010 (S.D. 0.097)

Hyperthyroid 0.785 (S.D. 0.028)

Hypothyroid 1.301 (S.D. 0.091)

The T_3 test has shown less discrimination in the diagnosis of hypothyroidism than of hyperthyroidism.

Elevated values

Infants and young children?

Hyperthyroidism

Severe hypoproteinemia with impaired synthesis of TBP—nephrosis, liver disease

TBP decrease—genetic, familial

Decreased synthesis of TBPA

Advanced metastatic malignancy

Hormones—thyroid preparations (except T_3), androgens, (?) corticosteroids

Drugs—diphenylhydantoin (Dilantin), phenylbutazone, anticoagulants, salicylates (large doses)

Chronic nonthyroidal illness

Acidosis—CO_2 retention, diabetes, uremia

Acute stress, immediate postoperative period

Congestive heart failure

Supraventricular tachycardia

Acute myocardial infarction (acute phase)

Decreased values

Hypothyroidism

Pregnancy

Systemic lupus erythematosus, acute intermittent porphyria

Hormones—estrogens, oral contraceptive compounds containing an estrogen, triiodothyronine

TBP increase—genetic, familial, or other causes

Use of heparinized plasma

Advantages of the T_3-^{131}I test

1. No radioactive material administered to patient (desirable in children and pregnant women and where repeated testing is done)

2. Patient need not be present—blood or serum samples suffice

3. Iodide contamination does not vitiate the results (Orografin may be an exception)

Free thyroxine index (FTI). The mathematical product of the T_3-^{131}I resin value and the serum PBI is called the "free thyroxine index." It shows a high correlation with free plasma T_4. The FTI equals PBI in $\mu g./100$ ml. × resin-T_3 uptake (expressed as a ratio of a pooled serum value; normal, 0.82 to 1.28). The normal range is 2.23 to 7.08.

Blood ^{131}I and the conversion ratio (CR)

In normal subjects the $PB^{131}I$ is less than 0.3% of the administered dose per liter of serum or plasma 72 hours after the I.M. administration of ^{131}I. The "conversion ratio" is determined 24 hours after an oral dose of ^{131}I by comparing the $PB^{131}I$ to total blood radioactivity as follows:

$$\frac{PB^{131}I \text{ (counts per second)}}{Total\ ^{131}I \text{ (counts per second)}} \times 100 =$$

Conversion ratio (CR)

This ratio is a measure of hormone discharged into the circulation and is usually above 50% in hyperthyroidism.

Thiocyanate or perchlorate "washout" test

A defect in the organification of iodide, that is, binding to tyrosyls, is found in certain types of goitrous cretins, is rarely found in adult goiter, and can occur because of the normal action of the antithyroid drugs used in the treatment of hyperthyroidism. As shown in Fig. 6-6, the

RAIU is performed and, usually at the fourth hour, 1 Gm. of potassium thiocyanate or perchlorate is administered orally either in capsule form or as a 25% solution. Where organification is inhibited, there is a very prompt discharge of ^{131}I from the thyroid, as indicated by a reduction in counts over the thyroid within several minutes. If organic binding is adequate, there is no change in the counting rate. The washout of ^{131}I may not necessarily be due to a blocking of organification but may indicate only that the thyroid gland's ability to organify iodine is overwhelmed by an excessive supply (Wolff, 1969).

Thyroid clearance

The volume of plasma cleared of RAI per unit of time by the thyroid gland may be determined by dividing the thyroidal ^{131}I by the plasma ^{131}I approximately 1 hour after the administration of a tracer dose. This technique avoids errors from inaccurate dosimetry, impaired gastrointestinal absorption, variations of renal excretion, or diffusion of RAI into extravascular tissues but is too time consuming for ordinary diagnostic work and has been more or less reserved for research studies. Normal values are 1.5 L./hour (0.5 to 3.5) or 20 ml./min.; in hyperthyroidism the clearance rate is increased five to ten times, but there may be overlapping with euthyroid subjects.

Measurement of the *urinary excretion of RAI* is rarely used today because of the inaccuracies inherent in the collection of urine specimens. However, some clinics find that the technical simplicity and elimination of the errors involved in counting over the thyroid gland make the urinary excretion test preferable.

Measuring *salivary RAI excretion* and the saliva/serum-^{131}I ratio has been of value particularly in the study of cretinism.

Absolute iodine uptake (AIU)

The absolute iodine uptake (AIU) is the quantity of iodide retained by the thyroid in a unit of time. It measures the amount of iodide trapped, in contrast to the RAIU, which is a proportion (in percent) of an administered dose. The AIU is the product of the thyroid clearance and the plasma inorganic iodide (PII):

$$\text{AIU (}\mu\text{g./hr.)} = \text{Thyroid clearance (ml./min.)} \times \text{PII (}\mu\text{g./100 ml.)} \times 0.6$$

The 0.6 is a factor to adjust for the difference in units. Normal values are 0.5 to 6 μg./hr. The AIU is a valuable index to measure when the results of the RAIU and thyroid clearance are equivocal.

Suppression tests

The ingestion of a sufficient dose of a thyroid hormone to inhibit pituitary TSH markedly reduces the RAIU in euthyroid subjects but does not appreciably alter the uptake in hyperthyroid patients. The feedback whereby TSH and thyroid hormone reciprocally regulate each other does not function in hyperthyroidism because TSH is continuously suppressed. The usual method is to perform a standard 24-hour RAIU test, then administer T_3 50 to 100 μg./day for 8 days, and repeat the RAIU. The second RAIU should be reduced to 50% of the baseline or to below 20%. Often 300 μg./day for 2 days will suffice (Dresner and Schneeberg, 1958), but Sisson, 1965, has suggested the following practical procedure:

1. After a baseline 24-hour RAIU, give 75 μg. of T_3 four times daily (300 μg./day) for 2 days and then 25 μg. four times daily (100 μg./day) for an additional 2 days.
2. Repeat the 24-hour RAIU between days 3 and 4.
3. If inadequate suppression is obtained, continue T_3 100 μg./day through day 8, and do a third RAIU.

The suppression test should be reserved for diagnostic problems. Elderly patients, particularly with cardiac disease, may be poor candidates for the test. If it is deemed vital, the minimum dose (50 μg.) should be used. The test is most useful when high borderline RAIU values are found (35%

to 55%) in doubtful cases, in patients with exophthalmos for whom the presence of Graves' disease is in doubt, and perhaps as a prognostic test after treatment of hyperthyroidism. Suppression implies a permanent remission of thyrotoxicosis; failure to suppress suggests a substantial probability of future recurrence.

Possible errors in suppression testing:

1. There may be an inadequate dose of T_3 or failure of the patient to take the hormone regularly.

2. In some euthyroid patients with nodular or adenomatous goiters TSH cannot be suppressed.

3. A "hot" nontoxic adenoma may not be suppressed.

4. Failure to suppress may occur in some euthyroid patients with exophthalmos; there is a strong likelihood that they have Graves' disease and may become clinically hyperthyroid in the future.

5. Suppression may occur in occasional patients with toxic nodular goiter ("hot nodule") leading to an erroneous diagnosis. However, if a 2-hour uptake is done, suppression does not occur as it may in some euthyroid patients.

Thyrotrophic hormone test (TSH test)

The TSH test is useful to differentiate pituitary from primary hypothyroidism or to diagnose equivocal hypothyroidism. It has been discussed on p. 50.

Thyroid scan (scintiscan)

An image of the thyroid gland can be reproduced by giving a tracer dose of RAI to the patient and using an automatic isotope detector (focusing collimator crystal detector and photomultiplier tube) with a recording device that moves across the patient's neck to map the distribution of RAI uptake. The present limit of discrimination is 1 cm. Since larger doses of RAI are required (25 to 50 μCi.) than for the usual RAIU, scans are not routinely employed and repeated scans are avoided unless absolutely required. ^{131}I is used most often, but other short-lived isotopes

such as ^{125}I, ^{128}I, and pertechnetate (technetium 99m) are being tested because they produce less thyroidal radiation. Color scanning may improve discrimination. Some of the uses of scanning, as illustrated in Fig. 6-10, are as follows:

1. To locate the thyroid gland where palpation of the neck is difficult or where it is essential to ascertain the morphologic character of the gland.

2. To recognize the "cold" nodule, that is, a nodule with little or no uptake of RAI (Fig. 6-10, *E* and *F*). Various workers have reported that 7% to 58% have been found to be malignant, and the remainder are caused by other lesions that reduce thyroid function (colloid adenoma [Fig. 6-10, *F*], cysts, fibrosis, necrosis, hemorrhage, focal thyroiditis, granuloma, calcified areas).

3. To recognize the "hot" nodule, that is, an area that accumulates considerably more RAI than the remainder of the gland. A "hot" adenoma may suppress the remainder of the thyroid by inhibiting pituitary TSH, as shown in Fig. 6-10, *D*.

4. To locate ectopic thyroid tissue such as the lingual thyroid shown in Fig. 6-10, *F*, the substernal goiter, or functioning thyroid metastases.

The uses of scanning are discussed in greater detail in Chapters 8 and 11.

Thyroid autoantibodies

The concept of autoimmunity in thyroid disease is discussed on p. 180. Essentially four types of antibodies have been described:

1. Precipitins and agglutinins to thyroglobulin
2. Complement-fixing antibodies to thyroid-cell microsomal fractions
3. Cytotoxic factor found in tissue cultures of thyroid cells
4. Fluorescent follicular-cell antibody

Method. The most commonly employed tests are the tanned red cell agglutination test (TRC) and the precipitin test. In the TRC test, tannic acid–treated erythrocytes are coated with thyroglobulin and aggluti-

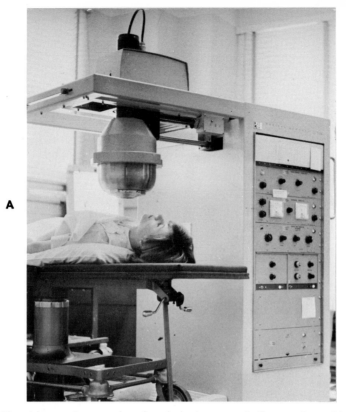

Fig. 6-10. Thyroid scans in normal and pathologic states. **A,** Scanner in position. **B,** Normal thyroid. **C,** Nontoxic nodular goiter with a prominent mass of the right neck and a large pyramidal lobe. **D,** "Hot" toxic autonomous nodule (Plummer's disease). **E,** "Cold" nodule due to carcinoma. **F,** "Cold" nodule due to a follicular colloid adenoma. **G,** Lingual thyroid (**A** courtesy Dr. M. Croll, Hahnemann Medical College, Philadelphia, Pa.; **B** to **G** from Radioisotope Department, Philadelphia General Hospital, Philadelphia, Pa.)

nate when exposed to the specific antibody. Very high titers (up to 5 million) are found in Hashimoto's thyroiditis and are diagnostic (over 1:250 or 1:500) in 70% to 80% of cases. When several different tests are used, antibodies have been found in 95% of patients. In spontaneous myxedema, thought by many to be the end stage of Hashimoto's thyroiditis, values almost as high are found. Other thyroid disorders may show positive reactions, though usually of low titer. Positive precipitin tests are found in patients with high TRC titers and are usually positive only in Hashimoto's thyroiditis. Antibodies have also been found in 6% of a normal population and in a substantial number of patients with elevated serum gamma globulins.

Diagnostic application

1. As an aid to establish the diagnosis of Hashimoto's thyroiditis.
2. In the differential diagnosis of goiter. A high titer almost assuredly indicates the presence of Hashimoto's thyroiditis and makes simple goiter and thyroid cancer unlikely. Chronic thyroiditis and thyroid cancer may coexist, however.
3. Where the diagnosis of myxedema is equivocal.
4. Postthyroidectomy hypothyroidism is a likely sequela in a thyrotoxic patient with a high antibody titer.

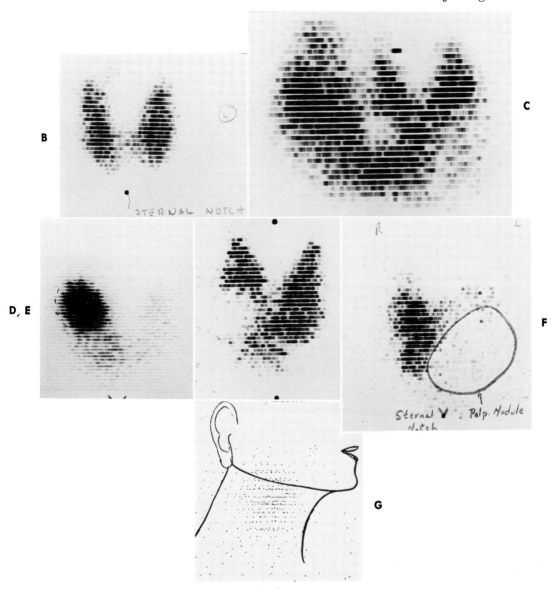

Fig. 6-10, cont'd. For legend see opposite page.

5. A high titer is found in primary thyroid myxedema but not in pituitary hypothyroidism.

Achilles reflex (ankle jerk) test

Prolongation of deep tendon reflexes ("hung-up reflex") is commonly found in myxedema, and a number of methods of measuring and recording the reflex have been introduced (kinemometer, photomotogram, etc.).

Normal values. Published values vary from 145 to 230 milliseconds tap to peak, from 240 to 340 msec. tap to half-relaxation, or from 230 to 280 msec. contraction time. Values are prolonged in hypothyroidism, CNS syphilis, and diabetic neuropathy. It has been suggested that most of the prolonged values in diabetic neuropathy are due to underlying hypothyroidism possibly related to oral hypoglycemic drug ingestion. Values tend to be shortened in hyperthyroidism.

A survey of recent publications reveals

a considerable divergence of opinion concerning the diagnostic value of this test. The most unfavorable opinions are voiced by those workers who have published the largest series of cases. In my experience the test was accurate in 90% of cases of full-blown myxedema but in only 65% of cases of hyperthyroidism. It was of little, if any, value in the borderline and equivocal case, and therefore its routine use did not appear to be justified.

Basal metabolic rate (BMR)

In older writings on thyroid testing, a description of the BMR occupied a considerable proportion of the text. Today we have come to rely on more direct and specific indices of thyroid function and no longer use the BMR as a routine procedure. It remains, however, one of the few studies that is proportional to the severity of hyperthyroidism or hypothyroidism and is usually included in any extensive diagnostic investigation. Normal values are from –15% to +15%. Standards have been reevaluated in recent years, and it has been suggested that the normal mean is more nearly –6% to –9% than 0%, so that a normal range of –20% to +5% is probably more accurate. Because the BMR measured total body metabolism, to which the thyroid contributes perhaps 40%, the BMR may vary markedly from the normal range in the presence of normal thyroid function. The nonthyroid factors that may alter the BMR are listed below:

1. *Elevated BMR*

   Nonbasal state—poor night's sleep, fear, nervousness, chilling, food ingestion, high protein intake night before testing

   Apparatus leaks, poorly fitting mask, perforated ear drums

   Dyspnea—asthma, cardiac failure, emphysema

   Hyperventilation and voluntary increase in expiratory chest volume

   Fever—BMR rises 7.2% per degree

   Acromegaly

   Androgen-producing tumors

   Aortic stenosis, aortic coarctation, hypertension

   Arteriovenous fistula

   Acidosis

   Chronic alcoholism

   Anemia, leukemia, polycythemia, lymphoblastoma

   Malignancy

   Osteitis deformans

   Pregnancy (last trimester)

   Parkinsonism

   Pheochromocytoma

   Drugs—thyroid hormone, aminophylline, dinitrophenol, testosterone, ephedrine, epinephrine, amphetamines, caffeine, nicotine

2. *Lowered BMR*

   Hypopituitarism, Addison's disease

   Eunuchoidism (slight fall)

   Nephrosis

   Severe malnutrition, starvation, anorexia nervosa, debility

   Drugs—sedatives, hypnotics, narcotics

   Incomplete absorption of exhaled CO_2 (old soda lime)

There is a wide range of overlap between euthyroid, hypothyroid, and hyperthyroid patients. The accuracy of the BMR is approximately 95% in hyperthyroidism and 60% to 80% in euthyroid subjects. Bartels and Bell, 1947, found that 8% of 1,000 hyperthyroid patients had BMR values below +20%.

Serum cholesterol

The serum cholesterol is elevated in hypothyroidism and lowered in hyperthyroidism, but exceptions are frequent and there is a wide normal range. In most patients with thyrotoxicosis, the cholesterol is below 220 mg./ml., and in most patients with myxedema, it is above 300 mg./ 100 ml. In pituitary myxedema the cholesterol is more likely to be normal. The cholesterol may be of some value in following the progress of thyroid diseases, rising with successful treatment of hyperthyroidism and falling with treatment of hypothyroidism.

Circulation time

The speed of circulation tends to be roughly proportional to the thyrometabolic status, being faster in hyperthyroidism and slower in myxedema. Measurement of the circulation time may be of value in diagnostic problems and provides an additional test when others are invalidated.

Calcium gluconate or magnesium sulfate is injected I.V. very rapidly. The end point consists of a sudden sensation of heat in the mouth, tongue, and cheeks. Decholin causes a bitter taste; saccharine, a sweet taste. Fluorescein causes facial fluorescence under ultraviolet light and is an objective measure of arm-to-face time. The average normal arm-to-tongue time is 12 seconds (range 8 to 16 seconds). Cardiac decompensation and myxedema prolong the time beyond 16 seconds, and hyperthyroidism shortens it to below 8 to 10 seconds.

Thyroid-stimulating hormone (TSH) and long-acting thyroid stimulator (LATS)

The determination of TSH, previously discussed on p. 35, may be of value in the differential diagnosis of primary thyroid myxedema and pituitary myxedema, but the method is difficult and expensive. LATS may be measured at the same time but is presently of interest only to the research worker. Since it has been detected in only some 60% of patients with Graves' disease, its value as a diagnostic test is limited. LATS will be discussed in greater detail in Chapter 8.

Miscellaneous laboratory findings

Several other tests (creatine tolerance, galactose tolerance, iodine tolerance) that once enjoyed popularity are no longer used. Hypertyrosinemia is found in hyperthyroidism, and blood levels are higher after an oral tyrosine load than they are in normal subjects. Serum total calcium is occasionally elevated in hyperthyroidism, and plasma-ionizable calcium has been found to be significantly elevated. In myxedema somewhat reduced levels were found. Total and ionized magnesium is reduced in hyperthyroidism and elevated in myxedema. The electrocardiogram, serum inorganic phosphorus and alkaline phophatase, x-ray examination of the epiphyses, serum uric acid, and erythrocyte sedimentation rate are especially useful in the diagnosis of hypothyroidism (Chapter 9).

CLINICAL EXAMINATION OF THE THYROID GLAND

There are three approaches to satisfactory palpation of the thyroid gland, and all three should be utilized.

Patient seated with examiner standing behind

The patient's head should be in a relaxed, level position so as to avoid tension of the neck muscles. Using the index and middle fingers of each hand, the examiner locates the isthmus, a thin ribbon of tissue found just below the lower border of the larynx, crossing the trachea at about the level of the second tracheal ring. The pyramidal lobe can be sought at this time, and tracheal deviation can be appreciated. Thickening or nodulation of the isthmus alerts the examiner to the probable presence of pathologic conditions of the lateral lobes. The delphian node, an enlarged lymph node (or nodes) just above the isthmus, is often the first manifestation of metastatic thyroid carcinoma. By sliding the fingers along the isthmus, the examiner can locate the medial borders of the lateral lobes. Thence by retracting the sternomastoid muscles laterally, the examiner can sweep the fingers over the surfaces of both lobes and attempt to locate the superior and inferior poles and the extreme lateral borders of the lateral lobes. In lean individuals the entire gland usually can be palpated and outlined, whereas in obese persons or those with a very muscular neck, the extent of the palpation is restricted. The examination is continued with the patient swallowing, which causes the gland to rise and fall. Sips of water may be necessary. Structures and masses that move with the larynx on swallowing are usually part of the thyroid or attached to it, whereas those that are immobile are generally outside the gland. Examination should then proceed with the patient's head markedly extended, flexed, and finally rotated to the right and left. If the inferior poles cannot be located, particularly in a patient in whom most of the gland is readily accessible, one must suspect substernal extension. Bruits should be sought by applying the bell of the stethoscope to each lateral lobe successively with the sternomastoids retracted, the head rotated right or left, and the patient suspending respiration for a few seconds. The entire neck should then be carefully explored, with the palpating fingers looking for enlarged lymph nodes or other masses. The jugular groove should be carefully palpated.

Anterior approach

The examiner sits in front of the seated patient and inspects the neck. The head is then markedly extended, a maneuver that may bring a previously hidden enlarged thyroid into view. The head is then brought back to a horizontal position, the anterior border of the right sternomastoid is retracted with the thumb of the left hand, and the right lateral lobe of the isthmus is examined with the right thumb. The process is repeated for the left lobe, examining with the left thumb and retracting with the right thumb. The right thumb then pushes the trachea and larynx to the patient's right, and the right lobe of the thyroid can be grasped between the thumb and index finger of the left hand. The process can be reversed to examine the left lobe. Each thyroid lobe can be thoroughly examined in this way. These maneuvers should be repeated when the patient swallows. Occasionally nodules that were not clearly palpated by the posterior approach may be more easily felt. When a substernal goiter is suspected, the examiner percusses through the first and second interspaces and over the upper manubrium. Coughing may cause a substernal goiter to rise partially into the neck.

Hyperextension with patient supine

The patient lies on an examining table, with the head in hyperextension, and the thyroid is palpated, with the examiner standing alongside the table at the level of the patient's chest. A useful additional maneuver is to have the examiner seated behind the patient, with the patient's head hanging over the edge in the bronchoscopy position.

REFERENCES

Barakat, R. M., and Ingbar, S. H.: J. Clin. Invest. 44:1117, 1965.

*Barker, S. B.: Physiological activity of thyroid hormones and analogues. In Pitt-Rivers, R., and Trotter, W. R., editors: The thyroid gland, vol. 1, Washington, D. C., 1964, Butterworth, Inc., p. 199.

Bartels, E. C., and Bell, G. O.: Lahey Clin. Bull. 5:70, 1947.

Braverman, L. E., and Ingbar, S. H.: J. Clin. Invest. 42:1216, 1963.

Cavalieri, R. R., and Searle, G. L.: The role of the liver in the distribution of ^{131}I thyroxine in man. In Cassano, C., and Andreoli, M., editors: Current topics in thyroid research, proceedings, International Thyroid Conference, Fifth, Rome, May 23-27, 1965, New York, 1965, Academic Press, Inc., p. 336.

Danowski, T. S., et al.: J. Clin. Endocr. 12:1572, 1952.

*De Groot, L. J.: New Eng. J. Med. 272:243, 297, 355, 1965.

*Deiss, W. P., Jr., and Peake, R. L.: Ann. Intern. Med. 69:881, 1968.

Dooner, H. P., et al.: Arch. Intern. Med. 120:25, 1967.

Dresner, S., and Schneeberg, N. G.: J. Clin. Endocr. 18:797, 1958.

Friend, D. G.: New Eng. J. Med. 263:1358, 1960.

Goodkind, M. J.: Unpublished research progress report, 1966.

*Grayson, R. R.: Amer. J. Med. 28:397, 1960.

*Greer, M. A., et al.: Antithyroid compounds. In Pitt-Rivers, R., and Trotter, W. R., editors: The thyroid gland, vol. 1, Washington, D. C., 1964, Butterworth, Inc., p. 357.

*Halmi, N. S.: The accumulation and recirculation of iodide by the thyroid. In Pitt-Rivers, R., and Trotter, W. R., editors: The thyroid gland, vol. 1, Washington, D. C., 1964, Butterworth, Inc., p. 71.

*Heimann, P.: Acta Endocr. 53:Suppl. 110:1, 1966.

*Herbst, A. L., and Selenkow, H. A.: New Eng. J. Med. 273:627, 1965.

*Significant reviews.

*Hoch, F. L.: New Eng. J. Med. **266**:446, 498, 1962.

Ingbar, S. H.: Endocrinology **63**:256, 1958.

*Ingbar, S. H., and Freinkel, N.: Recent Progr. Hormone Res. **16**:353, 1960.

*Johnson, N.: Brit. J. Surg. **42**:587, 1955.

Jorgensen, E. C.: Mayo Clin. Proc. **39**:560, 1964.

Luft, R., et al.: J. Clin. Invest. **41**:1776, 1962.

Man, E. B., et al.: Amer. J. Obstet. Gynec. **102**: 244, 1968.

Murphy, B. E. P., et al.: J. Clin. Endocr. **26**: 247, 1966.

Nadler, N. J.: Iodination of thyroglobulin in the thyroid follicle. In Cassano, C., and Andreoli, M., editors: Current topics in thyroid research, proceedings, International Thyroid Conference, Fifth, Rome, May 23-27, 1965, New York, 1965, Academic Press, Inc., p. 73.

Naumann, J. A., et al.: J. Clin. Invest. **46**: 1346, 1967.

Oppenheimer, J. H., et al.: J. Clin. Invest. **42**: 1769, 1963.

Oppenheimer, J. H., and Bernstein, G.: The metabolism and physiological significance of thyroxine-binding pre-albumin in man. In Cassano, C., and Andreoli, M., editors: Current topics in thyroid research, proceedings, International Thyroid Conference, Fifth, Rome, May 23-27, 1965, New York, 1965, Academic Press, Inc., p. 674.

Peter, J. B.: Biochem. Med. **2**:179, 1968.

*Robbins, J., and Rall, J. E.: Physiol. Rev. **40**: 415, 1960.

*Rosenberg, I. N., and Bastomsky, C. H.: Ann. Rev. Physiol. **27**:71, 1965.

Satoyoshi, E., et al.: Neurology **13**:645, 1963.

Silver, S., et al.: Amer. J. Med. **13**:725, 1952.

*Sisson, J. C.: J. Nucl. Med. **6**:853, 1965.

Sokoloff, L.: Amer. J. Dis. Child. **114**:498, 1967.

Sterling, K., and Brenner, M. A.: J. Clin. Invest. **45**:153, 1966.

*Tata, J. R.: Thyroid hormones and regulation of protein synthesis. In Karlson, P., editor: Mechanisms of hormone action, NATO advanced study institute, New York, 1965, Academic Press, Inc., p. 173.

Taurog, A., and Evans, E. S.: Endocrinology **80**:915, 1967.

*Werner, S. C., et al.: J. Clin. Endocr. **27**:1637, 1967.

*Werner, S. C., and Neuman, J. A.: Ann. Rev. Physiol. **30**:213, 1968.

Wiener, J. D.: New Eng. J. Med. **278**:738, 1968.

*Wissig, S. L.: Morphology and cytology. In Pitt-Rivers, R., and Trotter, W. R., editors: The thyroid gland, vol. 1, Washington, D. C., 1964, Butterworth, Inc., p. 32.

Wolff, J., and Chaikoff, I. L.: J. Biol. Chem. **174**:555, 1948.

*Wolff, J.: Physiol. Rev. **44**:45, 1964.

Wolff, J.: Amer. J. Med. **47**:101, 1969.

Chapter 7

Goiter

This discussion will be confined to thyroid enlargement (that is, goiter) not caused by hyperthyroidism, neoplasm, thyroiditis, or infiltrative or granulomatous lesions. Endemic goiter and sporadic goiter are considered separately even though such a dichotomy is arbitrary and is not accepted by all authorities.

ENDEMIC GOITER

Endemic goiter (simple, colloid, iodine-deficiency goiter) is a worldwide disorder found where iodine deficiency is so universal that at least 10% of a population is affected. The severest "endemic" is in the Himalayas, but endemics exist in the Andes, the Swiss Alps, the Congo, the Central Plains and Great Lakes regions of the United States, and in numerous scattered areas throughout the world. Recent investigations have uncovered areas of endemicity in England, Holland, Virginia, Kentucky, and the Mekong Delta and along the Pacific coast of South America. They are concentrated particularly in those mountainous and rural low-lying regions where the soil was deposited during the last great glacial period. The incidence in urban populations is less than in rural areas. An account of the world distribution is presented by Kelley and Snedden in a World Health Organization monograph (1960). It has been estimated that the goitrous population of the world numbers over 200 million.

Etiology

Iodine deficiency. Marine (Marine and Williams, 1908) clarified the role of *iodine deficiency* and the importance of prophylaxis. When the thyroidal iodide concentration was below 0.1 mg./gram dry weight, there was epithelial hyperplasia of the gland. The mean iodide concentration of goiters from a Himalayan goiter belt was 37 μg./gram compared to 330 μg./gram in nonendemic thyroid glands (Ramalingaswami, 1964). The studies of Stanbury's group (1954) in Mendoza, Argentina, firmly established the importance of iodine deficiency as the critical factor, though recognizing that other goitrogenic mechanisms may be operative. Acquired aberrations in thyroid biosynthetic mechanisms may play a role, as well as excessive spillage of iodine by the goitrous gland. The tendency for goiter to develop in young iodine-deficient rats is increased by the addition of calcium carbonate to the diet. Numerous observers have commented on the probable goitrogenicity of chalk, limestone, and fluorine in iodine-deficient regions. Even bacterial pollution has been suspected as a causative factor. Inconsistencies in the iodine-deficiency hypothesis have been discussed. Costa and Mortara, 1960, found a normal iodine intake and urinary iodide in endemic areas in Italy, and similar findings have been reported in other endemics. When the deficiency of iodide is minimal, the tendency to goiter formation is favored by hereditary factors or the presence of other goitrogens.

Familial, genetic, and constitutional factors. Heimann, 1966, noted a familial incidence in 42% of 401 patients with various thyroid conditions. There may be familial, genetic, constitutional, or unknown influences common to a population or segment of a population that render it particularly susceptible to iodine deficiency. Despite the severity of an endemic, goiter does not appear in all inhabitants. Malamos et al., 1965, studying the epidemiology of an endemic in Greece, noted that some families were affected more than others living in the same village. The goiter prevalence in children was related to the presence of goiter in the parents. When both parents were goitrous, 68.4% of their children had goiter. When only the father was affected, the incidence was 50%; only the mother, 42.2%; and when neither parent had a goiter, only 32.9% of the children were goitrous.

Goitrogenic foodstuffs. A goitrogenic substance in milk was responsible for an "epidemic" of goiter in school children in Tasmania despite a concurrent program of iodine prophylaxis. The source was a *Brassica* weed, called choumoellier, used in cattle feed; its elimination abolished the endemic. Other species of cruciferous weeds have been found to be goitrogenic. Cassava, containing a cyanogenetic glucoside, was a significant factor in an eastern Nigerian epidemic. Goiter can be produced in rabbits by feeding them cabbage. During the food shortage in World War II, most of the population in Holland and Belgium subsisted on turnips, carrots, cabbages, and other vegetables, and there was an increased incidence of goiter. The goitrogenic compound in rutabaga, turnip, cabbage, kale, and rape was found to be L-5-vinyl, 2-thiooxazolidone (goitrin), released by enzymatic action from its precursor "progoitrin." (Greer and Deeney, 1959). Goitrin completely blocks the organic binding of iodine. For a review of nutrition and goiter see Greer, 1950; for epidemiology see Vought, 1967.

Endemic iodide goiter. Approximately 1,000 cases of goiter induced by the ingestion of large amounts of seaweed have been observed in Hokkaido, the largest northern Japanese island (Suzuki et al., 1965). In contrast to other varieties of endemic goiter, all patients have remained euthyroid.

Pathophysiology

The following sequence of events leads to endemic goiter: iodine deficiency→reduction of circulating TH→TSH stimulation→thyroid hyperplasia and hypertrophy →restoration of circulating TH. The chronology of these changes has been studied in rats by Studer and Greer, 1965. Replenishing the iodine converts a hyperplastic thyroid to a colloid type of goiter in the rat, a change analogous to the human colloid goiter so prevalent in endemics and undoubtedly caused by severe iodine starvation alternating with intervals of less profound deficiency.

The physiology of the iodide-deficient gland is grossly disturbed. Serum TSH is increased, and the iodide trap is stimulated. There is a decreased ability to form T_4, usually combined with an increased concentration of MIT and DIT and a general reduction of thyroid hormone synthesis. The production of nonhormonal iodoprotein (butanol-insoluble) is a major pathway of iodine metabolism in nontoxic goiter that is sensitive to stimulation by TSH and suppressible by TH. The contribution of butanol-insoluble iodoproteins to the PBI, which is usually normal, may be counterbalanced by the preferential secretion of T_3, which does not add to the PBI, so that a euthyroid state can be maintained.

The disproportionate susceptibility of the female to goiter compared to that of the male remains unsolved. Dratman and Eskin, 1964, reported that injecting pooled human female serum obtained during the luteal phase of the menstrual cycle into rats enhanced the goitrogenicity of propylthiouracil, whereas serum from the follicular phase showed a tendency to inhibit goitrogenesis. Serum from male donors was without effect.

Pathology

The thyroid gland in endemic goiter progresses through three stages: hyperplasia, colloid formation, and nodule formation.

Hyperplasia. The cuboidal cells increase in number and become columnar. Hyperplasia produces infoldings with reduction of colloid content. The thyroid gland is increased in size and weight. In an endemic area the thyroid gland of the newborn is enlarged and shows intense epithelial hyperplasia.

Colloid formation. Hyperplasia is succeeded by involution in localized areas or throughout the gland, producing large colloid-filled follicles lined by a flattened epithelium. The cycle may be repeated in successive waves. The cause is unknown but has been attributed to various physiologic stresses encountered during growth, puberty, menstruation, and pregnancies but may be the result of transient improvements in the supply of iodine. In a severe "pure" endemic in the Himalayas where iodine has never been supplied, hyperplasia predominates, and colloid goiter is not encountered (Ramalingaswami, 1964).

Nodule formation. With recurrent waves of hyperplasia and involution occurring heterogeneously throughout the thyroid, the disproportion of growth and involution leads to the formation of nodules. Their number, size, and age of appearance correlate directly with the age of the patient and the severity of the endemic. The genesis of nodule formation has been studied by using autoradiographs. In simple and puberty goiters the RAI is uniformly distributed, indicating hyperplasia of the entire gland. In older patients most of the gland fails to concentrate RAI, and the isotope is confined to small discrete foci. Follicles capable of concentrating RAI are small in diameter, contain tall cells, and are grouped together. Later degenerative changes occur, and these previously active areas exhibit central necrosis, hemorrhage, and cyst formation. Frequent repetition of the above process converts the goiter into a multinodular mass wherein one or two nodules are active and the remainder are inactive. Occasionally a true adenoma with autonomous function is found.

Clinical features

Goiters usually appear in childhood and increase in prevalence up to puberty. The female is far more susceptible, though in the severest endemics, where a large proportion of the population is affected, the

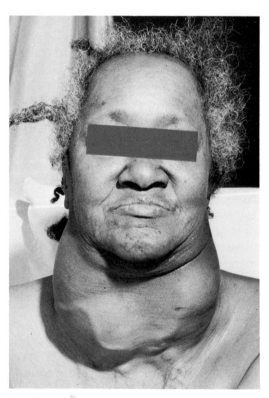

Fig. 7-1. Large sporadic multinodular goiter of 40 years' duration in a euthyroid asymptomatic 70-year-old female. (PBI 5.6, thyroxine 7.2, TBG 23.6 μg./100 ml., ET$_3$ 15.2%, RAIU 12% in 24 hours, no "washout" with KClO$_3$, TRC antibody titer negative.)

sex difference may be masked. After puberty, goiters in the male often regress and many will disappear unless the endemic is severe. In the female the goiters rarely regress significantly but tend to become large and nodular. Bulky goiters (Fig. 7-1) are not rare. Unless there is neck compression with respiratory obstruction, dysphagia, hoarseness, or cough, there may be no complaints. Goiter is a compensatory mechanism for impaired synthesis of thyroid hormone, and compensation may not always be adequate to prevent hypothyroidism. The prevalence of this complication has not been thoroughly explored in endemic goiter. Cretinism and deaf mutism are more common in severe endemics with a high prevalence of goiter. The cosmetic disfigurement is accepted in endemic regions as a normal anatomic finding.

The goiter may be so small as to be scarcely visible and discovered only by palpation or may be a huge bulky mass (Fig. 7-1). There may be substernal extension. The thyroid enlargement is usually smooth in the young, but by age 20 to 30 years, particularly in the female, nodulation is appreciable and increases progressively. True adenoma formation and cystic degeneration are not infrequent. During periods of stress in the female (menstruation, pregnancy, lactation), the gland may enlarge further and later regress somewhat after the stress is relieved or maintain its additional size. Neck compression is uncommon. Hemorrhage in a cyst causes sudden focal enlargement, pain, and perhaps fever. Thyrotoxicosis is an uncommon complication. Malignancy is probably no more frequent than in areas of sporadic goiter, though the subject is one of controversy.

Laboratory findings

The RAIU in euthyroid subjects is usually high and is inversely related to the iodide intake. The mean RAIU of the Mendoza patients (Stanbury et al., 1954) was 58.6%, compared to 37.5% in Bos-

tonians. The mean PBI in 104 subjects was 5.81±1.81 μg./100 ml. In the Greek endemic (Malamos et al., 1965) the mean PBI was 4.5 in males, 4.6 in females. Plasma inorganic iodide and urinary iodide excretion are both reduced.

Treatment

Prophylaxis. The provision of an adequate supply of iodine will abolish an endemic, provided that no other important factors are operative. In a worldwide survey conducted by the World Health Organization on the use of iodized salt, it was found that the goiter prevalence in highly endemic areas was reduced 40% to 95% in children and young adults. The most satisfactory prophylaxis is iodinization of table salt in a concentration of 1:10,000 to 1:200,000 depending on local estimates. Diets vary considerably in iodine content. The American diet averages 100 to 200 μg./day; that in Glasgow, Scotland, 290 μg./day (±19.3) (Wayne et al., 1964); an average hospital diet 65 to 529 μg./day (Vought and London, 1964). WHO recommends a minimum daily intake of 100 μg., whereas Wayne et al. suggest at least 160 μg./day. The official United States iodine content of table salt is 76.5 μg./gram. The daily ingestion of approximately 1.4 to 1.5 grams of iodized table salt should therefore prevent goiter. Prophylaxis by supplementing the water supply or administering iodine in a regular dose (that is, 1 drop of Lugol's solution per week) has not been as successful. A single I.M. injection of iodized oil may be effective for 2 to 3 years. Very rarely thyrotoxicosis may be precipitated by the administration of iodine ("jodbasedow").

Therapy of the goiter. Iodine administration will induce goiter regression if administered very early in the course of the disease when hyperplasia rather than colloid formation prevails. Effects are slow and require many months. Suppressive doses of TH may induce regression or even disappearance after prolonged administration. Thyroidectomy is rarely required to relieve neck compression or for cosmetic reasons. Replacement with TH is indicated for hypothyroidism. When other goitrogenic factors are discovered, their elimination is mandatory.

For a recent review of endemic goiter see Stanbury, 1969.

SPORADIC GOITER

Sporadic goiter (simple, nonendemic, colloid, nontoxic goiter) is a diffuse or nodular enlargement of the thyroid gland that occurs in a small proportion of a population and exhibits no particular geographic distribution. There is probably no fundamental difference between endemic and sporadic goiters other than the prevalence rate, the former involving more than, and the latter less than, 10% of a population. Sporadic goiter may be diffuse (simple) or nodular.

Simple (diffuse) goiter

Etiology. The cause is *unknown.* It cannot be attributed to iodine deficiency per se, though stress (puberty, menstruation, pregnancy, lactation) may increase iodine requirements and foster a relative deficiency. Wayne et al., 1964, found the mean daily iodine intake of patients with simple goiter in Glasgow, Scotland, a nonendemic area, to be at the lower end of a distribution curve for normal (nongoitrous) individuals. A number of *foods* possessing goitrogenic properties have been investigated (see discussion on endemic goiter, p. 117), but one can rarely elicit a history of excessive ingestion sufficient to be a significant factor. A growing list of *chemicals* and *drugs* (Table 6-1) can cause goiter but can only rarely be indicted. An inborn or genetically determined intrathyroidal enzymatic deficiency may cause subtle reductions in TH biosynthesis, eventuating in excessive TSH stimulation of the thyroid gland with resulting hyperplasia. That this situation may occur in adult sporadic goiter is suggested by the frequency of goiter in families and by the reports of a decreased thyroidal

T_4 content and an elevated MIT/DIT ratio. The enzymatic fault may be latent and impede hormonogenesis only in the face of a mild iodine deficiency or a goitrogenic substance. Goiter may occasionally be caused by the excessive ingestion of iodine itself (Wolff, 1969).

Pathophysiology. The pathophysiology is the same as that of endemic goiter.

Clinical features. Approximately 3% to 4% of the population in the eastern United States and 5% to 15% in the Midwest are goitrous. The female-to-male ratio varies from 4:1 to 8:1. Harden et al., 1964, studied 24 Scottish males with nontoxic goiter and found 7 tumors, 5 cases of iodine deficiency, 5 of thyroiditis, 4 due to drugs, and 3 unclassified. They concluded that goiter in the male is rarely "simple." Goiter is rarely manifest before puberty. Slight thyroid hyperplasia is not unusual in pubertal and adolescent girls and may regress in adulthood or progress to a larger goiter. With advancing age, goiters tend to enlarge and become nodular.

Symptoms and signs. Essentially the symptoms and signs are the same as those for endemic goiter. Hypothyroidism has been thought to be an unusual concomitant of goiter, though Cassidy found a prevalence of 15% and later described 234 patients with both conditions examined between 1953 and 1966 (Cassidy et al., 1968).

Laboratory findings. Studies usually fall within the euthyroid range unless there is hypothyroidism. The RAIU may be increased if there is diffuse thyroidal hyperplasia. An "iodide goiter" is suspected when the 2-hour RAIU is high, but the 24-hour value is low, the PBI is elevated, and the BEI or serum T_4 is normal. RAI scanning is useful to detect substernal extension or aberrant thyroid glands.

Differential diagnosis. A simple goiter must be differentiated from toxic goiter, chronic thyroiditis, and carcinoma. Other causes of thyroid enlargement are rare (thyroglossal cyst, abscess, granulomas).

TOXIC GOITER. In simple goiter the RAIU may be elevated but is suppressible with 75 to 100 μg. of T_3 daily for 8 days.

HASHIMOTO'S LYMPHADENOID GOITER (THYROIDITIS). Hashimoto's lymphadenoid goiter may present a diagnostic problem. Recent reports suggest that it is the major cause of goiter in children. The autoantibody titer is usually high, and the PBI/BEI ratio is more likely to be elevated than in goiter. Hashimoto's thyroiditis regresses more rapidly and usually more completely during TH therapy. Occasionally a thyroid biopsy is necessary to establish the correct diagnosis.

THYROID CARCINOMA. The differential from carcinoma rarely presents a problem as it does in nodular goiter.

Treatment. Any known goitrogen (food or drug) must be interdicted. When it is of paramount necessity to continue a particular therapy, such as para-aminosalicylate for tuberculosis, concomitant administration of thyroid hormone in suppressive doses may be effective. Very small goiters require no therapy but should be observed to detect progressive enlargement, nodular change, or the onset of hyperthyroidism. Suppressive therapy with thyroid hormone is effective in small diffuse goiters and may cause significant regression even in large goiters. If commenced when the goiter is diffuse, nodulation may be prevented. The daily dose is desiccated thyroid 120 to 240 mg. (2 to 4 grains) (or sodium L-thyroxine 0.2 to 0.4 mg.) and may be taken at one time each day. In unresponsive cases, if the 24-hour RAIU is not less than 10%, a larger dose of thyroid hormone is tested. Successful regression was achieved in 39 of 99 of our patients treated for 6 to 12 months (Schneeberg et al., 1962). In 15 of the 39, the goiter regression was complete.

If evidence of thyroid toxicity occurs during treatment (nervousness, sweating, dyspnea, palpitation, insomnia, or weight loss), the dose is reduced by 30 to 60 mg. of desiccated thyroid, or its equivalent, for 4 to 8 weeks. Later the original dose may be tolerated. Suppressive therapy should be avoided in cardiac, markedly hypertensive, or very elderly subjects. Rarely, when an unusually sensitive patient cannot tolerate adequate doses, a favorable response may be achieved with sodium D-thyroxine. If, despite suppressive therapy, a goiter continues to enlarge and particularly if it compromises respiration or deglutition, thyroidectomy is necessary. If the surgical risk is unacceptable, RAI therapy can reduce the size of a goiter. Iodides are of no value in the treatment of sporadic goiters and may rarely induce thyrotoxicosis ("jodbasedow").

Sporadic goiter of the newborn. Sporadic goiter has been found in newborn infants from thyrotoxic or hypothyroid mothers, or from mothers who have received thiouracil derivatives or iodides, or from normal mothers who have not received any drug. The goiter is usually small but may be large enough to cause tracheal compression. There can be neonatal hyperthyroidism if the mother is thyrotoxic. Since most of the nontoxic goiters regress spontaneously, therapy is necessary only if respiration is obstructed. Thyroidectomy with or without tracheotomy is performed.

Nodular goiter (adenomatous goiter)

Pathology. Nodules may be *nonneoplastic* due to degenerative, involutional, or inflammatory changes or may be *neoplastic (true adenomas)*. Classification may be difficult in some instances. They vary in size from microscopic to large masses. Mortensen et al., 1955, found the most common nodule, in the clinically normal thyroid, to be the nonneoplastic involutional nodule; this type has been called "adenomatous nodule," "colloid adenoma," or "degenerative-regenerative nodule." The adenomas are discrete, encapsulated, histologically homogeneous lesions that are classified as embryonal, fetal, microfollicular or macrofollicular, papillary cystadenoma, or Hürthle, depending on their microscopic characteristics (Fig. 7-2).

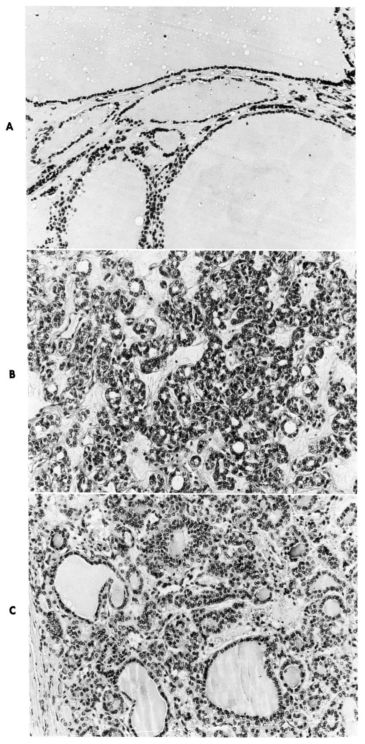

Fig. 7-2. Thyroid adenomas. **A,** Macrofollicular colloid adenoma. **B,** Fetal adenoma. **C,** Microfollicular and macrofollicular adenoma. (Courtesy Dr. Alexander Nedwich and the Department of Pathology, Hahnemann Medical College, Philadelphia, Pa.)

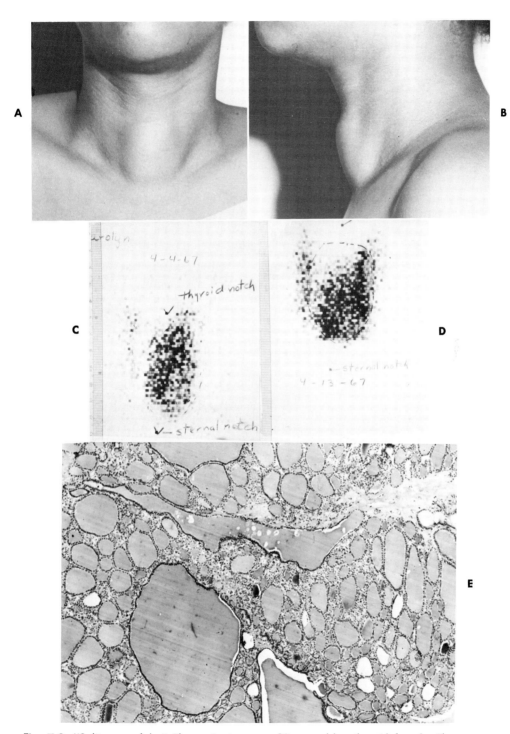

Fig. 7-3. "Solitary nodule." The patient was a 29-year-old euthyroid female. The mass, **A** and **B,** had been present since age 12 years but had shown recent enlargement. **C,** Radioiodine scan showing a "hot" nodule. **D,** Scan after TSH stimulation showing increased uptake of paranodular tissue. **E,** Histologic section of resected nodule showing a microfollicular and macrofollicular adenoma (X100).

Nodules may be solid or cystic, soft or hard, because of varying amounts of fibrosis with or without calcification.

Incidence. The two community-wide surveys of the prevalence of goiter in the United States (Vander et al., 1954, Framingham, Mass.; Matovinovic et al., 1965, Tecumseh, Mich.) showed a wide discrepancy (0.47% in Michigan, an area where goiter has been endemic; 4.1% in Massachusetts). Sokal, 1955, calculated the prevalence of nodular goiter in the United States to be 3.7%. Though the incidence probably varies somewhat from region to region, nodular goiter is not rare. It is more common in females than in males (4:1). Autopsy studies show a far greater prevalence than do clinical studies. The highest reported clinical incidence is 7%, whereas the reported autopsy incidence varies from 8% to 65%. Autopsy series will usually include more older persons in whom nodules are more common. Deeply placed, small, soft nodules may be easily missed. In obese, sthenic, and elderly patients with kyphosis and a short neck, accurate examination of the thyroid may be difficult. Very small nodules that would be impalpable are included in the autopsy series.

Clinical features. The discovery of a nodular goiter depends on the size and consistency of the nodules. Very small, soft nodules may be impalpable. In the Mayo Clinic series (Mortensen et al., 1955) of clinically "normal thyroid glands," 49.5% were histologically nodular, and the nodule diameter varied from 2 mm. to 7.5 cm. Nodular goiters are often classified as uninodular (solitary) (Fig. 7-3) or multinodular (Fig. 7-1). So-called solitary nodules are often dominant masses in goiters containing smaller impalpable nodules. The consistency varies from soft to very indurated masses, the latter usually being found in large bulky glands (Fig. 7-1). They may be mobile or fixed, cervical or substernal, and may or may not cause tracheal and/or esophageal deviation or compression of the recurrent laryngeal nerves. Nodular goiters may undergo cystic degeneration and may become partly calcified. Hemorrhage in a cyst may cause rapid enlargement, pain, fever, and rapid compression of neck structures. Firm, poorly defined nodules, particularly when the surface is bosselated, resemble chronic thyroiditis.

Laboratory findings. Tests of thyroid function are usually normal. Hypothyroid values obtain in approximately 15% of patients (Cassidy et al., 1968). Needle biopsy of a nodule may seed cancer cells or may miss the lesion. X-ray films of the neck and evaluation of swallowing function are utilized to study tracheal or esophageal deviation and/or compression. Chest films may reveal a substernal goiter. *RAI scanning (scintillation scanning, scintigram),* by providing information about the function of nodules, aids in the detection of cancer and may reveal aberrant thyroid tissue and substernal goiter. Nodules are classified as "hot," or hyperfunctioning, if they concentrate considerably more RAI than the non-nodular portions of the gland and "cold," or hypofunctioning, if they concentrate considerably less RAI than the remainder of the gland. "Warm" nodules concentrate the same as the remainder of the gland, and "cool" nodules concentrate less than the normal gland but more than the vascular background of the neck. Hot nodules are sharply delineated because, by inhibiting pituitary TSH, they suppress paranodular RAI concentration. After TSH stimulation the nonfunctional areas will accumulate RAI (Figs. 7-3 and 7-4). Occasionally a hot nodule may be more or less obscured by functioning thyroid tissue but can be revealed by suppressing the nonnodular TSH-dependent thyroid tissue with thyroid hormone (Fig. 7-5). Cold nodules have been found to contain cancer in from 7% to 58% of reported cases, whereas hot nodules have only rarely been cancerous. After TSH stimulation, approximately 25% of hypofunctional (cool) and nonfunctional (cold) nodules show a substantial augmentation

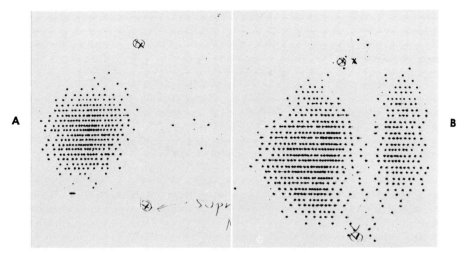

Fig. 7-4. A, "Hot" nodule in a euthyroid patient. The remainder of the thyroid is function-less because the nodular secretion of thyroid hormone inhibits endogenous TSH. **B,** TSH injection "lights up" the suppressed gland.

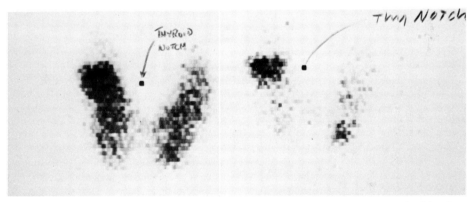

Fig. 7-5. Nontoxic autonomous "hot" nodule of the right upper pole is masked by func-tioning thyroid tissue. It is clearly revealed after suppression of the TSH-dependent gland by the administration of triiodothyronine (100 μg. daily for 5 days). A small autonomous focus was simultaneously uncovered at the left lower pole, but there was no palpable nodule in this region.

of RAI concentration, and in such instances malignancy is unlikely.

There are certain inherent errors in RAI scanning:

1. Nodules less than 1 cm. in diameter cannot be detected because they are below the limits of resolution of the scanner.

2. A hypofunctional or nonfunctional nodule may be completely missed if it is embedded in functioning thyroid tissue.

3. A hypofunctional, very large nodule may appear warm or slightly hot in comparison with normal tissue simply because of its bulk.

4. Total inactivity of a thyroid lobe may be attributed to cancer but is more likely from a benign lesion. Cancer rarely if ever causes total obliteration of a lobe.

Nodular goiter and thyroid cancer. Certain paramount questions plague the physician who encounters a nodular goiter.

1. *What are the probabilities of cancer residing in this nodule (or nodules)?*

The average published prevalence rate

is 5%. However, surgical statistics probably do not represent the nodular goiter population at large (Sokal, 1955). Thyroid cancer is rare, whereas nodular goiter is common. There were only 34 cases of thyroid cancer admitted to the Philadelphia General Hospital in the 10-year period 1936 to 1946 or 0.013% of 271,803 admissions (Perloff and Schneeberg, 1951). Similarly 17 cases were seen at Boston City Hospital from 1931 to 1942 and 27 cases at Massachusetts General Hospital from 1937 to 1944. The most representative study (Mustacchi and Cutler, 1956) surveyed 10 urban areas of the United States in 1947-1948 and found 336 cases in a population of 14,600,000 or 2.3 per 100,000 in the white population and 1.8 per 100,000 in the nonwhite population. When the prevalence of thyroid cancer is recalculated on the basis of the nodular goiter population rather than on the basis of cases coming to surgery, the incidence is less than 0.2% (Sokal, 1955). One of the most informative surveys is the Framingham Heart Study conducted by the National Heart and Cancer Institutes where a population of 5,127 subjects from 30 to 59 years of age was examined for a period of 15 years. The original report in 1954 (Vander et al.) described 218 nodules (4.2%). Nineteen were removed surgically and all were benign. The 15-year follow-up report (Vander et al., 1968) included 67 new lesions. Surgical removal of 45 lesions throughout the 15-year period failed to discover a single case of cancer, nor was cancer discovered in any of the original 218 cases of nodular goiter that were observed for 15 years. This study would tend to confirm the now widely accepted premise that thyroid cancer seldom develops in nodular goiters and is a rare disease in the population at large.

The Mayo Clinic autopsy study of 821 "clinically normal" thyroids uncovered 17 unexpected thyroid cancers (Mortensen et al., 1955) for an incidence of 4.2% of the histologically nodular goiters, a value similar to the 5% reported in surgical statistics. One might therefore justify wholesale removal of normal thyroids to eliminate cancer. Finally, thyroid cancer causes only 0.6% or less of all deaths from cancer in the United States.

2. Can I differentiate the benign nodular goiter from thyroid cancer?

Since only a small number of nodular goiters come to surgery, some selectivity has always been exercised by physicians. How accurate is this screening process? Sokal, 1957, found that 16% of patients selected for surgery had cancer, whereas only 1 of 140 patients selected for nonsurgical treatment ultimately proved to have thyroid cancer. "The deaths from thyroid cancer among the conservatively treated cases have been so few that they would almost certainly have been exceeded by operative deaths had all patients with nodular goiter been subjected to surgery."

The *criteria used for advocating surgery* are generally agreed upon:

a. Single or dominant hard or very firm fixed lesions particularly if enlarging or appearing *de novo*.

b. Enlarged cervical lymph nodes or other signs of metastasis, particularly the Delphian node found just above the thyroid isthmus.

c. Nodules in children, adolescents, young adults, or males of any age are viewed with suspicion. Approximately 65% of thyroid cancers are found in women. Thyroid nodules are uncommon in men and carry a threefold probability of being malignant compared to similar nodules in women. Almost 50% of nodules in children are malignant. Because of the known relationship between prior x-ray irradiation of the neck and subsequent thyroid cancer, such a positive history should heighten one's suspicion of malignancy.

d. Nodules that fail to concentrate RAI, that is, cold or cool nodules.

e. Compression of neck structures.

f. A nodule that fails to regress after

suppressive therapy or a gland that becomes enlarged or more indurated.

g. Soft tissue films of the thyroid showing psammoma bodies.

h. Coexistence of a pheochromocytoma.

The so-called solitary nodule has always been viewed as potentially cancerous, whatever its character. However, one third to one half of these are multinodular with a single palpable dominant mass. The incidence of malignancy in solitary and multinodular goiters does not differ significantly.

3. *Will prophylactic thyroidectomy prevent cancer?*

The question of prophylactic thyroidectomy assumes that nodules are precancerous lesions, but the evidence is not convincing. More than half of all thyroid cancers are found in otherwise nonnodular glands. The incidence of thyroid cancer is unchanged or perhaps increasing slightly, whereas the worldwide incidence of nodular goiter is decreasing as areas of endemicity are being eradicated. To be truly prophylactic, total thyroidectomy is required, and this is a well-nigh impossible task. After partial thyroidectomy the remnants are under TSH stimulation, which in itself may favor carcinogenesis. Thyroid cancer has been found after prophylactic thyroidectomy in a number of reported cases.

The following plan is recommended in patients with nodular goiter: Surgery is advised in high-risk cases (p. 126). The remainder of patients with small, soft, mobile nodules whose consistency does not differ from the remainder of the thyroid are observed for several years either without therapy or preferably on suppressive thyroid medication (180 mg. desiccated thyroid daily). Small nodular goiters may regress after 3 to 18 months but will recur if thyroid hormone is omitted. Though regression implies a benign lesion, some papillary adenocarcinomas do respond. Very few patients ultimately require thyroidectomy because of the appearance of findings suggesting malignancy. Suppres-

sive thyroid hormone treatment should be maintained permanently after surgery to block TSH and prevent recurrence of nodules. Delay in surgery probably entails no added risk to the patient, since the majority of thyroid cancers are low grade, are rarely fatal, and have a high rate of cure. The highly malignant lesions tend to be rapidly fatal despite early radical surgery. Crile, 1966, found that 15% of all thyroid nodules were cystic and aspirated them. Thirty-six of 50 of his patients were cured by such aspiration therapy.

Patients cognizant of the possibility of cancer or those who have been already advised to have surgery should probably not be deterred, for obvious psychologic reasons, unless the lesion is so obviously benign that removal would not warrant the surgical risk. The medicolegal problems of advising for or against surgery have never been delineated.

There are no clearly defined or universally accepted rules of procedure in handling the nodular goiter, and each problem requires individual evaluation. Statistical surveys are of limited value. The concepts presented by the author are not universally accepted, and the conservative approach is decried in many quarters by those who advocate wholesale surgery.

The natural history of *hyperfunctioning adenomas* or *euthyroid "hot" nodules* (Fig. 7-3) is largely unknown, but such nodules have been viewed as a potential source of clinical hyperthyroidism or of masked thyrotoxicosis with cardiac manifestations. See p. 152 for further discussion.

REFERENCES

Cassidy, C. E., et al.: Goiter and hypothyroidism. In Astwood, E. B., and Cassidy, C. E., editors: Clinical endocrinology, New York, 1968, Grune & Stratton, Inc., p. 210.

Costa, A., and Mortara, M.: Bull. WHO 22:493, 1960.

Crile, G., Jr.: Surgery 59:210, 1966.

Dratman, M. B., and Eskin, B. A.: Amer. J. Obstet. Gynec. 89:646, 1964.

°Greer, M. A.: Physiol. Rev. 30:513, 1950.

°Significant reviews.

Greer, M. A., and Deeney, J. M.: J. Clin. Invest. **38**:1465, 1959.

Harden, R. M., et al.: Brit. Med. J. **1**:1419, 1964.

Heimann, P.: Acta Med. Scand. **179**:113, 1966.

Kelly, F. C., and Snedden, W. W.: Prevalence and geographical distribution of endemic goiter, WHO Monogr. Ser. **44**:27, 1960.

Malamos, B., et al.: Epidemiologic and metabolic studies in the endemic goiter areas of Greece. In Cassano, C., and Andreoli, M., editors: Current topics in thyroid research, proceedings, International Thyroid Conference, Fifth, Rome, May 23-27, 1965, New York, 1965, Academic Press, Inc., p. 851.

Marine, D., and Williams, W. W.: Arch. Intern. Med. **1**:349, 1908.

Matovinovic, J., et al.: J.A.M.A. **192**:234, 1965.

Mortensen, J. D., et al.: J. Clin. Endocr. **15**:1270, 1955.

Mustacchi, P., and Cutler, S. J.: New Eng. J. Med. **255**:889, 1956.

Perloff, W. H., and Schneeberg, N. G.: Surgery **29**:572, 1951.

*Ramalingaswami, V.: Endemic goitre. In Pitt-Rivers, R., and Trotter, W. R., editors: The thyroid gland, vol. 2, Washington, D. C., 1964, Butterworth, Inc., p. 71.

Schneeberg, N. G., et al.: Metabolism **11**:1054, 1962.

Seljelia, R., and Nakken, K. F.: Scand. J. Clin. Lab. Invest. Suppl. **106**:125, 1969.

Sokal, J. E.: Conn. State Med. J. **19**:718, 1955.

Sokal, J. E.: Arch. Intern. Med. **99**:60, 1957.

*Stanbury, J. B., et al.: Endemic goiter. The adaptation of man to iodine deficiency, Harvard Univ. Monogr. Med. Public Health, No. 12, 1954.

Stanbury, J. B., editor: Endemic goiter, Pan-American Health Organization, WHO, Scientific publication no. 193, Washington, D. C., 1969.

Studer, H., and Greer, M. A.: Acta Endocr. **49**:610, 1965.

Suzuki, H., et al.: Acta Endocr. **50**:161, 1965.

Vander, J. B., et al.: New Eng. J. Med. **251**:970, 1954.

Vander, J. B., et al.: Ann. Intern. Med. **69**:537, 1968.

Vought, R. L., and London, W. T.: Amer. J. Clin. Nutr. **14**:186, 1964.

*Vought, R. L.: Epidemiology of goiter. In Bloomfield, R. A., and Senhauser, D. A., editors: Second Midwest Conference on Thyroid, Columbia, Mo., 1967, University of Missouri Press, p. 75.

Wayne, E. J., Koutras, D. A., and Alexander, W. D.: Clinical aspects of iodine metabolism, Philadelphia, 1964, F. A. Davis Co., p. 83.

*Wolff, J.: Amer. J. Med. **47**:101, 1969.

Chapter 8

Hyperthyroidism

Hyperthyroidism is a hypermetabolic disorder resulting from the excessive secretion of thyroid hormone (TH). Synonyms include toxic goiter (diffuse or nodular), Graves' disease, Plummer's disease, exophthalmic goiter, Basedow's or Parry's disease, and thyrotoxicosis. There are two principal varieties—Graves' disease and Plummer's disease.

Graves' disease. A *triad* comprising diffuse thyroid hyperplasia, hyperthyroidism, and ophthalmopathy, with the occasional addition of pretibial myxedema and/or acropachy.

Plummer's disease or toxic adenomatous goiter. There may be one or more adenomas that are functioning autonomously (hot nodule or nodules), though occasionally they may be more or less TSH-dependent. This variety is clearly a different disease from Graves', lacks ophthalmopathy, and undoubtedly has a different cause. The clinical picture of Graves' disease, being by far the more common entity, will dominate the ensuing discussion, and Plummer's disease will be treated separately.

Etiology

The cause of Graves' disease is unknown. It is not a consequence of heightened tissue reactivity, nor is there evidence of the production of a qualitatively abnormal or "toxic" TH. The following theories have been entertained.

Thyroid-stimulating hormone (TSH). The hypothesis that excessive pituitary TSH is responsible for hyperthyroidism is no longer tenable. Plasma TSH levels are decreased and the TSH→thyroid feedback is permanently suppressed by the high concentration of circulating TH. The elevated RAIU and thyroidal secretion cannot be inhibited by very large doses of TH because the thyroid stimulator is not TSH. Hyperthyroidism has been observed in hypophysectomized patients and in panhypopituitarism. There is both histologic evidence of regressive changes and absence of TSH excess in the anterior pituitary.

Harris and Woods, 1956, found that electrical stimulation of the tuber cinereum consistently increased thyroid activity in adrenalectomized, but not in intact, rabbits. Evidence of adrenocortical hypofunction in some cases of human thyrotoxicosis was cited as clinical corroboration of the validity of this experimental approach.

Severe emotional stress in patients with Graves' disease is a common occurrence and is cited as evidence that CNS→hypothalamic TRF→ TSH + EPS→thyroid hyperactivity is the pathway causing hyperthyroidism. Gibson, 1962, in a critical review, found little evidence to suggest that thyroid activity was significantly affected by acute physical or emotional trauma.

Long-acting thyroid stimulator (LATS). When newer methods for assaying TSH became available, an unusual thyroid stimulator was discovered in the blood of hyperthyroid patients (Adams and Purves, 1956). The index of response was the TSH-induced augmentation of circulating ^{131}I in mice (p. 35), which was maximal at 2 hours. The rise was delayed to 8 to 12 hours when serum from hyperthyroid patients was used—thus the designation "long-acting thyroid stimulator," or LATS. LATS has been identified in the blood of 25% to 70% of patients with Graves' disease and in 85% when concentrated gamma globulin is used in the assay; it is usually absent in toxic adenomatous goiter and in normal subjects. It exhibits a high correlation with localized myxedema (dermopathy) and ophthalmopathy. LATS has been found both in the serum of infants with congenital hyperthyroidism and in the serum of their mothers, thus implying transplacental transfer of the mother's LATS with passive induction of thyrotoxicosis in the infant. The injection of sera from hyperthyroid patients into mice or into humans provokes a direct increase in thyroid function that is independent of the anterior pituitary. McKenzie, 1968, found LATS in the sera of rabbits immunized with human thyroid. Although the animals did not appear hyperthyroid, both the RAIU and the rate of release of ^{131}I was increased and was not suppressed by T_4 administration. Although LATS is probably a thyroid stimulator, it may act by inhibiting a thyroid repressor. It is chemically and immunologically distinct from TSH and has been identified as a 7S immunogammaglobulin (IgG) with a molecular weight of approximately 150,000, consisting of two pairs of polypeptide chains (H = heavy, L = light) linked by disulfide bridges (Munro et al., 1967). It has not been recovered from pituitary extracts of hyperthyroid patients but has been detected in the serum of hypopituitary hyperthyroid patients. It may originate in lymphoid or reticuloendothelial tissue and may, in fact, be an antibody.

Graves' disease may therefore be an autoimmune disorder with LATS being an immunoglobulin antibody and some unknown agent of thyroidal or nonthyroidal origin being the antigen, or it may be found without an antigenic precursor. Present evidence strongly suggests that LATS is the cause of Graves' disease, but disturbing discrepancies are the absence of detectable LATS in many patients with Graves' disease and the failure of LATS titers to parallel the severity of thyrotoxicosis or its clinical course, to regress with improvement of the disease, or to disappear when the thyroid gland is ablated. These discrepancies may be resolved when more sensitive assay methods become available.

Older literature described lymphoid and thymic hyperplasia and hypertrophy in hyperthyroidism. Gunn, 1964, found small medullary lymph follicles in the thymus glands of patients with Graves' disease, which correlated with lymphoid follicles in their thyroid glands but did not correlate with the presence of circulating thyroid antibodies. Antigastric antibodies, related to impaired gastric acid secretion, have been found in 37.5% of hyperthyroid patients, compared to 10% of controls (Williams, 1966), lending further weight to the suggestion that there is a basic disturbance of immunologic tolerance in Graves' disease. A short-acting thyroid stimulator, dubbed "SATS" and distinct from TSH and LATS, has been found occasionally in the serum of hyperthyroid patients, but its significance remains unknown.

Exophthalmos-producing substance (EPS). The role of EPS (p. 36) as a distinct entity of anterior pituitary origin separable from TSH and of etiologic importance in the ophthalmopathy of Graves' disease remains unsettled.

Neoplastic origin of hyperthyroidism (ectopic TSH). Increased thyroid function, associated with minimal clinical signs, has been reported in 7 cases of choriocarcinoma with elevated RAIU, serum PBI, and

BMR and decreased serum cholesterol (Odell et al., 1963). Bioassay of plasma and of the tumor revealed elevated TSH-like material. Other neoplasms, including choriocarcinoma in a male and a metastasizing bronchial carcinoma, have elaborated a TSH-like factor (McKenzie, 1967). A rare TSH-secreting pituitary tumor can induce thyroid hyperfunction.

Other causes of hyperthyroidism. Secretion of stored TH resulting from radiation damage to the thyroid or subacute thyroiditis may produce a transient state of hyperthyroidism. Rarely hyperthyroidism may be precipitated in humans (jodbasedow) and occasionally in rabbits with experimental goiter by the administration of iodides. *Strumae ovarii* are rarely the cause of hyperthyroidism and inhibit the function of cervical thyroid tissue.

Pathophysiology

Total thyroid mass is increased, cellular function is augmented, and the thyroidal iodide space is expanded. Thyroidal blood flow is increased, providing more iodide for hormone synthesis and substrate to satisfy the augmented metabolic requirements of the hyperplastic gland. Hormonal stores are depleted because of the rapid rate of secretion. There is enhanced iodide accumulation, turnover rate, organic binding, and secretion rate. The disappearance rate of injected T_4 is accelerated. Both TBG and TBPA are usually diminished, and the free T_4 fraction is increased. TSH induces an increase in serum PBI, T_4, and thyroidal clearance of plasma iodide, but no apparent augmentation of RAIU. A disproportionate increase of T_3 compared to T_4 has been suggested, and rarely the major circulating hormone is T_3. The majority of studies, however, have revealed no qualitative differences in the circulating iodinated compounds in euthyroid and hyperthyroid subjects and have found T_4 to be the major constituent.

Most of the clinical features of hyperthyroidism have been attributed to the effects of excessive TH. Some, or perhaps all, of the cardiovascular and sympathomimetic signs may be from either excessive *catecholamine* secretion or heightened end-organ sensitivity to normal catecholamine levels. Thyroid hormone may simply modify the response of the catecholamine receptors. Some clinical features may be wholly or in part due to various *vitamin deficiencies* caused by the heightened cellular metabolism with greater requirements for all vitamins (p. 95). Oxidative reactions of most tissues (skeletal, muscle, heart, liver, kidney) and the total basal metabolism are increased. The alterations in tissue and organ metabolism have been discussed on p. 94.

Pathology
Diffuse toxic goiter (Graves' disease)

The thyroid gland is enlarged, weighs from 30 to 150 grams, is hypervascular, and presents a dense meaty appearance with a relatively smooth surface. Histologic examination (Fig. 8-1) reveals hypertrophy and hyperplasia of the follicular epithelium. The follicle increases from the normal average diameter of 300 μ to over 400 μ. Thyroid-cell height increases from a normal of 5 to 15 μ, and the cells become heaped in layers that fold into the follicular lumen in papillary projections. The nucleus is enlarged, and numerous droplets fill the cytoplasm. The electron microscope reveals changes of intense physiologic activity as compared to the normal gland (Fig. 6-2). The follicular lumen appears smaller because of epithelial cellular encroachment and contains scanty, pallid, vacuolated colloid. Lymphoid hyperplasia, fibrosis, and increased vascularity fill the interfollicular spaces. The administration of iodine to the patient induces partial involution, a more normal-appearing, single-layered, flat-to-cuboidal epithelial lining of many follicles, increased colloid content, reduction of lymphoid hyperplasia, and decreased vascularity. Antithyroid drugs tend to increase the intensity of the hyperplastic changes, but involution can

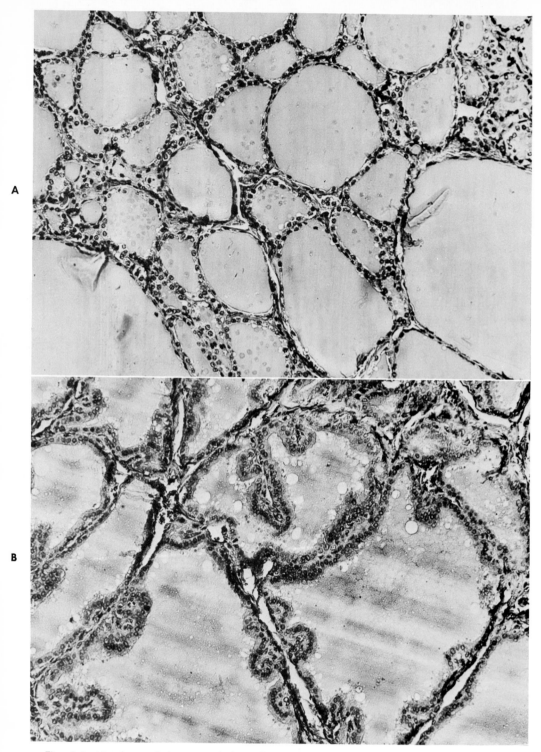

Fig. 8-1. Histology of the normal thyroid, **A,** contrasted with Graves' disease, **B.** Note epithelial hyperplasia, increased cell height, papillary infoldings, and marginal vacuolization of colloid. There is partial involution from 15 days of preoperative iodide preparation. (Courtesy Dr. William Ehrich [deceased], Department of Pathology, Philadelphia General Hospital, Philadelphia, Pa.)

still be induced by the subsequent administration of iodine.

Extrathyroidal pathology of Graves' disease. The following are various pathologic extrathyroidal changes:

1. *Orbit*—cellular infiltration with lymphocytes, macrophages, plasma, and mast cells. Accumulation of mucopolysaccharide, edema fluid and retro-orbital fat.

2. *Extraocular muscles*—atrophy (in some cases hypertrophy), interstitial myositis with cellular infiltration and late fibrosis, and fatty infiltration.

3. *Lymphoid hyperplasia, enlarged spleen* and *thymus.*

4. *Skeletal muscle*—cellular atrophy, vacuolization, loss of striations, fatty infiltration, and mucopolysaccharide deposition have been found. Occasionally similar lesions occur in the myocardium.

5. *Bone*—osteoporosis and osteitis fibrosa.

Toxic adenomatous (nodular) goiter

Adenomas, or a single adenoma, function autonomously to secrete excessive TH. The tumorous nodules consist of microfollicles or macrofollicles presenting the histologic picture described in Graves' disease. Surrounding thyroid parenchyma is usually atrophic. The true adenomatous or toxic nodular goiter can be distinguished from the multinodular goiter with hyperthyroidism, a condition that is probably the result of successive waves of hyperactivity and involution rather than of true adenoma formation and is really Graves' disease with incidental nodulation.

Clinical features

Incidence. The true incidence of this relatively common worldwide disorder is unknown. The prevalence rate published by Wilensky, 1943, was 2.2 per 1,000, by Halliday, 1945, 2.2 per 100,000 in England and 2.8 in the United States, and by Logan and Cushion, 1958, 1.1 per 1,000 in representative general practices in Britain.

Age. The greatest incidence appears from 20 to 40 years of age, whereas toxic adenomatous goiter is encountered chiefly from 40 to 60 years. It is rare before puberty.

Sex. The female to male ratio is 4:1 to 10:1, though the sex differences are less striking in children and in the elderly.

Epidemiology. Whether endemic goiter predisposes to hyperthyroidism has been the subject of disagreement. Iverson, 1949, noted a rise in prevalence in Denmark starting in 1941 and reaching a maximum in 1944, literally an "epidemic wave of thyrotoxicosis," which coincided with the 1941 to 1945 German occupation. By 1947 the incidence had declined to the prewar level. He also noted a seasonal variation with a peak incidence in the summer. Use of the word "epidemic" suggests an infective factor, a notion that may not be far-fetched in view of current speculation about the immune aspects of the disease and the fact that a viral agent might stimulate an autoimmune response.

Familial and genetic factors. A strong familial tendency is well known and has been ascribed to genetic factors that sensitize the predisposed individual to the inciting agent. Ingbar et al., 1956, found an accelerated peripheral turnover of T_4 in the euthyroid relatives of patients with Graves' disease.

The clinical features of hyperthyroidism may vary from minimal to florid toxicity. This variation may be the net result of the hyperactivity of the thyroid gland and the end-organ responsiveness of the individual. It has been observed that schizophrenic patients and some pregnant women can tolerate large doses of thyroid hormone. Refetoff et al., 1967, described a familial syndrome of deaf mutism, stippled epiphyses, goiter, and high circulating levels of T_4 in which all the subjects were euthyroid, and they suggested a possible target organ refractoriness to thyroid hormone. Males seem to tolerate hyperthyroxinemia better than females and tend to have fewer subjective symptoms. The triad of Graves' disease is (1) goiter, (2) hyperthyroidism, and (3) ophthalmopathy. In most patients all three have a coincidental onset, but occasionally only one or two may be present (p. 155).

Onset. The onset varies considerably but is more likely to be insidious, with a gradual waxing of the clinical signs. Occasionally symptoms appear precipitately, particularly after a traumatic or shocking incident.

Symptoms and signs

NERVOUSNESS. There is tension, restlessness, irritability. The patient is unable to relax, paces the floor, is prone to crying spells, is unable to concentrate, and becomes loquacious and argumentative. Activity is almost purposeless, and motor maneuvers may be rapid but clumsy. Insomnia is frequent. The startle reaction is exaggerated. In children, failing school work or poor behavior may be the first indication. Rarely apathy, lethargy, or depression may mask the disease and may be a forerunner of crisis. An apathetic facies may be combined with restlessness or tremor. "Apathetic hyperthyroidism" may be transient, and the patient may later become hyperkinetic. Rarely a frank psychosis may become manifest. The *tremor* of Graves' disease is a fine fibrillation of the outstretched fingers or tongue, which must be distinguished from the coarser tremor of nervousness, senility, or Parkinson's disease.

SWEATING. Sweating is continuous; when it occurs sporadically or in waves, one must suspect the menopause. The patient may be unaware of hyperhidrosis, but the examiner can appreciate the slightly sticky skin present even in cool weather. A sweaty warm neck is characteristic of thyrotoxicosis, whereas sweaty axillae and a dry neck are found in anxious euthyroid patients. The hands are warm and moist in hyperthyroidism, cold and clammy in the neurotic. Cold hands are so rare in hyperthyroidism that their presence renders the diagnosis doubtful.

SKIN AND HAIR. The skin is warm and often *satin smooth*, even in men, from a loss of much of the keratin layer. Pruritus, dermographia, urticaria, hyperpigmentation, or vitiligo, and erythema of the palms or elbows occasionally occur. The hair becomes very soft, smooth, often straight and does not retain a permanent wave.

HEAT INTOLERANCE. The patient prefers cool weather, dislikes summer or warm rooms, and feels excessively warm and uncomfortable after exertion. He wears fewer clothes and requires fewer bedclothes than he used to.

CARDIOVASCULAR CHANGES. There is an increased blood volume, erythrocyte mass, and peripheral blood flow in order to satisfy the heightened tissue requirements for oxygen of the hyperthyroid individual. The following cardiovascular changes that occur in hyperthyroidism represent the organism's adjustments to meet these demands:

Heart rate	
Cardiac index	
Pulse pressure (systolic ↑, diastolic ↓)	
Mean systolic ejection rate	
Cardiac output (resting)	
Cardiac output (exercise) (disproportionate increase)	Increased
Right heart and pulmonary pressure	
Coronary blood flow	
Stroke oxygen consumption	
Peripheral blood flow	
Plasma volume	
Cardiac work efficiency	
Peripheral vascular resistance	Decreased
Digitalis glycoside response	
Capillaries	Dilated
Stroke output	Same or slightly elevated
Circulation time	Rapid

Palpitation, especially with emotional tension and upon effort, is common. Tachycardia (rate over 90 beats per minute) tends to be proportional to toxicity. The cardiac rate, however, may show considerable lability and occasionally may be normal. The only formal study of the sleeping pulse rate (Crooks and Murray, 1958) showed that 53.7% of hyperthyroid and 2.8% of euthyroid subjects had sleeping pulse rates greater than 80 beats per minute. In euthyroid subjects premature atrial contractions tend to disappear with exercise, but in hyperthyroidism they persist. The pulse pressure is increased because of a systolic rise and a diastolic fall. The apex beat is exaggerated and the heart sounds are hyperactive, forceful, or pounding. The accentuated split mitral first sound, together with a midsystolic pulmonic flow murmur, may suggest mitral stenosis. If one then observes the prominent pulmonary conus on a chest x-ray film (Fig. 8-2), this erroneous diagnosis may appear confirmed. Cardiovascular abnormalities other than sinus tachycardia are more common after age 40; paroxysmal or sustained atrial fibrillation is the dominant arrhythmia and may occasionally be the sole clinical sign. Resistance to the action of digitalis is in part due to an increased rate of digitalis degradation. Whether hyperthyroidism can be the sole cause of heart disease has been the subject of a long-standing controversy. Favoring the concept are several published series on patients who had no other intrinsic cardiac pathology to account for cardiac hypertrophy, heart failure, or arrhythmia. Notwithstanding, a careful search for underlying organic heart pathology should be made. The electrocardiogram often displays tachycardia, prolonged P-R interval, various non-specific ST-T wave abnormalities with T terminal inversion, shortened Q-T interval, and premature atrial contractions. Myocardial infarction is rare.

WEIGHT LOSS. Most hyperthyroid patients lose weight despite an excellent appetite and an increased caloric intake. Anorexia

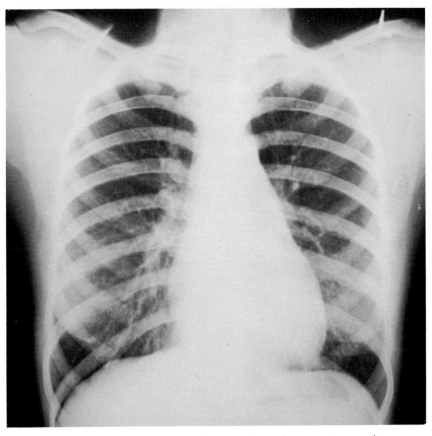

Fig. 8-2. Cardiac silhouette in Graves' disease. Note the prominent pulmonary conus resembling mitral stenosis.

is more common in the aged. The decline in weight is rarely major unless the disease has been neglected. Occasionally the caloric intake exceeds caloric expenditure, resulting in weight gain. One may suspect underlying hyperthyroidism in the cardiac patient who loses an inordinate amount of weight during diuresis or the obese subject who seems to lose weight without effort on a dietary program.

FATIGUE AND WEAKNESS. Early in thyrotoxicosis there may be increased energy and lessened fatigue, but most patients report that they tire more readily. Weakness of the quadriceps muscles on step climbing is a common symptom. Lahey, 1926, described a quadriceps test to demonstrate muscle weakness. The normal subject can hold a leg in a forward horizontal position while seated in a chair for more than 60 seconds, whereas the hyperthyroid subject can maintain this position for only up to 25 seconds. Recognizable muscle atrophy is unusual. Grip strength and trunk power were measured with hand and back dynamometers in 240 hyperthyroid patients (Satoyoshi et al., 1963). In 61% moderate or severe weakness was found particularly in patients over 40 years of age. Some reduction of muscle mass was common, but significant proximal atrophy was found in only 7%. However, muscle wasting was noticeable in 28% of patients in whom the disease had been present for over 3 years.

Goiter. If the thyroid gland is not palpably enlarged, the diagnosis is in doubt. Occasionally because of obesity or rigid hypertrophied neck muscles, the gland may be hidden. A deeply placed, partly substernal gland may elude the examiner's fingers but can be discovered by RAI scanning. Thyroid enlargement may be confined to one or more nodules. The gland has a characteristic rubbery firmness. A pathognomonic sign is the *bruit,* a whirring systolic or to-and-fro murmur best appreciated with the bell of the stethoscope applied to each lateral lobe successively with the head turned to the opposite side. Experience is necessary to differentiate the bruit from the audible pulsation of the carotids. A bruit is rarely heard even in large goiters in the absence of hyperthyroidism and is not found in the toxic nodular goiter.

OPHTHALMOPATHY. The term "ophthalmopathy" refers to all of the eye disorders of Graves' disease. *Exophthalmos* refers to forward displacement (proptosis) of the globe, often associated with certain pathologic changes of the oculomotor muscles and the orbital tissues. Readings with the exophthalmometer usually exceed 18 to 20 mm., but lower readings may be found in patients with distressing symptoms. Two clinical varieties are recognized (Werner, 1961): (1) the *benign* (noninfiltrative) form (Fig. 8-3, *A* to *D*), which probably corresponds to Mulvaney's "thyrotoxic" form (Mulvaney, 1944), usually accompanies hyperthyroidism and consists of a stare with infrequent blinking (Stellwag's sign), widened palpebral fissures (Dalrymple's sign), lid lag (von Graefe's sign), lag of the globe on upward gaze, and upward gaze without wrinkling of the forehead (Joffroy's sign). There may also be weakness of convergence (Möbius' sign) and proptosis of the globe (exophthalmos). (2) The *severe* infiltrative form (Fig. 8-3, *E* to *G*), corresponding to Mulvaney's "thyrotrophic" type, is associated with proptosis of the globe, which of itself may be no more advanced than in the benign form. However, serious infiltrative changes accompany the exophthalmos and may threaten vision. There is an increase in retro-orbital fat, fluid, mucopolysaccharides, and fibrous tissue. The extraocular muscles are hypertrophic, hypotonic, and infiltrated with lymphocytes and mucopolysaccharides. Fibrosis eventually replaces degenerated muscle. The total orbital contents and pressure are increased, exerting a forward thrust upon a globe that is inadequately anchored by weakened extraocular muscles. In time, excess retro-orbital fibrosis prevents the globe from returning solidly into the orbit. The prominence of

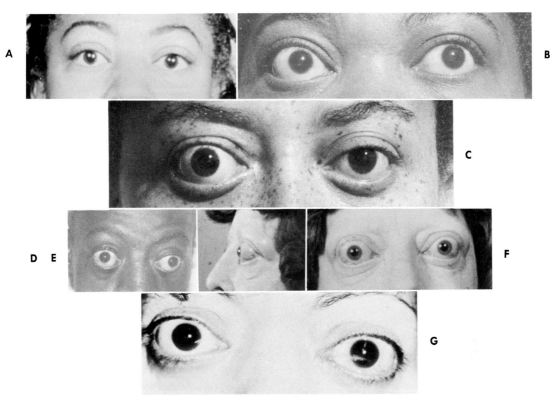

Fig. 8-3. Ophthalmopathy in Graves' disease. **A,** Minimal retraction of lower lids, no exophthalmos. **B,** Lid retraction with mild exophthalmos (18 to 19 mm.). **C,** Asymmetrical exophthalmos (O.D. 24 mm., O.S. 18 mm.). **D,** Ophthalmoplegia (partial paralysis, left lateral gaze, O.D.). **E** and **F,** Infiltrative ophthalmopathy with severe exophthalmos. **G,** Residual corneal scar in left eye after unilateral malignant exophthalmos.

the eyes may be asymmetrical. There may be periorbital edema with extrusion of orbital fat, conjunctivitis with edema of the ocular conjunctiva (chemosis), excessive lacrimation, decreased resiliency of the eyeball, and lagophthalmos. Diplopia may be severe, and there may be other oculomotor weaknesses (ophthalmoplegia). The patient complains of excessive eye fatigue, pain, tearing, and irritation, occasionally photophobia, and reduced visual acuity. Vision may be reduced or lost from optic neuritis, retinal hemorrhage, or corneal ulceration and its sequelae. The severe form bears no relationship to the severity of the hyperthyroidism and, indeed, is often found in milder or "masked" thyrotoxicosis or may appear after hyperthyroidism is cured, in euthyroid subjects, or even with myxedema.

Most of the phenomena of the benign form are caused by lid retraction because of heightened sympathetic stimuli upon the levator palpebrae superioris (Müller's muscle), which can be alleviated by the instillation of guanethidine eye drops and by control of thyrotoxicosis. Lid lag may occasionally persist. Lid retraction can usually be distinguished from exophthalmos by careful examination and by observing that the sclera is exposed above the cornea, whereas in exophthalmos it is exposed above and below. If one places the examining finger vertically over the eye from the supraorbital to the infraorbital ridge, one can just touch the globe, but in exophthalmos the globe will protrude and prevent this maneuver. The most objective measure of exophthalmos is by means of an exophthalmometer. Serial observations will detect improvement or worsening of the proptosis. A causal relationship between LATS, EPS, and ophthalmopathy is still conjectural.

GASTROINTESTINAL PHENOMENA. Exaggerated peristalsis and smooth muscle tone stimulate hyperdefecation. Occasionally there is watery diarrhea. Hyperperistalsis may be so intense as to cause abdominal pain, which may rarely simulate peptic ulcer, biliary colic, pancreatitis, or appendicitis. Nausea and vomiting was the sole symptom of Graves' disease in one of my patients. Slight polyuria and dry mouth with thirst may lead to a suspicion of diabetes mellitus, and this may appear to be confirmed by the diabetogenic effects of hyperthyroxinemia. Indigestion may be a consequence of gastric anacidity particularly in older patients.

MENSTRUATION. More than half of all women with Graves' disease experience hypomenorrhea, though the menstrual cycle usually remains regular. Amenorrhea is less common. There is a direct relationship between the decrease in flow and the severity of hyperthyroidism. Amenorrhea is more common in severely toxic patients and occurs usually when exophthalmos is present. Successful treatment relieves the menstrual disorder promptly. Infertility is common, but full-term pregnancy is compatible with untreated hyperthyroidism. There is a greater incidence of stillbirth and abortion.

Unusual clinical phenomena

ONYCHOLYSIS (PLUMMER'S NAILS, "UNDERMINED NAILS"). Separation of the distal fingernail from its bed converts the normal convexity of the nail-bed junction to a concavity, a condition that permits dirt to accumulate deeply under the nail in a concave line (Fig. 8-4). The fingernails are often soft and friable and may show fine prominent linear striations. Though not absolutely pathognomonic of Graves' disease, its presence is an important diagnostic clue. It has been described after local nail trauma and in syphilis, hypothyroidism, and chronic arthritis, and in fur workers but apparently does not occur in toxic adenomatous goiter. Onycholysis regresses when Graves' disease is controlled.

PRETIBIAL ("LOCALIZED," "CIRCUMSCRIBED") MYXEDEMA. There are small, brownish or violaceous, plaquelike, rubbery-firm swel-

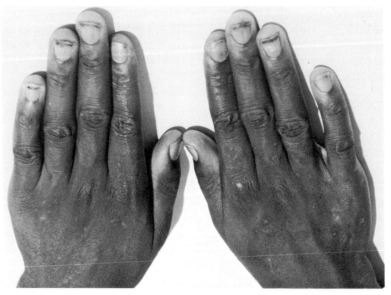

Fig. 8-4. Onycholysis in Graves' disease. The fifth finger of the left hand shows the typical reversal of the normal distal convexity.

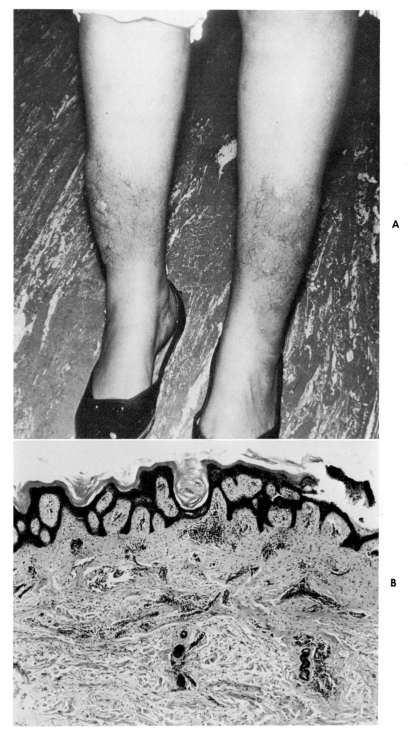

Fig. 8-5. Pretibial myxedema. **A,** The small keloid on the right leg is the site of a biopsy. **B,** The histologic section shows hyperkeratosis and moderate acanthosis. Deposits of mucopolysaccharide separate the collagen bundles and appear as the darker gray areas in the corium. The deeper layers show edema.

lings of the skin and subcutaneous tissues that symmetrically involve the pretibial area of both lower legs (Fig. 8-5) and/ or the dorsum of the feet, but they may be multilateral or asymmetrical, may rarely surround the leg or spread to the thigh, or may even appear on the hands or scalp. The lesions are painless, do not pit, heal after biopsy or trauma, albeit sometimes with keloid formation (Fig. 8-5), and are usually no more than a cosmetic inconvenience. Rarely they may become extensive enough to resemble elephantiasis. Infiltrative ophthalmopathy is a constant associated finding. The microscopic appearance (Fig. 8-5) resembles myxedema, and chemical analysis shows a high content of hyaluronic acid and other mucopolysaccharides. It is pathognomonic of Graves' disease but usually is manifest after active hyperthyroidism has been controlled with treatment. The cause is unknown. LATS was present in the plasma of each of 7 patients studied by Kriss et al., 1964, and they suggested that the lesions represented a local inflammatory response to some local antigen, with LATS as the antibody. They later reported that topical application of 0.2% fluocinolone acetonide under an occlusive dressing induced regressions and suppressed LATS formation in each of 11 patients. There is, however, a high incidence of spontaneous regression. Many other therapeutic modalities (applied locally or generally) have been explored, including thyroid hormones, TSH, ACTH, other corticosteroids, and hyaluronidase.

SPLENOMEGALY. Splenomegaly, as well as generalized lymphadenopathy, has been encountered in a small percentage of patients.

GYNECOMASTIA. Gynecomastia is an unusual finding in hyperthyroid males; the breasts usually regress after the patient becomes euthyroid.

ACROPACHY. Clubbing of the fingers and

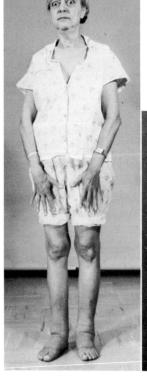
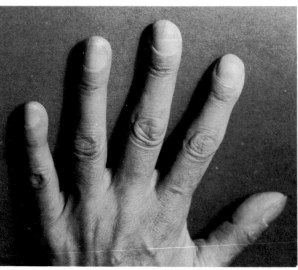

Fig. 8-6. Acropachy, with localized myxedema of the lower legs, ankles, and dorsum of the feet, and infiltrative ophthalmopathy in a patient with Graves' disease. (Courtesy Drs. K. and G. Chalal, Philadelphia, Pa.).

swelling of the soft tissues of the fingers and dorsum of the hands with diaphysial periosteal new bone proliferation is a rare accompaniment of past or present Graves' disease (Fig. 8-6). It is more prevalent in males and is usually associated with localized myxedema and exophthalmos. Acropachy is usually the last of the three to appear and may indeed develop years later.

OSTEOPOROSIS. Overt osteoporosis is rarely encountered. Occasionally, particularly in postmenopausal females, it is the principal manifestation and can be associated with vertebral compression or other fractures. In children there may be accelerated linear bone growth and epiphysial maturation.

CENTRAL NERVOUS SYSTEM. Psychosis is a rare complication. Encephalopathy with coma, hemiparesis, or bulbar palsy may mask underlying thyrotoxicosis; rarely there are epileptiform seizures. A high incidence of EEG abnormalities has been found, especially in young women.

MYOPATHY. Hyperthyroidism may be overlooked when dramatic muscle atrophy and weakness, particularly involving large muscle groups and the pelvic and shoulder girdles, interfere with motor function and, in extreme examples, invalid the patient. Myopathy is more common in older patients and in long-standing hyperthyroidism. Occasionally severe weakness develops in a few days, and deaths, probably from respiratory failure, have been reported. Apathetic hyperthyroidism may coexist. The disease must be differentiated from progressive muscular atrophy and myasthenia gravis. Successful amelioration of hyperthyroidism results in complete regression of the myopathy.

PEDAL EDEMA. Mild edema of the lower extremities without kidney, heart, liver, or severe nutritional disease may be a presenting symptom.

Clinical course of hyperthyroidism. One can become familiar with the natural history of Graves' disease today only by consulting Sattler's *Basedow's Disease,* pub-

lished in 1909, long before the modern era of early diagnosis and treatment. The disorder is usually chronic but may be subject to cyclic waxing and waning of considerable degree so that shorter or longer periods of comparative well-being alternate with those of more or less severe illness. The most extreme type of exacerbation is crisis. Occasionally hyperthyroidism is short lived and permanently remits after a few months; in such instances toxicity is minimal. In long-standing cases a state of thyroid exhaustion was described in the older literature when the disease had "burned itself out" and sometimes ended in myxedema. One may rarely observe an acute form often following an emotional shock and not infrequently exhibiting a self-limited course. Though the modern clinician tends to view hyperthyroidism as a benign disease, Sattler found a mortality rate of 11%.

Laboratory findings

For a discussion of thyroid laboratory tests see p. 100. Tests are grouped according to the particular conditions pertinent to the case.

1. Routine studies

PBI. Usually the PBI is above 7.5 or 8 μg./100 ml. but may fall within the normal range in 2% to 12% of cases. High normal values or minimal elevations are often found in toxic nodular goiter. Values above 18 μg./100 ml. are unusual and suggest iodine contamination.

RAIU. In hyperthyroidism the 2-hour uptake is 15% or greater, and the 24-hour uptake is 50% or greater. In 95% of cases it will be above 35% in 24 hours and in 82% above 50%. In toxic nodular goiter (hot nodule) the RAIU is frequently normal. The numerous factors that may vitiate the RAIU are discussed in Chapter 6.

T_3-RESIN TEST. Values above 18% (erythrocyte test) or above 35% (resin test) or above 130% by the pooled serum method are found in most cases. The test is not vitiated by iodine.

SCINTISCAN. Thyroid scanning is essential

in nodular goiter in order to reveal a toxic adenoma (hot nodule) (Figs. 7-3, 7-4, and 7-5).

2. Studies of value when PBI and RAIU are rendered invalid by prior iodine (T$_3$-resin belongs in both 1 and 2)

BEI. In hyperthyroidism values are above 6.4 µg./100 ml. The BEI is not vitiated by inorganic iodide but *is* by organic iodide (x-ray dyes, etc.). See p. 102.

SERUM THYROXINE. When done by column chromatography, values are similar to the BEI. Normal values by competitive protein-binding analysis (Murphy and Pattee, 1968) range from 4 to 11 µg./100 ml. Ninety-five percent of hyperthyroid values are above 10.8 µg./ml. (See p. 103.) Determination of serum thyroxine is rapidly supplanting the PBI in many laboratories.

BMR. Values above 10% are found in more than 95% of hyperthyroid patients.

CIRCULATION TIME. Values below 10 seconds arm-to-tongue are typical of hyperthyroidism. See p. 112.

3. Studies used when RAIU is equivocally elevated and in other diagnostic problems

T$_3$-SUPPRESSION TEST. Significant suppression (that is, below 10% RAIU or a 50% reduction from the baseline) is almost invariably found in Graves' disease. (See p. 108.)

CONVERSION RATIO. Values are above 50%. The plasma PB^{131}I at 72 hours is usually greater than 0.3%/L. (p. 107).

THYROID CLEARANCE. In hyperthyroidism, clearance is augmented 5 to 10 times the normal (20 ml./min.) and is usually above 3.5 L./hour.

FREE THYROXINE. The proportion of free T$_4$ is 0.104±0.026%, and the absolute value is 13.08±3.42 mµg./100 ml. in hyperthyroidism (Sterling and Brenner, 1966). The free thyroxine index is above 7.0.

ABSOLUTE IODINE UPTAKE (AIU). The AIU is above 6 µg./hr. in hyperthyroidism (see p. 108).

4. Other laboratory findings

BLOOD COUNT. Leukopenia (3,500 to 5,000), relative lymphocytosis and/or monocytosis is encountered frequently. Plasma volume is increased, and there may occasionally be a mild anemia.

ENZYMES DECREASED. Creatine kinase and lactic dehydrogenase are decreased.

LIVER FUNCTION TESTS. Various liver function tests have been found to be abnormal in 10% to 40% of cases.

SERUM PROTEINS. Albumin may be decreased, and gamma globulin may be increased.

SERUM CALCIUM. A mild but significant elevation has been found in the absence of hyperparathyroidism. Hyperphosphatemia is an occasional feature.

Differential diagnosis

In most patients the diagnosis is obvious, but occasionally one of the hypermetabolic states, previously shown in part 1 of the outline on p. 112, may be confused with hyperthyroidism.

Psychoneurosis with anxiety and tension. Patients having psychoneurosis may present clinical features that resemble hyperthyroidism such as hyperkinesis, sweating, tremulousness, stare, tachycardia, systolic hypertension, weight loss, weakness, and fatigue. Their symptoms are usually lifelong, whereas the hyperthyroid can assign a beginning, however vague. Of importance is the absence of ophthalmopathy, despite a slight stare, and the absence of bruit if there is thyroid enlargement. The neurotic patient is more likely to have gained than to have lost weight, and if weight loss obtains, it is usually attributable to anorexia. Excessive sweating is axillary and palmar rather than generalized. The hyperthyroid has a sweaty neck, an unusual finding in an anxious patient. The hands of the euthyroid, tense subject are cold and clammy, the feet are often cold, and he prefers a warm environment. The tremor of the tense individual tends to be coarse in contrast to the fine tremors of the hyperthyroid. The tachycardia is inconstant; the pulse exhibits greater lability and is normal during sleep or under sedation.

Menopause. Climacteric women may experience sweating, heat intolerance, insomnia, nervousness, tachycardia, systolic hypertension, and tremors and may resemble patients with thyrotoxicosis. The sweats are cyclic and generally follow a vasomotor flush. A trial of estrogen therapy will usually resolve the question in 2 or 3 weeks.

Heart disease. Hyperthyroidism should always be suspected in the cardiac patient with congestive failure who has lost weight, particularly if there is atrial fibrillation. Heart disease masking hyperthyroidism is not a rare phenomenon.

Thyrotoxicosis factitia. Excessive ingestion of thyroid hormone may reproduce all of the clinical phenomena of hyperthyroidism except goiter and exophthalmos. The diagnosis is ordinarily not suspected until one finds a high PBI with a low RAIU. If liothyronine is the culprit, the PBI will be low. When the patient is hospitalized, evidences of thyrotoxicosis subside unless there is access to the hormone.

Pheochromocytoma. Pheochromocytoma may rarely be confused with thyrotoxicosis because of sweating, tachycardia, tremor, weight loss, hyperglycemia, and an elevated BMR. Goiter and ophthalmopathy are absent, and the PBI and RAIU are normal. Occasionally there is mild thyroid hyperfunction because of the effects of the catecholamines.

Thyroiditis. Subacute (De Quervain's) thyroiditis may be mistaken for hyperthyroidism because of sweats, tachycardia, nervousness, enlarged thyroid, and occasional elevation of the PBI and BMR. However, the gland tends to be very tender and firm, and the RAIU is usually depressed.

Exophthalmos. Unilateral proptosis of the eyes is unusual in Graves' disease and should suggest an orbital tumor, infiltrative

Table 8-1. Distinctive features of Graves' disease and Plummer's disease

	Toxic diffuse goiter (Graves')	Toxic nodular goiter (Plummer's)
Age	Young—under 40 years	Over 40 years
Onset	More rapid, sometimes acute	Insidious, very slow
Goiter	Diffuse	Nodular
Bruit	Usually present	Usually absent
Clinical phenomena	Usually clear-cut	May be vague, masked; less tremor; apathetic
Thyroid crisis	Yes	Rare or never
Myopathy	May occur rarely	Never
Heart disease	Sinus tachycardia, occasionally atrial fibrillation	More common; thyrotoxic heart disease, arrhythmias, congestive failure
Exophthalmos	Common	Rare (or never)
Onycholysis, pretibial myxedema, acropachy	May occur rarely	Never
Response to iodine	Prompt	Poor, if at all
Laboratory	Usually diagnostic; RAIU usually elevated	Borderline, frequently equivocal; RAIU normal or elevated
LATS	Present in many cases	Absent
Response to antithyroid drug	Good; 54% "permanent" remission	Fair; 35% or less permanent remission
Surgery	Recurrence 2-15%	Recurrence rare

lesion, or intracranial tumor or aneurysm. Familial prominence of the eyes is not unusual in Negroes. Mild bilateral exophthalmos has been reported in acromegaly, Cushing's syndrome, and liver cirrhosis.

Miscellaneous. Hyperthyroidism is rarely, if ever, confused with certain hypermetabolic disorders such as malignancy, lymphoblastoma, polycythemia vera, leukemia, or tuberculosis. Certain features of diabetes mellitus such as weight loss, despite a good appetite, and polyuria may resemble hyperthyroidism, but laboratory studies should provide a clear-cut differentiation. Hyperthyroidism may sometimes coexist with acromegaly. Thyrotoxic myopathy may be confused with myasthenia gravis. Specific tests (using neostigmine) for the latter ordinarily are negative in hyperthyroidism, but occasionally the two disorders coexist. Periodic paralysis complicating hyperthyroidism has been reported, but differentiation from thyroid myopathy is not difficult.

In equivocal cases more prolonged observation of the patient together with repetition of key laboratory tests will usually establish the correct diagnosis. Delay in treatment is not critical. A therapeutic trial with an antithyroid compound may be valuable, but iodine is rarely employed today.

Toxic nodular goiter (Plummer's disease)

The distinctive features of toxic nodular goiter are outlined in Table 8-1. Signs of thyrotoxicity may be minimal, and unless the index of suspicion is high, the diagnosis will be missed. The shiny eye, alertness, loquaciousness, and slightly sticky skin may be all the clues offered. A poor response to digitalis and diuretics and perhaps excessive weight loss are sometimes the sole manifestations in a thyrocardiac. Borderline and equivocal laboratory values are frequent.

Treatment of hyperthyroidism

Criteria useful in selecting individual treatment are outlined below, but the choice depends to a large extent on the experience of the physician, local surgical skills and isotope facilities, and the convenience, comfort, and wishes of the patient.

1. Antithyroid drugs (long-term)
   a. Small diffuse goiter, recent onset, mild
   b. Children, adolescents, young adults*
   c. Pregnancy†
   d. Recurrent (mild) hyperthyroidism in young patients‡
   e. Small nodular goiters (occasionally)
2. Thyroidectomy
   a. Most nodular goiters (unless small)
   b. Plummer's disease‡
   c. Moderate-to-large goiters
   d. Most substernal goiters unless small
   e. Neck compression (dyspnea, dysphagia, aphonia, marked tracheal deviation and/or narrowing)
   f. Drug-sensitive young patients in group 1
   g. Suspicion of thyroid malignancy
   h. Recurrent hyperthyroidism after group 1 treatment in young patients
3. Radioactive iodine (RAI)
   a. Most patients with diffuse goiter from 30 to 40 years of age or older
   b. Thyrocardiacs
   c. Small nodular goiter from 30 to 40 years of age or older
   d. Drug-sensitive group 1 patients from 30 to 40 years of age or older
   e. Group 2 patients with contraindications for surgery or failure to control thyrotoxicity preoperatively with antithyroid drugs
   f. Recurrent or persistent hyperthyroidism from 30 to 40 years of age or older
   g. Young patients with reduced life expectancy

The intelligence and future cooperation of the patient and/or his family, particularly in the case of a child, represent important influences in making a choice.

Antithyroid drugs

Antithyroid drugs (Table 8-2) inhibit the synthesis of TH and, by increasing the excretion of iodide, may reduce the

---

*Some authorities favor thyroidectomy.
†Some authorities favor thyroidectomy in the first two trimesters.
‡RAI is preferred in many quarters.

Table 8-2. Antithyroid compounds for the treatment of hyperthyroidism (parent compounds shown at bottom)

Compound	Trade name	Chemical structure	Daily dose in mg. Initial	Daily dose in mg. Maintenance
6-n-Propyl-2-thiouracil*	Propylthiouracil Propacil Propycil Prothyran Procasil Propyl-thyracil (50 mg. tablets)	[ring structure: H–N–C=O, S=C, CH, N–H, $CH_2CH_2CH_3$]	200-400	50-150
1-Methyl-2-mercapto-imidazole* (methimazole)	Tapazole Mercazole Thiamazole (5 and 10 mg. tablets)	[ring structure: N–CH, HS–C, N–CH, CH_3]	20-60	10-20
6-Methyl-2-thiouracil*† (methylthiouracil)	Methiacil Muracil Thimecil Methicil (25 and 50 mg. tablets)	[ring structure: H–N–C=O, S=C, CH, N–H, CH_3]	300-600	100-200
1-Methyl-2-carbe-thoxythio-imidazole† (carbimazole)	Neo-mercazole (5 and 10 mg. tablets)	[ring structure: $COOC_2H_5$, N–CH, S=C, N–CH, CH_3]	20-60	10-20
Parent compounds		[Thiourea: $S=C$ with two NH_2; Thiouracil: ring structure H–N–C=O, S=C, CH, N–C, H H]		

Thiourea   Thiouracil

*Available in United States; only 6-propyl-2-thiouracil and methimazole have been included in the U.S.P. XVII.
†Popular in Great Britain.

quantity of this essential precursor for the production of thyroid hormones. They may induce an alteration in antibody formation, with resulting reduction in the synthesis of LATS or other inciting agents. The thyroid gland is not permanently damaged, so that the synthesis of hormone is resumed when the drug is omitted. Drugs can reliably maintain a euthyroid state for any prescribed period of time.

Potassium perchlorate causes gastrointestinal irritation and has induced agranulocytosis and fatal aplastic anemia. Propylthiouracil (PTU) and methimazole are popular in the United States; carbimazole is used principally in Great Britain. The choice of methimazole or PTU is largely one of habit and experience, since in proper dosage (Table 8-2) the antithyroid effects are similar, though on a weight basis methimazole has 10 or more times the effectiveness of PTU and appears to act more rapidly.

Long-term therapy. Individuals with mild Graves' disease of recent onset with a small diffuse goiter and young persons with recurrent hyperthyroidism are ideal subjects. I favor drug treatment for *children* and *adolescents*, but surgery has its proponents. The *pregnant hyperthyroid* can be safely carried to term, and after delivery the therapeutic regimen can be reevaluated. Long-term antithyroid drug therapy is reserved for the cooperative patient who understands the need for follow-up visits, the length of time the treatment is likely to require, the dangers of omitting medication, and the prognosis.

The usual initial daily dose of PTU is 300 to 400 mg., and methimazole 30 to 40 mg., but patients with mild toxicity may be started on 200 mg. of PTU or 20 mg. of methimazole, and patients with large or nodular goiter and very severe cases may require 600 mg. of PTU or 60 mg. of methimazole. The daily dosage is divided into three equal portions and given every 8 hours by mouth. There is no parenteral preparation because of poor solubility. Clinical response appears within 2 weeks, and a completely euthyroid state is achieved in 4 to 8 weeks in patients with mild toxicity and small goiters but may require several months in patients who are severely toxic. Improvement is delayed until stored hormone has been secreted and metabolized, and this process will require a longer time in patients with a large goiter. The preceding or concomitant use of iodine also favors hormone storage and may delay the clinical response. If the initial dose proves ineffective, a larger dose is used until control is achieved. Sometimes the dose need not be increased but merely subdivided and taken at more frequent intervals, that is, instead of 100 mg. of PTU every 8 hours, 50 mg. is given every 4 hours, with a final bedtime dose of 100 mg. In rare instances up to 1,200 mg. of PTU or 100 mg. of methimazole is required to control hyperthyroidism. If large doses induce hypothyroidism, the dose is reduced, or maintained and TH is added. The concomitant use of full dosage of an antithyroid drug with 120 to 180 mg. of desiccated thyroid is a logical and effective program to control thyrotoxicity and to prevent hypothyroidism and thyroid hyperplasia. Almost every patient will respond if therapy is continued for at least 4 months. Apparent refractoriness can ordinarily be attributed to abandoning treatment too quickly, or to prior iodine administration that may delay a therapeutic response for several weeks or to failure of the patient to take the drug as prescribed. True refractoriness to antithyroid therapy is extraordinarily rare. Since the thiourylenes themselves undergo metabolic change within the thyroid, an exaggeration of this phenomenon might so rapidly inactivate the drug as to interfere with the maintenance of effective concentrations. The patient is examined at 2-week intervals for the first 2 months and thereafter at longer intervals. He is instructed to omit medication and report to the physician in case of skin rash, sore throat, stomatitis, fever, or other untoward event. Frequent determinations of the white blood count are impractical because it fails to anticipate the onset of agranulocytosis, the most serious complication. Progress is judged by weight gain, slowing of the pulse, and recession of thyrotoxic symptoms. Although clinical appraisal is primary, repetition of the PBI or T_4 is a valuable criterion of the patient's progress. The PBI can be misleading occasionally, since it is only a measure of circulating hormone and does not necessarily reflect thyroid-secretion rates or the metabolic status.

Once the patient is euthyroid, the dose is reduced in increments of 50 to 100 mg. every 4 to 6 weeks for PTU, and 5 to 10 mg. for methimazole, until the maintenance dose has been determined (Table 8-2). One strives to find the minimum dosage consistent with complete control, since the incidence of toxic reactions tends to vary directly with the dose. If the dosage is reduced too quickly and hyperthyroid phenomena recur, it is raised again to the previously successful level. If the patient becomes hypothyroid, and this may be accompanied by further enlargement of the thyroid gland, the dosage may be reduced, or preferably maintained, but desiccated thyroid 60 to 120 mg. daily or more is added. By this means the underlying hyperthyroidism does not escape control, the goiter regresses, and hypothyroidism is relieved.

Duration of therapy. Duration of therapy has become established, more by custom than by objective criteria, as about 1 year after the attainment of a euthyroid state. Using Astwood's criterion, if a goiter shrinks appreciably in size, treatment can probably be terminated at that time. The ability to suppress RAIU with T_3 during therapy has been suggested as a guide to determine the optimum time to stop treatment and as a prognostic signpost. The assumption is that if the RAIU can be suppressed, Graves' disease has regressed and the patient will remain well.

What criteria will help us recognize the patient who will remain permanently euthyroid after termination of treatment? Astwood's group (Hershman et al., 1966) recently evaluated their results in 176 patients. The minimum period of observation for patients in remission was 6 years after the conclusion of treatment, and 95 (54%) remained well. In 75% the duration of remission was 10 to 20 years, and in 25% it was 6 to 9 years. Most recurrences (70%) were within the first year without treatment. Recurrences after 6 years of euthyroidism occurred in only 2.8%. A short duration of symptoms and reduction of the size of the goiter correlated well with a favorable outcome. Willcox, 1962, reported remissions in 72% of 152 patients followed for 1 to 12 years, half of whom were observed from 5 to 19 years. The marked differences in the reported rate of relapse by various workers may depend on the iodine intake. Alexander et al., 1965, found that if they added only 200 μg. of iodide per day following 18 months of antithyroid therapy, the relapse rate was doubled. The chances of permanent remission are less likely in the patient who is difficult to control and requires larger than average doses, or in the patient whose symptoms recur promptly with reduction of the dose. The incidence of "permanent" remission in patients with nodular goiter is 35% or less. Patients will omit medication as soon as they feel better unless the necessity for continuance has been carefully explained.

The therapeutic program should be reappraised if a patient relapses after a course of antithyroid therapy. One may attempt a second course, but the chances of a permanent cure are reduced. I have treated a number of these patients for periods of several years. Surgery has been rejected, and the patients were too young to receive RAI. Asper, 1960, has stated that "There may be some patients who can never be withdrawn from treatment without having a recurrence of hyperthyroidism." One of his patients who rejected thyroidectomy and RAI has been taking 100 mg. of PTU almost daily for 14 years. Prolonged therapy subjects the thyroid gland to unremitting TSH stimulation, which conceivably favors nodule formation and perhaps even carcinoma. After 1 year it is wise to add 120 to 180 mg. daily of desiccated thyroid so as to inhibit TSH.

Toxic reactions. The following are the toxic reactions to antithyroid drugs (the most prevalent are italicized):

Blood—*leukopenia*, agranulocytosis, aplastic anemia, acute thrombocytopenic purpura, hypoprothrombinemia
Skin—*urticaria, dermatitis, pruritus*, folliculitis, exfoliative dermatitis, subcutaneous nodules, loss of hair

Fever

Gastrointestinal tract—nausea, vomiting dyspepsia, diarrhea, stomatitis, loss of taste, toxic hepatitis, jaundice

Neurologic conditions—paresthesias, neuralgias, amnesia, confusional states

Musculoskeletal conditions—arthralgia, joint swelling, myalgia

Miscellaneous conditions—polyarteritis, conjunctivitis, lupuslike reaction, yellow discoloration of hair, nail changes, lymphadenopathy, serum-sickness syndrome

Toxic reactions occur in 2% to 5% of patients and are usually mild. Most reactions are of the hypersensitivity type that are dose related and appear early in the course of treatment. Some patients may exhibit intolerance rather than allergic hypersensitivity as manifested particularly by gastrointestinal symptoms. The most common reactions are mild macular or morbilliform rashes, with or without pruritus, or urticaria that subside when the drug is withdrawn or the dose reduced. If the blood count is normal, an antihistamine may be employed and the antithyroid drug continued cautiously or a different compound substituted. If the hyperthyroidism is mild, the drug is stopped and thyrotoxicity is controlled with reserpine and phenobarbital. When the reaction has subsided, a different antithyroid drug is cautiously tested in low dosage. If no reaction occurs within 2 to 3 days, the dose may be increased. More severe skin reactions may require corticosteroid therapy.

Agranulocytosis is an acute fulminating complication seen in 0.1% of cases, but mild leukopenia with relative lymphocytosis is characteristic of untreated hyperthyroidism and is not a contraindication to drug therapy. Agranulocytosis does not develop gradually as in drug-induced bone-marrow depression but is an explosive anaphylactoid reaction. Its onset signals the need for immediate withdrawal of the drug and hospitalization of the patient. Therapy is the same as for agranulocytosis from other causes. Though the mortality rate has been reported to be high, prompt recognition and early treatment will save most patients.

Among the reactions listed in the outline above, deaths have been rare. Fatalities have been reported from agranulocytosis and polyarteritis. Intrahepatic cholestatic jaundice subsides promptly when the drug is stopped.

Thyroidectomy

Surgery effects the most rapid cure but is associated with certain ineradicable complications (Table 8-3). In toxic nodular goiter surgical complications and postsurgical hypothyroidism are rare because a more conservative thyroidectomy suffices. The cosmetic effects of the operation cannot be ignored in a female patient, and a small incidence of keloid formation must be accepted. Latent parathyroid hypofunction with minimal or no symptoms has been demonstrated by using EDTA or sodium phytate. The effects of the loss of thyrocalcitonin upon fine calcium regulation remains to be investigated. The mortality rate in the past two decades approaches zero, the morbidity rate is low, and thyroid crisis is rare. Permanent cure is accomplished in 90% to 92% of adults and 85% of children in the most expert hands. The risk of postsurgical hypothyroidism is greater in patients whose sera

Table 8-3. Complications of thyroidectomy for hyperthyroidism*

Complication	Percent
Mortality	0 - 3.1
Hypothyroidism	4 -29.7
Recurrence or persistence	2 -17.9
Hypoparathyroidism	
Permanent	0 - 3.6
Transient	1.2- 8
Vocal cord paralysis	0 - 4.4
Vocal cord paresis	0.8- 5
Wound problems	4.0-15.5

*Based on data from Hershman, J. M.: Ann. Int. Med. 64:1306, 1966.

contain thyroid antibodies. The incidence of serious complications is undoubtedly less with other methods of therapy; nevertheless, in certain cases (see outline on p. 144) surgery is mandatory.

An antithyroid drug is given in full dosage (Table 8-2) until the day before surgery. The patient can usually be ambulatory and may even continue light or sedentary work unless he is very toxic. He is examined at 2- to 4-week intervals until he is euthyroid and has a normal PBI. A normal or subzero BMR is desirable before thyroidectomy. If there is any suspicion of hypothyroidism, it is preferable to prescribe TH rather than reduce the dose of the antithyroid drug and risk losing control of the hyperthyroidism. Any convenient date may be selected for the operation. Once the patient is euthyroid and the date of surgery is known, Lugol's solution (5% I_2 and 10% KI) or saturated potassium iodide solution is given in a dose of 0.3 ml. daily for another 2 to 3 weeks to ensure involution of the gland and reduction of its vascularity. The patient is then admitted to the hospital when he is ready for surgery. Preoperative preparation requires 1 to 3 months, occasionally less, not infrequently more. The physician in charge must not permit coercion from the patient or the surgeon to influence his judgment. There is no excuse today to permit an inadequately prepared patient to be hurried to surgery. A serum or plasma calcium and inorganic phosphate should be obtained to serve as a baseline in case of suspected postoperative hypocalcemia.

In severely toxic individuals, elderly patients, and those who have lost considerable weight—bed rest, sedation, attention to diet, and the use of vitamin supplements are of value. If a mild toxic reaction to the antithyroid drug occurs, an antihistamine may be added for a time or another antithyroid agent substituted. In patients intolerant to antithyroid drugs, preparation with iodide alone can be attempted as in the days before these drugs were available. If the trial of iodinization is unsuccessful, RAI treatment must be substituted. Preparation for surgery with corticosteroids and/or reserpine and guanethidine must be viewed as experimental.

Radioactive iodine

Radioactive iodine (RAI) is the most popular therapy in adults from 30 to 40 years of age or older because it is inexpensive, simple, convenient, and effective. There are none of the surgical complications and only rare recurrences. Admission to the hospital is usually unnecessary. The chief disadvantages are the delay in achieving a cure and the high incidence of posttherapy myxedema. RAI, traversing the same biosynthetic pathway as iodine (^{127}I), is deposited in the follicular colloid where it precisely bombards the adjacent epithelium with beta radiation as the isotope disintegrates. Since its penetration is only 2 mm., it exerts no appreciable effect on extrathyroidal tissue but causes inflammatory destruction of acini, which are then replaced by fibrous healing. Selection of patients is outlined on p. 144. Despite its widespread use, not a single case of thyroid cancer from previous RAI administration has been reported in an adult, but there have been two malignancies among approximately 120 children who had been treated before they were 18 years of age. Most thyroidologists prefer not to treat young people with RAI, whereas others have elected to treat any patient over age 20. Though a number of cases of leukemia have been reported, a recent survey (Saenger et al., 1968) showed the incidence to be no higher than in patients treated surgically. However, the observed mortality from leukemia for hyperthyroid patients was 50% higher than that from leukemia for the United States population, suggesting an association between hyperthyroidism and leukemia. The possibility of activating acute leukemia in susceptible subjects has been voiced. The finding of persistent chromosomal aberrations in peripheral leukocytes of RAI-treated patients lends further support to a conservative approach in the young. Pregnancy, lactation, and the possibility of thyroid malignancy are absolute contraindications. RAI traverses the placenta and may damage the fetal thyroid when it commences to function at 12 to 14 weeks; so one must be certain that a woman about to receive RAI is not pregnant. Since RAI is secreted into the mother's milk, a nursing infant must be weaned prior to treatment of the mother. There is no proof of genetic damage from thyroid or gonadal irradiation, but theoretical implications suggest that the possibility cannot be completely discounted. Progeny of females treated with RAI have been normal.

Methods of therapy with RAI. The major obstacle is the difficulty in choosing a therapy dose with a predictable effect. The response of patients with similar thyrotoxic syndromes to identical doses of RAI may vary considerably so that one individual remains toxic and requires a second treatment and another becomes hypothyroid. Various dosimetry regimens have been advocated:

1. Calculated from formulas that take into account gland size, thyroid uptake of a tracer dose, and effective half-life and aim to deliver 6,000 to 10,000 rads or approximately 150 μCi. /gram; Quimby's (1962) formula is an example:

$$\text{Average dose} = \frac{\mu\text{Ci. administered}}{\text{Weight of thyroid in grams}} \times$$

$$\frac{\%\ \text{retained}}{100} \times \frac{\text{Effective}}{\text{half-life}} \times 15, \text{ in rads}$$

A large error can be introduced by palpatory estimation of thyroid weight.

2. Arbitrarily determined dose varying from 3 to 15 mCi., depending on some of the factors in 1.

3. Fixed dose to all patients (approximately 3 to 4 mCi.) with repeated doses as required.

4. Large dose sufficient to produce hypothyroidism followed by lifelong therapy with thyroid hormone.

The dose tends to be proportional to the size of the gland and to the severity of thyrotoxicity. Larger doses are required for nodular goiters, for older patients, and for those who have received previous RAI.

RAI is given orally in capsule form washed down with water or dissolved in water, and given either in the fasting state or after a light breakfast. Antithyroid medication must be omitted for 3 to 5 days before treatment. In severely toxic older patients, particularly if heart disease is present, prior treatment with antithyroid drugs is recommended to render the patient euthyroid so as to obviate a post-irradiation exacerbation of thyrotoxicity. Prior iodine administration may control toxicity, but blocks the uptake of ^{131}I and thus delays treatment. This may be for a short interval because the thyrotoxic gland utilizes iodide rapidly. Immediate reactions (that is, within 10 days) are rare, but particularly when large doses are employed, sore throat and mild thyroid swelling with tenderness and/or radiation sickness may occur. Corticosteroid therapy relieves the symptoms from immediate reactions. In the case of a large goiter, tracheal compression can occur from thyroid swelling. Post-therapy exacerbation of hyperthyroidism, once feared, has been a rare occurrence but may add some risk in cardiac patients. The elevated PBI that is found after RAI therapy is largely the result of biologically inactive iodoproteins and intact thyroglobulin diffusing into the circulation, though rarely, active hormone is released. Hypoparathyroidism after RAI treatment is a rare curiosity, though evidences of transient disturbances in parathyroid function have been found. The earliest evidence of improvement is in 3 to 4 weeks, so that toxic patients need antithyroid drugs or reserpine to tide them over. If toxicity persists after 4 to 6 months, a second dose of RAI is given, but if it is mild, drug therapy is repeated for another 3- to 4-month course and then omitted to evaluate the response. Second doses of

RAI should be withheld as long as possible because additional improvement can occur throughout the first posttherapy year. It is desirable to attain a cure with the minimal radiation dose. A euthyroid state is observed in 2 to 4 months in diffuse toxic goiter and 4 to 6 months or longer with nodular goiter. About 60% to 85% of patients are cured by one dose; the remainder require one or more additional doses. Effectiveness is 99% if one continues to give successive doses until a permanent remission is achieved. Recurrence after a complete remission is unusual. The goiter regresses completely if it was originally small, and incompletely but significantly, if large. If regression results in a nodule coming into prominence, it should be viewed as a potentially malignant lesion and studied and treated appropriately.

Hypothyroidism after RAI therapy. The complication of hypothyroidism after RAI therapy has assumed major proportions in recent years. It is more common in patients with small diffuse goiters and in those who have had previous thyroid surgery and is rare after treatment of a nodular goiter. Cassidy and Astwood reviewed the literature up to 1959 and found an overall incidence of 12% in 4,468 total cases. With longer follow-up, myxedema has been reported in 26.5% in 7 years (Beling and Einhorn, 1961), 29 to 43% in 10 years (Green and Wilson, 1964; Dunn and Chapman, 1964), 50% in 14 years (Dunn and Chapman), and 51% up to 16 years (Nofal et al., 1966). A yearly increase of 2% to 3% has shown no tendency to level off after 15 years, so that the incidence of myxedema may theoretically reach 100% in time. The University of Michigan group (Nofal et al., 1966) treated 848 patients and estimated a 10-year posttherapy incidence of 70%. Hypothyroidism probably results from radiation-induced obliterative endarteritis and interference with DNA synthesis and with thyroid cellular division and replication, so that colonies of thyroid cells fail to reproduce over the years and thyroid-cell mass succumbs to a process of slow attrition. Transient hypothyroidism may occur in perhaps 5% to 10% of cases. It usually lasts several weeks, rarely many months, so that replacement therapy should be interrupted at least once in every patient to ascertain that it must be continued. Hypothyroidism appearing after 1 year is usually permanent. Myxedema during the first posttherapy year is rarely overlooked, but if the onset is delayed, the disorder may go undetected. *The need for prolonged observation must be explained to every patient who receives RAI therapy.*

Various measures are being explored to reduce the incidence of hypothyroidism. A large dose of RAI controls hyperthyroidism more rapidly than a small dose but is more likely to induce hypothyroidism. Smith and Wilson, 1967, halved the conventional dose of 7,000 rads to 3,500 rads and reduced the prevalence of hypothyroidism from 29% to 7% in 5 years. Hagen et al., 1967, reported that 6% of patients who received 80 μCi./gram ^{131}I became hypothyroid compared to 33% who had received 160 μCi./gram after an average follow-up of 19 months. The smaller dose delays cure of hyperthyroidism considerably and necessitates the use of an antithyroid drug during the uncontrolled interval, but the long-term percent of cures appears equal for the large dose and the small dose of RAI. Posttherapy myxedema is seen as well after surgery (28% in Nofal's report, 1966) and should not be marshaled as an argument for abandoning RAI therapy.

Thyroid physiology is often grossly distorted after RAI treatment. The thyroidal accumulation of RAI may be increased, leading to a false diagnosis of persistent or recurrent hyperthyroidism. This accumulation of RAI may be due to a reduced mass of tissue under increased TSH stimulation with a rapid turnover rate ("thyroid remnant") or to impaired organic binding of the trapped iodide.

Ancillary measures

Bed rest. Bed rest is required only for the very toxic patient or for the thyrocardiac, but remarkable benefits may accrue. The average patient can be ambulatory, though adequate rest periods should be advised.

Nutrition. Patients who have lost much weight should receive a high protein–high calorie diet and supplemental vitamins. Many patients, however, require no special dietary instruction.

Drugs. Sedatives may be of value, especially early in treatment. *Reserpine* depletes catecholamines both peripherally and centrally and exerts extrathyroidal peripheral effects that promote decreased sweating, nervousness and tremor, reduction of tachycardia, amelioration of atrial fibrillation, and reduction of systolic blood pressure and of the BMR. The oral dosage is 0.25 to 0.5 mg. every 6 to 8 hours. In severely toxic patients and in crisis, reserpine may be given I.M. with dramatic results. *Guanethidine* blocks the release of a hormonal transmitter from the postganglionic adrenergic nerves and induces catecholamine depletion but does not act upon the brain or adrenal medulla. Its effects are similar to those of reserpine when given in an average daily dose of 80 mg. It relieves eyelid retraction and may cause ptosis. Neither drug has shown any significant effect on thyroid-gland size, vascularity, RAIU, or PBI. Drugs causing catecholamine depletion should not be used for a week or more before surgery because of the danger of hypotension during anesthesia. *Propanolol,* a beta adrenergic blocker, is being studied for its ability to reduce tachycardia and increased cardiac output and to control atrial arrhythmias in hyperthyroid patients.

Iodine. Iodine exerts rapid but usually incomplete and transient control of Graves' disease. Its effects in nodular toxic goiter, in older patients, and in thyrocardiacs are minimal or nil. Prior to 1943 this was the standard method of preparing a patient for thyroidectomy, and occasionally under extraordinary circumstances it may still be used without antithyroid drugs. It had occasionally been employed in the treatment of mild hyperthyroidism, particularly in patients intolerant to antithyroid drugs, but the availability of reserpine, guanethidine, and corticosteroids has rendered iodide therapy, except as preparation for thyroidectomy, superfluous. Its use is not without danger, since it can cause aggravation of thyrotoxicosis. Iodine promotes involution of the hyperplastic gland, increases the quantity of stored hormone, and decreases the release of hormone.

Treatment of toxic nodular goiter

When a nodular goiter is large, and particularly if it produces neck compression or there is reason to suspect cancer, thyroidectomy is the treatment of choice. Nodular glands are less radiosensitive, tend to be larger than diffuse goiters, and often require repeated doses of RAI, but myxedema is not a common sequela. Controversy exists as to the wisdom of treating any but the very smallest nodular goiter with RAI. RAI scanning should be performed in all cases to detect the autonomously functioning adenoma (hot nodule). Since quite large doses of RAI are usually, though not invariably, required to ablate a hot nodule, partial thyroidectomy is carried out in patients under 40 years of age, whereas RAI ablation may be used in older patients. No one is yet certain that the removal of a hot nodule in a hyperthyroid patient negates the possibility of subsequent hyperfunction of the remaining thyroid tissue as part of an unsuspected diffuse process, so that simple enucleation of the nodule is not recommended. The probability of an autonomous ("hot") nodule in a euthyroid subject eventually producing hyperthyroidism is unknown. Thyrotoxicity seems to bear a direct relationship to the size of the nodule, so that growing nodules appear likely to eventually elaborate sufficient hormone to cause hyperthyroidism. Cancer occurring in a hot nodule is a rarity, but any nodule, regardless of its scanning characteristics, that presents hardness, rapid growth, or other signs of possible malignancy should be removed.

Treatment of thyroid heart disease

RAI is employed almost exclusively in thyroid heart disease unless there are specific reasons for surgery. Antithyroid drug therapy is given initially to control toxicity, followed, after a 3-day interruption, by RAI. One may tend to err on the side of overtreatment so as to achieve rapid control; in some patients slight hypothyroidism may be desirable. During the lag between commencing antithyroid therapy and amelioration of thyrotoxicosis, cardiac treatment is particularly important. Bed rest, sedation, and the use of diuretics provide considerable benefit. Resistance to digitalis is expected, but response is often achieved with large doses. Quinidine is usually ineffective in relieving atrial arrhythmias when the patient is hyperthyroid. Reserpine aids in controlling tachycardia and toxic manifestations and can therefore help to relieve the metabolic burden being imposed on the circulation. Propanolol is being investigated for its ability to relieve the hyperkinetic circulatory state of thyrotoxicosis.

Special problems in hyperthyroidism
Juvenile hyperthyroidism

The merits of surgical versus long-term antithyroid drug therapy have been debated for years. RAI is interdicted in children. Those favoring surgery point to the high incidence of relapse after drug treatment and the ultimate need for surgery. The medical proponents believe that a salvage rate of 50% is justification for avoiding the complications of surgery that might be more critical in the child than in the adult. Antithyroid drugs can be used initially and continued for 24 to 30 months. The dose of PTU is 120 to 175 mg./m.^{2} body surface (Means et al., 1963) or 6 to 7 mg./kg. body weight (Root et al., 1963) divided into three equal doses every 8 hours. Subsequent reductions are similar to those employed in adults. If relapse occurs after medication is stopped, a second course is recommended. If a second relapse occurs, surgery is advised.

Neonatal Graves' disease is a rare but fascinating example of the transference of a thyroid activator, LATS, from a thyrotoxic mother across the placental membrane to induce hyperthyroidism in the fetus. The neonate shows goiter, exophthalmos, and hyperthyroidism. Associated concomitants have been congestive heart failure, hepatosplenomegaly, thrombocytopenia, and jaundice. The disorder is self-limited, with regression to normal within 1 to 3 months, apparently correlating with the 6- to 7-day half-life of LATS in neonatal serum. The hyperthyroidism may, however, be due to maternal transfer of excessive TH rather than LATS, in which case the toxicity will regress more rapidly. Antithyroid drug therapy is employed until the disorder remits.

Pregnancy and hyperthyroidism

Certain symptoms that occur during normal pregnancy may resemble those of hyperthyroidism, such as dyspnea, palpitation, hyperhidrosis, heat intolerance, flushes, hyperorexia, polyuria, nervousness, and amenorrhea. The pregnant euthyroid patient may show goiter, tachycardia, increased pulse pressure, and warm skin. Laboratory values must be carefully interpreted, since most are elevated in normal pregnancy (p. 99). The early recognition of hyperthyroidism complicating pregnancy is mandatory because of an increased rate of spontaneous abortion, premature delivery, and stillbirth. Antithyroid drug therapy can be employed, provided that maternal hypothyroidism is avoided. Many authorities favor surgery during the first 6 months and antithyroid drugs, iodides or expectant therapy in the final trimester. To avoid fetal and neonatal complications, one can combine antithyroid drugs to control the hyperthyroidism with thyroid hormones to prevent maternal and fetal hypothyroidism. The following regimen is suggested: (1) PTU 100 mg. or methimazole 10 mg. every 8 hours (thrice daily) until thyrotoxicity is controlled; (2) add U.S.P. desiccated thyroid 120 to 180 mg. (2 to

3 grains) daily or its equivalent; (3) later taper the antithyroid drug gradually to a maintenance dosage of 50 to 150 mg. of PTU or 10 to 20 mg. of methimazole daily, combined with the TH throughout the the remainder of the pregnancy. The patient should be examined and the PBI, BEI, or T_4 measured every 4 to 6 weeks; the goal is to maintain the level within the normal range for pregnancy, that is, PBI 7 to 12 μg./100 ml. and occasionally much larger daily doses of thyroid than 180 mg. may be necessary. T_3 administration may be preferable to T_4 because of its ready diffusibility and can be given in doses of 50 to 100 μg. or more daily. It is essential to employ the smallest possible dose of the antithyroid drug compatible with adequate control; too large a dose is dangerous, but too little may engender the complications of hyperthyroidism and even, albeit rarely, neonatal thyrotoxicosis. After parturition the physician may elect to continue the medical regimen or substitute RAI or surgery. If the baby is nursed, antithyroid drugs and RAI are interdicted because these agents are transmitted in the milk.

For reviews of pregnancy and hyperthyroidism, see Herbst and Selenkow, 1965, and Werner, 1967.

Severe ocular changes and infiltrative ophthalmopathy

Treatment with TH, corticosteroids, ACTH, iodides, estrogens, reserpine, guanethidine, hypophysectomy or radiation destruction of the hypophysis or pituitary stalk section, x-ray irradiation of the orbits, or the retro-orbital injection of hyaluronidase have been advocated, but no standard therapy has emerged. Severe ophthalmopathy pursues a prolonged course characterized by an unpredictable and often stepwise increase, attainment of a plateau of indeterminate duration, and usually slow spontaneous remission. Fear of aggravation of the oculopathy by adequate control of hyperthyroidism because of a hypothetical increase of TSH is no longer voiced, and today it is considered mandatory to control

the hyperthyroidism. The severe eye changes exhibit an independent course, whereas the milder noninfiltrative form improves when hyperthyroidism regresses.

Rest, usually with long periods in bed, combined with sedation may be of benefit. Local measures to protect the cornea and globe, particularly when there is lagophthalmos, are necessary. These measures include tinted eyeglasses, perhaps with side-shields during the day and goggles at night, protective eye drops of a corticosteroid or 1% to 2% methylcellulose, and a lubricating ointment to the eyelids. Elevating the head of the bed 1 to 2 inches and the use of diuretics reduces edema. Guanethidine and reserpine are of doubtful value, though the instillation of 1 or 2 minims of a 5% solution of guanethidine has been suggested. Taping the eyelids closed at night is sometimes effective. Early tarsorrhaphy is a useful procedure. The sutured lateral eyelids can be parted when the ophthalmopathy improves. Prednisone in small doses in less advanced forms and in massive doses in severe ophthalmopathy may successfully halt rapid progression. Finally, when all measures have failed and the disorder is threatening loss of vision, surgical decompression of the orbit to provide space for the orbital contents to expand without forcing the globe farther out becomes necessary. Three methods are available: The transcranial Naffziger procedure unroofs the orbit and is advocated in the most serious cases. The simpler Krönlein-Moran operation, used in less serious cases, removes the lateral orbital wall and allows the globe to decompress into the zygomatic soft tissues. A transantral procedure removes the floor of the orbit and the ethmoid plates.

Thyroid crisis ("storm")

Thyroid crisis as a complication is rare; although prior to the use of antithyroid drug preparation for thyroidectomy, it was continually feared as an immediate postoperative catastrophe. Today thyroid crisis is most often encountered in previously undiagnosed hyperthyroidism and appears to be precipitated by infection, particularly pneumonia, or by other stressing events. McArthur's review, 1947, described 36 crises among 2,033 patients in 25 years and thus includes the preantithyroid drug era. The precipitating factor was thyroidectomy in 14, pneumonia in 7, iodine withdrawal in 4, postoperative hemorrhage and secondary suture in 3, wound sepsis in 2, and digitalis intoxication in 1. In all cases thyrotoxicosis was severe, the nutritional status was poor, and serious complicating diseases were frequent. Statistics concerning the prevalence of crisis differ because of varying diagnostic criteria, but any severe life-threatening fulminating exacerbation associated with marked tachycardia and fever may be defined as a crisis. Some authors confine the diagnosis to patients with fever over an arbitrary value (102° to 103° F.) and pulse rate above 140 beats per minute. The pathogenesis is poorly understood, but the disorder seems to be due to an excessive response to the sudden release of TH into the circulation. Whether there is a disproportionate ratio of T_3 to T_4 or an excessive catecholamine release has not been established.

The onset is acute, and clinical phenomena include high fever, marked tachycardia and/or atrial fibrillation, drenching sweats, extreme hyperkinesis verging on hysteria and delirium, marked tremor, vomiting, diarrhea, dehydration, and finally prostration, delirium, coma, and death. Psychosis, apathy, heart failure, jaundice, azotemia, and intercurrent infections may occur. The mortality rate, always high, has been reduced to 25% to 50%.

Treatment ideally is prophylactic. Thyroidectomy for hyperthyroidism should be reserved for the completely euthyroid patient. Treatment of crisis is heroic and tends to be "shotgun", with employment of all available antithyroid measures simultaneously, since there is no firmly established regimen. Treatment of thyroid crisis is as follows:

1. Bed rest; parenteral barbiturate or morphine Stat.; chlorpromazine has a hypothermic effect; isolation from external stimuli.
2. Reserpine 2 mg. Stat. I.M. or I.V., followed by 0.5 to 3 mg. every 6 hours; change to oral reserpine with improvement.
3. I.V. 5% glucose-saline solution containing 100 mg. hydrocortisone; requirements vary from 2,500 to over 5,000 ml./24 hours and 150 to 300 mg. hydrocortisone; add vitamin B-complex solutions to one infusion per day.
4. Lugol's solution (or saturated solution KI), 0.5 ml., added to I.V. infusion/24 hours.*
5. Methimazole, 30 mg. orally or by gastric tube every 6 hours.
6. Hypothermic measures: hypothermic blanket or ice bags, alcohol sponges.
7. Oxygen.
8. Digitalization for congestive heart failure, and atrial fibrillation; propanolol, 20 mg. t.i.d., for cardiac hyperirritability or marked tachycardia.
9. Antibiotics for intercurrent or precipitating infection.
10. Tube or oral feedings after acute emergency is controlled.
11. Plasmaphoresis for intractable cases (Ashkar, 1968).

Graves' disease without hyperthyroidism

Graves' disease without hyperthyroidism has been called the "ophthalmic form of Graves' disease" because the patient exhibits ophthalmopathy but lacks the clinical phenomena of hyperthyroidism. The disorder is being recognized more frequently, and though the true incidence is not known, the disorder was reported in 12 of 345 cases of Graves' disease (Hall et al., 1967). The ophthalmopathy is frequently asymmetrical so that a space-taking lesion in the orbit may be suspected. The PBI and RAIU are usually in the euthyroid range, but the RAIU is not suppressed by liothyronine administration. Hall et al., 1967, collected 54 patients from three other series plus their own; in 15 there was full suppression, and in 39, absent or partial suppression, so that normal suppression does not eliminate the diagnosis. Serum

---

*Some authorities believe that iodides are contraindicated.

assays for thyroid antibodies and LATS are frequently positive. The absence of hyperthyroidism has been attributed to a lack of thyroid reserve, so that the stimulation of LATS is ineffective (Liddle et al., 1965). This hypothesis is supported by evidence of Hashimoto's thyroiditis in 24 of 28 euthyroid patients with ophthalmic Graves' disease. Infiltrative ophthalmopathy may even rarely occur in hypothyroid patients with no prior history of hyperthyroidism (Fox and Schwartz, 1967). The proportion of patients who eventually become clinically hyperthyroid is unknown.

REFERENCES

Adams, D. D., and Purves, H. D.: Proc. Univ. Otago Med. School **34**:11, 1956.

Alexander, W. D., et al.: Lancet **2**:866, 1965.

Ashkar, F. S.: A.M.A. Clinical Convention, Dec. 4, 1968.

Asper, S. P.: Arch. Intern. Med. **106**:878, 1960.

Beling, U., and Einhorn, J.: Acta Radiol. **56**: 275, 1961.

Cassidy, C. E., and Astwood, E. G.: New Eng. J. Med. **261**:53, 1959.

Crile, G., and Schumacher, O. P.: Amer. J. Dis. Child. **110**:501, 1965.

Crooks, J., and Murray, I. P. C.: Scot. Med. J. **3**:120, 1958.

Dunn, J. T., and Chapman, E. M.: New Eng. J. Med. **271**:1037, 1964.

Fox, R. A., and Schwartz, T. B.: Ann. Int. Med. **67**:377, 1967.

*Gibson, J. G.: J. Psychosom. Res. **6**:93, 1962.

Green, M., and Wilson, G. M.: Brit. Med. J. **1**:1005, 1964.

Gunn, A., et al.: Lancet **2**:776, 1964.

Hagen, G. A., et al.: New Eng. J. Med. **277**: 559, 1967.

Hall, R., et al.: Ophthalmic Graves' disease. In Irvine, W. J., editor: Thyrotoxicosis, Baltimore, 1967, The Williams & Wilkins Co., p. 210.

Halliday, J. L.: Psychosom. Med. **7**:135, 1945.

Harris, G. W., and Woods, J. W.: Brit. Med. J. **2**:737, 1956.

*Herbst, A. L., and Selenkow, H. A.: New Eng. J. Med. **273**:627, 1965.

Hershman, J. M.: Ann. Intern. Med. **64**:1306, 1966.

Hershman, J. M., et al.: J. Clin. Endocr. **26**: 803, 1966.

Ingbar, S. H., et al.: J. Clin. Invest. **35**:714, 1956.

Iversen, K.: Amer. J. Med. Sci. **217**:121, 1949.

Kriss, J. P., et al.: J. Clin. Endocr. **24**:1005, 1964.

Lahey, S. C.: J.A.M.A. **87**:754, 1926.

Liddle, G. W., et al.: Amer. J. Med. **39**:845, 1965.

Logan, W. P. D., and Cushion, A. A.: Studies on medical and population subjects. In Morbidity statistics from general practice, vol. 1, London, 1958, H.M.S.O.

*McArthur, J. W., et al.: J.A.M.A. **134**:868, 1947.

McKenzie, J. M.: Studies in the production and mode of action of LATS. In Irvine, W. J., editor: Thyrotoxicosis, Baltimore, 1967, The Williams & Wilkins Co., p. 12.

*McKenzie, J. M.: Physiol. Rev. **48**:252, 1968.

Means, H. J., et al.: The thyroid and its diseases, ed. 3, New York, 1963, Blakiston Division, McGraw-Hill Book Co., pp. 184, 230, 247.

Mulvaney, J. H.: Amer. J. Ophthal. **27**:612, 693, 820, 1944.

Munro, D. S., et al.: Chemical structure of LATS and influence on thyroid function in thyrotoxicosis. In Irvine, W. J., editor: Thyrotoxicosis, Baltimore, 1967, The Williams & Wilkins Co., p. 1.

Murphy, B. E. P., and Pattee, C. J.: The measurement of thyroxine in blood. In Astwood, E. B., and Cassidy, C. E., editors: Clinical endocrinology, vol. 2, New York, 1968, Grune & Stratton, Inc., p. 296.

Nofal, N. M., et al.: J.A.M.A. **197**:605, 1966.

Odell, W. D., et al.: J. Clin. Endocr. **23**:658, 1963.

Overall, J. E., and Williams, C. M.: J.A.M.A. **183**:307, 1963.

Quimby, E. H.: Physical aspects of radioiodine use. In Werner, S. C., editor: The thyroid gland, ed. 2, New York, 1962, Paul B. Hoeber, Inc., Medical Book Department of Harper & Bros., p. 181.

Refetoff, S., et al.: J. Clin. Endocr. **27**:279, 1967.

Root, A. W., et al.: J. Pediat. **63**:402, 1963.

Saenger, E. L., et al.: J.A.M.A. **205**:855, 1968.

Satoyoshi, E., et al.: Neurology **13**:645, 1963.

*Sattler, H.: Basedow's disease, New York, 1952, Grune & Stratton, Inc. (translated by Marchand, G. W., and Marchand, J. F.).

Smith, R. N., and Wilson, G. M.: Brit. Med. J. **1**:129, 1967.

Sterling, K., and Brenner, M. A.: J. Clin. Invest. **45**:153, 1966.

Werner, S. C.: J.A.M.A. **177**:81, 1961.

*Werner, S. C., moderator: Panel discussion, J. Clin. Endocr. **27**:1637, 1967.

Wilensky, A. O.: Amer. J. Surg. **60**:221, 1943.

Willcox, P. H.: Postgrad. Med. J. **38**:275, 1962.

Williams, M. J.: Brit. Med. J. **1**:388, 1966.

*Significant reviews.

Chapter 9

Hypothyroidism

Hypothyroidism is the clinical expression of a deficiency of circulating thyroid hormone (TH). Myxedema is the most extreme variety.

Etiology

The causes of adult hypothyroidism are as follows*:

Deficiency of thyroid tissue
    Spontaneous "idiopathic" atrophy (43%)
    Destruction by thyroidectomy (8.7%), RAI (22%), or external x-ray irradiation
    Chronic thyroiditis (7.7%), Riedel's struma, subacute thyroiditis, "burned-out" Graves' disease
    Aberrant thyroid gland
    Agenesis of thyroid gland
    Infiltration by primary or metastatic cancer, granuloma, or chronic infection
Deficiency of hormone synthesis
    Hypopituitarism (4%) ⎫ Loss of pituitary
    Deficiency of TRF   ⎬   TSH
    Intrathyroidal enzymatic deficiencies—goitrous, nongoitrous, genetic
    Antithyroid agents (drugs, foods, iodides)
    Iatrogenic (after withdrawal of thyroid hormone therapy)
    Endemic and sporadic goiter

Deficiency of thyroid tissue

Spontaneous "idiopathic" atrophy, spontaneous idiopathic myxedema. The idiopathic variety is the most common, accounting for almost half of all cases. The cause remains obscure but may be related to Hashimoto's thyroiditis.

---

*Percent values in brackets are from Watanakunakorn, C., et al.: Arch. Int. Med. 116:183, 1965.

Destruction of thyroid parenchyma. Postsurgical hypothyroidism is proportional to the completeness of thyroidectomy and is more common in patients whose glands showed considerable lymphoid infiltration and who exhibited a significant titer of circulating thyroid antibodies particularly of the complement-fixing variety (C.F.T.). The widespread use of RAI in the treatment of hyperthyroidism is promoting an increased prevalence of hypothyroidism.

Chronic thyroiditis. Chronic thyroiditis (Hashimoto's and nonspecific varieties) accounts for a small proportion of cases. Current thinking, however, views "idiopathic myxedema" as the end stage of Hashimoto's lymphadenoid thyroiditis. Rarely Graves' disease with ophthalmopathy may occur in hypothyroid patients and is probably explained by the presence of Hashimoto's thyroiditis, which destroys sufficient thyroid tissue so that there is no target for a thyroid stimulator such as LATS. Hypothyroidism rarely follows subacute thyroiditis. "Burned-out" Graves' disease was often included as a cause in the early literature.

Agenesis, aberrant thyroid. See discussion of cretinism and juvenile hypothyroidism below.

Deficiency of hormone synthesis

Hypopituitarism. Hypopituitarism with loss of TSH and/or TRF accounts for less than 5% of cases.

Intrathyroidal enzymatic deficiencies. Intrathyroidal enzymatic deficiencies with

Table 9-1. Iatrogenic hypothyroidism (from withdrawal of thyroid hormone therapy)

M. B., female, 48 years old, self-medication with thyroid pills, 3 to 6 grains daily for 25 years, for a "low metabolism"

Date	Clinical status	RAIU 24 hours	PBI μg./100 ml.	Medication
4/25/57	Euthyroid	5%	6.2	Thyroid, 180 mg./day, discontinued 4/26/57
5/31/57	Hypothyroid (10 lb. weight gain, sluggish, sleepy)	—	3.1	None
6/14/57	Slight improvement	—	3.2	None
7/19/57	Euthyroid	—	5.0	None
9/ 3/57	Euthyroid; weight returned to original	26%	5.4	None
11/12/65	Euthyroid	—	5.7	None

defective hormonal synthesis is a rare cause of goitrous cretinism but may prove to be a factor in the causation of "simple" goiter. In areas of both endemic and sporadic goiter, decompensation may occur particularly in older individuals when the thyroid has attained its limits of compensatory hyperplasia and can no longer produce sufficient hormone from the scanty supply of iodine. About 15% of goitrous patients are hypothyroid (Cassidy et al., 1968).

Antithyroid agents. Various drugs or foods may interfere with TH synthesis and can lead to hypothyroidism in rare instances. They may aggravate some inherent defect in thyroid biosynthetic mechanisms. Iodide myxedema, an even rarer condition, encountered in patients subjected to prolonged iodide-containing medicaments, probably causes hypothyroidism by a similar mechanism.

Iatrogenic ("Farquharson effect") deficiency. Transient hypothyroidism may follow the withdrawal of thyroid therapy in euthyroid subjects (Table 9-1) until the suppressed endogenous TSH recovers and is able to stimulate the dormant thyroid gland.

Defect in peripheral utilization

A hypothetical mechanism and unlikely as an explanation for all but the rare case is a defect in peripheral utilization. Hutchison et al., 1957, described a case of sporadic cretinism that responded only to T_3 and not to desiccated thyroid. They suggested a peripheral defect in the utilization of T_4. De Groot et al., 1968, studied three siblings with an inherited resistance to the action of thyroid hormone as evidenced by clinical euthyroidism, deaf-mutism, delayed bone age, stippled epiphyses, goiter, and a PBI of 13 to 17 μg./100 ml.

Pathology

The pathologic findings are based on surprisingly few published autopsies, since the first report by Ord in 1878. The following discussion is based principally on the 9 cases described by Douglass and Jacobson, 1957.

Thyroid. The weight varied from 5 to 30

grams. It was replaced by dense, partly hyalinized fibrous tissue interspersed with a few focal accumulations of lymphocytes and plasma cells. There were residual foci of degenerated follicular epithelium with Hürthle-cell and squamous-cell metaplasia, often without lumens, and scanty, poorly staining colloid; occasional multinucleated giant cells were seen.

Anterior pituitary. A significant increase in TSH-secreting gamma cells and a decrease in alpha cells were reported by Ezrin et al., 1959.

Adrenal cortex. The adrenal cortex is often normal but lipid depletion and atrophy occasionally are seen. The coexistence of myxedema with Addison's disease (usually nontuberculous), called Schmidt's syndrome, may be an example of a multiple autoimmune endocrinopathy.

Testes. In 5 patients with prepuberal onset of thyroid failure there were various degrees of Leydig cell and tubular degeneration with basement-membrane thickening (de la Balze et al., 1962). In subjects with adult onset the alterations are less marked.

Brain. The brain is often edematous, with atrophic cortex and neuronal degeneration. The cerebellum may be enlarged, with degeneration and hemorrhage.

Peripheral nerves. The peripheral nerves undergo interstitial mucoid infiltration of the endoneurium and perineurium with fibrosis, metachromasia, and axon-cylinder and myelin-sheath degeneration (Nickel and Frame, 1963a).

Heart. There is hypertrophy, dilatation, and interstitial edema with mucinous material and fibrous tissue replacement. There is also swelling of muscle cells with loss of transverse striations, vacuolization, and basophilic degeneration.

Skeletal muscle. Skeletal muscle is edematous, pale, and flabby, with loss of striations. Myofibrils show sarcoplasmic degeneration; increased number of nuclei with prominent nucleoli and displacement to a central position within the fiber; basophilism of the sarcoplasm, endomysi-

um, and perimysium; interstitial-tissue edema, and mucoid degeneration and fibrosis (Nickel and Frame, 1963b). Similar changes are found in muscle of heart, esophagus, colon, gallbladder, urinary bladder, and uterus.

Arteries. Reports of coronary, cerebral, and/or aortic atherosclerosis are frequent, but the patients are usually elderly.

Intestinal tract. Muscle changes similar to those of skeletal muscle. Colon particularly shows accumulation of mast cells and mucoid substance.

Skin. Extracellular interfibrillar (connective tissue) accumulation of a metachromatic material quantitatively proportional to degree and duration of hypothyroidism and consisting of combinations of protein with mucopolysaccharides (hyaluronic acid, chondroitinsulfuric acid) (Gabrilove and Ludwig, 1957). Collagen fibers become loosened and fibrillar, and there is dermal edema, hyperkeratosis with plugging of hair follicles and sweat gland ducts, and atrophy of the epithelial layer.

Clinical features

The prevalence is unknown, but statistics based on hospital admissions probably underestimate the frequency, since most victims are treated as outpatients. In a geriatric unit, 1.7% of 3,417 new patients were hypothyroid (Lloyd and Goldberg, 1961). The majority are middle aged. The female to male ratio is from 4:1 to 8:1. A familial predisposition has been suspected. Genetic influences have been related principally to Hashimoto's thyroiditis.

Onset. Progress of hypothyroidism is so slow and insidious that the patient can rarely date even the approximate onset. Occasionally, after thyroid ablation by RAI or surgery, the disorder develops more rapidly and is recognized more promptly. The thyroxine decay curve, measured by the fall of the BMR after withdrawal of replacement therapy from a patient with myxedema, reaches its nadir in an average of 80 days.

The clinical features of myxedema will

be considered in detail. Milder states of hypothyroidism may elude recognition but should be suspected when any of the following conditions obtain: a history of previous RAI therapy or the presence of a thyroidectomy scar, chronic fatigue, muscle cramps, paresthesias, arthralgias, neuralgias, mild ataxia, unexplained weight gain, edema, somnolence, asthenia, cold sensitivity, hypothermia, dry skin and hair, hoarseness, constipation, vague indigestion, flatulence, resistant anemia, growth retardation, delayed puberty, menstrual disorders, infertility, and habitual abortion. Various combinations of these phenomena may exist for several years, with the eventual and gradual metamorphosis into full-blown myxedema.

Body build and habitus. The patient is typically short in stature, is stocky and sthenic without appearing obese, and has a short thick neck. A small goiter may be a sign of Hashimoto's thyroiditis. These phenomena almost suggest an increased susceptibility of a characteristic type of individual.

Facies. The face (Fig. 9-1) is waxy pale, albeit sometimes there is a malar flush, puffy with blepharoptotic eyelids, suborbital "bags," and an often translucent edema of the upper lids. Although the personality is often pleasant, the expression is dulled and heavy, sometimes apathetic. The features appear thickened, the lips puffy, and the tongue somewhat large. Occasionally the tongue may be greatly hypertrophied because of mucinous infiltration.

Voice. The voice is hoarse, leathery, croaking, or froglike. The speech is slow and deliberate, and the patient appears to enunciate with great effort; speech is thick and sometimes slurred. The vocal cords are thickened.

Skin. The skin is coarse, dry, doughy thick, scaly and flaky, cool, and often mottled and cyanotic. There is a faint yellowish pallor due to a combination of decreased

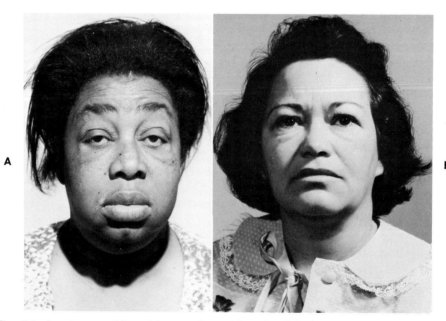

Fig. 9-1. Spontaneous idiopathic myxedema. Note the dulled expression, puffy face, and periorbital edema. Patient in **A** shows typical blepharoptosis. **A**, 46-year-old woman (PBI 0.8, cholesterol 424, RAIU 3%, TSH 2.5%). **B**, 43-year-old woman. Duration, 3 years (PBI 1.2, BEI 0.9, Hb 10.9 grams, RAIU 4.5%, TSH 4.1%).

dermal circulation, mild anemia, and carotenemia. Sweating and sebaceous and ceruminous secretions are diminished. The axillae are dry and odorless. Pruritus may lead to scratch dermatitis. There is slow healing of cuts and bruises. The knees and elbows become particularly coarsened and appear dirty. There may be pitting edema of the lower extremities.

Hair. The hair is coarse, dry, and brittle, ends break off easily, and scalp hair becomes thin. The growth rate is markedly retarded so that shaving and haircuts are less frequent. There is marked loss of axillary hair and thinning of pubic hair, and the eyebrows become sparse.

Nails. The rate of growth of nails is slowed, and the nails are thickened, brittle, and cracked.

Mucous membranes. The mucous membranes may appear pale, puffy, and somewhat dry.

Cardiovascular system. Typical findings include slow pulse, low blood pressure, cardiac enlargement, feeble pulsations by fluoroscopy, distant heart sounds, prolonged circulation time, and normal venous pressure. Perhaps one third of the patients have hypertension which sometimes regresses with thyroid therapy. The cardiac output, reduced because of diminished stroke volume, is usually proportional to the decreased O_2 consumption. Systemic peripheral resistance is increased. Exercise augments the cardiac output and decreases the systemic resistance in contradistinction to findings in congestive heart failure. The ECG changes are shown in Fig. 9-2. Pericardial effusion contributes to the physical signs, enlarged cardiac silhouette, and ECG alterations. In long-standing cases there may be exertional dyspnea and orthopnea, but this is more likely caused by increased pericardial effusion, often together with pleural effusions and ascites than by congestive heart failure. Serous cavity transudates are a result of increased capillary permeability, aggravated by reduced plasma albumin and increased mucoproteinaceous tissue content. True con-

gestive heart failure is rare and probably indicates associated cardiovascular pathology. Cardiac pain may be from effort angina and only rarely relieved by thyroid or may be a precordial ache unrelated to effort that regresses with thyroid therapy. Whether atherosclerosis is accelerated in myxedema is still controversial, but there is considerable evidence to the contrary. Coronary heart disease is increased in prevalence only in hypertensive patients.

Gastrointestinal tract. Complaints of distention, flatulence, constipation, and indigestion are related to reduced intestinal motility, slowed gastric emptying, and gall bladder hypotonicity. Rarely fecal impactions or paralytic ileus occurs. There is reduction of gastric acid, and this combined with some interference with the absorption of foodstuffs contributes to anorexia, fermentation, and borborygmus. Atrophy of the intestinal mucosa, mucinous and fatty infiltration of the peritoneum and intestinal wall, and dilatation and/or lengthening of the colon have been found at autopsy.

Nervous system. Slowed cerebration, poor memory, decreased emotional tone with mental torpor and complacency, drowsiness, and personality changes may be attributed to reduced cerebral blood flow, O_2 and glucose uptake, deficiency of cerebral enzyme systems, and possibly cerebral edema. The electroencephalogram shows low frequency and low voltage. Occasionally nervous hyperirritability and tension may mask the diagnosis of myxedema. Myxedema may be overlooked in an organic *psychosis* ("myxedema madness"), and the patient may be subjected to shock therapy or be incarcerated in a mental institution. A proportion of such patients can be rehabilitated with thyroid therapy. Signs of *cerebellar* involvement (ataxic gait, dysarthric speech, dysdiadochokinesis, and nystagmus) may be caused by myxedema.

Peripheral neuropathy is reflected by paresthesias, pain in the extremities, and burning of the hands and feet. The symp-

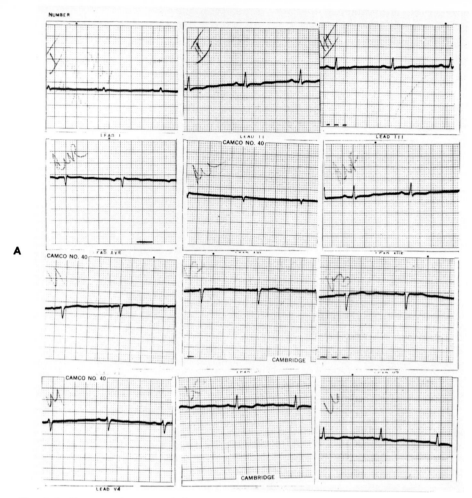

Fig. 9-2. Electrocardiogram of the patient shown in Fig. 9-1, *B*. The tracing in **A** shows typical bradycardia, low voltage, S-T segment flattened, and T waves inverted or of low amplitude. Tracing in **B** shows amelioration of the abnormal findings after thyroid therapy.

toms are usually out of proportion to any objective findings.

Deafness may be nerve and/or middle ear in origin; tinnitus may accompany the hearing loss. Myxedematous tissue under the transverse carpal ligament can cause a *"carpal-tunnel syndrome"* with distal sensory and motor disturbances that may be episodic, are frequently nocturnal, and are relieved by thyroid therapy.

Gonadal changes. Menstrual disturbances are frequent and are usually characterized by menorrhagia and metrorrhagia, a consequence of anovulation with

failure to elaborate LH. Occasionally severe vaginal hemorrhage may be the presenting complaint. A subnormal level of several coagulation factors was reported by Simone et al., 1965. Infertility, habitual abortion, and diminished libido are common. Instances of full-term pregnancy in untreated cases are sufficiently rare to be reported. The importance of mild, subclinical, or borderline hypothyroidism causing sterility and accidents of pregnancy has probably been overemphasized and empirically overtreated. In the male, diminution of libido, impotence, and vari-

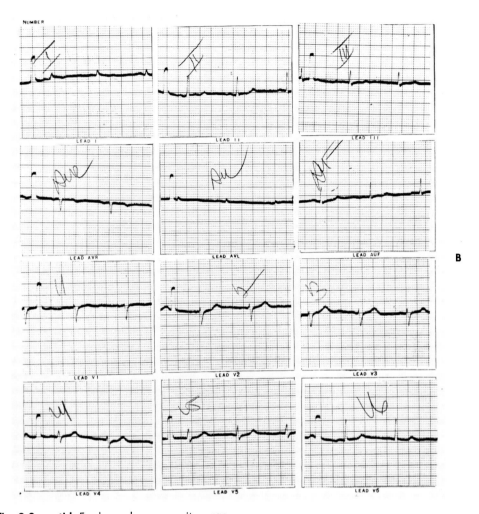

Fig. 9-2, cont'd. For legend see opposite page.

ous degrees of hypospermatogenesis are proportional to the severity of the myxedema.

Muscles. In severe myxedema there is muscle weakness, loss of tone, pain, and stiffness. Rarely there may be marked myotonia particularly affecting the shoulder and pelvic girdle. Transient local swelling of directly percussed or pinched muscles, called "myoedema" or "mounding phenomenon," is a neglected physical sign. Pseudomyotonic and muscle spasm reactions to muscular activity occur. Hypertrophic muscles that are firm and inelastic may involve the arms and legs and inhibit normal function (pseudomuscular hyper-

trophy, Hoffman's syndrome; in children it is known as the Kocher-Debré-Semelaigne syndrome). The electromyogram shows low voltage, short duration motor units, hyperirritability, repetitive discharge after reflex motion, and polyphasicity. The abnormality in the contractile mechanism is probably related to enzyme and electrolyte abnormalities, a decrease in number of cell mitochondria, and a decrease in uncoupling phosphorylation activity. Prolonged or "hung-up" (pseudomyotonic) deep-tendon reflexes are pathognomonic (p. 111), though they have been described in CNS syphilis and diabetes mellitus. When the Achilles tendon is sharply tapped, the relaxation phase of the reflex is prolonged; at times it can be demonstrated only with reinforcement. The foot extends quite promptly but then slowly drifts back to its resting position. Repetitive tapping of the tendon can convert a myxedema reflex to a normal pattern.

Clinical course

The patient experiences a general loss of his sense of well-being, a gradual slowing down of all physical and mental processes, and a torpor that may be brought to his attention by family or friends. Eventually he withdraws more and more from daily activities and begins to vegetate, to neglect personal hygiene, and to sleep a great deal. If the diagnosis is overlooked, treatment for edema, resistant anemia, stubborn constipation, nephritis, degenerative arthritis, "neuritis," deafness, or psychosis is carried on by a succession of physicians who may employ tonics, stimulants, diuretics, digitalis, vitamin B_{12}, iron, or antidepressant drugs, all to no avail. If serous effusions produce respiratory difficulties, the patient may be hospitalized, at which time the correct diagnosis is usually made. Unfortunate is the poor soul who lapses into coma and is treated as a case of cerebrovascular accident in an emergency ward. Death due to intercurrent infection may occur at any time. Spontaneous cure is rare but can occur. Transient hypothyroidism may follow RAI treatment for hyperthyroidism, and regression of myxedema will occur if an antithyroid compound or food that interfered with thyroid function is withdrawn. On the average the correct diagnosis is made about 5 years after the patient first consults a physician.

Laboratory diagnosis

PBI. Values of PBI are usually less than 3.5 μg./100 ml. and rarely exceed 4 μg./ml., unless there is iodine contamination or an abnormally elevated TBG. The BEI and serum T_4 are less than 3 μg./ml. Serum T_4 by competitive protein-binding analysis is below 4 μg./ml., and values less than 1.4 μg./ml. are invariably

diagnostic (Murphy and Pattee, 1968). The free thyroxine proportion (Sterling and Brenner, 1966) is 0.028±0.008%. The free thyroxine index is less than 2.

RAIU. The 24-hour uptake rarely exceeds 10% and is often less than 5%. Values up to 20% occasionally occur in pituitary myxedema. Normal, low, or even somewhat elevated values, despite definite hypothyroidism, are found in Hashimoto's thyroiditis.

TSH test. The TSH test serves to differentiate primary thyroid myxedema from pituitary myxedema (p. 50). When the diagnosis of hypothyroidism is questionable, lack of PBI and RAIU increase after TSH stimulation should establish its presence, whereas a significant response is indicative of a euthyroid state or pituitary hypothyroidism (Schneeberg et al., 1954). Failure to respond to TSH is also seen in states of "low thyroid reserve," in which a remnant of thyroid tissue, usually remaining after subtotal thyroidectomy or RAI therapy, is already under maximal endogenous TSH stimulation and cannot increase its function.

Serum cholesterol. Usually the value for serum cholesterol is above 300 mg./100 ml. but the very wide range of normal renders a single determination valuable only if greatly elevated. Normal values are more common in pituitary myxedema. Cholesterol ester, beta-lipoprotein, phospholipids, and total lipids are elevated.

BMR. Usually the BMR is below −15% and in severe cases below −35% to −40%. Any of the numerous extraneous factors that may elevate the BMR (see outline on p. 112), may produce a false normal value in myxedema.

T_3-resin test. Usually the value is low, but there is considerable overlap with euthyroid values. The T_3-RBC test is below 11%, and the T_3-resin test is below 23%. The pooled serum method is less than 0.8, or 80%, and the thyrobinding index is above 1.3.

Achilles reflex. Prolongation beyond 230 msec. occurs in clear-cut myxedema, but there is considerable overlap with normal subjects in milder states of thyroid deficiency.

Hematopoietic system. Anemia occurs in somewhat more than 50% of advanced cases and is usually normocytic and normochromic. Macrocytic anemia may occur, and the coexistence of primary pernicious anemia must be considered. The anemia may be due to the combined effects of reduced O_2 tension in bone marrow, diminished vitamin B_{12} absorption from gastric achlorhydria, and menorrhagia. The bone marrow is often hypocellular. Blood coagulation may be defective from a deficiency of factors VIII and IX.

Miscellaneous. The blood volume and hematocrit are reduced, whereas extracellular fluid is increased. There is low serum iron and decreased iron-binding capacity. An elevated uric acid and a rapid sedimentation rate are commonly found. Blood carotene is usually elevated. Total serum proteins, particularly the beta globulins, are commonly increased, whereas serum albumin and gamma globulins are decreased. There is an increased TBG-binding capacity. Spinal fluid proteins are often elevated. Serum creatine phosphokinase is high, normal creatinuria is lacking, and creatine tolerance is increased. Water diuresis after a fluid load is impaired. Urinary 17-KS and 17-OHCS are low. Values for serum inorganic phosphorus and alkaline phosphatase are likely to be reduced, particularly in children. Electrolyte values are normal in uncomplicated cases, though hyponatremia with inappropriate ADH secretion has been described. *Thyroid antibodies* are commonly found in high titer (p. 109) in primary thyroid failure, whereas they are absent in pituitary hypothyroidism. The ECG, previously discussed, may be classic, and occasionally the electrocardiographer is the first to suggest the diagnosis.

Differential diagnosis

The following patients may present problems in diagnosis.

Pallid, puffy facies. Severe anemia, the nephrotic syndrome, and Cushing's syndrome sometimes resemble myxedema. Nephrosis and myxedema may closely resemble each other, and the low BMR, hypercholesterolemia, and slightly low PBI in nephrosis may cause confusion. However, the nephrotic patient is more active and alert, the skin is not as dry, cool, or scaly, the voice is not hoarse, there is heavy proteinuria, and the RAIU is usually normal. In Cushing's syndrome the PBI and RAIU may be low, but the usual signs of the disorder predominate. In severe anemia the failure to respond to any therapy other than TH is diagnostic, but pernicious anemia and myxedema may occur in the same patient.

Neurasthenic female. Complaints of fatigue, lack of energy, mild depression, constipation, dry skin and hair, brittle nails, cold sensitivity, and weight gain are usually not accompanied by any physical findings indicative of hypothyroidism. Hypometabolism is frequent and must not be accepted as proof of thyroid failure without confirmatory evidence. The administration of TH may be followed by improvement, but it is rarely clear cut and, despite increasing doses, is quickly dissipated. The patient may become habituated to thyroid medication and is resistant to weaning.

Low thyroid tests. Not infrequently a patient with chronic fatigue is labeled hypothyroid on the basis of a single low PBI, BMR, RAI, or T_3 test. The possible effects of drugs mut be considered (for example, a low T_3 test from an oral contraceptive compound).

Old age. The general slowing down of metabolic processes in old age may induce a superficial resemblance to myxedema. It is important not to overlook hypothyroidism in the geriatric patient.

Therapeutic trial as a diagnostic aid

When the diagnosis remains in doubt despite careful study, a therapeutic trial may be helpful. To be completely objective, a placebo trial would be desirable but, in practice, is usually not conducted.

The patient with hypothyroidism shows unequivocal and maintained improvement, whereas the neurotic often reports an initial vague response that soon dissipates, and augmentation of the dose is then explored, possibly with a repetition of the cycle of improvement followed by recurrence. The neurotic may report a return of symptoms within 1 day of omitting thyroid medication, whereas the true hypothyroid will note symptoms of returning thyroid deficiency after an interval of 1 to 3 weeks.

Treatment

Replacement therapy with thyroid hormone must be maintained for the duration of the patient's life. Five compounds are currently available:

Thyroid hormone compounds

Thyroid U.S.P. (desiccated thyroid) is powdered, defatted, whole gland prepared from bovine and/or porcine thyroid and compressed into tablets. The U.S.P. XVII requires an iodine content of 0.17% to 0.23%, but most preparations contain more and are diluted with an inert powder. Porcine thyroid is biologically more active, has a greater total iodine content, a higher concentration of active iodothyronines and more T_3 than thyroid of beef origin. The T_3 and T_4 contents were 52% and 41% higher, respectively, and the molar ratio of T_4/T_3 was 2.96 for active porcine compared to 3.71 for active bovine desiccated thyroid (Kologlu et al., 1966). Despite variations in activity and chemical composition and the occasional finding of an inert preparation, dry desiccated thyroid exhibits great stability for long periods of time. It is available in the following doses: 15 mg. (¼ grain), 30 mg. (½ grain), 60 mg. (1 grain), 130 mg. (2 grains), and 180 mg. (3 grains).

Thyroglobulin (Proloid, Endothyrin) is described by Warner-Chilcott Laboratories as "purified thyroglobulin extracted from fresh animal thyroid glands." Its action is similar to equivalent amounts of desiccated thyroid; its T_4 content is the same, but it contains one third more T_3. It is available in the same doses as desiccated thyroid. Proloid also is offered in a 90 mg. (1½-grain) tablet and a 300 mg. (5-grain) tablet.

Sodium L-thyroxine (Synthroid, Levoid, Letter, Titroid, Thyroxin Fraction) is the synthetic crystalline monosodium salt of levothyroxine. Available in (1) tablets of 0.025, 0.05, 0.1, 0.15, 0.2, 0.3 mg., (2) 10 ml. vials containing 500 μg. of lyophilized active ingredient and 10 mg. of mannitol N.F. and a 5 ml. vial of sodium chloride diluent for injection.

Sodium D-thyroxine (Choloxin) is the synthetic crystalline monosodium salt of dextrothyroxine. Available in 2 and 4 mg. tablets. It is effective in the treatment of myxedema (Schneeberg, 1964).

L-Triiodothyronine, liothyronine sodium (Cytomel) is the sodium salt of L-triiodothyronine. Available as 5, 25, and 50 μg. tablets.

Approximate equimetabolic doses of these preparations are as follows:

Desiccated thyroid U.S.P.	60 mg. (1 grain)
Thyroglobulin	60 mg. (1 grain)
Sodium L-thyroxine	0.1 mg.
Sodium D-thyroxine	2.0 mg.
Liothyronine	0.050 mg. (50 μg.)

All five products have the same qualitative action when given in equivalent doses and will consistently relieve myxedema. Desiccated thyroid U.S.P. is the least expensive compound for long-term therapy and is usually reliable and quite uniform in its action. The cost of the product may be of prime importance to some patients. At the time of writing, the following comparison was made of the cost of 100 tablets:

	Wholesale	Approximate retail
Armour's thyroid U.S.P., 60 mg. (1 grain)	$0.53	$ 1.80
Proloid, 60 mg. (1 grain)	0.75	1.90
Synthroid, 0.1 mg.	1.27	2.60
Cytomel, 25 μg.	2.28	4.00
Choloxin, 2 mg.	—	15.00

Because various whole thyroid products differ in potency, it is well to employ thyroid prepared by a reliable pharmaceutical house and to use the same preparation in a given patient. One encounters an inactive product only rarely. Hardening of old tablets or wetting of tablets may also reduce physiologic activity. Most endocrinologists have encountered or heard of at least one patient who failed to respond to desiccated thyroid but was responsive to sodium L-thyroxine or liothyronine. Whether such cases represent a true end-organ resistance, failure of intestinal absorption, or the use of an inactive preparation is not clear.

Many authorities prefer to use sodium L-thyroxine because it is a pure synthetic product that requires no standardization to ensure uniformity. Since it lacks T_3, its onset of action may be somewhat slower than that of desiccated thyroid or thyroglobulin, and it may lack some subtle effects at present unknown. To better mimic the biologic characteristics of the natural product, a synthetic mixture of L-thyroxine and liothyronine has been marketed recently.*

Liothyronine (T_3) (p. 84) is the most rapidly acting of the thyroid hormones. Very little is bound to plasma protein, and it is rapidly diffusible into body tissues. Clinical and laboratory evidence of its action often becomes manifest in 12 to 24 hours, as compared to 3 to 7 days with other products. Its action is transient, however, so that omission of medication for a couple of days is followed by a more rapid recurrence of hypothyroidism than one observes after stopping desiccated thyroid or sodium L-thyroxine. Liothyronine may be preferable to initiate therapy in certain cases such as in myxedema coma, but it is not recommended for long-term administration. It is an excellent choice for a therapeutic trial because of its transient effect. It must be employed with particular caution in elderly patients and in those with heart disease because the rapid increase in metabolism may impose a burden on the cardiovascular system. Par-

*Euthroid, or Liotrix, from Warner-Chilcott Lab. and Thyrolar, from Armour Pharmaceutical Co.

enteral solutions of sodium L-thyroxine are available and can be prepared for liothyronine.

Method of treatment

The entire daily dose of the preparation selected may be taken at one time, since thyroxine action is slow in waxing and waning and has a carry-over of many days if medication is omitted. Such is not true for liothyronine, of which divided doses may be preferable. The initial dose and the speed of increasing the dose tend to vary inversely with the severity of thyroid deprivation and with the age of the patient. In advanced cases and particularly in older individuals and in those with complicating hypertension or coronary heart disease, one commences with 8 to 15 mg. daily (1/8 to 1/4 grain) of desiccated thyroid or its equivalent and increases the dose at intervals of 14 days in increments of 8 to 15 mg. Once the patient's metabolism has been appreciably increased, the extraordinary sensitivity of the thyroidless subject to thyroid medication is reduced, and the danger of serious toxic effects becomes less. In milder cases the initial daily dose is 15 to 30 mg. (1/4 to 1/2 grain) and is increased by 15 to 30 mg. every 10 to 14 days. The *maintenance dose* is the minimal effective amount that abolishes all clinical evidences of myxedema. It is also desirable, though not essential, to restore abnormal laboratory values to the euthyroid range. The most readily available laboratory guide is the PBI. One must be cognizant of the differing PBI responses to the various thyroid preparations in equimetabolic doses (Lavietes and Epstein, 1964) in hypothyroid patients:

	Maintenance dose	
Preparation	Effect on PBI	Illustrative PBI (µg./100 ml.)
Liothyronine	None	1
Thyroglobulin	Minimal	3
Desiccated thyroid U.S.P.	Moderate	4
Sodium L-thyroxine	Slightly high	6
Sodium D-thyroxine	Very high	10

There is a substantial fall in cholesterol and elevation of the BMR to a normal value. The pseudomyotonic tendon reflex becomes normal quite early and is too sensitive as a criterion of adequate therapy. It is important to reiterate that the *clinical response is the most reliable guide to therapy*. Notwithstanding, patients are more likely to be undertreated than overtreated. This may be serious in children and young individuals but is often desirable in patients with coronary heart disease. It usually requires about 3 months to find the optimum maintenance dose, though some further trial and error at other dose levels may be necessary. The following is the daily maintenance dose range that is effective in the majority of cases:

Desiccated thyroid U.S.P. Thyroglobulin	90 to 180 mg. (1½ to 3 grains)
Sodium L-thyroxine	0.15 to 0.3 mg.
Sodium D-thyroxine	2 to 4 mg.
Liothyronine	50 to 150 μg.

The patient should be reexamined thereafter every 2 to 3 months for the first year and twice yearly thereafter, provided no complications arise. It is essential that the patient clearly understand the serious and potentially lethal nature of the disorder and the need for therapy for the duration of his life.

Patients with so-called myxedema heart disease associated with serous effusions show little or no response to digitalis or diuretics. Thyroid alone is capable of mobilizing the edema fluid. Pleural, pericardial, or abdominal paracenteses may be necessary when accumulations of fluid restrict heart action or seriously compromise respiration.

Similar to the victim of Addison's disease, the patient with untreated myxedema is *extraordinarily sensitive to sedatives, narcotics, antihistamines, and barbiturates*. In myxedema the cortisol secretion rate may not increase promptly or adequately in response to stress, probably because of a deficiency in the secretion and/or release of ACTH. Thus some degree of ad-

renocortical insufficiency accompanies myxedema, and the administration of cortisol with TH at the beginning of treatment has been advocated.

Response to therapy

Within 2 to 4 days diuresis begins, with loss of fluid weight, a beginning loss of the puffiness particularly of the face, and a general feeling of warmth. The patient begins to revive from a long hibernation and becomes more conscious of heartbeat, pulse, and motor activity. Physical activity increases and may lead to temporary restlessness. Appetite and bowel action improve, cold sensitivity regresses, and mental function and speech improve. Menstrual disorders are ameliorated before a euthyroid state is attained. Hair, skin, and nail improvement takes place more slowly. Anemia may require many weeks of therapy to be corrected. Usually within 2 to 4 months, depending on its original severity, the patient is restored to a euthyroid state.

Side effects. Patients with hypothyroidism are very sensitive to thyroid therapy. They should be forewarned of the possible onset of headaches, throbbing in the temples, palpitation, dyspnea, excessive warmth, joint pain, and muscle cramps. The dosage is reduced or treatment omitted for several days and then increased more slowly. Occasionally angina pectoris may occur in patients with coronary heart disease. It may subside only when therapy is suboptimal. Palpitation and tachycardia occur in some patients who seem to be tolerant only to a very small dose of thyroid. In these and in some of the patients with angina, sodium D-thyroxine in adequate dosage will be accepted. Allergy to thyroid medications is rare.

Myxedema coma is a serious complication that sometimes first brings the diagnosis to medical attention. The onset may be without apparent cause, but the common precipitating factors are infections, especially pneumonia, exposure to cold, or the stress of an injury. Most patients are elderly. Coma may occur rapidly or follow a period of extreme lethargy. Profound hypothermia is common and correlates with a poor prognosis. Shock, hyponatremia, hypochloremia, elevation of the BUN, and hypoglycemia are common findings. Gastrointestinal bleeding has been observed. A high spinal-fluid protein content may raise the suspicion of a brain tumor. Respiratory acidosis with CO_2 retention has been incriminated as a cause of death. The impaired respiratory mechanics and alveolar hypoventilation resemble those found in extreme obesity (Pickwickian syndrome).

Treatment of coma. The aim for coma treatment is to replace the deficiency of TH as rapidly as possible without overwhelming the patient's capacity to respond. In recent years intravenous liothyronine has been employed because of its rapidity of action and rapid diffusion into tissues. Two approaches have been pursued, the one using quite large amounts to raise the level of circulating hormone rapidly, whereas the other utilizes smaller doses because of the danger of causing cardiac arrhythmias, coronary insufficiency, or a cerebrovascular accident. Frequent ECG tracings should be done at the beginning of therapy. Initial doses varying from 12.5 to 100 μg. have been advocated, with subsequent doses depending on the patient's condition. When parenteral preparations are not available, administration by stomach tube is necessary, but because of the probability of poor gastrointestinal absorption, considerably larger doses are necessary. The mortality rate is high; the best reported results are those of Holvey et al., 1964, who administered an initial estimated total replacement dose of 500 μg. of sodium L-thyroxine intravenously to 7 patients, all of whom survived. Catz and Russell, 1961, reported that 7 of 12 patients survived with the use of liothyronine. If CO_2 narcosis is present, artificial respiration, with tracheotomy if necessary, can rapidly induce consciousness. The use of a respirator for a time thereafter may be required. Electrolyte and fluid replacement, the use of I.V. glucose to combat hypoglycemia, vasopressor agents for shock, and blood transfusions for severe anemia are important elements of therapy. Intravenous hydrocortisone during the first 24 hours in a dose of 100 to 300 mg. may be lifesaving. In some cases pituitary myxedema may be an unrecognized cause of coma, and cortisol therapy is mandatory. Combating the hypothermic state by body warming is recommended by some, decried as harmful by others.

PITUITARY MYXEDEMA

Hypothyroidism is an integral part of the clinical picture of most patients with anterior pituitary insufficiency. Occasionally the signs of myxedema may predominate and may resemble classical thyroid myxedema. Since in the latter condition there is often gonadal and adrenocortical insufficiency secondary to myxedematous involvement of the pituitary and/or the target organ, the differential may be difficult and the pituitary origin of the disorder may be overlooked. The administration of TH to a patient with hypopituitarism can precipitate adrenocortical insufficiency and death, so that the accurate differentiation between primary thyroid and pituitary myxedema is of more than academic interest. Some of the clinical and laboratory findings of value in making this differential have been outlined in Table 5-1. The response to TSH (p. 50) is the best diagnostic test. In rare instances monotrophic loss of TSH with preservation of other anterior pituitary hormones is encountered and can be recognized only by using the TSH test or by measuring plasma TSH. Therapy of pituitary myxedema should be initiated with hydrocortisone for the first 48 hours, followed by small (8 mg. daily) and slowly augmented doses of thyroid.

Metabolic insufficiency and pseudohypothyroidism. I have encountered many patients who, though clearly euthyroid after careful study, have been taking various thyroid preparations for years. Treatment was originally started because of fatigue, lethargy, or a variety of vague complaints combined with hypometabolism. The benefits of therapy have been as vague as the original complaints. Those who seemed to respond best to T_3 were often labeled as having "metabolic insufficiency" or "nonmyxedematous hypometabolism," but most of these individuals suffered from an anxiety neurosis or masked depression. The syndrome was originally suggested by Kurland et al., 1955, who described 4 patients with hypothyroid-like complaints, low BMR, and normal thyroid function who failed to respond to desiccated thyroid but did improve when T_3 or T_3 plus T_4 was administered. Patients who conformed to these criteria have been designated as having "metabolic insufficiency," but they must be extraordinarily rare. Two double-blind studies (Levin, 1960, Sikkema, 1960) have failed to confirm the existence of this entity. The diagnosis "pseudohypothyroidism" is probably more accurate.

CRETINISM (CONGENITAL HYPOTHYROIDISM) AND JUVENILE HYPOTHYROIDISM

Prepubertal hypothyroidism presents problems that are unique from the adult form of the disease because of the critical role of the thyroid hormones in growth and maturation. The age of onset will determine the clinical manifestations and the response to therapy.

Cretinism

Cretinism is a consequence of thyroid hormone deprivation of the fetus. It has been suggested that the word "cretin" be applied only to the severe endemic form and the term "congenital hypothyroidism" be reserved for sporadic cretins, but the diagnosis "cretinism" is so generally used and universally understood that it will probably survive all attempts at change.

Etiology and classification

Endemic cretins are the offspring of goitrous parents in areas of endemic goiter, whereas sporadic cretins have normal fore-bears and rarely have goiters. The most extreme examples show imbecility, severe neurologic disturbances, and deaf-mutism possibly because the mother is hypothyroid as well. *Pendred's syndrome* is an entity combining goiter and deaf-mutism in an individual who may be hypothyroid or euthyroid; it is inherited as a simple recessive trait. Occasionally in endemic areas dwarfed, mentally retarded patients who resemble cretins and may be goitrous are found to be euthyroid and have a normal PBI. It seems possible that, though these individuals were once severely hypothyroid, remnants of thyroid tissue commenced functioning in adult life.

The varieties of cretinism and juvenile hypothyroidism are outlined below:

Endemic
Sporadic
   Developmental fault
      Athyreosis (agenesis, aphasia)
      Thyroid dysgenesis
         Ectopic thyroid (maldescent)
         Hypogenesis
   "Goitrous cretinism"—inborn error of biosynthesis, "dyshormonogenesis"
      Trapping (concentration) defect
      Organification defect
      Coupling defect
      Deiodination defect
      Synthesis of abnormal nonhormonal iodoprotein
   Idiopathic hypothyroidism (Hashimoto's thyroiditis?)
   Loss of TSH (hypopituitarism)
   Maternal ingestion of goitrogens—cretinism
   Juvenile ingestion of goitrogens—postnatal

Athyreosis has been well known as a cause, but not so well recognized is the frequency of *ectopic foci* of thyroid activity found from the base of the tongue to the normal cervical location by RAI scanning. The ectopic thyroid is functionally inadequate but apparently capable of sufficient hormone synthesis to prevent the most extreme forms of hypothyroidism. Recognition may thus be delayed well into postnatal infancy. Although Hutchison, 1963, studied 51 cases in Scotland with RAI and found 27 "definite ectopic," 11 "possible ectopic," and 11 athyreotic, others have found the majority to be athyreotic.

Most cases of thyroid dysgenesis and athyreosis are free of other congenital somatic defects. The familial incidence is quite low. Blizzard and his group (Chandler et al., 1962) found agglutinating, complement-fixing, and thyrocytotoxic antibodies in 24.8% of mothers of athyreotic cretins and in only 6% of mothers of normal offspring and suggested that fetal thyroid damage could be sustained as part of an autoimmune process transmitted across the placental barrier. A higher proportion of nontasters of phenylthiocarbamide (PTC) has been found among cretins and their families than among the general population. An excess of nontasters has been found in nontoxic goiter, so that inability to taste PTC suggests some basic thyroid defect of unknown significance.

Inborn errors of hormone biosynthesis. Sporadic familial goitrous cretinism, or dyshormonogenesis, is uncommon but has evoked great interest because its unique biochemical disturbances may provide a clue to the cause of simple (sporadic) goiter. Because of a high familial incidence it is believed that they are genetically determined, may result from the inherited loss of a single intrathyroidal enzyme or enzyme system, and are transmitted by a recessive autosomal gene. It is not necessarily manifest in early infancy, does not necessarily exhibit a goiter, and may be associated with varying degrees of hypothyroidism. In fact, the disorder is not incompatible with euthyroidism.

The following sites of the biosynthetic errors can be better appreciated by reference to Figs. 6-4 and 6-5.

TRAPPING DEFECT. Apparently only 1 case of a trapping defect has been described (Stanbury and Chapman, 1960)—that of a 14-year-old male whose thyroid and salivary glands did not concentrate RAI. Iodine administration was effective in relieving hypothyroidism and reducing the size of the goiter.

ORGANIFICATION DEFECT. The most common variety is the organification defect. There is failure to bind iodide to tyrosine because of a deficiency either in the peroxidase enzyme system, so that active iodine [I^+] is not released from iodide [I^-], or in the enzyme system responsible for the iodination of tyrosine, or to a combination of both. The defect can be demonstrated by the thiocyanate washout test (Fig. 6-6). The accumulation of RAI is rapid as in thyrotoxicosis, may reach normal or even high levels, and may show a rapid decline. The same defect has been described in euthyroid goitrous individuals with congenital deafness inherited as a simple recessive.

COUPLING DEFECT. MIT and DIT accumulate because of a defect in the coupling enzyme, and the MIT/DIT ratio tends to be increased. The finding of iodotyrosines in blood and urine, together with the ability to trap iodide, organify tyrosine, and deiodinate iodotyrosine, has suggested that the fault must be in the coupling mechanism. The loss of iodotyrosines in the urine leads to a continuous depletion of iodide, resulting in goiter and hypothyroidism.

DEIODINATION DEFECT. A dehalogenase deficiency was recognized in a group of goitrous cretins by demonstrating that they were unable to deiodinate administered MIT-^{131}I both in vivo and in vitro. Iodotyrosines accumulate in the blood, are excreted in the urine, and become a source of iodide loss.

SYNTHESIS OF NONHORMONAL IODOPROTEIN. McGirr, 1963, studied 20 patients who secreted a butanol-insoluble iodoprotein that was physiologically inert. Twelve were hypothyroid, 8 were euthyroid, and the goiters were sometimes very large. He suggested that there was either abnormal protein synthesis due to a change in the thyroglobulin molecule or a defect in the proteolytic enzymes that hydrolyze thyroglobulin.

The brain in cretinism

The brain (Eayrs, 1960) is small and retains infantile proportions. Neurons are smaller than normal, are closely packed, show defective myelination, and impaired dendritic growth. There is increased cerebral capillary permeability, reduction in extent of the capillary bed, and capillary enlargement so that the brain is served by a relatively small number of dilated capillaries. Whereas adult brain tissue metabolizes carbohydrate almost exclusively, the developing brain favors the synthesis of proteins and lipids, a function that may be partially thyroxine dependent. The electro-encephalogram shows sporadic slow activity, little or no alpha rhythms, and small amplitude.

Clinical features of cretinism

Hypothyroidism is the most common endocrine disorder found during childhood.

The characteristic features of the cretin (Fig. 9-3) are rarely present at birth because maternal TH, transferred to the fetus across the placental membrane, persists for several weeks. The clinician must therefore be alert to the following early clues exhibited during the neonatal period.

1. Poor feeding. Lethargy, anorexia, somnolence, a large tongue, and respiratory difficulties all contribute to slow nursing and weak sucking. There is a *failure to gain weight.*

2. Lethargy. The baby is quiet and relatively immobile, sleeps a great deal, cries little and then hoarsely, and shows little response to stimulation. He is often described as a "good" baby.

3. Constipation. Constipation is persistent, resistant to all measures, and often associated with flatulence and abdominal distention. The stools are hard and dry.

4. Respiratory distress. There are episodes of choking and cyanosis especially during feeding. Respiration is noisy, and the parents complain that the baby always has a head cold.

5. Skin. The skin is dry, somewhat thickened, cool, grayish pallid with mottled cyanosis, and with prolongation of icterus neonatorum. Carotenemia may be evident. There may be signs of myxedema with periorbital and facial puffiness. Infantile hair tends to persist.

6. Umbilical hernia.

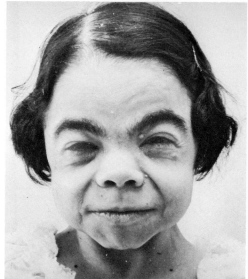

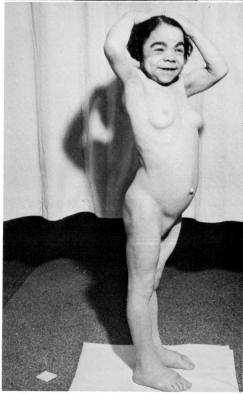

Fig. 9-3. Adult cretin (age 33, untreated). Note characteristic cretinoid features, dwarfism (height 44 in.), absent axillary and scant pubic hair, poorly developed breasts, pot belly, and small umbilical hernia. Primary amenorrhea. (PBI 5.9, BEI 0, RAIU 0, TSH response 0). The increased PBI/BEI ratio suggests that this patient was a goitrous cretin in early life and the goiter regressed.

7. *Tongue.* The tongue is enlarged and often protruding.

8. *Hypothermia.*

9. *Bradycardia and low pulse pressure.*

10. *Goiter.* There is goiter in the goitrous cretin and impalpable thyroid in the agenetic and dysgenetic cretin.

In the months following birth, all of these manifestations become more florid, and cretinoid features appear with the typical coarsened physiognomy, profusion of black, sometimes brittle hair with a low hairline, short thick neck, and broad, saddle-type nose (Fig. 9-3). More profound changes of myxedema appear, and there is failure to achieve normal linear growth, delayed closure of the fontanelles, diminished physical activity, muscle hypotonicity, and prolonged tendon reflexes. All of the usual developmental signposts are delayed, such as teething, sitting, crawling, walking, and talking. Evidence of mental deficiency appears at an early age, and a normal I.Q. is rarely attained. The child is placid, shows little awareness of his surroundings or companions, plays little or not at all with toys, and tends to be good natured and easy to handle. Evidence of more profound defects in the nervous system may appear, such as spasticity, tremors, or clumsy and uncoordinated movement. The usual preponderance of females, peculiar to most thyroid disorders, is found in the athyreotic variety, whereas in the goitrous cretin there is no sex dominance.

An example of untreated adult cretinism is shown in Fig. 9-3. Cretins bear such a close resemblance to each other that they appear to be members of the same family. The completeness of the syndrome depends on the degree of hormonal deprivation. In less severe cases the gross features of the cretin are absent, and the infant may simply be short, small, and somewhat retarded. As he grows older, the most striking manifestation is the very slow rate of growth, so that the height may be equal to that of a healthy child several years younger.

Laboratory studies

X-ray studies. At birth there is absence of the distal femoral, proximal tibial, humeral, and cuboid epiphyses. Thereafter the radiologist surveys other epiphyses appropriate to the age of the patient. Epiphysial cartilaginous ossification, instead of being an orderly homogeneous process, appears in irregular scattered foci and later coalesces to form an irregular epiphysial center (stippled epiphyses, epiphysial dysgenesis). It may be present in some centers and not in others or may become evident only after therapy is started. It is pathognomonic of hypothyroidism, and its presence in certain epiphyses helps to date the onset of thyroid failure.

PBI. PBI is almost invariably low, except in some goitrous cretins secreting an abnormal iodinated protein (Fig. 9-3). In such instances a low *BEI* and serum T_4 will be found.

RAIU. The RAIU uptake is very low in athyreotics and in goitrous cretins with a trapping defect. In other goitrous cretins the RAIU may be normal or elevated. *TSH* will cause a marked rise if hypothyroidism is due to hypopituitarism. In ectopic thyroids, *RAI scanning* may reveal areas of uptake anywhere from the base of the tongue down to the normal cervical position. The thiocyanate or perchlorate washout test is done in goitrous cretins with a defect of organification. Very small doses of RAI (0.1 to 0.5 μCi.) should be employed in infants and young children. If instrumentation of maximum sensitivity is not available, the study should be omitted.

Serum cholesterol. Elevations of serum cholesterol are rare at birth but tend to appear after 2 to 3 years.

Alkaline phosphatase and inorganic phosphate. Usually the alkaline phosphatase and inorganic phosphate are below the normal value for the age of the patient.

Blood count. Somewhat more than 50% of patients are anemic.

ECG. The ECG may show characteristic

changes (Fig. 9-2). Chest films show an enlarged heart.

BMR. The BMR is an unreliable test in infants when performed by ordinary clinical methods and a difficult test to perform and interpret in young children.

Serum carotene. Serum carotene may be elevated.

Glucose-6-phosphate dehydrogenase. The activity of glucose-6-phosphate dehydrogenase is decreased.

Differential diagnosis

Cretins must be differentiated from other individuals presenting deficient growth, retarded bone age, and physical and mental retardation. The mongolian idiot (Down's syndrome) can be recognized at birth more readily than the cretin, is more physically active, shows no evidences of hypothyroidism or myxedema, and has the characteristic epicanthic fold, deformed ears, incurving of the fifth finger, and normal bodily proportions. The karyotype shows trisomy-21, and the child does not respond to thyroid therapy. The much rarer *hypopituitary dwarf* may exhibit signs of less severe hypothyroidism but not the typical stigmas of the cretin. Bodily proportions are normal, the bone age is retarded, but there is no epiphysial dys-

genesis, growth may be only temporarily, or not at all, stimulated by thyroid therapy, and a positive response to TSH is obtained. Other forms of *dwarfism* do not resemble cretins, do show normal thyroid tests, and do not respond to thyroid therapy.

Treatment

Any of the five preparations described on p. 166 may be used; the author favors initiating therapy with liothyronine because of its rapid action and later substituting desiccated thyroid or sodium L-thyroxine. An approximate dose schedule according to age is shown in Table 9-2. After 2 weeks of liothyronine therapy, add the prescribed dose of desiccated thyroid for about 1 week and then discontinue the liothyronine. Desiccated thyroid is then increased every 2 weeks in 15 to 30 mg. increments. The daily maintenance dose (Table 9-2) should be that amount of replacement therapy consistent with clinical euthyroidism and a maximum rate of growth and development.

If there is profound myxedema, distant heart sounds, and ECG changes, the initial dose and the size and speed of dosage increase should be somewhat less. Occasional unexplained deaths have occurred in severe cretinism usually 2 to 4 weeks

Table 9-2. Guide to thyroid hormone replacement therapy in cretinism and juvenile hypothyroidism

Age	Initial dose			Maintenance dose	
	Desiccated thyroid or thyroglobulin (mg./day)	Sodium L-thyroxine (mg./day)	Liothyronine (μg./day)	Desiccated thyroid or thyroglobulin (mg./day)	Sodium L-thyroxine (mg./day)
0- 6 months	8-15	0.006-0.025	5-15	30-65	0.05-0.1
6-12 months	8-15	0.006-0.05	10-20	30-90	0.05-0.15
1- 2 years	15-30	0.025-0.05	10-25	65-130	0.1 -0.2
2- 6 years	15-30	0.025-0.05	10-25	65-195	0.1 -0.3
6 years to puberty	15-45	0.05 -0.15	15-25	65-260	0.1 -0.4

after therapy has been started. Nevertheless, one should usually err on the side of aggressive overtreatment to ensure a maximal response and not be deterred by mild symptoms of overdosage. The dose should be augmented as rapidly as the infant's tolerance permits so as to reach maintenance levels as quickly as possible and prevent prolongation of the hypothyroid state. The amount of TH replacement to repair hypometabolism and gross physical deficiencies may not be adequate to ensure normal skeletal and central nervous system growth and development. If signs of thyroid toxicity (restlessness, insomnia, tachycardia, vomiting, diarrhea) appear, the dose must be reduced. The PBI should be brought within the normal range, with full realization of the varying effects of different preparations (p. 167). The low serum alkaline phosphatase rises and the cholesterol, if elevated, falls. New ossification centers appear, and coalescence of areas of epiphysial dysgenesis occurs with adequate treatment. The patient must be protected against needless x-ray exposure by the use of a minimum number of follow-up studies, by the use of properly maintained equipment, and by proper shielding of adjacent areas. Psychometric evaluation at regular intervals provides an objective measure of mental response.

Prognosis

Mental achievement in cretins is best when therapy is started in very early infancy and maintained without interruption. It is unlikely that significant TH deprivation occurs in utero if the mother was euthyroid. Athyreotic infants begin to suffer from hypothyroidism about 1 to 3 weeks after birth, at a time when central nervous system damage is particularly critical. Approximately 75% of total brain growth is extrauterine, and about half of that occurs in the first 5 to 6 months. Significant mental retardation is rare if hypothyroidism originates after 2 years of age.

Physical improvement can be expected even when therapy is somewhat delayed. In the series reported from Wilkins Clinic (Smith, 1957), 10 of 22 severe cretins treated adequately before 6 months of age and 12 of 29 patients treated before 1 year of age achieved an I.Q. of over 90. None of the 50 inadequately treated patients or patients treated after 1 year of age attained a comparable I.Q. If older cretins are treated, there is little or no improvement in mental function, but there will be some stimulation of growth, dental maturation, and reversal of the clinical signs of hypothyroidism. Occasionally the patient may become unmanageable when the metabolic state is improved, and the dose of thyroid must be reduced.

Juvenile hypothyroidism

Juvenile or "acquired" hypothyroidism presents clinical features (see outline below and Fig. 9-4) that vary, depending on the age of onset and the severity of thyroid hormone deprivation.

Growth retardation
    Short stature, retarded bone age, infantile skeletal proportions
    Infantile nasal bones
    Epiphysial dysgenesis
    Slow growth of hair and nails
Dental retardation
    Prolonged retention of deciduous teeth
    Delayed appearance of permanent teeth
Delayed puberty
    Female—late menarche, breast budding
    Male—delayed testicular enlargement, pubic hair, voice deepening
Cerebration
    Slowed—deficient school performance, torpor, placidity, amiability
Other hypothyroid stigmas
    Fatigue, lethargy, cold intolerance, constipation, poor appetite, cool dry pallid skin, carotenemia, dry brittle coarse hair, puffy face, bradycardia, hypothermia, hoarse voice, weight gain, poor muscle tone

Sporadic familial goitrous hypothyroidism, when not severe, may become manifest in late childhood following the slow development of a goiter. If hypothyroidism begins during the first 2 years, the effects on cerebration and growth may be severe enough to resemble the congenital

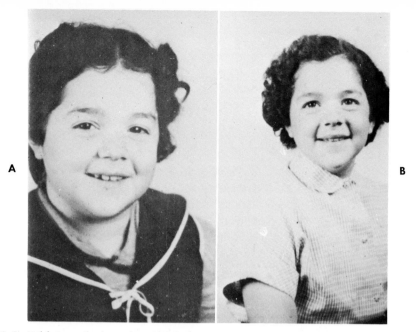

Fig. 9-4. Mild juvenile hypothyroidism characterized solely by growth retardation. This patient illustrates one of the consequences of inadequate therapy from the age of diagnosis (7 years) to age 12 years, **A**, and the beneficial effects of adequate and sporadic treatment thereafter; compare **B**, which was taken 6 months after therapy. She had no symptoms or other signs of hypothyroidism. She had an I.Q. of 112. Further data are contained below:

Age (years)	Height (inches)	Weight	PBI	
7	41	—	—	Inadequate interrupted treatment
10	46	—	2.3	Bone age retarded 4 years
11	48¾	—	—	Bone age retarded 4 to 5 years
12	50	94	3.5	Thyroid U.S.P. 15 to 30 mg./day
12⅙	50½	87	—	Thyroid U.S.P. 60 to 120 mg./day
12⅔	52⅛	85	5.8	Thyroid U.S.P. 120 mg./day
13	56⅛	95	4.5	Thyroid U.S.P. 120 mg./day
17	60½	125	5.5	Thyroid U.S.P. 120 to 180 mg./day
23	61	130	5.2	Married, delivered full-term healthy infant

variety. After 2 years of age the child's mental potential is probably not seriously threatened. The most striking features are the marked slowing or cessation of growth and the retardation of epiphysial and dental maturation. One can often date the approximate age of onset by careful assessment of these features. Serial height measurements are of great value in the diagnosis. The onset may be insidious and the clinical features so minimal that the diagnosis may be seriously delayed. The onset of puberty is retarded in most cases, but rare examples of precocious menstruation have been reported. Probably a considerable proportion of the goitrous and a majority of the athyreotic cases are examples of chronic lymphocytic thyroiditis (Hashimoto's struma). Winter et al., 1966, found circulating antithyroglobulin antibodies in 16 of 18 juvenile hypothyroid patients and complement-fixing antibodies to a thyroid microsomal antigen in 50%. A few of the goitrous patients will be found to be examples of inborn errors of thyroid hormone synthesis.

The *laboratory diagnosis* is the same as in adults, though RAI scanning is useful in the search for ectopic foci of thyroid tissue.

Treatment

The initial dose of thyroid varies with the age of onset and the severity of thyroid failure. The tolerance of children to thyroid therapy is, in general, quite high. If therapy is commenced near the age of puberty, the acceleration of bone age may be rapid and premature epiphysial maturation can occur if therapy is pursued too vigorously. Means, 1963, has witnessed the onset of a psychosis "if the return to the normal metabolic level is too abrupt." The tendency, however, is to undertreat rather than overtreat. An approximate dose schedule according to age of onset is shown in Table 9-2. The lowest initial dose is for the severely myxedematous subject and for the patient with ECG abnormalities or an enlarged heart.

REFERENCES

Cassidy, C. E., et al.: Goiter and hypothyroidism. In Astwood, E. B., and Cassidy, C. E., editors: New York, Clinical endocrinology, vol. 2, Grune & Stratton, Inc., 1968, p. 210.

Catz, B., and Russell, S.: Arch. Intern. Med. **108:**129, 1961.

Chandler, R. W., et al.: New Eng. J. Med. **267:** 376, 1962.

DeGroot, L. J., et al.: Clin. Res. **16:**264, 1968 (abst.).

de la Balze, F. A., et al.: J. Clin. Endocr. **22:** 212, 1962.

Douglass, R. C., and Jacobson, S. D.: J. Clin. Endocr. **17:**1354, 1957.

*Eayrs, J. T.: Brit. Med. Bull. **16:**122, 1960.

Ezrin, C., et al.: J. Clin. Endocr. **19:**958, 1959.

Gabrilove, J. L., and Ludwig, A. W.: J. Clin. Endocr. **17:**925, 1957.

Holvey, D. N., et al.: Arch. Intern. Med. **113:** 89, 1964.

*Hutchison, J. H.: The aetiology and diagnosis of nongoitrous hypothyroidism in childhood. In Mason, A. S., editor: The thyroid and its diseases, proceedings of a conference held at the College of Physicians of London, March 15-16, 1963, Philadelphia, 1963, J. B. Lippincott Co., p. 39.

Hutchison, J. H., et al.: Lancet **2:**314, 1957.

Kologlu, S., et al.: Endocrinology **78:**231, 1966.

Kurland, G. S.: J. Clin. Endocr. **15:**1354, 1955.

Lavietes, P. H., and Epstein, F. H.: Ann. Intern. Med. **60:**79, 1964.

Levin, M. E.: J. Clin. Endocr. **20:**106, 1960.

Lloyd, W. H., and Goldberg, I. J. L.: Brit. Med. J. **2:**1256, 1961.

Means, J. H., et al.: The thyroid and its disease, ed. 3, New York, 1963, Blakiston Division, McGraw-Hill Book Co., p. 365.

*McGirr, E. M.: Defects of thyroid hormone synthesis. In Mason, A. S., editor: The thyroid and its diseases, proceedings of a conference held at the Royal College of Physicians of London, March 15-16, 1963, Philadelphia, 1963, J. B. Lippincott Co., p. 52.

Murphy, B. E. P., and Pattee, C. J.: The measurement of thyroxine in blood. In Astwood, E. B., and Cassidy, C. E., editors: Clinical endocrinology, New York, 1968, Grune & Stratton, Inc., p. 296.

*Nickel, S. N., and Frame, B.: Nervous system in myxedema. In Crispell, K. R., editor: Hypothyroidism, New York, 1963, The Macmillan Co., (a) p. 166, (b) p. 178.

Ord, W.: Medico-Chirugica Transactions **61:**57, 1878.

Schneeberg, N. G.: Amer. J. Med. Sci. **248:** 399, 1964.

Schneeberg, N. G., et al.: J. Clin. Endocr. **14:** 223, 1954.

Sikkema, S. H.: J. Clin. Endocr. **20:**546, 1960.

Simone, J. V., et al.: New Eng. J. Med. **273:** 1057, 1965.

*Smith, D. W.: Pediatrics **19:**1011, 1957.

Stanbury, J. B., and Chapman, E. M.: Lancet **2:**1162, 1960.

Sterling, K., and Brenner, M. A.: J. Clin. Invest. **45:**153, 1966.

Winter, J., et al.: J. Pediat. **69:**709, 1966.

*Significant reviews.

Chapter 10

Thyroiditis

A classification of the types of thyroiditis is shown in the following outline:

Subacute thyroiditis—"acute," De Quervain's, granulomatous, pseudotuberculous
Chronic thyroiditis
    Struma lymphomatosa, Hashimoto's, lymphadenoid goiter, lymphocytic
    Chronic nonspecific thyroiditis
    Riedel's struma—sclerosing, invasive fibrous, ligneous
Acute suppurative thyroiditis

SUBACUTE THYROIDITIS

Subacute thyroiditis, also known as acute, De Quervain's, granulomatous, or pseudotuberculous thyroiditis, is a nonsuppurative, inflammatory disorder of the thyroid gland. The etiology is unknown, but a virus has been implicated because of its association with acute upper respiratory infections, the occasional occurrence after influenza and cat-scratch disease, and an unusual frequency during mumps epidemics. Eylan et al., 1957, isolated mumps virus from the thyroid in 2 cases and found positive complement-fixation titers in 10 cases.

Pathology

The thyroid is diffusely enlarged, or there may be unilateral or focal involvement. The involved areas are firm and whitish or yellowish white. There is progressive destruction of thyroid parenchyma with loss of follicles, a granulomatous "tuberculoid" reaction with giant cells,

histiocytosis, interstitial inflammation, and fibrosis. Cellular exudates contain polymorphonuclear leukocytes, lymphocytes, plasma cells, and occasional microabscesses.

Pathophysiology

The inflammatory process impedes the thyroidal accumulation of iodide and the synthesis of thyroid hormones. Only small amounts of hormone continue to be formed and, because of the inflammatory disruption of the follicle, are rapidly discharged into the circulation, together with thyroglobulin and various butanol-insoluble nonhormonal, iodinated proteins. The latter may result from disordered synthetic mechanisms and the presence of leukocytic proteases and peptidases. The thyroid is unresponsive to exogenous TSH, another indication of its functional inactivity. Regeneration of thyroid follicles occurs as recovery proceeds, and iodide accumulation may rebound to elevated levels.

Clinical features

The disorder is uncommon, but is frequently overlooked. Cassidy, 1968, examined 215 cases from 1956 through 1965, and there were 372 cases at the Mayo Clinic in the period 1952 through 1961 (Woolner, 1964). The female/male ratio is 3 or 4 to 1. It may occur at any age but is most common from 30 to 50 years. The disease is self-limited, lasts from a few days to several months (average 1 to 3 months), regresses without causing any permanent damage to the thyroid, but has a tendency to recur. Temporary hypothyroidism may be observed because of exhaustion of hormone stores in a protracted inflammatory process, but permanent hypothyroidism is rare. Examination of thyroid tissue years after recovery shows only residual fibrosis. Hyperthyroidism has been observed as a coincidental disorder.

The disease can be divided into two varieties with full recognition that there is a spectrum of clinical states merging from the acute to the subacute or more chronic forms.

Acute thyroiditis. There is the rapid onset of swelling and tenderness of the thyroid gland with radiation of pain to the ears, mastoid, jaw, cheeks, or pharynx. Occasionally the initial complaint predominates in these areas, and the patient may first consult an otolaryngologist or dentist. Fever, tachycardia, chills, sweats, malaise, dysphagia, neck pain, and headache are characteristic. The temperature may reach 104° F. and then subside to a more prolonged low-grade elevation. Occasionally there are signs suggesting hyperthyroidism. The thyroid is symmetrically enlarged, firm, and exquisitely tender; rarely there is erythema of the overlying skin. In some cases there is involvement of one lobe, or one or more tender nodules appear, and the inflammatory process later migrates throughout the gland.

Subacute thyroiditis. The more common variety is subacute thyroiditis and is characterized by a less dramatic onset and features that are often vague and subject to remissions and recurrences. Occasionally there are no complaints and a tender enlarged thyroid is discovered during a physical examination. Subacute thyroiditis is frequently misdiagnosed as fever of unknown origin, dental abscess, pharyngitis, chronic sinusitis, otitis media, or influenza. The more chronic forms may be confused with thyroid adenoma, goiter, thyroid carcinoma, globus hystericus, or neurasthenia. Occasionally Hashimoto's thyroiditis may resemble De Quervain's when it runs a subacute course and the thyroid is tender. Constitutional symptoms, so prominent in the more acute variety, may be absent or minimal. The patient may complain of no more than some malaise, "a deep sore throat," and anorexia. Focal involvement of the thyroid is more common in the beginning, with areas of tender nodulation and eventual spread to involve an entire lobe and then both lobes.

Laboratory findings

Characteristic laboratory findings are as follows:

1. Rapid sedimentation rate and a normal white cell count. Occasionally there is slight leukocytosis.

2. Low RAIU, except in the localized varieties where there may be uninvolved thyroid parenchyma, which can be delineated by RAI scanning. Cassidy, 1968, found the RAIU to be below 15% in 27 cases, normal in 35, and above normal in 10.

3. Normal or elevated PBI and increased PBI/BEI, and PBI/T_4 ratios. Circulating thyroid autoantibodies are absent or found in low titer. Serum protein electrophoresis has shown low albumin and elevation of alpha-1, alpha-2, beta, and gamma globulins. The BMR is elevated.

Differential diagnosis

Subacute thyroiditis is only rarely confused with nodular goiter or thyroid carcinoma. The recovery of function in thyroiditis, as shown by RAI scanning, may aid in the differentiation of "cold" nodules. There may rarely be slight tenderness in Hashimoto's thyroiditis. Occasionally a hypersensitive thyrotoxic subject may complain of a tender thyroid. Hemorrhage into a thyroid cyst or adenoma may resemble subacute thyroiditis with local swelling, severe, albeit localized, pain, and failure to accumulate RAI in the area. Subacute thyroiditis is rarely so well localized, and the onset is not so precipitate. Acute suppurative thyroiditis (see p. 184) is usually a more rapidly progressive disease with inflammation of the overlying skin, pointing of an abscess, fluctuation of a mass, and a high polymorphonuclear white cell count. If thyroid carcinoma is suspected, open biopsy or partial thyroidectomy becomes mandatory. A frozen section may prevent an unnecessary operation.

Treatment

In mild cases aspirin or other analgesics, cold applications, and suppressive doses (75 to 150 μg.) of liothyronine may suffice. A corticosteroid affords relief in 24 to 48 hours and serves as a diagnostic aid in doubtful cases. We favor large doses initially to achieve rapid amelioration of symptoms. Prednisone is used in a dosage of 10 mg. four times daily for 48 hours, then three times a day for 3 to 5 days, and twice daily thereafter. After 10 to 14 days, relief may be maintained with 5 to 10 mg. twice a day. One seeks the smallest effective maintenance dose. After 3 or 4 weeks, treatment can often be terminated. If symptoms recur as the dosage is tapered, the previously effective dosage is repeated for another week or two, and again dosage reduction is attempted. Corticosteroids seem to afford only symptomatic relief while the self-limited inflammatory process runs its course of several weeks to 2 to 4 months. Recurrences usually occur within several days but may appear months after apparent subsidence. If corticosteroids are contraindicated and thyroid suppressive therapy is not effective, local x-ray irradiation, the method of choice prior to the cortisone era, relieves symptoms. Normal, or nearly normal, thyroid function is restored within 4 weeks of clinical cure.

HASHIMOTO'S THYROIDITIS

A variety of chronic thyroiditis, first described by Hashimoto in 1912 and called Hashimoto's thyroiditis, has been the object of great interest in the past decade because of its apparently increasing frequency and evidence suggesting that it is an autoimmune disease.

Etiology

Rose and Witebsky, 1956, immunized rabbits against homologous thyroid tissue extracts combined with Freund adjuvant and found in the rabbit thyroid both circulating antithyroid antibody and inflammatory lesions that resembled human chronic thyroiditis. The subsequent discovery of circulating antibodies to human thyroglobulin and thyroid cell constituents in patients with Hashimoto's disease suggested that an antigen-antibody reaction might be the basic cytotoxic insult provoking the destructive process. Henceforth the term "autoimmune thyroiditis" became synonymous with Hashimoto's thyroiditis. The demonstration of thyroid-cell basement-membrane damage and its correlation with the level of antibody titer seemed to prove that there was an avenue of antigen escape from the cell to provoke the initial immune reaction, though whether this was a primary change was uncertain. Small amounts of thyroglobulin were regularly found by Daniel et al., 1967, in the lymph draining from the thyroid gland of normal monkeys so that the substrate for an immunologic reaction may be constantly available. The evidence for a cause-and-effect relationship remains unproved, particularly in view of the failure to always correlate the thyroid lesion with the antibody titer, to achieve passively transferred thyroiditis with serum antibody, and to explain the presence of thyroid antibodies in a small but significant percent of normal individuals. The disease may be a reaction of the delayed-hypersensitivity type, a hypothesis supported by the production of thyroiditis in guinea pigs by transfer of lymphoid cells (Felix-Davis and Waksman, 1961). A genetic predisposition has been noted. Hall et al., 1960, found circulating autoimmune antibodies in 22 of 39 relatives of patients.

Pathology

The gland is diffusely enlarged, rubbery firm, and with a bosselated lobulated surface. Nodules of focal disease may predominate early. Three major histologic changes are observed (Fig. 10-1):

 Dense lymphoid infiltration, often with lymph follicles and germinal centers

 Follicular disruption and *atrophy* with loss of colloid, often side by side with regenerative hyperplasia and hypertrophy; fibrosis, though usually evident, is rarely severe

 Askanazy cells represent characteristic oxophilic changes in the thyroid cell cytoplasm and are considered to be pathognomonic. Plasma cells and histiocytes are seen occasionally.

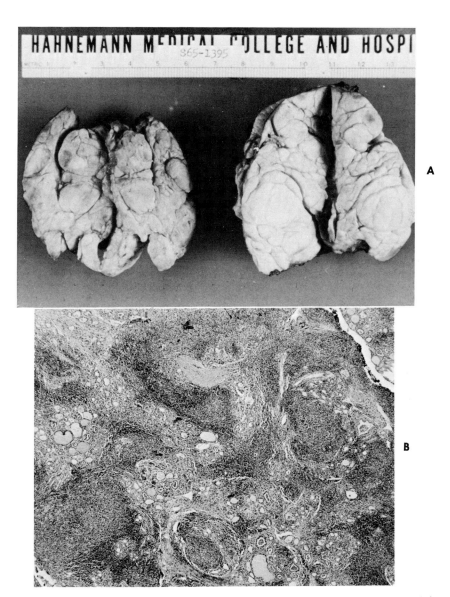

Fig. 10-1. Hashimoto's thyroiditis. **A,** The two thyroid lobes weighed 65 grams; the lobulated bosselated surface is typical. **B,** The histologic section (×20) shows distorted architecture, lymphocytic proliferation with germinal centers and intervening connective tissue, and residual follicles (lined by large eosinophilic cells not discernible at this magnification). (Courtesy Dr. Alexander Nedwich and Department of Pathology, Hahnemann Medical College, Philadelphia, Pa.)

The disorder progressively destroys thyroid parenchyma and results in hypothyroidism. The gland may be enlarged, normal, or decreased in size and weight, a state described as "asymptomatic atrophic thyroiditis" by Bastenie et al., 1967. The current hypothesis views most cases of "spontaneous idiopathic myxedema" as the end stage of this slow process of parenchymal attrition. Nevertheless, serial biopsies have shown no progressive histologic changes in half of the patients in one series (Vickery and Hamlin, 1961) and progressive, though minimal, advances in the other half.

Pathophysiology

Thyroid parenchymal destruction compromises hormone biosynthesis and secretion. The reduced level of circulating T_4 and T_3 evokes continuous TSH stimulation, with resultant regenerative changes and goiter formation. Eventually exhaustion atrophy due to chronic overstimulation may result. Although high TSH levels have not been demonstrated, the fault may lie in the lack of sensitivity of the bioassay methods. Elevated TSH has been assumed because of the evidence of follicle stimulation, by the regression of the goiter with suppressive TH therapy, by the failure to augment the RAIU or PBI with TSH injections, and by the rapid turnover rate of RAI with a high $PB^{131}I$ and conversion ratio. The PBI/BEI ratio rises because of leakage of thyroglobulin through the damaged or increasingly permeable basement membrane, perhaps to the formation of other iodinated proteins and to the reduction in circulating hormone as measured by the BEI and T_4. Defective tyrosine organification has been demonstrated by positive washout tests with thiocyanate or perchlorate (p. 107). The blocking effect of iodide on RAIU is increased as in hyperthyroidism. Intrathyroidal exchangeable iodine and the biologic half-life of RAI are reduced. These changes have been reviewed by Skillern, 1964.

Clinical features

Incidence. An increase seems likely in this not uncommon disorder. At the Mayo Clinic (McConahey et al., 1962) only 2 cases were recorded in 1930, but there were 185 cases in 1959.

Age and sex. Hashimoto's thyroiditis occurs at all ages and constitutes the principal cause of pediatric goiter. The highest incidence is from 30 to 60 years of age, and 90% are women.

Symptoms. The goiter evokes few symptoms and is usually first discovered during a physical examination. Symptoms caused by neck compression are rare. The patient may be euthyroid or hypothyroid. Hyperthyroidism ("hashitoxicosis") is an unusual concomitant.

Signs. There is a painless, moderate-sized, rubbery, firm goiter with a lobulated smooth surface and a bosselated edge. The pyramidal lobe is often enlarged. In the early stages, nodules or gross asymmetry due to unilateral involvement may occur. When the goiter is large, it assumes a horseshoe shape and is quite nodular. In rare instances it may be slightly tender. Occasionally the gland is normal or decreased in size.

Association with Graves' disease or thyroid carcinoma

Graves' disease. Circulating thyroid autoantibodies are found in many patients with Graves' disease. The two disorders may coexist, suggesting a common factor. Enlargement of the thymus and the presence of medullary lymphoid follicles in patients with hyperthyroidism, together with the recognition of the role of the thymus in immune mechanisms has further strengthened the autoimmune hypothesis (Michie et al., 1967). Patients with high antibody titers and thyroid gland lymphoid infiltrates (focal thyroiditis?) often become hypothyroid after surgery.

Thyroid carcinoma. A more-than-chance association of Hashimoto's thyroiditis and thyroid malignancy has been suggested by some workers but denied by others.

Woolner et al., 1959, found 18 carcinomas and 12 lymphosarcomas in 605 cases of thyroiditis.

Laboratory studies

There are no specific tests, and those listed below must be evaluated in the light of the clinical data. Results of PBI, BEI, T₄, and RAIU will vary, depending on the extent of thyroid destruction versus follicular regeneration and on whether the patient is euthyroid or hypothyroid.

PBI, BEI, T₄. The PBI/BEI ratio is elevated in about 50% of patients. The BEI and T_4 are normal or low.

RAIU. The RAIU may be normal, low, or high, but the uptake can be suppressed by TH and fails to increase when TSH is injected. If localized thyroiditis is suspected, an RAI scan is performed. A response to TSH may be unilateral and will not be apparent unless differential lobe counting is done. A normal TSH response is diffuse throughout both lobes. In somewhat less than 50% of patients there is a positive washout test with perchlorate or thiocyanate. There is often increased sensitivity to the blocking effect of small doses of iodides (less than 2 mg.). A high level of PB¹³¹I has been found.

Autoimmune antibodies. The *tanned red cell hemagglutination test* (TRC) is positive in high titer (over 1:2,500) in 50% to 80% of cases. It is of diagnostic significance only if the titer is high and if there is clinical substantiation, because low titers are not uncommon in other thyroid disorders and in some normal subjects. Occasionally a high titer is found in Graves' disease or granulomatous thyroiditis, albeit probably in some of these there is focal Hashimoto's disease. *Complement-fixing antibody* to thyroid microsomal antigen is also found in a titer of over 1:64 in many patients. A combination of several antibody tests will yield positive results in up to 95% of patients.

Serum flocculation tests. Abnormal thymol, cephalin-cholesterol, zinc sulfate, and colloidal gold tests are commonly found in Hashimoto's thyroiditis but are not specific. The erythrocyte-sedimentation rate is frequently accelerated. All of these changes are attributed to alterations in serum proteins, that is, mild hypoalbuminemia and elevated total and gamma globulin.

Needle biopsy. Enthusiasm for needle biopsy depends to a large extent on local experience. We have employed this procedure only when the diagnosis is in doubt and have tended to prefer open biopsy if there is an indurated nodule. Needle biopsy, however, is a safe procedure, and because the process is usually diffuse, the specimen obtained is representative of the entire gland. The specimen is usually easy to obtain, in contrast to the difficulty often experienced in nodular goiter, and Skillern, 1964, considers this a useful diagnostic feature.

Differential diagnosis

The diagnosis is almost certain if one finds the combination of mild hypothyroidism, a small- to medium-sized goiter of rubbery firmness exhibiting diffuse involvement with lobulated surface and bosselated edges, autoimmune antibodies in high titer, increased PBI/BEI ratio, and a normal or slightly elevated RAIU. The diagnosis is more certain if the RAIU is suppressed by TH and fails to increase after TSH. A therapeutic trial with 180 mg./day of desiccated thyroid or its equivalent will produce regression of the goiter in most cases within 1 to 3 months. Hashimoto's is most often confused with simple goiter, and the differential may be so difficult, when atypical laboratory results are obtained, that a biopsy is necessary. Thyroid cancer only rarely causes confusion, but occasionally the two may coexist. If apparent chronic thyroiditis regresses with suppressive thyroid therapy but a submerged nodule becomes prominent, thyroid malignancy should be suspected. One must recall that high titers of thyroid antibodies have been found in thyroid cancer, particularly in children, but ordinarily the titer is low. Graves' disease can be ruled out by failure to suppress the RAIU with TH. Subacute thyroiditis deserves consideration only when one finds slight tenderness of the gland, but the history is usually typical even in very mild cases, and the laboratory results are quite different.

Treatment

Suppressive therapy with TH (120 to 180 mg./day desiccated thyroid or its equivalent) causes significant goiter regression in the majority of cases and constitutes almost a specific therapy. It must be maintained indefinitely because interruption is followed by a rapid recurrence of the goiter. Early treatment is desirable to prevent further enlargement and nodularity and may avoid fibrous scarring that can interfere with the response to suppressive treatment in later years. Whether therapy is palliative or curative cannot be answered, though the evidence suggests that the underlying disorder continues. Very small goiters require no treatment, but the patient must be reexamined at intervals because some goiters become progressively larger, and most patients eventually become hypothyroid and require replacement therapy. Mild neck compression is usually relieved by thyroid therapy; surgery is rarely necessary. In older patients with considerable fibrosis of the thyroid, little or no regression can be expected. Corticosteroid therapy has been used in attempts to disrupt the autoimmune mechanism, but it exerts only a transient effect.

CHRONIC NONSPECIFIC THYROIDITIS

Many pathologists insist upon the presence of certain histologic changes (see p. 180) before accepting a diagnosis of Hashimoto's thyroiditis and have named cases not clearly conforming to these criteria "chronic nonspecific thyroiditis" or "chronic thyroiditis." Others believe that the Hashimoto spectrum should be broadened to include all varieties of chronic thyroiditis, excepting Riedel's struma.

RIEDEL'S STRUMA

Riedel's struma (invasive fibrous thyroiditis; sclerosing, woody, or ligneous thyroiditis) is a clinical curiosity. Only 20 cases (16 females, 4 males) were encountered in 36 years among 42,000 thyroidectomies at the Mayo Clinic (Woolner et al., 1957). The patients' ages ranged from 30 to 67 years. The thyroid is destroyed by a chronic inflammatory process of unknown etiology that bears no relationship to either De Quervain's or Hashimoto's thyroiditis. There is replacement by dense fibrous tissue that destroys thyroid parenchyma and extends beyond the thyroid capsule into adjacent structures. Patients complain of a painless unilateral or bilateral neck mass. Obstructive symptoms are not usual. The thyroid is stony hard and rigidly anchored to surrounding structures. Hypothyroidism has been found in about 20% of patients. Because of its resemblance to thyroid malignancy, a biopsy is mandatory. If neck compression occurs, palliative splitting or wedge resection of the isthmus and medial portions of the lateral lobes is done. Extensive thyroidectomy is technically impossible and usually unnecessary. Thyroid replacement therapy is required only if the patient is hypothyroid. Riedel's struma appears to be a benign nonprogressive or at least self-limited disease that bears a good prognosis.

ACUTE SUPPURATIVE THYROIDITIS

There is bacterial invasion of the thyroid by staphylococci, streptococci, or pneumococci from a contiguous or distant focus. The onset is usually abrupt with local pain, swelling, chills, fever, dysphagia with pain on swallowing, and pain on flexion or extension of the head on the neck, such pain being referred to the jaw, ear, or occipital region. The inflammation may be localized or diffuse and may either resolve or cause suppuration. The process may be subacute, with symptoms lasting from 1 to 8 weeks before the patient's admission to the hospital. Unless the manifestations are typical of cellulitis or abscess, the diagnosis may be difficult and the disorder confused with subacute thyroiditis. Thyroid function studies are normal unless the gland is extensively involved. Therapy consists of appropriate antibiotics, immobilization of the neck, local hot saline soaks, and analgesics. Surgical drainage of an abscess may be necessary. The patient must be observed carefully for possible extension of the inflammation into the mediastinum.

REFERENCES

Bastenie, P. A., et al.: Lancet 1:915, 1967.

*Cassidy, C. E.: The diagnosis and treatment of subacute thyroiditis. In Astwood, E. B., and Cassidy, C. E., editors: Clinical endocrinology, vol. 2, New York, 1968, Grune & Stratton, Inc., p. 220.

——————

*Significant reviews.

Daniel, P. M.: Immunology 12:489, 1967.

Eylan, E., et al.: Lancet 1:1062, 1957.

Felix-Davis, D., and Waksman, B. H.: Meeting of the American Rheumatism Association, Atlantic City, N. J., June 22-23, 1961 (quoted by De Groot et al., 1962).

Hall, R.: Lancet 2:187, 1960.

Hashimoto, H.: Arch. Klin. Chir. 97:219, 1912.

McConahey, W. M., et al.: J. Clin. Endocr. 22:542, 1962.

Michie, W., et al.: Lancet 1:691, 1967.

Rose, N. R., and Witebsky, E.: J. Immunol. 76:417, 1956.

*Skillern, P. G.: Thyroiditis. In Pitt-Rivers, R., and Trotter, W. R., editors: The thyroid gland, Washington, D. C., 1964, Butterworth, Inc., vol. 2, p. 130.

Vickery, A. L., and Hamlin, E. J.: New Eng. J. Med. 264:226, 1961.

*Woolner, L. B., et al.: J. Clin. Endocr. 17:201, 1957.

*Woolner, L. B., et al.: J. Clin. Endocr. 19:53, 1959.

*Woolner, L. B.: Thyroiditis: classification and clinicopathologic correlation. In Hazard, J. B., and Smith, D. E., editors: The thyroid, Baltimore, 1964, The Williams & Wilkins Co., p. 123.

Chapter 11

Thyroid cancer

Thyroid cancer accounts for only 0.5% of all cancers and slightly less than 0.5% of deaths from malignancy. It is an unusual cause for admission to a hospital. Vanderlaan, 1947, reviewed 18,668 autopsies performed at the Boston City Hospital from 1896 to 1945 and found only 5 cases. The small number of cases seen at autopsy (0.08%) is increased by 20 times, however, when special attention is paid to the thyroid gland. Silverberg and Vidone, 1966, reviewed several such series, including their own, and found an overall average of 1.79%. Sokal, 1953, estimated the incidence to be 25 patients per million population per year. Mustacchi and Cutler, 1956, surveyed representative urban centers of the United States and found 336 cases in a population of 14,600,-000. Many authorities believe that there has been a true increase in the past two decades. In areas of endemic goiter, thyroid carcinoma is often said to be more common, but the malignant foci are paranodular rather than intranodular. However, conflicting opinions concerning the incidence in endemics have been voiced (Pendergrast, 1961). Thyroid cancer differs in biologic characteristics and clinical course from malignancies of other tissues, being generally less lethal. There is evidence that some thyroid cancers are dependent on pituitary-TSH stimulation and can be controlled by TSH suppression.

Etiology

Thyroid tumors can be produced in laboratory animals by several methods, including a low-iodine diet, an antithyroid compound or partial thyroid destruction to induce excessive TSH stimulation of the thyroid with or without the addition of a carcinogen, or the use of RAI alone or in combination with a thiourea or a carcinogen. Fully 75% of children with thyroid cancer have a history of prior x-ray irradiation to the neck region. Irradiation of the adult thyroid gland can cause cancer, and an increase was found among survivors of the 1945 atomic bombing of Hiroshima and Nagasaki. The apparent rising incidence of thyroid carcinoma, particularly among children, may be attributed to testing of nuclear weapons in the 1950's, though conclusive evidence is lacking.

Thyroid cancer may stem from two sources. The first is pituitary-TSH stimulation, with the production of a hormonally dependent tumor that later may or may not become autonomous. Greenspan et al., 1967, using a new immunofluorescent assay, found significantly elevated TSH levels in all cases. The second is either prior radiation that injures the thyroid cell and may induce mutations in the genes or the exhibition of a carcinogenic compound. Children are more susceptible to carcinogenic agents, probably because "the

gene alterations leading to cancer formation presumably require cell division for
their expression" (Robbins et al., 1967)
and cell division occurs infrequently in
the adult gland. Whether thyroid carcinomas arise *de novo* or originate from preexisting adenomas is unresolved. The majority of endocrinologists believe that most
lesions, however old, are probably cancerous from their inception.

Classification and pathology

The histologic diagnosis is often arbitrary and fraught with difficulty, so that
one encounters various classifications. In
the outline below, a classification of thyroid
malignancy is presented, and in Table

11-1 some of the predominant characteristics of the main groups are outlined.

Papillary
Mixed papillary-follicular } (Differentiated)
Follicular

Anaplastic (undifferentiated)—small, giant, or
spindle cell; medullary

Miscellaneous—Hürthle, sarcoma, lymphoma,
epidermoid

Metastatic to thyroid

The papillary and follicular carcinomas
contain elements of each other and are
named according to the predominant pattern. In fact, the mixed papillary-follicular
thyroid carcinoma comprises the largest
single group.

Papillary adenocarcinoma. Papillary ad-

Table 11-1. Types of thyroid malignancy and some of their characteristics

	Papillary	*Follicular*	*Anaplastic*
Predominant age of patient	20-25 years	50-59 years	Elderly females
Histology	Unencapsulated Papillary formation on fine vascular-connective tissue stalks Large pale-staining nuclei Psammoma bodies Blood vessel invasion rare	Encapsulated Follicle formation—microfollicular, trabecular Small nuclei containing abundant coarse chromatin Blood vessel invasion	Undifferentiated (no papillary or follicle formation) Sheets of bizarre epithelial cells, large, multinucleated or elongated, spindle shaped Areas of necrosis Invasion beyond capsule
Approximate frequency	60%	20%	10%-20%
Predominant route of metastases	Lymphatics Contralateral thyroid Regional lymph nodes	Distant (bone, brain, lung)	Local and distant
Mortality	Low Death rare before age 45 Becomes more lethal after chronic prolonged course	Low to moderate Depends on characteristics outlined in text	Rapidly fatal Respiratory obstruction common
Average 5-year mortality	20%	30%	80%-90%

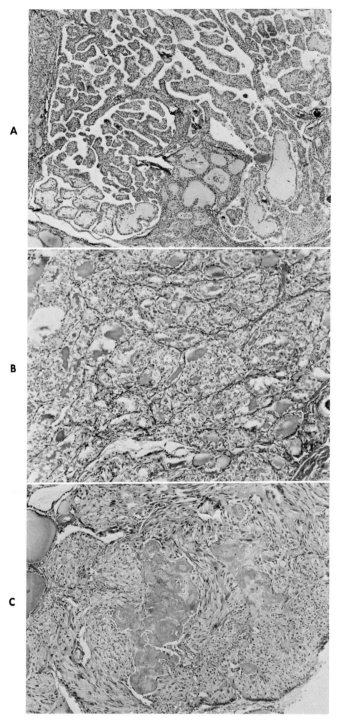

Fig. 11-1. Thyroid carcinoma. **A,** Papillary adenocarcinoma. Note psammoma bodies (calcified areas). **B,** Follicular carcinoma showing follicles lined with large neoplastic cells, some containing colloid. **C,** Medullary carcinoma showing masses of amyloid. The patient also had a pheochromocytoma. (Courtesy Dr. Alexander Nedwich and Department of Pathology, Hahnemann Medical College, Philadelphia, Pa.)

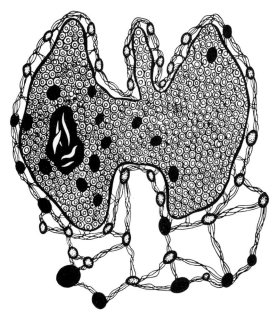

Fig. 11-2. Diagram of intraglandular thyroid lymphatics. The lymph vessels are united in a network around the follicles, penetrate the capsule, and merge with the pericapsular lymph nodes, forming a plexus on the surface of the gland. A focus of carcinoma is shown in the right lobe and spreads via the lymphatics to all parts of the gland and to the pericapsular and deep cervical lymph nodes, represented by the black areas. (From an original photograph kindly supplied by Dr. William O. Russell, University of Texas, M. D. Anderson Hospital and Tumor Institute, Houston, Texas. With permission of Cancer, Journal of the American Cancer Society **16:**1425, 1963.)

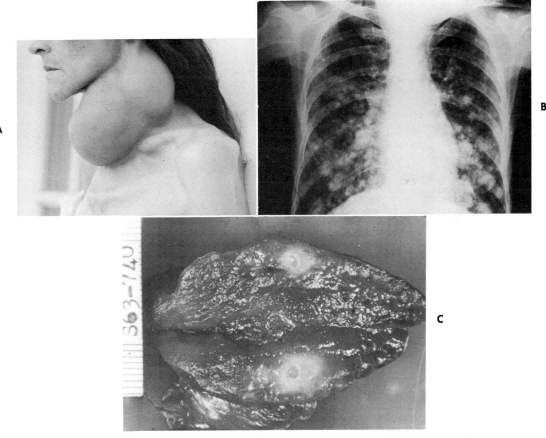

Fig. 11-3. Follicular carcinoma of thyroid. **A** and **B,** Bulky goiter with extensive pulmonary metastases. **C,** Malignant nodule with calcified rim. (**A** and **B** courtesy Dr. Carlos Minnig, Cali, Colombia, S. A.; **C** courtesy Dr. Alexander Nedwich and Department of Pathology, Hahnemann Medical College, Philadelphia, Pa.)

enocarcinoma (Fig. 11-1, *A*) is a low-grade malignancy that progresses slowly. Untreated patients have survived for years with metastases, and death is rare before age 45. Spread is via intrathyroidal lymphatics to the contralateral lobe and to regional lymph nodes (Fig. 11-2). Distant metastasis occurs in less than 10% of cases. The primary lesion may be microscopic (occult papillary carcinoma), and the diagnosis is made by biopsy of an enlarged cervical lymph node, the so-called lateral aberrant thyroid. Though usually a benign lesion, it may exhibit delayed aggressive behavior.

Follicular carcinoma. The following is Lindsay's (1964) classification of follicular carcinoma (Figs. 11-1, *B*, and 11-3): (1) *follicular variant of papillary carcinoma,* which has an identical natural history and cytologic characteristics as does papillary carcinoma; (2) *localized follicular carcinoma,* the angioinvasive encapsulated form outlined in Table 11-1; and (3) *invasive follicular carcinoma,* a more malignant lesion that probably arises in a preexisting benign adenoma and becomes an encapsulated angioinvasive adenoma. *Medullary* (Fig. 11-1, *C*) *or solid carcinomas* with a relatively solid epithelial pattern and a few microfollicles are included in this group. The solid lesions with amyloid stroma comprise a distinct entity and spread to regional lymph nodes. They are characterized by prolonged survival, despite their anaplastic histologic appearance. The amyloid is probably derived from thyroglobulin secreted by the neoplastic cells, apparently circulates in the blood, and may be deposited in the renal tubules as casts. Medullary carcinomas are often associated with pheochromocytomas, gastrointestinal mucosal neuromas, and a familial incidence. The syndrome has been transmitted over two and three generations and may be inherited as an autosomal dominant trait. Associated parathyroid adenomas have been attributed to a compensatory parathyroid response to thyrocalcitonin, a thyroid hormone that has been found in large amounts in medullary thyroid tumors. There is evidence suggesting that the medullary carcinoma cell arises from the thyroid parafollicular cell, the probable site of origin of thyrocalcitonin.

Anaplastic carcinoma. Anaplastic carcinomas are undifferentiated, highly malignant lesions found predominantly in older women; they grow rapidly and are fatal within a year. They may evolve from low-grade papillary or follicular carcinoma and exhibit residual foci of papillary and/or follicular structures. Lindsay, 1964, suggests that the giant-cell variety represents the end stage or dedifferentiated form of papillary carcinoma. The natural history of the more benign forms of thyroid carcinoma is that of metamorphosis to a highly malignant form after 20 to 25 years.

Secondary (metastatic) thyroid carcinoma. Secondary thyroid carcinomas are generally thought to be uncommon, but in a series of 28 of our cases (Perloff and Schneeberg, 1951), 6 were metastatic. Silverberg and Vidone, 1966, found that of 62 patients dying with metastasizing malignancies, 24.2% had lesions in the thyroid. The breasts, kidneys, and lungs are the most common primary sites. The histologic differentiation of primary from secondary lesions may be difficult, especially by frozen section.

Pathophysiology

Although most thyroid tumors do not retain the functions of normal tissue, some papillary and follicular adenocarcinomas concentrate iodide, respond to TSH stimulation, and can be suppressed by TH. It is not always possible, however, to correlate iodide concentration with the histologic characteristics, though, in general, anaplastic undifferentiated lesions do not accumulate iodide and follicular lesions appear to be more likely to secrete T_4. The turnover rate of iodide is usually increased, as would be expected in the presence of small acinar structures. The iodine is not discharged by perchlorate or thiocyanate, thus indicating organic binding. Thyroid cancers may produce biologically inert butanol-insoluble iodoproteins. One of these, called compound X, has been found in 60% of patients with thyroid malignancy, was partly soluble in butanol, and resembled serum albumin (Robbins et al., 1955). After therapy with RAI, thyroglobulin may be found in serum and iodotyrosines in urine.

Clinical features

Females predominate by approximately 2:1, a ratio considerably lower than for other thyroid disorders. The age of occurrence is shown in Table 11-1.

Symptoms and signs. The principal finding is an *asymptomatic mass in the neck.* Well-differentiated cancers tend to present as a localized nodule, whereas undifferentiated lesions frequently exhibit a bulky goiter with early symptoms of neck compression (Fig. 11-3). Malignancy is suspected if a nodule or mass is found in a previously normal gland or if a known nodule begins to enlarge and becomes indurated, irregular in outline, and fixed. Carcinomatous nodules are usually firmer than adjacent normal thyroid tissue, though they can become soft from necrosis. Spread beyond the thyroid capsule can produce hoarseness, dysphagia, or dyspnea. Tracheal deviation is more common with benign goiters, but tracheal fixation is an important sign. Thyroid cancers are ordinarily painless unless they enlarge rapidly. Occasionally one finds an enlarged cervical lymph node containing papillary thyroid elements with an apparently normal thyroid gland, a situation that was called "lateral aberrant thyroid," but foci of papillary adenocarcinoma are usually found when the homolateral thyroid lobe is explored. Only rarely do these lateral masses prove to be sequestered, benign, thyroid nodules or true lateral, aberrant, ectopic, thyroid tissue. Enlargement of the Delphian nodes, found just above and below the isthmus, is evidence of metastatic thyroid cancer. Lymph nodes may be the site of metastases in the supraclavicular areas and can be found by x-ray examination in the mediastinum and hilar regions of the lungs. Axillary metastases are so rare that their presence should suggest a secondary thyroid carcinoma. Rarely the initial complaint is bone pain or a pathologic fracture from osseous metastases, cough from pulmonary metastases, or transverse myelitis from vertebral metastases. The malignancy rarely destroys enough of the gland to induce hypothyroidism. The presence of thyrotoxicosis tends to reduce any suspicions of coexisting thyroid cancer, but recent statistics from the Armed Forces Institute of Pathology (Olen and Klinck, 1966) reported an incidence of cancer with hyperthyroidism of 2.5%. Coexisting parathyroid adenomas have been observed. Diarrhea may occur with medullary carcinoma.

Laboratory findings

The laboratory offers limited assistance. The value of RAI scanning of thyroid nodules has been discussed in Chapter 7. Seven percent to 58% of cold nodules are cancerous, and the remainder are the site of inactive colloid nodules, adenomas, cysts, and hemorrhagic or necrotic areas, or are foci of thyroiditis (Fig. 11-4). The enhanced uptake of radiophosphorus (^{32}P) has not proved sufficiently reliable for diagnostic purposes. Soft tissue x-ray films of the neck may reveal the crescentic calcifications of psammoma bodies. The finding of various butanol-insoluble iodoproteins may arouse suspicion of cancer, though the finding lacks specificity. The presence of high titers of circulating antithyroid antibodies establishes the presence of Hashimoto's thyroiditis, though they may rarely be found in thyroid cancer. The coexistence of both conditions has been noted. Needle biopsy of thyroid nodules may spread the disease or may miss the lesion. Unilateral thyroidectomy combines diagnosis and therapy in one procedure and is preferable to open biopsy. A frozen section is usually performed at the time of surgery.

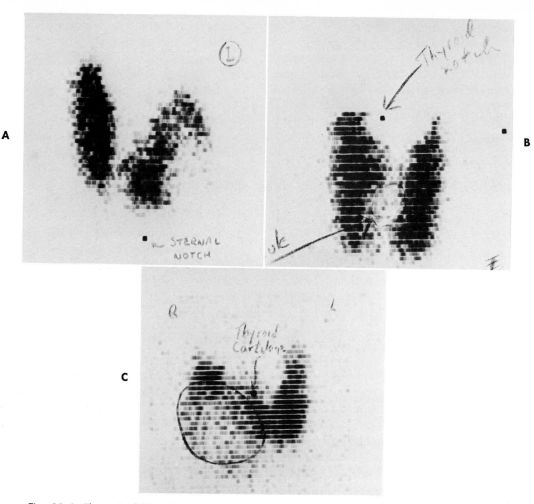

Fig. 11-4. Three "cold" nodules suspected of harboring thyroid cancer. **A,** Large, hard nodule in left lower lobe that was a follicular carcinoma. **B,** Small, firm, mobile isthmus nodule that appeared during pregnancy and continued to enlarge slowly. Diagnosis: papillary carcinoma. **C,** Firm large mass in right neck that was a benign follicular adenoma.

Differential diagnosis

Thyroid cancer must be differentiated from benign thyroid nodules, goiter, cysts, and thyroiditis. Rapid progressive thyroid enlargement may occur in amyloid goiter, a rare cause of thyroid enlargement. The management of the solitary nodule is discussed on p. 127.

Treatment

Surgery. Surgical excision is the keystone of therapy and combines eradication of the primary lesion with ample excision of surrounding tissue. In the management of the solitary nodule, one never enucleates the nodule per se but performs unilateral thyroidectomy (lobectomy), together with excision of the isthmus. If the nodule is located in the isthmus, total thyroidectomy is required. Because of the frequency of contralateral dissemination, many authorities recommend total thyroidectomy in all cases, but this method remains controversial. Russell, 1963, has graphically illustrated (Fig. 11-2) the abundant network of intralobar lymphatics, which may channel tumor cells from one lobe to the other. Among his 80 patients, 70 had spread of tumor cells to the isthmus, to the other lobe, to the pericapsular lymph nodes of the opposite lobe, or to more than one of these structures. Others, however, less frequently find bilateral involvement. The more radical the operation, the more likely is recurrent laryngeal nerve damage or inadvertent parathyroidectomy. Since total extirpation is a necessary preparation for subsequent RAI therapy of metastases, this need may be considered an additional reason for total thyroidectomy. Certainly the opposite lobe should be explored in all cases. The neck must be carefully inspected and involved lymph nodes excised. In the latter instance total thyroidectomy is necessary. Routine prophylactic radical neck dissection on the involved side, though advocated by some authorities, is considered by Crile an unnecessary and mutilating procedure, particularly in young patients. He removes only involved lymph nodes. If other metastatic lymph nodes appear at a later date, they are removed as they appear. Neck dissection is done where there is wide dissemination of invasive papillary carcinoma (Crile, 1964). A solitary distant metastasis may be excised in the hope of totally eradicating cancer. The value of postoperative x-ray treatment, especially where local metastases have been excised, is not established, though reasonably good results have been reported. Complete surgical eradication is not always possible, especially in anaplastic cancers, and radical surgery is often abandoned in favor of palliative excision followed by radiation therapy.

Radioiodine (RAI). RAI is used in the treatment of surgically inaccessible metastatic lesions or in inoperable cases. Its value is limited to lesions that will, or can be induced to, accumulate sufficient RAI to exert a destructive effect. This method requires prior eradication of all functioning thyroid tissue by surgery or RAI. Undifferentiated tumors rarely concentrate RAI

and, in the main, are not amenable to treatment. Notable exceptions have been observed sufficiently often to suggest that complete reliance on histologic characteristics may be misleading. The quantity of RAI accumulated by the tumor can be determined by administering a large tracer dose of ^{131}I and (1) scanning appropriate areas, (2) gauging the total body retention by measuring the 48- to 72-hour urinary excretion, (3) performing autoradiography of a metastatic lesion subjected to biopsy, or (4) by all three. Usually one must depend on the urinary excretion study, though neck and body scans are valuable. The patient is given 0.5 to 1.0 mCi. ^{131}I, and if the excretion is 60% or less, one infers the presence of functioning thyroid tissue. A cancericidal dose (100 to 150 mCi.) of ^{131}I is administered. Doses that are too small or administered in divided aliquots are not effective and may induce subsequent radioresistance or increase the degree of malignancy. If there is insufficient retention to justify treatment, residual tissue is stimulated by TSH injections, or endogenous pituitary-TSH is increased by the administration of antithyroid drugs. Catz et al., 1959, attempt to eliminate every remnant of normal thyroid tissue and all potentially cancerous cells by periodic TSH administration, 10 units daily for 5 to 7 days, followed by tracer doses of 1 to 2 mCi. ^{131}I. If total body and neck scans then reveal any residual thyroid tissue, 40 to 100 mCi. ^{131}I is administered. Suppressive doses of liothyronine (75 to 150 μg. daily) are then given to render the patient euthyroid and to suppress endogenous TSH. After a therapeutic dose the patient is restudied monthly. If therapy need not be repeated, the patient is restudied every 3 to 6 months. If an antithyroid drug is used to increase the uptake of RAI, one gives propylthiouracil 1,000 mg., or methimazole 100 mg., daily for 1 to 3 months and then omits the drug for 3 to 5 days and determines the RAI retention by measuring the 48- to 72-hour urine excretion. Disadvantages of these methods of increasing the concentration of ^{131}I in metastases are sensitivity reactions to TSH, stimulation of tumor growth, drug reactions, and the prolonged hypothyroid state necessary for success with antithyroid drugs, together with the inevitable delay in treatment that this involves. In the interval, endogenous TSH may stimulate the malignancy to further growth or metamorphosis to a more malignant state. Methods to deplete the patient of iodine, such as the use of an iodine-deficient diet combined with intravenous mannitol, may prove to be of help in increasing the RAI uptake.

Toxic reactions to radioiodotherapeusis include mild radiation sickness, bone marrow depression, and amenorrhea. Less common untoward effects, increased in frequency with very large dosages, are pancytopenia, aplastic anemia, leukemia, liver dysfunction, and pulmonary fibrosis (in patients with extensive pulmonary metastases). Precautions against the radiation hazards from the patient and his excreta must be supervised by the therapist.

Suppression with thyroid hormone. Well-differentiated thyroid cancers may be TSH-dependent and can be suppressed by 180 mg. or more of desiccated thyroid per day. Lesions may regress and recurrences may be prevented. It has recently been shown (Greenspan et al., 1967) that larger doses of TH are required to suppress TSH in cases of thyroid cancer than in other thyroid disorders. Treatment should be maintained for the duration of life.

Prognosis

The natural history of thyroid malignancy is characterized by a prolonged course commonly with late metamorphosis to a more malignant type, so that clear-cut evaluation of the various therapeutic modalities is not presently possible. The outlook for prolonged survival is greatest for the differentiated, predominantly papillary types and becomes less favorable for the follicular, solid, and Hürthle cell carcinomas. Crile reported that 10 of 107 pa-

tients with papillary carcinoma died of the disease but found that if a patient was free of cancer 5 years after surgery, recurrence was rare. The small papillary lesions first discovered because of nodal metastasis or found incidentally during thyroid operations for other conditions ("occult papillary carcinoma") are, in the main, not lethal. The undifferentiated anaplastic carcinomas are fatal in less than a year. Halnan, 1966, found a consistent inverse correlation between age at the time of diagnosis and survival within the groups of differentiated and undifferentiated tumors and suggested that "existing methods of treatment may have much less influence on survival than often is thought." In Crile's series, 1964, of papillary cancers, the mortality rate in the group over 48 years of age was 31% compared to 2% in the group less than 48 years. McDermott et al., 1954, published the following cumulative survival rates:

	5 years	10 years	20 years
Papillary	73%	60%	45%
Follicular	71%	48%	24%
Undifferentiated	17%	17%	17%

Subsequent pregnancy has no apparent deleterious effect on the course of the disease.

REFERENCES

Catz, B., et al.: Cancer **12**:371, 1959.
Crile, G., Jr.: Ann. Surg. **160**:178, 1964.
Greenspan, F. S., et al.: American Thyroid Association meeting, 1967, Ann Arbor, Mich.
Halnan, K. E.: Cancer **19**:1534, 1966.
*Lindsay, S.: Pathology of the thyroid gland. In Pitt-Rivers, R., and Trotter, W. R., editors: The thyroid gland, vol. 2, Washington, D. C., 1964, Butterworth, Inc., p. 255.
McDermott, W. V., Jr., et al.: J. Clin. Endocr. **14**:1336, 1954.
Mustacchi, P., and Cutler, S. J.: New Eng. J. Med. **255**:889, 1956.
Olen, E., and Klinck, G. H.: Arch. Path. **81**: 531, 1966.
Pendergrast, W. J.: J. Chronic Dis. **13**:22, 1961.
Perloff, W. H., and Schneeberg, N. G.: Surgery **29**:572, 1951.
Robbins, J., et al.: J. Clin. Endocr. **15**:1315, 1955.

*Significant reviews.

Robbins, J., et al.: Ann. Intern. Med. **66**:1214, 1967.

Russell, W. O., et al.: Cancer **16**:1425, 1963.

Silverberg, S. G., and Vidone, R.: Pacif. Med. Surg. **73**:175, 1966.

Silverberg, S. G., and Vidone, R. A.: Ann. Surg. **164**:291, 1966.

Sokal, J. E.: New Eng. J. Med. **249**:393, 1953.

Vanderlaan, W. P.: New Eng. J. Med. **237**:221, 1947.

Chapter 12

The adrenal cortex

ANATOMY OF THE ADRENAL CORTEX

The adrenal glands are composed of an outer *cortex* surrounding a small core, the *medulla*. They cap the upper poles of the kidneys at the level of the eleventh dorsal vertebra. The right is triangular, whereas the left is more oblong or crescentic. They are encapsulated, invested in renal fascia, and embedded in perirenal adipose tissue. In guinea pigs, after intracapsular adrenalectomy, the connective tissue capsule is capable of regenerating the complete adrenal cortex. On sectioning, most of the cortex is yellow except for the brown zona reticularis. The average weight of the normal single adrenal removed at surgery is 3.5 to 4 grams in the female and 4 to 4.5 grams in the male, whereas the weight of a gland removed at autopsy averages 6 to 6.5 grams (Symington, 1962). The difference may be explained by antemortem stress.

Blood supply. Considerable variation of the blood supply exists, but usually there are three suprarenal arteries: the superior, middle, and inferior, originating, respectively, from the inferior phrenics, the aorta, and the renal arteries. The suprarenal arteries traverse the gland surface (capsular plexus) and divide into 20 to 50 small branches that encircle the gland and penetrate the capsule to form a subcapsular arterial plexus from which sinusoidal capillaries (Fig. 12-1) traverse the zona glomerulosa, widening as they reach the zona fasciculata. Free anastomoses between adjacent capillaries increase as the capillaries proceed through the deeper layers of the zona fasciculata. The capillaries are lined by reticuloendothelium and are therefore more accurately called "sinusoids." Venous drainage is via a single main central vein that empties on the right into the inferior vena cava and on the left into the renal vein. The adrenal vein in man contains longitudinal, irregularly spaced muscle bundles whose functional significance is unknown, though Symington, 1962, suggested that they may represent a means of control of adrenocortical secretion. The arterial supply of the adrenal medulla is independent of the cortex and consists of medullary arteries that traverse the cortex radially without giving off any cortical branches. Epinephrine constricts the medullary arteries and diverts blood flow into the sinusoids of the cortex. This shift is a probable physiologic response to stress, for the purpose of increasing adrenocortical activity. For a description of the blood supply see Dobbie et al., 1968.

Innervation. A suprarenal plexus derived from the splanchnic nerves richly innervates the adrenal medulla. The adrenal cortex is devoid of innervation except for nerve fibrils in relation to the vasculature. Postganglionic fibers innervate the longitudinal muscle of the adrenal vein.

Embryology. The fetal cortex arises from the mesoderm of the ventral coelomic epithelium and is ten to twenty times the size of the adult gland, relative to body weight.

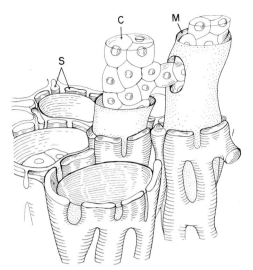

Fig. 12-1. Structure of the adrenal cortex (zona fasciculata). Stereogram of parenchymal cords, **C,** surrounded by "basement membranes," **M,** and sinusoids or capillaries, **S.** (From Elias, H., and Pauly, J. E.: Endocrinology **58:**714, 1956.)

The fetal zone comprises 80% of the fetal gland at term and consists of large cells with large pale-staining nuclei and abundant eosinophilic cytoplasm. In the outer 20% (definitive, permanent, or preadult cortex), fascicular and glomerulosa zones become the adult cortex when the fetal adrenal gland involutes soon after birth. The adrenal loses about 50% of its weight within 2 to 3 weeks without any signs of adrenal insufficiency appearing in the infant, and the gland gradually assumes an adult architecture.

The fetal zone is absent in anencephalic monsters, indicating its dependence on pituitary ACTH. It is a functioning organ that produces active steroids, with the exception of aldosterone. Fetal blood contains a high level of the estrogen precursors, Δ^5-3β-hydroxysteroids, such as dehydroepiandrosterone. These compounds disappear as the fetal cortex undergoes involution. Excessive destruction of fetal corticosteroids by the placenta has been suggested (Lanman, 1962) as an explanation of the marked hypertrophy of the fetal cortex.

The adrenal medulla originates from ectodermal cells of the neural crest, which form two cell types, the sympathoblast or stem cells of the mature sympathetic ganglia and the pheochromoblasts, which give rise to the chromaffin cells of the adrenal medulla. The latter migrate, at the 20 mm. stage of the embryo, to the mesoderm that forms the cortex and penetrate the cortical anlage in cordlike masses, finally uniting within the cortex. The two cell types also may be found along the sympathetic nerve ganglia and plexuses and the organ of Zuckerkandl near the aortic bifurcation. These paraganglionic masses are large in the newborn but involute rapidly, though they may be a source of tumor growth.

Accessory adrenocortical tissue, often containing chromaffin tissue, is usually found in close apposition to the adrenal glands but may occur within the kidney parenchyma or anywhere from the diaphragm to the pelvis. Although its physiologic importance in man is doubtful, it has been found in some 30% of autopsies.

Histologic structure of the adrenal cortex (Fig. 12-1). The adrenocortical parenchyma is composed of delicate connective tissue supporting a continuum of three zones of epithelial cells bounded by capillaries so that each cell is in contact with circulating blood. In the outer, thin, subcapsular *zona glomerulosa* the cells are arranged in clusters, U-shaped nests, or ovoid masses exhibiting a great variety of structural types. It is rarely prominent and may be undefinable or present only focally as a few groups of cells. The *zona fasciculata* constitutes a large portion of the cortex and is the middle zone forming a broad belt of parallel radially directed cords and strands of cells adjacent to thin capillaries extending from the zona glomerulosa to the zona reticularis. The *zona reticularis* is sharply defined as a pigmented network of irregularly arranged, compact cells adjacent to the adrenal medulla. The relative volumes of the three zones as determined by Swinyard, 1940, are as follows: zona glomerulosa 15%, zona fasciculata 78%, and zona reticularis 7%. Cell proliferation is greatest in the zona glomerulosa and least in the zona reticularis. Three hypotheses have been advanced to account for adrenocortical growth and repair (Deane, 1962b): (1) *cell-migration hypothesis*—cells arise in the capsule or by glomerulosa cell division and migrate to the medullary border, where they die and disappear; (2) *zonal hypothesis*—cells remain in situ and replicate as required; and (3) *transformation field hypothesis*—cells of the zona fasciculata predominate in function and cell duplication; the zona glomerulosa and zona reticularis are reserve zones capable of transforming into fasciculata-like cells during adrenal hyperfunction. Regeneration from the capsule of the guinea pig adrenal has been previously alluded to.

The zona glomerulosa is relatively independent of pituitary ACTH, is not stimulated by injected ACTH, and survives hypophysectomy, whereas the remainder of the gland atrophies (Fig. 5-1). It is the probable source of aldosterone. The zona fasciculata and zona reticularis are ACTH-dependent, undergoing atrophy in its absence, and are the probable source of the corticosteroids, the androgens and the estrogens. They comprise a unit with the clear cells of the zona fasciculata serving as a storage depot for steroid precursors. Possibly the most active biosynthetic site is the clear cells at the interface between the zona fasciculata and zona reticularis. See Symington, 1962, and Dobbie et al., 1968, for discussions of the structure of the adrenal cortex.

Electron microscopy. Studies reveal abundant tubulovesicular mitochondria that are probably of primary importance in steroidogenesis. In the zona glomerulosa the mitochondria are elongated with laminar cristae; in the zona fasciculata they are larger and ovoid with vesicular cristae, and in the zona reticularis the cristae are variable in size, shape, and structure. The adrenocortical cells are separated from subendothelial spaces by a basement membrane and send numerous microvilli into these spaces. Whether cytoplasmic projections that are seen to penetrate the basement membrane and the capillary endothelium are the mechanism of secretion into the circulation is a matter of speculation. Fenestration of the endothelial cells may represent a route for secretory products. For a review see Luse, 1967, and Long and Jones, 1967.

ADRENOCORTICAL HORMONES
Steroid chemistry

The cyclopentanophenanthrene nucleus forms the carbon skeleton of the adrenocortical steroids. It consists of 17 carbon atoms comprising three 6-carbon rings (A, B, C) and one 5-carbon ring (D) arbitrarily numbered from ring A to ring D as shown below.

Sterane nucleus

Carbons at positions 18 and 19 arise from carbons at positions 13 and 10, respectively, to form the "sterane" nucleus. Each carbon has attached hydrogens that are customarily not shown. The CH_3 at C^{18} and C^{19} is omitted and is usually shown as a projecting line. When a hydrogen is absent (that is, unsaturated), a double bond is inserted and its origin is designated by the prefix "delta" (Δ) or the suffix "ene." The number following the Δ indicates the first carbon of the double bond. Thus in the formula below the designation is "Δ^4."

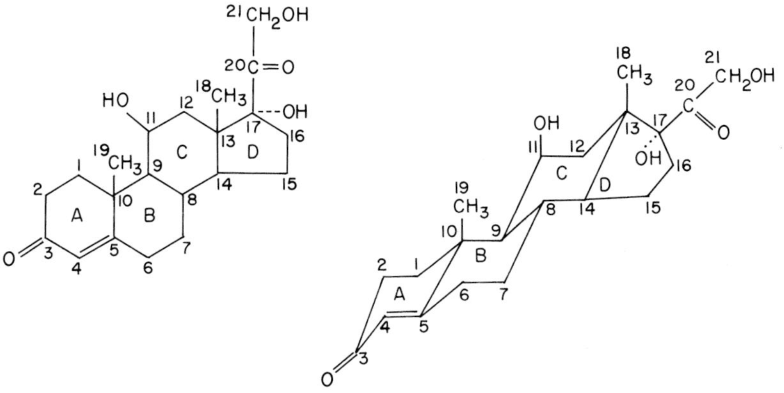

Fig. 12-2. Stereochemical structure of cortisol. On the left is the conventional two-dimensional structure, and on the right is a side view showing the three-dimensional configuration. (From Travis, R. H., and Sayers, G.: In Goodman, L. S., and Gilman, A. Z.: The pharmacologic basis of therapeutics, ed. 3, New York, 1965, The Macmillan Co.)

Two double bonds are denoted by "diene" with the Δ followed by two numerals indicating the origin of each double bond. Thus a double bond between C^4 and C^5 and one between C^6 and C^7 would be "$\Delta^{4,\,6}$-diene."

An important side chain, the C^{20} and C^{21}, arises from C^{17}, forming the C_{21} *compounds*. The parent nucleus is called "pregnane," from which all of the corticosteroids are derived.

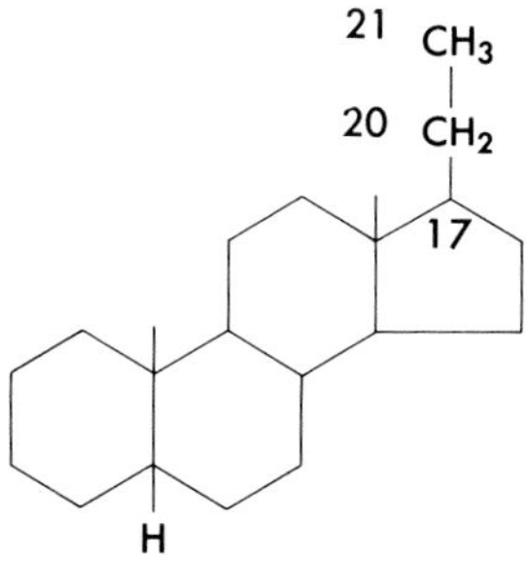

Pregnane

Cortisol (hydrocortisone) is the principal corticosteroid and has 21 carbons, the important C^{21} side chain, the C^{4-5} double bond and oxygenation at C^{11} and C^{17} (Fig. 12-2).

The C_{19} *compounds*, derived from the parent nucleus androstane, are androgens and 17-ketosteroids (17-KS).

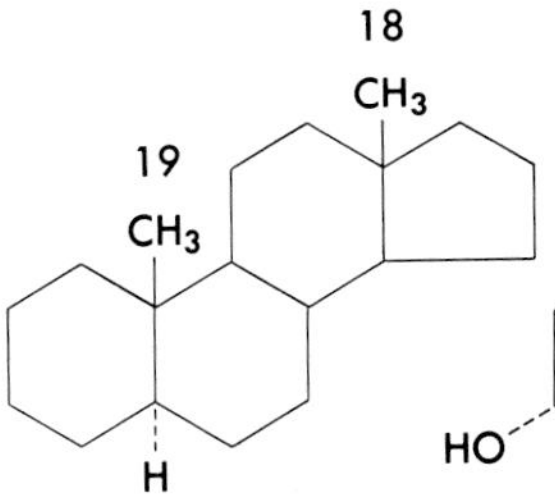

Androstane 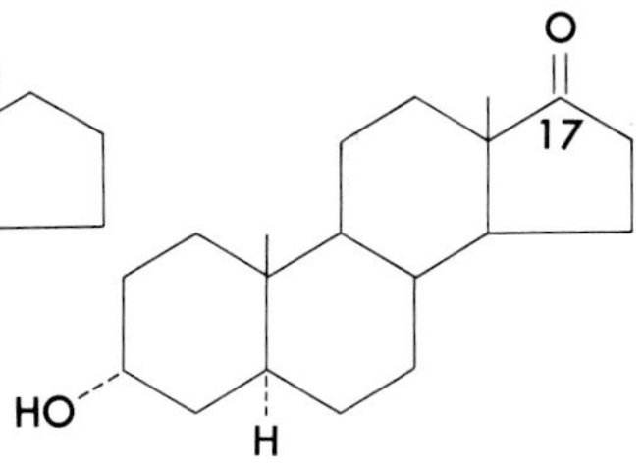   Androsterone

They have 19 carbons and a ketone on C^{17}. Androsterone is a typical 17-KS.

The C_{18} *compounds*, derived from estrane, are estrogens. Estradiol is the most potent of the group.

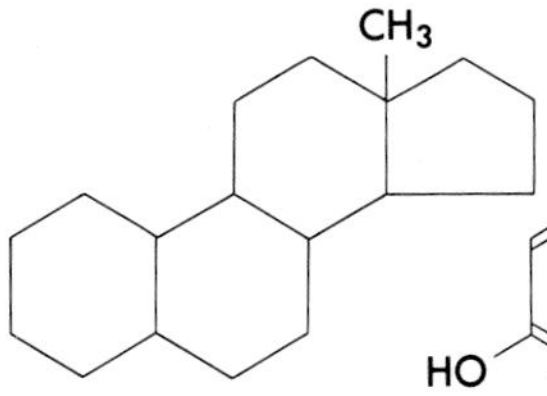

Estrane 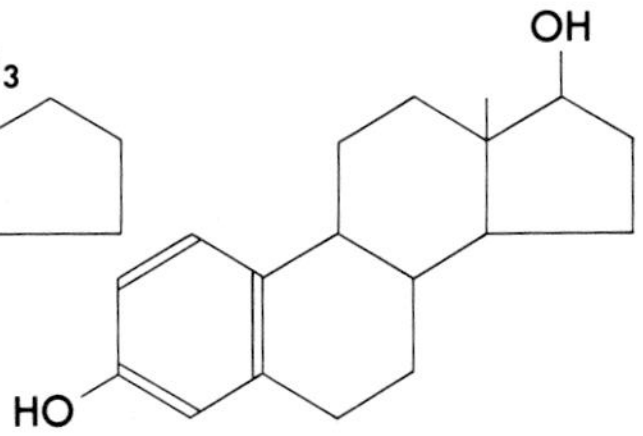   Estradiol-17β

Nomenclature of some of the substitutions and additions is as follows:

1. *Hydroxyl*, —OH; prefix, hydroxy-; suffix, -ol; two hydroxyls = dihydroxy.
2. *Ketone*, or *carbonyl*, =O; prefix, keto- or oxo-; suffix, -one.

The more commonly used designation "keto-" may also be called "oxo-." Thus 17-keto-steroids and 17-oxosteroids are synonyms. Two carbonyl groups are called "dione."

3. *Desoxo-*, or *deoxo-*, indicates hydrogenation of a ketone group $\left(C=O \rightarrow C \begin{smallmatrix} H \\ \\ H \end{smallmatrix} \right)$.

4. *Desoxy-*, or *deoxy-*, indicates hydrogenation of a hydroxyl group (C—OH→C—H₂).

5. *Dehydro-* indicates loss of adjacent hydrogens to form a double bond joining 2 carbons (CH—CH→C=C).

6. *Tetrahydro-* indicates hydrogenation of ketone and double bonds, as commonly occurs on ring A:

Formation of a tetrahydro compound

An example of the naming of a compound is the C_{18} estrogen called "estrone."

$\Delta^{1,3,5(10)}$-Estratriene-3-ol-17-one,
3-hydroxy-$\Delta^{1,3,5(10)}$-estratriene-17-one
(estrone)

The Δ names the double bonds between carbons 1-2, 3-4, and 5-10. In order to show the ending of the 5-10 double bond, which does not follow numerical sequence, the number 10 is inserted. "Triene" indicates three double bonds. "3-ol" shows the hydroxy group at C^3, and "17-one" indicates a ketone at C^{17}. An alternative chemical name is shown in the illustration. Because the chemical name is too cumbersome, compounds are usually designated by shorter *trivial names* such as "estrone" in the compound shown. The first adrenocortical hormone to receive a trivial name was corticosterone, and the other adrenocortical compounds were named as derivatives.

Stereochemistry

Steroids exist in three dimensions as shown in Fig. 12-2. The designation "alpha-" (α), shown by a *dotted* valence bond, indicates an atom behind the plane of the molecule. The position is called "trans-" and compounds of this configuration are called "allo-." "Beta-" (β) projects above or in front of the plane, is shown by a *solid* valence bond, and is in the "cis-" position, and compounds of this configuration are celled "etio-." "Epi-" refers to an unusual radical. Thus in cortisol one hydroxyl is 11β; the 11α variety is called 11-epicortisol. The four 6-carbon rings A, B, C, and D are locked into a three-dimensional stable conformation corresponding to the general shape of a chair (Moore and Heftmann, 1962):

In cortisol all the attached groups are in the β position except the hydroxyl at C^{17}, which is in the α position (Fig. 12-2). The biologic activity of a steroid compound can be greatly changed by altering its configuration. The 11β-hydroxyl, the C^{19} β-methyl, and the C^4-C^5 double bond appear to be essential. Reduction of C^{20} to a hydroxyl causes a major loss of potency. Cortisol is the most potent of the naturally occurring corticosteroids; conversion of the C^{11} hydroxyl to a ketone, the structure of cortisone, reduces glucocorticoid potency by about 20%. Removal of the 17α-OH from cortisol, the structure of corticosterone, causes considerable loss of potency in humans but not in small animals. Added substituents to the cortisol molecule may considerably enhance its biologic potency. These substituents are the "cortisol analogues." In Table 12-1, seven of these substituted compounds are shown, together with their relative potencies.

Table 12-1. Synthetic analogues of cortisol and cortisone

Compound	Trade name	Formula	Relative potency	Equivalent dose in mg.	Salt retention
Cortisol (hydro-cortisone)	Cortef Cortril	CH₂OH / C=O / HO ...-OH / C D / A B / O	100	20	Moderate
Cortisone	Cortisone Cortone Cortogen	O= C	80	25	Moderate
Predniso-lone (Δ¹-corti-sol)	Meticorte-lone Delta-Cortef Hydeltra	A / O	400	4	Slight
Prednisone (Δ¹-corti-sone)	Meticorten Deltra Deltasone Paracort	O / C / A B / O	300	5	Slight
6α-Methyl predniso-lone	Medrol	A B / O / CH₃	500	4	None
Fludro-cortisone (9α-fluor-ocortisol)	Florinef F-Cortef Aflorane	A F / O	1,000 to 2,500	0.1*	Marked (100 × corti-sone)

*Usual dose for mineralocorticoid effect.　　　　　　　　　　　　　　*Continued.*

Table 12-1. Synthetic analogues of cortisol and cortisone—cont'd

Compound	Trade name	Formula	Relative potency	Equivalent dose in mg.	Salt retention
Triamcinolone (16α-hydroxy-9α-fluoroprednisolone)	Kenacort Aristocort	CH_2OH, $C{=}O$, HO, ---OH, ---OH, D, F, O	500	4	None
Dexamethasone (16α-methyl-9α-fluoroprednisolone)	Decadron Dexameth Deronil Hexedrol Gammacorten	CH_2OH, $C{=}O$, ---OH, ---CH_3, D	3,000	0.5-0.75	None
Betamethasone (16β-methyl-9α-fluoroprednisolone)	Celestone	CH_2OH, $C{=}O$, ---OH, CH_3, D	2,600	0.6	None

Types of adrenocortical steroids

The adrenal cortex produces three types of steroid compounds—corticosteroids, mineralocorticoids and sex steroids.

Corticosteroids. Corticosteroids ("sugar" or "metabolic" hormones, corticoids, glucocorticoids, 11,17-oxysteroids, 17-hydroxycorticoids) are produced principally by the zona fasciculata and have widespread metabolic effects. *Cortisol* comprises 80% of the corticosteroids found in adrenal venous blood. The daily production varies from 15 to 30 mg. in the resting state to 150 to 250 mg. when maximally stimulated.

Chemical name—11β,17α,21-trihydroxy-Δ4-pregnene-3,20-dione; or Δ4-pregnene-3,20-dione-11,17α, 21-triol

Trivial names—cortisol, hydrocortisone, Kendall's compound F

Corticosterone is the principal secretory product in many animals. About 2 to 5 mg./day is secreted in man. It differs from cortisol only in its lack of hydroxyl at C^{17} and is considerably less active in humans.

Chemical name—11β,21-dihydroxy-4-pregnene-3,20-dione; or 11β,21-dihydroxypregn-4-ene-3,20-dione

Trival names—corticosterone, Kendall's compound B

Mineralocorticoid. Mineralocorticoid ("salt-retaining hormone"), or aldosterone, derived from the zona glomerulosa, is the principal electrolyte-regulating hormone.

Its sodium-retaining activity is 100-fold greater than that of other corticosteroids. It is believed to exist in two forms in equilibrium:

11,18-Hemiacetal form   Open form

11β,21-Dihydroxy-3,20-diketo-4-pregnen-18-al
(aldosterone)

Chemical name—11β,21-dihydroxy-3,20-diketo-4-pregnen-18-al; or Δ⁴-pregnene-11β,21-diol-3,20-dione-18-al

Trivial name—aldosterone

The normal secretion rate on an unrestricted diet averages 250 μg./day, up to 1,000 μg. with salt restriction and as low as 50 μg. with sodium chloride administration.

Sex steroids. The sex steroids consist of androgens, estrogens, and progesterones.

Androgens are C_{19} steroids derived from the zona fasciculata and zona reticularis, as well as from the testes, and have biologic effects resembling those of testosterone, though of considerably less potency. Most have a carbonyl group at C^{17} and are excreted in the urine as 17-ketosteroids (17-KS). Dehydroepiandrosterone (DHEA) constitutes about 70% of the 17-KS of adrenal origin. The adrenal secretion rate of DHEA is 25 to 30 mg./day. The following compounds have been isolated from adrenal tissue: dehydroepiandrosterone, androstenedione, androstenolone, 11β-OH-androstenedione, testosterone, androsterone, 11β-OH-epiandrosterone, 6β-OH- and 6α-OH-androstenedione. The first four have been isolated from adrenal vein blood, and 11β-OH-androstenedione and androsterone are formed exclusively in the

adrenal cortex. Other steroid-producing tissues lack the essential 11β-hydroxylase enzyme. Testosterone, the most potent androgen, can be synthesized by adrenocortical tissue and is probably produced in small quantities in normal individuals. The C_{19} steroids are often divided into the stronger androgens containing 2 oxygen atoms ($C_{19}O_2$) and the weaker ones containing 3 oxygen atoms ($C_{19}O_3$).

Estrogens. The adrenal cortex is not a physiologically important source of estrogens. Most of the data concerning adrenal estrogen production are derived from studies of pathologically hyperfunctioning glands. Nonetheless, small amounts have been found in the urine of castrated women and disappear after adrenalectomy. Estrone has been isolated from ox adrenals.

Progesterone, a C_{21} compound, is a key intermediate in the synthesis of the corticosteroids, and a number of its metabolic products may appear in the urine. The progestational effects of adrenal progesterone are antagonized by the corticosteroids.

Biosynthesis of adrenocortical steroids

Corticosteroids. Adrenocortical steroids are derived from a small pool of adrenal cholesterol via acetate → acetyl coenzyme A → mevalonic acid → squalene → lanosterol → zymosterol → desmosterol → cholesterol. Cholesterol loses its side chain, possibly through a number of steps involving intermediates of dihydroxycholesterol, to form Δ^5-pregnenolone:

Cholesterol Δ^5-Pregnenolone

The latter is converted into progesterone by the enzyme 3β-dehydrogenase, which replaces the 3-hydroxy with a 3-carbonyl, and by a 3-keto-isomerase enzyme to transfer the double bond from the 5-6 position to the 4-5 position.

Δ^5-Pregnenolone   Progesterone

Progesterone occupies a key position in the subsequent transformations leading to the formation of cortisol, other corticoids, and aldosterone. The synthesis of cortisol involves three sequential hydroxylating-enzyme reactions at C^{17}, C^{21}, and C^{11} as follows:

Progesterone 17α-Hydroxyprogesterone

Cortisol can also be formed from 17-OH-pregnenolone. Some progesterone is converted to 11-desoxycorticosterone (DOC) by hydroxylation of C^{21} and thence to corticosterone by 11β-hydroxylation:

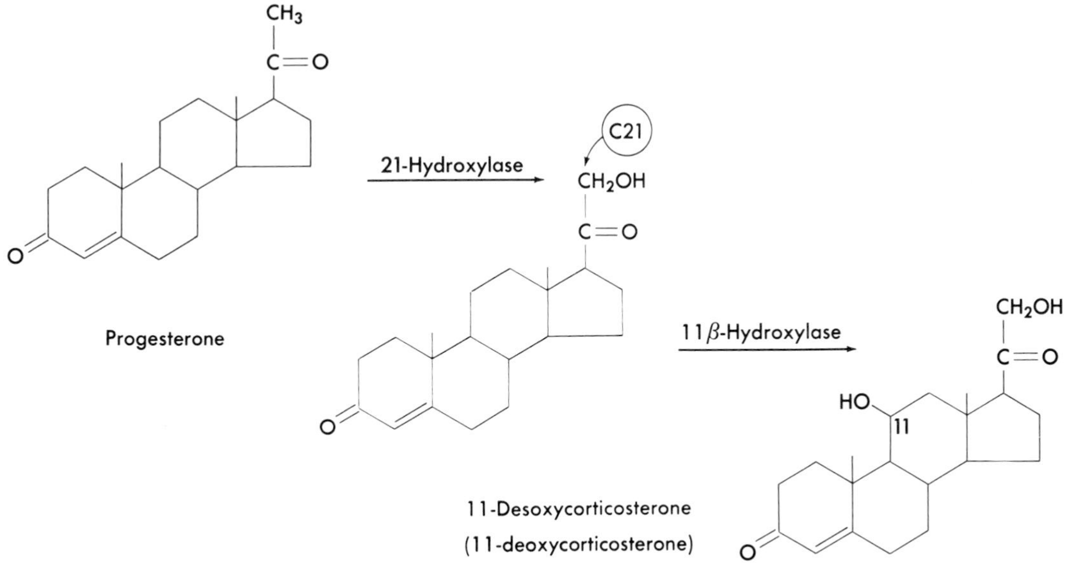

Progesterone

11-Desoxycorticosterone
(11-deoxycorticosterone)

Corticosterone

This conversion is the major pathway in mice and rats, species in which corticosterone, rather than cortisol, is the major corticosteroid.

The enzymes governing these synthetic reactions are located in various parts of the adrenocortical cell. Those that remove the cholesterol side chain and the 11β-hydroxylase enzyme are in the mitochondria; 3β-dehydrogenase is found in the microsomal fraction; and the 17- and 21-hydroxylases are found in the soluble fraction.

Thus steroid compounds are apparently transferred from one intracellular structure to another during the biosynthetic process.

Aldosterone. There is as yet no complete agreement concerning the major pathway for aldosterone synthesis. Corticosterone and/or desoxycorticosterone were thought to be the chief intermediaries, but recently

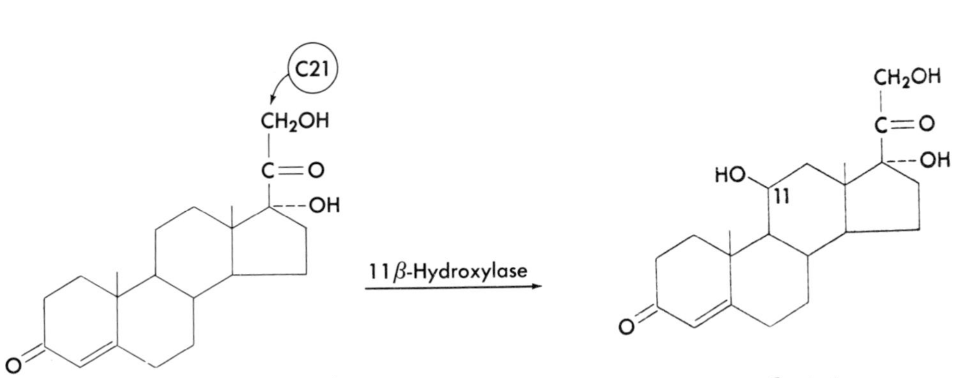

11-Desoxycortisol
(11-deoxycortisol)

Cortisol
(hydrocortisone)

18-hydroxycorticosteroid compounds seem the most likely immediate precursors (Samuels and Uchikawa, 1967). The following is a possible pathway:

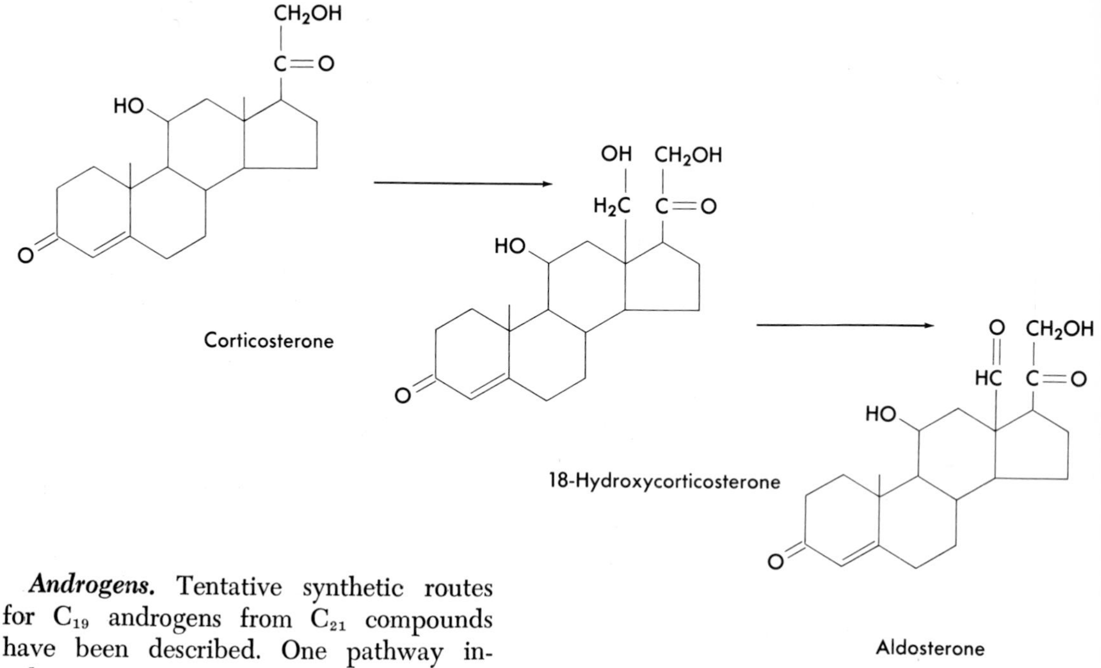

Corticosterone

18-Hydroxycorticosterone

Aldosterone

Androgens. Tentative synthetic routes for C_{19} androgens from C_{21} compounds have been described. One pathway involves the conversion of 17-OH-progesterone to androstenedione and thence to testosterone.

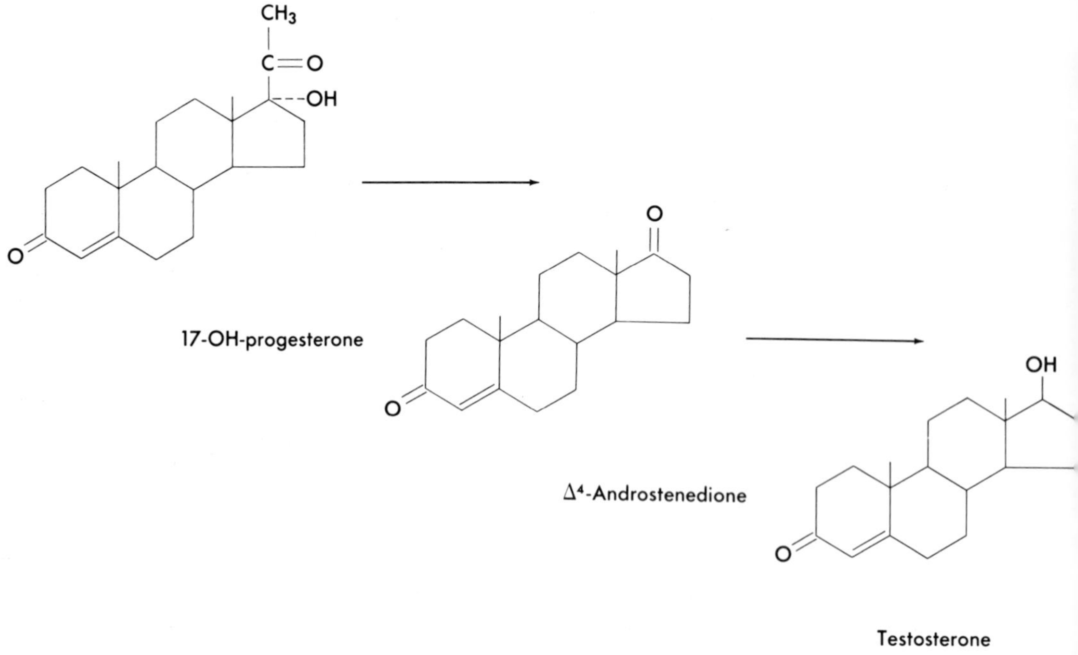

17-OH-progesterone

Δ^4-Androstenedione

Testosterone

Androstenedione has about 10% of the androgenic potency of testosterone. Dehydroepiandrosterone (DHEA) apparently is not a product of progesterone but appears to arise from Δ^5-pregnenolone → 17-OH-pregnenolone, and it is converted into Δ^4-androstenedione. *Steroid sulfates* are presently thought to be secretory products rather than degradation products of the adrenal cortex, and the possibility has been entertained that the biosynthetic sequence may be as follows: cholesterol sulfate → Δ^5-pregnenolone sulfate, 17-OH-pregnenolone sulfate → dehydroepiandrosterone sulfate (Lieberman, 1967).

Estrogens. The adrenocortical synthesis of estrogens is still a subject of controversy. The synthetic pathways at the present time are hypothetical, and there is as yet no unequivocal proof that estrone can be derived from 19-OH-Δ^4-androstenedione or that estradiol-17β stems from testosterone via 19-OH-testosterone.

Ascorbic acid. ACTH induces a rapid discharge of adrenal ascorbic acid, but the function of the vitamin in adrenocortical physiology remains a mystery. It may enhance biosynthesis by some action in the mitochondrial electron-transport chains (Bransome, 1968).

Regulation of adrenocortical steroid synthesis-secretion

Corticosteroids. The hypothalamic corticotrophin-releasing factor (CRF) evokes pituitary ACTH secretion, and this axis comprises the chief regulator of corticosteroid production. The likely focus of ACTH is upon the conversion of cholesterol to pregnenolone facilitated by TPNH (Haynes-Berthet theory). In fact, ACTH may itself play a role in regulating the supply of TPNH. Koritz and Hall, 1964, found that pregnenolone could inhibit cholesterol hydroxylation in adrenal mitochondria in vitro. They hypothesized that ACTH might stimulate the release of pregnenolone from mitochondria and thus stimulate steroidogenesis by relieving the inhibition of cholesterol hydroxylation. Cir-

culating free cortisol is the physiologically active steroid fraction, whereas cortisol bound to plasma protein (transcortin) is inert. The free cortisol level maintains a fairly constant circadian (24-hour) rhythm under unstressed conditions (Fig. 14-1). Any physiologic circumstance that depletes free cortisol stimulates the secretion of CRF → ACTH and increases the level of circulating ACTH and the adrenocortical secretory rate. The level of free cortisol is restored. One can turn off the extremely sensitive CRF–ACTH–adrenal secretory axis rapidly by the administration of a corticosteroid in a dose exceeding the normal production. Long-term administration induces adrenocortical atrophy. A direct action of cortisol upon the adrenal cortex may exert some additional regulatory control. Under various conditions of *stress* corticosteroid inhibition may or may not constitute an ACTH inhibiting signal. Yates, 1967, found that dexamethasone blocked ACTH release under certain stressful stimuli (ether, epinephrine, burn, abdominal incision, electric shock) but not under others (vasopressin, intestinal traction, hemorrhage, cervical dissection, exposure to 100% nitrogen, and a larger dose of epinephrine). The level of circulating cortisol necessary to inhibit the CRF-ACTH mechanism is higher during stress than under normal conditions. Suppression does not readily occur even when relatively large doses of corticosteroids are administered. The control of adrenocortical activity has been reviewed by Yates.

Though epinephrine and norepinephrine may evoke a discharge of ACTH, these agents are probably of minimal physiologic importance. Vasopressin indirectly provokes corticotrophin release by evoking a CRF response and may have a direct stimulating action on the adrenal cortex.

Aldosterone. The complex regulation of aldosterone secretion has been attributed to a number of factors. There is no unique aldosterone-stimulating hormone.

RENIN-ANGIOTENSIN SYSTEM. Renin is secreted by the juxtaglomerular apparatus, a renal secretory unit consisting of two parts: (1) *juxtaglomerular cells* (JG), highly specialized myoepithelial cells that form a cuff about the walls of the renal afferent arteriole just before it enters the glomerulus; the JG cells contain granules that are the site of renin formation or storage; and (2) *macula densa,* consisting of specialized epithelial cells in the first segment of the distal convoluted tubule. These cells are in contact with the JG cells and may signal the tubular electrolyte content to the JG apparatus. A decrease in mean pressure in the renal afferent arteriole (by assuming the upright posture or by salt depletion) → decreased stretch of the arteriolar wall → JG cells form renin granules and secrete renin into blood-lymph → angiotensin I $\xrightarrow[\text{enzyme}]{\text{hydrolyzing}}$ angiotensin II → stimulation of zona glomerulosa of adrenal cortex to secrete aldosterone (as well as cortisol and corticosterone) → retention of Na + H_2O by renal tubules → increase of blood volume, blood pressure, and renal blood flow → rise of mean arteriolar pressure → increased stretch of arteriolar wall → reduction of renin secretion. The reverse effects will result from an increase in mean afferent arteriolar pressure (by salt loading), resulting in inhibition of aldosterone secretion. Davis, 1967, believes the above sequence constitutes a negative feedback system that functions physiologically to maintain homeostasis in the face of wide variations of sodium intake. The increase in circulating aldosterone found in pregnancy may be attributed to increased renin-angiotensin activity and to the high concentration of estradiol and estriol.

ELECTROLYTE. Sodium restriction is a potent stimulus to aldosterone secretion. A second extra-adrenal sodium–retaining factor has been postulated that is necessary to prevent the escape from aldosterone-induced sodium retention. Aldosterone, plus this factor, appears to be necessary for maintaining Na + H_2O retention by the kidney. Potassium loading increases and depletion reduces aldosterone secretion, probably by its influence on the movement of sodium. The potassium ion has a direct but minor effect on the adrenal cortex; the Na^+/K^+ ratio may be important. Bartter, 1966, induced a decreased aldosterone secretion in the face of hyponatremia and hyperkalemia by expanding extracellular fluid volume, leading him to doubt the importance of electrolyte changes. Hypomagnesemia can increase aldosterone secretion.

BARORECEPTORS. A decrease in extracellular fluid volume reduces intravascular volume and evokes a rise in aldosterone. A number of receptor sites (baroreceptors) sensitive to volume changes and to alterations in the stretch of vascular walls has been described in the carotid artery and right atrium. Constriction of the inferior vena cava constitutes a stimulus to aldosterone secretion.

NEURAL REGULATION. A number of workers have searched for evidence of diencephalic and midbrain control of aldosterone secretion, and Farrell, 1959, described a pineal extract, "adrenoglomerulotropin," that elicited aldosterone secretion. Recent evidence, however, from Farrell's laboratory has implicated ubiquinone, found in pineal lipid fractions, as an inhibitor, rather than a stimulator, of aldosterone secretion (Fabre et al., 1965). Emotional stimuli and stress may increase the aldosterone secretion rate. Sympathetic nerve control may play a mediating role in the aldosterone response to assumption of the upright posture and sodium depletion.

ACTH. Pituitary ACTH plays a subsidiary role in the regulation of aldosterone secretion but appears to be a prerequisite for maximal production. In some instances ACTH stimulates aldosterone secretion, whereas in others, such as secondary hyperaldosteronism, its role is supportive. Its effect is enhanced by sodium depletion, reduced by sodium loading, and self-limited after several days even when its action on cortisol persists. Pituitary ablation in humans is associated with low urinary aldosterone excretion and reduced secretion rate. Suppressive corticosteroid administration decreases the aldosterone secretion rate and reduces the adrenal response to angiotensin.

HEPATIC REGULATION. Impaired liver metabolism and clearance of aldosterone may induce hyperaldosteronism, and homeostatic mechanisms must be brought into play to restore the normal level. The biologic half-life of aldosterone is prolonged in severe liver disease.

Whether the above six regulatory mechanisms involve a common denominator or act singly or in concert must await further exploration. It seems likely that electrolyte and volume alterations function as signals to the renin-angiotensin system and that the other factors are subsidiary.

Circulating adrenocortical hormones

In man approximately 80% of the circulating corticosteroids is composed of cortisol. The normal plasma concentration of 17-OHCS ranges from 4 to 30 μg./100 ml. with a diurnal variation. About 50% is unconjugated and 50% metabolized to the glucuronidated tetrahydro derivative. The biologic half-life is 100 to 115 minutes in normals and is markedly prolonged in liver disease and myxedema and shortened by hypoglycemia and hyperthyroidism. The liver metabolizes circulating steroids, converts them to more unsaturated and more water-soluble compounds (such as tetrahydrocortisol) and conjugates them mainly with glucuronic acid. Aldosterone is present in amounts less than a hundredth of the cortisol level.

Protein binding. Ninety percent of the circulating cortisol is bound to an alpha globulin formed chiefly in the liver called "corticosteroid-binding globulin," "CBG," or "transcortin." At higher plasma-cortisol levels, CBG becomes saturated and binding to albumin increases. Cortisol and corticosterone have the highest affinity and aldosterone the lowest for CBG. However, an aldosterone-binding protein different from CBG may be involved. The cortisol-binding capacity of CBG varies from 15 to 26 μg. of cortisol bound per 100 ml. of plasma. It is increased by estrogens, pregnancy, and fasting and decreased in liver cirrhosis, nephrosis, multiple myeloma; in the newborn infant; in boys with gynecomastia or cryptorchidism; and in women with hirsutism, hypertension, obesity, diabetes, and menstrual disorders (de Moor et al., 1965). Though the total plasma-corticosteroid level is altered in these conditions, the cortisol bound to CBG is biologically inactive and the free cortisol remains unchanged. However, free cortisol values in apparently eucorticoid subjects treated with estrogen may be somewhat elevated. Protein binding acts as a buffer against rapid changes in free cortisol and may protect it from liver destruction. The renal excretion of cortisol depends on the net effect of glomerular filtration of the unbound steroid and tubular resorption. Urinary free cortisol is therefore directly related to circulating free cortisol. For a review see Cope, 1964b, and Daughaday, 1967.

Diurnal rhythm. A *circadian* or *diurnal* (24-hour) *rhythm* of circulating cortisol with a peak at 8 A.M. and a gradual fall commencing at noon and continuing to the lowest point at midnight is a normal physiologic phenomenon (Fig. 14-1). Doe et al., 1960, found the percent of the mean cortisol value to be 126% at 6 A.M., 123% at 9 A.M., 88% at 3 P.M., and 54% at 9 P.M. Urinary 17-OHCS values exhibit a similar rhythm. These diurnal patterns are controlled by a circadian cycle of plasma ACTH. The circadian ACTH and cortisol patterns maintain homeostasis and do not reflect changes in cortisol production rate. These physiologic rhythms are disturbed or abolished by Cushing's syndrome, by various forms of stress, and by brain damage involving the cerebral cortex or reticular-activating system and are diminished in hypothyroidism and obesity. Reversal of the time of sleep and physical activity of several days' duration leads to an appropriate reversal of the circadian pattern. An apparent circadian rhythm for aldosterone may be governed by day-night postural changes. See Nichols and Tyler, 1967, for a review.

Metabolism, transformations, and excretion

The liver is the principal site of metabolic enzymatically controlled transforma-

tions of adrenocortical steroids. The kidney effects minor changes.

Cortisol to cortisone. An early reversible transformation is the oxidation of the C^{11} hydroxyl to a ketone, with conversion of cortisol to the probably biologically inactive cortisone. Some of the latter is excreted unchanged in small amounts.

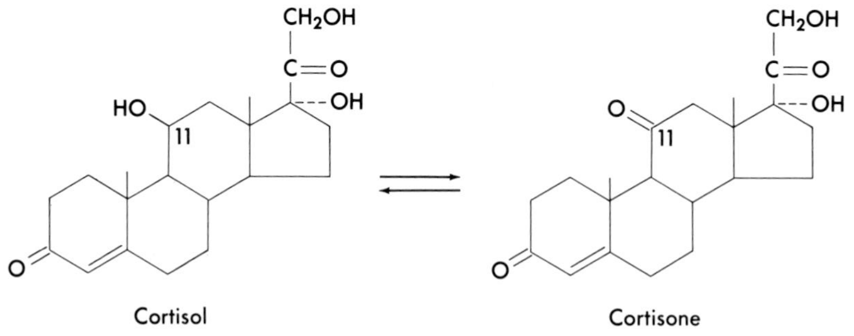

Cortisol

Cortisone

Reduction in ring A to form tetrahydro compounds

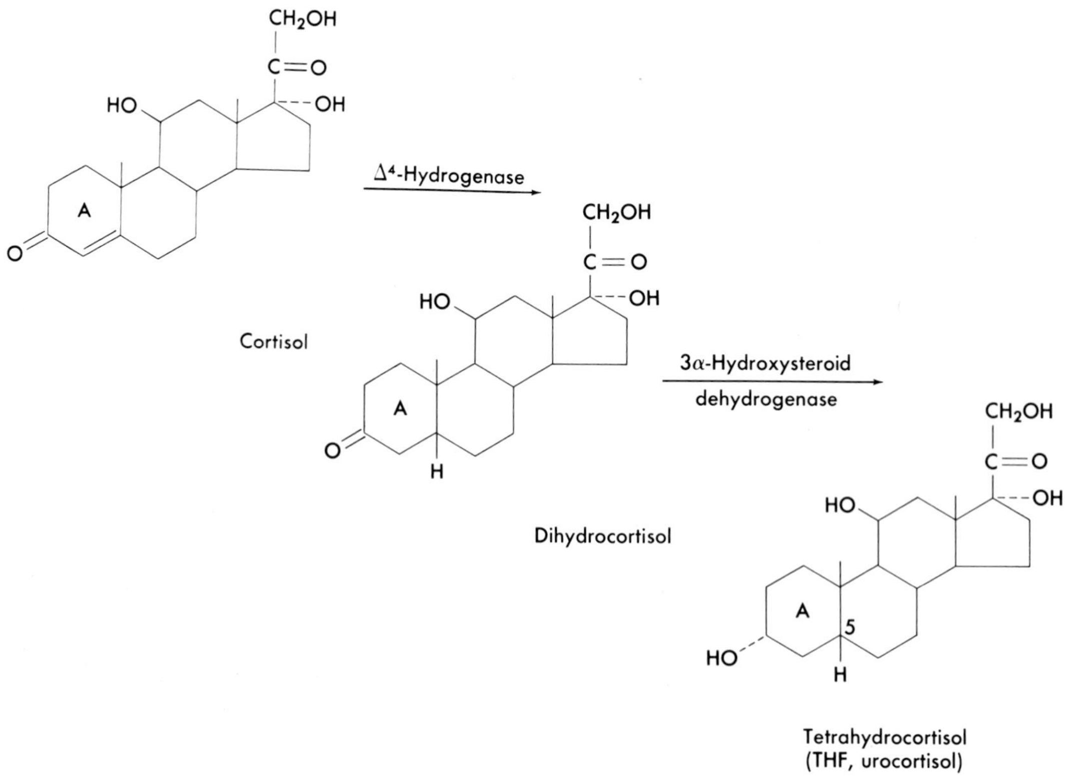

Cortisol

Δ^4-Hydrogenase

Dihydrocortisol

3α-Hydroxysteroid dehydrogenase

Tetrahydrocortisol
(THF, urocortisol)

Cortisone, aldosterone, and other corticosteroids undergo these same transformations to tetrahydro derivatives. Aldosterone is metabolized to tetrahydroaldosterone and a 3-oxoconjungate aldosterone.

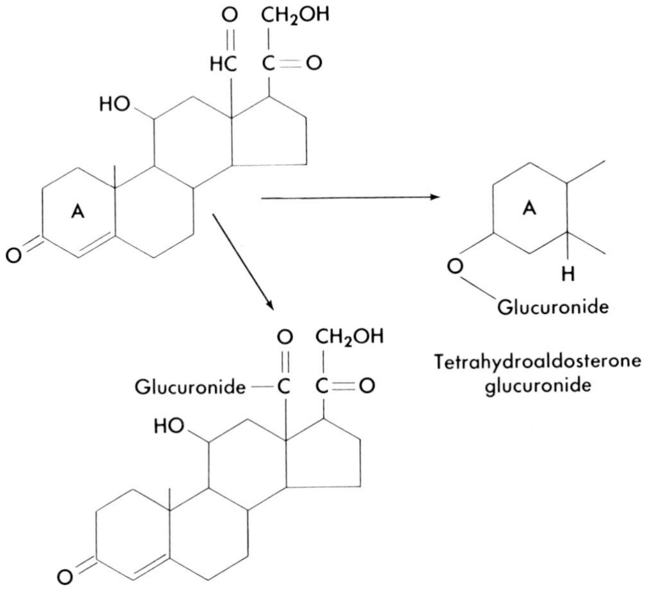

Tetrahydroaldosterone glucuronide

3-Oxoconjugate aldosterone glucuronide

Thus tetrahydrocortisol (urocortisol), allotetrahydrocortisol, and tetrahydrocortisone (urocortisone) make up half of the metabolites of cortisol. In *allo*tetrahydrocortisol the hydrogen at C^5 is in the α position, whereas in the other two compounds it is in the β position. About half the secreted aldosterone is reduced to the tetrahydro derivative and excreted as a glucuronide. These metabolic products comprise most of the 17-OHCS found in urine. The daily excretion of cortisol is 40 to 50 μg., of tetrahydrocortisol 0.5 to 1.5 mg., and of tetrahydrocortisone 1 to 6 mg. (Cope, 1964c). These compounds are combined with glucuronic acid at the C^3 position to form glucuronides.

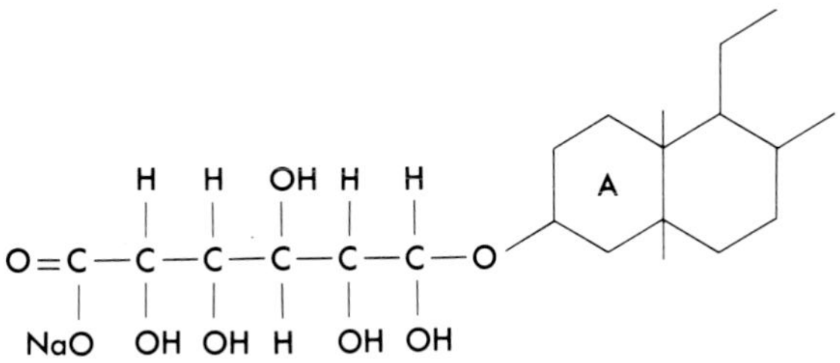

Tetrahydrocortisol glucuroniside sodium

Small amounts of sulfuric acid conjugates may be formed, especially in newborn infants. Glucuronidation renders the conjugates water soluble and promotes renal excretion. The tetrahydro compounds are biologically inactive, and the reactions shown above are irreversible.

Formation of cortols and cortolone. Cortols and cortolone constitute about one fourth the cortisol metabolites and are formed by reduction of the C^{20} ketone with the addition of hydrogen to form a C^{20} hydroxyl.

Tetrahydrocortisol   β-Cortol

Tetrahydrocortisone is transformed into a cortolone. Cortols and cortolones are conjugated with glucuronic acid and are excreted in the urine.

Formation of 6β-hydroxycortisol. 6β-hydrocortisol is a compound formed by hydroxylation of cortisol at C^6 and is a minor metabolic product of cortisol, particularly in infants. It may be synthesized in small amounts by the adrenal cortex.

Formation of 17-ketosteroids. There may be removal of the entire C^{21} dihydroxyacetone side chain to form 17-KS of the 5β series such as 3α, 11β-dihydroxyetiocholane-17-one and 3α-hydroxyetiocholane-11,17-dione (Rosenfeld et al., 1967).

Biologic effects of corticosteroids

Corticosteroids exhibit a wide diversity of both stimulatory and inhibitory effects and influence the metabolism of most body tissues. The adrenal cortex is indispensable for life and necessary for the metabolic response to stress. Death results in several days if the adrenal glands of animals are removed.

A "permissive" role of cortisol was described by Ingle, 1943, wherein the hormone establishes a necessary milieu or conditioning process so that certain biologic actions that remain dormant in the adrenalectomized animal may be expressed. For example, Ingle found that small doses of adrenocortical extract induced a full-blown restoration of the diabetes of an adrenalectomized, partially depancreatized rat given estrogen, whereas the estrogen was not effective in the absence of the adrenal hormone.

Carbohydrate metabolism. Corticosteroids increase the production of glucose; hence the term "glucocorticoids," or "sugar hormones." They augment the concentration of hepatic glycogen by stimulating gluconeogenesis and, in excessive doses, induce hyperglycemia, glycosuria, an anti-insulin effect, and some inhibition of the peripheral utilization of glucose, alterations described as "steroid diabetes." There is suppression of glucose phosphorylation and altered membrane transport of glucose. The block is between extracellular glucose and intracellular glucose-6-phosphate (Munck and Brinck-Johnsen, 1967). Adrenalectomy leads to diminished mobilization of protein and amino acids, decreased gluconeogenesis, depletion of hepatic and to a less extent muscle glycogen, insulin hypersensitivity, low blood sugar levels, fasting hypoglycemia, and hypoglycemia unresponsiveness. All these phenomena are corrected by the administration of cortisol.

Protein metabolism. Corticosteroids restore the diminished nitrogen excretion of fasting adrenalectomized rats and increase nitrogen excretion in intact fasted animals. The plasma urea and amino acids are increased and the hepatic uptake of the latter is accelerated, suggesting that the liver may trap amino acids and shunt them to pyruvate and glucose. The adrenal cortex is essential for the normal turnover of protein; corticosteroids exert a protein catabolic, an antianabolic, or a combined effect. Most of the evidence suggests that the major effect is antianabolic. Cortisol causes a rapid net decrease in the synthesis of mRNA leading to reduced synthesis of structural protein.

Fat metabolism. The mobilization of fatty acids from adipose tissue and their transport to the liver is under corticosteroid control and is closely linked to glucose metabolism. Ketosis is minimal in adrenalectomized animals and the mobilization of fatty acids induced by catecholamines or growth hormone is restricted. Excessive cortisol leads to hyperlipidemia and an increase of total body fat, together with a reduction of protein.

Water and electrolytes. Cortisol promotes Na and H_2O retention and K excretion. Adrenalectomy lowers the glomerular filtration rate, effective renal plasma flow and tubular excretion, promotes renal and extrarenal salt loss and delays the excretion of a water load. Salt wasting leads to hyponatremia, dehydration, hypotension, and azotemia. These alterations are restored by the administration of corticosteroids. Some of the improvement in the excretion of a water load may be ascribed to a reversal of the tendency of water to shift from the extracellular to intracellular space noted in adrenal insufficiency.

Blood and lymphoid tissues. Corticosteroids cause thymic and lymphoid involution, lympholysis, lymphopenia, and eosinopenia, with a relative increase in polymorphonuclear leukocytes. There is a reduction of mRNA and protein synthesis in lymphoid tissues, though the opposite effect has been found for liver (White et al., 1967). Polycythemia, thrombocytosis, shortening of the clotting time and of the partial thromboplastin time, and an increase in antihemophilic factor have been described.

Bone and calcium metabolism. Osseous and cartilaginous epiphysial synthesis and proliferation are impeded, leading to inhibition of linear skeletal growth. The protein matrix and subsequently the mineral content of bone are reduced, resulting in osteoporosis. Corticosteroids have a hypocalcemic effect probably because of the combined action of reducing calcium absorption from the gut, antagonizing the effects of parathyroid hormone and of vitamin D, and inhibiting excessive bone resorption. They reverse the hypercalcemia of most conditions except hyperparathyroidism. They increase urinary phosphate excretion and reduce the $TmPO_4$ and the plasma inorganic prosphate.

Immunologic effects and hypersensitivity. Glucocorticoids suppress antibody production in some experimental animals but not invariably in monkey or man. Although people who are overdosed with corticosteroids and patients who have Cushing's syndrome exhibit impaired resistance to infection, the union of antigen and antibody is not inhibited. Corticosteroids relieve the acute manifestations of hypersensitivity reactions such as asthma, allergic rhinitis, urticaria, and serum sickness, but the mechanism is unknown. A number of chemical mediators have been implicated (histamine, serotonin, bradykinin), but histamine has been considered the chief offender. The pharmacologic action of histamine such as the immediate wheal and flare phenomenon is not altered, though the transformation of histidine to histamine is depressed and tissue histamine is depleted.

Inflammation and infection (Grant, 1967). Corticosteroids exhibit an antiinflammatory effect. The mechanism is obscure, but the prevention of the formation of vasoactive kinins, agents that may be in part responsible for the inflammatory reaction, has been suggested. They prevent lysosome disruption and thus prevent the release of endogenous proteases and other enzymes. There is suppression of vascular permeability, of lymphocyte and phagocyte migration and accumulation, and endothelial sticking of leukocytes. Bactericidal and phagocytic potency of white blood cells appears to be impaired, though there is considerable conflicting evidence. There is inhibition of fibroblastic proliferation and suppression of hyaluronic acid formation and collagen production. Wound healing and the formation of granulation tissue may be impaired.

Gastrointestinal effects. Hypochlorhydria frequently follows adrenalectomy, whereas cortisol administration may lead to increased hydrochloric acid and pepsin secretion and gastric ulcer formation in susceptible individuals. The mechanism may be due to the excessive acid secretion, combined with a decrease of the protective gastric mucous coating. The inflammatory reaction is minimal, and healing is retarded.

Cardiovascular effects. A normal level of circulating corticosteroids is essential to permit a normal pressor response to catecholamines and other vasoconstrictors in adrenal insufficiency and to ensure adequate myocardial function. Schayer, 1967, has postulated an intrinsic stress- or inflammation-activated microcirculatory dilator, probably histamine, that is antagonized by corticosteroids. Thus the dilator tends to open capillaries, and corticosteroids tend to close them. The blood pressure–maintaining effect of corticosteroids is probably due to a combination of the above factors and a tendency to increase angiotensin.

Central nervous system effects. Prolonged administration of corticosteroids to susceptible individuals can induce reversible psychic changes, including depression, euphoria, irritability, insomnia, and psychosis. They increase the excitability of the central nervous system. The electroencephalogram is altered in adrenal insufficiency and restored by replacement therapy. In subjects with normal adrenal function, pharmacologic doses of corticosteroids produce EEG changes. The detection sensitivity for taste, smell, and hearing is greatly enhanced in patients with adrenocortical insufficiency and returned to normal by corticosteroid replacement therapy.

Muscle effects. Adrenalectomy is followed by muscle weakness that is relieved in part by correction of electrolyte changes and restoration of blood pressure but is completely ameliorated only by glucocorticoids. "Steroid myopathy" is associated with mitochondrial swelling, an increase in glycogen, lipid deposition, vacuolization, fraying of filaments, and areas of necrosis (Ritter, 1967). Corticosteroids inhibit muscle glucose utilization.

For a review of the physiologic effects of cortisol, see Beck and McGarry, 1962.

Biologic effects of aldosterone

Hypoaldosteronism causes Na depletion, K retention, dehydration, hemoconcentration, hypotension, and, ultimately, shock (Addisonian crisis).

Renal effects. Aldosterone increases Na and Cl reabsorption in the distal convoluted tubule but promotes a loss of hydrogen, ammonium, and possibly magnesium. Water is retained, leading to an increase of extracellular fluid volume and a decrease of renin secretion by the juxtaglomerular apparatus. After several days the sodium-retaining effect subsides, but potassium excretion continues. The mechanism of this "escape" is unknown. Large doses of progesterone and the spironolactones inhibit the effects of aldosterone on the renal tubule.

Saliva and sweat. Aldosterone reduces the Na/K ratio of saliva and the Na content of sweat. The renal "escape" phenomenon does not occur.

Blood pressure. Blood pressure tends to be elevated indirectly by means of an increase of total exchangeable Na and extracellular fluid volume and apparently not by means of the renin-angiotensin effect, since renin levels tend to decrease.

Relation to other endocrine glands and hormones

Thyroid gland. Glucocorticoids tend to suppress thyroid function (p. 98).

Growth hormone (GH). Corticosteroids block the physiologic effects of GH as evidenced by retardation of growth in children, in experimental animals, and in juvenile Cushing's syndrome. There is interference with the proliferation of epiphysial cartilage and with the production of cartilaginous matrix, and there is suppression of the normal rise of plasma GH that is evoked by hypoglycemia.

Gonadotrophins. Corticosteroids exert variable effects on urinary gonadotrophins, though a marked transient rise has usually been found. Oligomenorrhea or amenorrhea is almost the rule in Cushing's syn-

drome and frequently occurs in women treated with cortisol in pharmacologic doses. The mechanism may be related to effects on the hypothalamic–anterior pituitary axis and also to the frequent concomitant hypersecretion of adrenal androgens. Gross ovarian atrophy results from prolonged cortisol therapy.

Antidiuretic hormone (ADH). Hypersecretion of ADH has been postulated to explain the delayed excretion of a water load found in patients with adrenocortical insufficiency; an ADH-corticosteroid feedback relationship has been suggested, but the evidence has been conflicting.

LABORATORY TESTS OF ADRENOCORTICAL FUNCTION

Most tests of adrenocortical function involve the measurement of plasma and/or urinary 17-OHCS. The completeness of 24-hour urine collections should be veri-

Table 12-2. Drugs that can interfere with the determination of urinary 17-hydroxycorticoids (17-OHCS), 17-ketogenic steroids (17-KGS), or 17-ketosteroids (17-KS)*

Drug	Effect on: 17-OHCS	17-KS	17-KGS
Meprobamate (Equanil, Miltown) Triacetyloleandomycin (Cyclamycin, TAO) Spironolactone	↑	↑	↓
Phenaglycodol Penicillin Nalidixic acid (NegGram)		↑	↑
Chlordiazepoxide hydrochloride (Librium) Etryptamine acetate (Monase)	↑	↓	
Chlorpromazine (Thorazine)	↓	↑	
Hydroxyzine (Atarax)	↑		
Reserpine	↓	↓	
Diatrizoate meglumine and iodipamide (Duografin)			↓
Progestins (contraceptive agents)	↓	↓	

*Based on data from Llerena, O., and Pearson, O. H.: New Eng. J. Med. **279**:983, 1968; Nelson, J. C., et al.: J. Clin. Endocr. **28**:1515, 1968; and Borushek, S., and Gold, J. J.: Clin. Chem. **10**:41, 1964.

Table 12-3. The two principal methods for "group" estimations of corticosteroids

		Side chain		
		(21) CH_2OH (20) $C=O$ ----OH Dihydroxy-ketone side chain (α-ketol)	All other C^{21} side chains originating at C^{17}	
	Corticosteroid compounds measured	Cortisol Cortisone 11-Desoxycortisol Tetrahydrocortisol Tetrahydrocortisone Tetrahydro-11-desoxycortisol	Cortol Cortolone 17-OH-progesterone Pregnanetriol	
1. *Porter-Silber (PS) chromagens*	Reaction with phenylhydrazine in $H_2SO_4 \rightarrow$ yellow color	+	−	*Normal daily urinary excretion:* 3-12 mg. (male) 2- 8 mg. (female)
2. *17-ketogenic (oxygenic) steroids (17-KGS)*	Removal of dihydroxyketone side chain by oxidation with sodium bismuthate producing 17-ketosteroids, which are then measured by the Zimmerman reaction	+	+	*Normal daily urinary excretion:* 7-16 mg. (male) 5-12 mg. (female)

fied by the simultaneous measurement of urinary creatinine. Drugs that may interfere with the determination are listed in Table 12-2.

Corticosteroids (17-OHCS) in urine

Methods that estimate the concentration of groups of steroids, rather than a single compound, are sufficiently accurate for diagnostic studies. Two principal techniques are used (Table 12-3):

The *Porter-Silber (PS) reaction* measures corticosteroids and their conjugated metabolites that have the 21-dihydroxyacetone side chain. This grouping reacts with the Porter-Silber reagent (phenylhydrazine in ethanolic sulfuric acid) to form a yellow chromogen that is read in a colorimeter. The term "Porter-Silber chromogens" indicates their lack of specificity. Most of the chromogens formed are produced by cortisol, but non-steroidal substances contained in various drugs, bilirubin, ascorbic acid, and certain sugars may contribute to the color reaction. Published modifications are based principally on the Glenn-Nelson, 1953, or Reddy method, 1954. Normal values are shown in Table 12-3.

17-Ketogenic steroids (17-KGS) in urine (Norymberski, 1953) are determined by the cleavage and removal of the C^{21} side chain and oxidation of the hydroxyl (OH) at C^{17} to a ketone ($=O$), thus converting a 17-hydroxycorticosteroid (17-OHCS) to a 17-ketosteroid (17-KS). In addition to those compounds measured by the PS reaction, the 17-KGS measures cortol, cortolone, 17-hydroxyprogesterone, and pregnanetriol (Table 12-3). It therefore lacks the specificity of the PS reaction in assessing cortisol concentration but may uncover disorders characterized by elevated pregnanetriol excretion, such as congenital adrenal hyperplasia. The 17-KGS give a closer approximation of cortisol production than do the PS chromogens. About 50% of secreted cortisol appears in the urine as 17-KGS. 17-KGS values are about 4 mg. higher than 17-OHCS values. An approximation of pregnanetriol excretion can be made by measuring the difference between the PS and the 17-KGS determinations.

The excretion of urinary 17-OHCS is directly proportional to body size. This proportion may be negated by relating 17-OHCS excretion to urinary creatinine. Normal subjects excrete 3 to 7 mg. 17-OHCS/gram creatinine. Urinary 17-OHCS is reduced in patients with a creatinine clearance of less than 10 ml./min., despite a normal plasma 17-OHCS.

Plasma corticosteroids (17-OHCS)

The term "plasma cortisol" is often used synonymously with "plasma 17-OHCS," but determination of the former entails a more complicated technique. Since 90% of the plasma 17-OHCS represents corticosteroid bound to cortisol-binding globulin (CBG, transcortin), factors that elevate CBG, such as pregnancy and estrogens, raise the 17-OHCS to levels found in Cushing's syndrome. However, the biologically active free cortisol is relatively unchanged. Most methods are based on the Porter-Silber (PS) reaction and are therefore "PS chromogens." Normal 8 A.M. values range from 4 to 30 μg./100 ml. Values are elevated during stress, in Cushing's syndrome, in pregnancy, and because of estrogens and smoking. Low values may be found in adrenocortical and anterior pituitary insufficiency, in congenital adrenal hyperplasia, and during corticosteroid-induced adrenal suppression by certain synthetic compounds (that is, dexamethasone, triamcinolone, etc.).

Fluorescent methods are more sensitive than chromogenic techniques. Cortisol and corticosterone in a strong solution of sulfuric acid fluoresce intensely with ultraviolet light. The procedure of Mattingly, 1962, is the simplest and eliminates the need for column chromatography. Plasma samples of 1 to 2 ml. suffice; the determination can be completed in about 1 hour, and a technician can perform 40 to 50 determinations in a day. Background fluorescence contributes about 3 μg./100 ml.

Mean normal values vary from 12.9±3.45 to 22.3±0.29 (de Moor and Steeno, 1963). Although problems of nonspecific fluorescent substances in plasma or in reagents have not been solved, fluorescent methods will undoubtedly enjoy a wider trial because of their simplicity. Both the PS and the fluorescent methods primarily measure cortisol, but the former also detects 11-desoxycortisol (Reichstein's compound S) and the latter corticosterone (Kendall's compound B). For a more precise estimate of plasma 17-OHCS, both methods are employed simultaneously and their close agreement would eliminate the possibility of any appreciable amount of desoxycortisol or corticosterone.

A dialysis method that depends on the steroid-binding properties of plasma has been described (Murphy and Pattee, 1963). Only 1 ml. of plasma is required, and the determination is not affected by many of the substances and conditions that interfere with colorimetric and fluorescent methods. As increasing amounts of cortisol are added to plasma containing a fixed amount of cortisol-4-^{14}C, a proportional decrease in the percentage of cortisol-4-^{14}C bound to plasma protein occurs. The cortisol content of plasma can then be read from a standard curve. See Braunsberg and James, 1961, for a review of corticosteroids in blood.

Free cortisol. Unconjugated urinary "free" cortisol or plasma-free cortisol may be measured by isotopic labeling methods or by subtracting the plasma protein–bound fraction from the total 17-OHCS. Plasma-free cortisol is filtrable by the glomerulus. In Cushing's syndrome the rise of plasma 17-OHCS is composed almost entirely of the free fraction, and there is consequently a marked rise of urinary free cortisol. As the plasma concentration of 17-OHCS rises, the proportion of unbound cortisol increases disproportionately. For an eight-fold increase in plasma 17-OHCS, the free fraction rises 112-fold. Normal subjects excrete 5 to 50 μg./24 hr., whereas in Cushing's syndrome, values of 50 to over 500 μg. are found.

Cortisol secretion rate (CSR). The CSR is determined by the intravenous injection of isotopically labeled cortisol (cortisol-^{3}H or cortisol-^{14}C), its dilution by unlabeled cortisol, and the measurement of its unique isotopically labeled urinary metabolite. The secretory rate is then calculated from the formula:

Daily secretion rate $=$

$$\frac{\text{Urine radioactivity (counts per minute)}}{\text{in 24-hour urine}}{\text{Specific activity of tetrahydrocortisol}}$$

The determination should be carried out in the unstressed state, and the daily excretion of urinary 17-OHCS must be relatively steady. Normal values published by Cope, 1964d, were 16.2±5.7 mg. and by Migeon et al., 1963, 17.4 mg. (women), 20.4 mg. (men). In obesity, values are moderately elevated; in Cushing's syndrome the range is 35 to 420 mg. daily. Reduced rates have been found in pregnancy, Addison's disease, congenital adrenal hyperplasia, pituitary insufficiency, hypothyroidism, and liver cirrhosis. The secretion rate may be slowed in liver disease, in which hepatic cortisol metabolic degradation is deficient, or accelerated in hyperthyroidism, in which the peripheral utilization of cortisol is increased.

Measurement of tetrahydrodeoxycortisol (THS). THS can be measured directly in urine. It is increased during the metyrapone test, in the hypertensive variety of congenital adrenal hyperplasia, and in adrenocortical carcinoma causing Cushing's syndrome.

Urinary total neutral 17-ketosteroid (17-KS, 17-oxosteroids)

The urinary 17-KS's are metabolic, usually inert, products of androgenic (C_{19}) testicular and adrenocortical steroids. They are measured by the Zimmerman reaction (Callow et al., 1938), a condensation reaction in an alkaline medium between metadinitrobenzene and the 17-KS's. The resultant reddish purple (permanganate)

Zimmerman compound can be quantitated colorimetrically with an absorption peak at 520 mμ.

17-KS + Metadinitrobenzene $\longrightarrow$ Zimmerman compound

The determination involves certain inherent deficiencies because of nonspecific interfering substances (contaminants, chromogenic substances, drugs). Ketone groups at other than the C^{17} position may alter the color reaction. The 17-KS value can be employed only as a crude estimate of androgen excretion because most of the products are weak androgens and because testosterone, the most potent androgen, is not a 17-KS. Various conditions that elevate or lower the total neutral urinary 17-KS's are outlined below. Normal values, shown in the following outline, are for adults 20 to 50 years of age. In children, less than 2 mg. per day is excreted until about 8 years of age, when the output commences to rise and reaches a maximum at about the age of 25 years. After 45 to 50 years of age there is a gradual fall, so that by age 70 values are about one half the adult concentration.

Conditions that elevate urinary 17-KS
  Adrenocortical hyperplasia, tumor
  Congenital adrenal hyperplasia
  Cushing's syndrome (hyperplasia, carcinoma)
  Stress
  ACTH stimulation
  Late pregnancy
  Corticosteroid administration (large doses)
Conditions that lower urinary 17-KS
  Adrenocortical insufficiency, Addison's disease
  Adenohypophysial insufficiency (ACTH deficiency)
  Male hypogonadism
  Myxedema
  Advanced liver disease
  Corticosteroid suppression
  Severe malnutrition, inanition

Normal values
  Adult males   10-22 mg. (average, 16 mg.)
  Adult females   5-15 mg. (average, 10 mg.)

Fractionation (separation) permits evaluation of groups or of individual 17-KS's and though technically difficult, provides more useful information. Some form of chromatography is employed (paper, glass fiber paper, absorption on different media, thin-layer, countercurrent distribution, or gas-liquid) to accomplish the final separation. The enzymatic separation of steroids is a sensitive specific technique currently under investigation. The 11-oxygenated ketosteroids (11-oxy-17-ketosteroids, $C_{19}O_3$) are derived only from the adrenal cortex, whereas the 11-desoxy-17-ketosteroids ($C_{19}O_2$) originate from the adrenals and testes (Table 12-4). In children, total urinary 11-oxy-17-KS's are higher than 11-desoxy-17-KS's, the reverse of the adult ratio. In adrenocortical androgenic hyperplasia and after ACTH stimulation, there is a disproportionate elevation of the 11-oxy-17-KS. Separation of the β-ketosteroids (mainly DHEA) (Table 12-4) is valuable in the diagnosis of adrenal carcinoma. The ratio of beta/alpha is normally less than 0.2, whereas in carcinoma it is usually considerably higher. The adrenal cortex accounts for approximately 65% of the total 17-KS and the testes account for 35%. Some laboratories fractionate the 6 or 7 major 17-KS compounds or separate the $C_{19}O_2$ from the $C_{19}O_3$; others report the DHEA alone or the DHEA + androsterone as "DHEA" or report the beta/alpha ratio. There is a remarkable

Table 12-4. Urinary 17-ketosteroids

Origin	Compound	Normal values in mg./24 hr. mean and range*	
		Male	*Female*
Adrenal cortex and testes	Dehydroepiandrosterone (DHEA) (10%-15%)	2.8 (0.4-9.3)	1.23 (0-6.4)
	Androsterone (25%)	4.3 (1.8-6.7)	2.7 (0.4-5.4)
($C_{19}O_2$, 11-desoxy)	Etiocholanolone (25%)	2.95 (0.8-6.5)	3.7 (0.6-5.8)
Adrenal cortex	11-OH-androsterone	1.36 (0.27-3.5)	0.9 (0.2-2.2)
($C_{19}O_3$, 11-oxy, 20%)	11-Ketoandrosterone	0.3 (0.07-0.8)	0.24 (0.02-0.65)
	11-Ketoetiocholanolone	0.7 (0.12-2.2)	0.63 (0-1.97)
	11-OH-etiocholanolone	0.54 0.2-1.71)	0.5 (0-1.63)

†Total $C_{19}O_2$—3.9 mg./24 hr. (1.5-6.1)　　　　　　β-17 KS/α-17KS less than 0.2
Total $C_{19}O_3$—3.8 mg./24 hr. (1.8-6.6)

*Bull. Lab. Med. **13**:1, 1964. Variable depending on technique.
†Perloff, W.: J.A.M.A. **167**:2041, 1958.

constancy of the fractionation pattern for each individual.

ACTH stimulation. Responsiveness to exogenous ACTH is the most valuable diagnostic method of assessing adreno-cortical reserve. The test is discussed on p. 49.

Metyrapone test (Metopirone, SU-4885). Metyrapone, a 11β-hydroxylase inhibitor, induces a compensatory rise in ACTH and is used to gauge pituitary-ACTH reserve. The test is described on p. 46.

Suppression test. The normal feedback control of ACTH-cortisol can be inhibited rapidly by the administration of a corticosteroid in doses just above the physiologic range. In Cushing's syndrome this homeostatic mechanism is no longer responsive, because cortisol is inappropriately hypersecreted and suppression of ACTH can be accomplished only by large doses of a corticosteroid. If an adrenocortical tumor is the cause, it autonomously secretes cortisol and will resist inhibition even with large doses. Suppression tests are therefore a reliable laboratory aid to diagnose Cushing's syndrome and to distinguish adrenocortical hyperplasia from tumor, though occasional discrepancies are encountered. The synthetic corticosteroids dexamethasone or triamcinolone, potent ACTH inhibitors, are used because they do not of themselves measurably add to the plasma or urinary 17-OHCS values. Liddle's test (1959) has become the standard. Dexamethasone is given orally in a dose of 0.5 mg. every 6 hours for 48 hours. In normal subjects the urinary 17-OHCS's fall to less than 3 mg./day by the second day, whereas in patients with Cushing's syndrome the 17-OHCS's remain elevated. If the dose is increased to 2 mg. every 6 hours for 48 hours, suppression to at least 50% of the control value is achieved in Cushing's syndrome caused by adrenocortical hyperplasia but not by adenoma or carcinoma. Plasma corticosteroid levels are similarly reduced by dexamethasone. A single dose dexamethasone suppression test was presented by Nugent et al., 1963, and has become popular as a screening test for Cushing's syndrome. One milligram of dexamethasone is given at 11 or 12 P.M., and a fasting plasma 17-OHCS is obtained the next morning at 8:00. Normal values are below 11 μg./100 ml., whereas in patients with Cushing's syndrome the values remain above 13 μg./100 ml. Poor suppression has been observed in some patients with pituitary adenoma, in acutely stressed subjects, in patients receiving contraceptive or anticonvulsive drugs, and in anorexia nervosa. A partial response was observed in some cases of juvenile diabetes. Tucci et al., 1967, claim to have increased the test's specificity by also measuring the urinary 17-OHCS excreted from 7 A.M. to 12 noon. The urinary steroid-creatinine ratio (mg. of 17-OHCS/mg. of creatinine $\times$ 1,000) should normally be suppressed to less than 4. The urinary 17-KS is reduced by dexamethasone or other potent corticosteroids in androgenic adrenocortical hyperplasia but not in virilizing adrenal tumor.

Aldosterone. Since the aldosterone production rate is about 0.1 to 0.2 mg./day, measurement of the very small quantities in plasma (0.001 to 0.01 μg./100 ml.) is performed only in research centers. Urinary aldosterone levels can be determined by several methods, but all are exacting and tedious, requiring several days of work. Normal values by various methods are from 0.5 to 18 μg./24 hr. (mean 10 μg.). Biglieri et al., 1967, found the normal aldosterone secretory rate to be in the range of 60 to 168 μg./24 hr. Elevated urinary values are typical of primary aldosteronism and may occur in patients on a low-salt or high-potassium intake, in edematous states (cirrhosis of the liver, nephrosis, congestive heart failure), in malignant hypertension, in adrenal carcinoma, and in pregnancy. Values are low or not detectable in Addison's disease.

Pregnanetriol. A urinary metabolite of 17-OH progesterone, pregnanetriol, is found in the urine of most patients with congenital adrenal hyperplasia (CAH), whereas only small quantities (less than 4 mg./day in adults, 0.5 in children) are found in normal subjects.

Pregnanetriol
(5β-pregnane-3α,17α,20α-triol)

Levels tend to fluctuate with the menstrual cycle, rising at midcycle to a maximum during the secretory phase. Bongiovanni et al., 1964, found that plasma levels in normal infants did not exceed 5 μg./100 ml., whereas in CAH the range was 80 to 550 μg./100 ml.

Indirect tests of adrenocortical function

In the years before more direct methods of measuring adrenocortical function were available, the clinician had to depend on indirect tests that gauged the peripheral effects of adrenocortical steroids. Some of these are still employed as screening procedures.

Eosinophil (Thorn) test. Cortisol evokes a fall in circulating eosinophils. If an injection of ACTH is followed by a marked drop in the total eosinophil count, a responsive adrenal cortex is present. Total eosinophil counts are often incorporated in the routine ACTH test. Normal counts vary from 100 to 400 eosinophils/cu. mm. and decrease 90% or more during adequate ACTH stimulation.

Water excretion test. Subjects with adrenocortical insufficiency fail to excrete a water load as promptly as normal individuals. This defect is also shared by some patients with pituitary insufficiency, myxedema, and renal and liver disease. The original procedure of Robinson et al., 1941, was improved by Soffer and Gabrilove, 1952. Breakfast is withheld; the patient empties his bladder and then drinks 1,500 ml. of tap water in 15 to 45 minutes. Because of the remote possibility of water intoxication, some workers prefer to administer 20 ml./kg. body weight. The volume of urine collected from the beginning of the test to the fifth hour should be greater than 800 ml. If the test is abnormal, it is repeated following 1 day of cortisol administration (20 mg. four times daily). Impaired water diuresis will be corrected in adrenocortical insufficiency and pituitary insufficiency but not in myxedema and renal or liver disease. In the original Robinson-Power-Kepler test, a second part is performed if water diuresis is impaired. One calculates the A value as the urea and chloride clearance, along with the urine output collected in hourly aliquots and compared to an overnight specimen collected between 10:00 in the evening and 7:00 the next morning.

$$A = \frac{\text{Urine urea (mg.\%) night specimen}}{\text{Fasting BUN mg./100 ml.}} \times$$

$$\frac{\text{Fasting plasma chloride mEq./L.}}{\text{Night urine chloride mEq./L.}} \times$$

$$\frac{\text{Largest hourly day urine (ml.)}}{\text{Night urine volume (ml.)}}$$

In normal subjects the A value is greater than 30; values less than 25 are considered indicative of adrenocortical insufficiency in the absence of severe renal disease.

Serum electrolytes. In adrenocortical insufficiency the normal serum Na/K ratio of approximately 32 is often reduced. The serum chloride and CO_2 may also decrease. Urinary and sweat sodium concentrations may increase. The mean normal salivary Na/K ratio reported by Frawley, 1967, was 1.3 (0.33 to 2.1), whereas in Addison's disease it was 5 (2.2 to 8.1) and in Cushing's

syndrome 0.5 (0.2 to 1.2). In Cushing's syndrome the plasma potassium and chloride may fall and the CO_2 may rise (hypochloremic hypokalemic alkalosis).

Carbohydrate tests. In adrenal insufficiency one frequently finds a low fasting blood sugar, hypoglycemia after 24 hours of fasting or after intravenous glucose administration, and a flat oral glucose tolerance curve. The once popular insulin tolerance test may provoke profound hypoglycemia and hypoglycemia unresponsiveness and has been supplanted by the more specific tests already outlined. In Cushing's syndrome a diabetic glucose tolerance curve or frank diabetes mellitus may obtain.

REFERENCES

*Bartter, F. C.: Control of aldosterone secretion. In Gual, C., editor: Proceedings of the Sixth Pan-American Congress of Endocrinology, Mexico City, Oct. 10-15, 1965, Amsterdam, 1966, Excerpta Medica Foundation, International Congress ser. no. 112, p. 97.

*Beck, J. C., and McGarry, E. E.: Brit Med. Bull. **18:**134, 1962.

Biglieri, E. G., et al.: J.A.M.A. **201:**510, 1967.

Bongiovanni, A. M., et al.: J. Clin. Endocr. **24:** 1312, 1964.

*Bransome, E. D., Jr.: Ann. Rev. Physiol. **30:** 171, 1968.

*Braunsberg, H., and James, V. H. T.: J. Clin. Endocr. **21:**1146, 1961.

Callow, N. H., et al.: Biochem. J. **32:**1312, 1938.

*Cope, C. L.: Adrenal steroids and disease, Philadelphia, 1964, J. B. Lippincott Co., (a) p. 20, (b) p. 60, (c) p. 89, (d) p. 161.

*Daughaday, W. H.: The binding of corticosteroids by plasma protein. In Eisenstein, A. B., editor: The adrenal cortex, Boston, 1967, Little, Brown & Co., p. 385.

*Davis, J. O.: The regulation of aldosterone secretion. In Eisenstein, A. B., editor: The adrenal cortex, Boston, 1967, Little, Brown & Co., p. 203.

*Deane, H. W.: The anatomy, chemistry, and physiology of adrenocortical tissue. In Deane, H. W., editor: The adrenocortical hormones, their origin, chemistry, physiology, and pharmacology, Berlin, 1962, Springer-Verlag, (a) p. 22, (b) pp. 45-47.

*Dobbie, J. W., et al.: The structure and functional zonation of the human adrenal cortex.

*Significant reviews.

In James, V. H. T., and Landon, J., editors: The investigation of hypothalamo-pituitary-adrenal function, London, 1968, Cambridge University Press, p. 103.

Doe, R. P., et al.: J. Clin. Endocr. **20**:1484, 1960.

Fabre, L. F., Jr., et al.: Amer. J. Physiol. **208**: 1275, 1965.

Farrell, G.: Recent Progr. Hormone Res. **15**:275, 1959.

Frawley, T. F.: Adrenal cortical insufficiency. In Eisenstein, A. B., editor: The adrenal cortex, Boston, 1967, Little, Brown & Co., pp. 443-444, 482-483.

Glenn, E. M., and Nelson, D. H.: J. Clin. Endocr. **13**:911, 1953.

°Grant, N.: Metabolic effects of adrenal glucocorticoid hormones. In Martini, L., Fraschini, F., and Motta, M., editors: International Congress on Hormonal Steroids, proceedings of the second congress, Milan, May 23-28, 1966, Amsterdam, 1967, Excerpta Medica Foundation, International Congress ser. no. 132, p. 269.

°Hechter, O., and Pincus, G.: Physiol. Rev. **34**: 459, 1954.

Henkin, R. I., et al.: J. Clin. Invest. **46**:429, 1967.

Ingle, D. J.: Amer. J. Physiol. **138**:577, 1943.

Koritz, S. B., and Hall, P. F.: Biochemistry **3**: 1298, 1964.

Lanman, J. T.: An interpretation of human fetal adrenal structure and function. In Currie, A. R., Symington, T., and Grant, J. K., editors: The human adrenal cortex, Baltimore, 1962, The Williams & Wilkins Co., p. 547.

Liddle, G. W., et al.: J. Clin. Endocr. **19**:875, 1959.

Lieberman, S.: Steroid sulfates as biosynthetic intermediates. In Martini, L., Fraschini, F., Motta, M., editors: International Congress on Hormonal Steroids, proceedings of the second congress, Milan, May 23-28, 1966, Amsterdam, 1967, Excerpta Medica Foundation, International Congress ser. no. 132, p. 22.

Long, J. A. and Jones, A. L.: Lab. Invest. **17**: 355, 1967.

°Luse, S.: Fine structure of adrenal cortex. In Eisenstein, A. B., editor: The adrenal cortex, Boston, 1967, Little, Brown & Co., pp. 1-59.

Mattingly, D.: J. Clin. Path. **15**:374, 1962.

Migeon, C. J., et al.: Metabolism **12**:718, 1963.

Moor, P. de, and Steeno, O.: J. Endocr. **28**:59, 1963.

Moor, P. de, et al.: Ann. Endocr. **26**:488, 1965.

Moore, J. A., and Heftmann, E.: Chemistry of the adrenocortical steroids. In Deane, H. W., editor: The adrenocortical hormones, Berlin, 1962, Springer-Verlag, pp. 192-193.

°Munck, A., and Brinck-Johnsen, T.: Specific metabolic and physiochemical interactions of glucocorticoids in vivo and in vitro with rat adipose tissue and thymus cells. In Martini, L., Fraschini, F., and Motta, M., editors: International Congress on Hormonal Steroids, proceedings of the second congress, Milan, May 23-28, 1966, Amsterdam, 1967, Excerpta Medica Foundation, International Congress ser. no. 132, p. 472.

Murphy, B. E., and Pattee, C. J.: J. Clin. Endocr. **23**:459, 1963.

°Nichols, C. T., and Tyler, F. H.: Ann. Rev. Med. **18**:313, 1967.

Norymberski, J. K., et al.: Lancet **1**:1276, 1953.

Nugent, C. A., et al.: J. Clin. Endocr. **23**:684, 1963.

°Pincus, G.: Ann. N. Y. Acad. Sci. **61**:283, 1955.

Reddy, W. J.: Metabolism **3**:489, 1954.

Ritter, R. A.: Arch. Neurol. **17**:403, 1967.

Robinson, F., et al.: Proc. Staff Meet. Mayo Clin. **16**:577, 1941.

Rosenfeld, R. A., et al.: Metabolism of adrenal cortical hormones. In Eisenstein, A. B., editor: The adrenal cortex, Boston, 1967, Little, Brown & Co., pp. 105, 106.

°Samuels, L. T., and Uchikuwa, T.: Biosynthesis of adrenal steroids. In Eisenstein, A. B., editor: The adrenal cortex, Boston, 1967, Little, Brown & Co., p. 72.

Schayer, R. W.: Perspect. Biol. Med. **10**:409, 1967.

Soffer, L. J., and Gabrilove, J. L.: Metabolism **1**:504, 1952.

Swinyard, C. A.: Anat. Rec. **76**:69, 1940.

°Symington, T.: Brit. Med. Bull. **18**:117, 1962.

Tucci, J. R., et al.: J.A.M.A. **199**:129, 1967.

°White, A., et al.: Mode of action of adrenal steroids in lymphoid tissue. In Martini, L., Fraschini, F., and Motta, M., editors: International Congress on Hormonal Steroids, proceedings of the second congress, Milan, May 23-28, 1966, Amsterdam, 1967, Excerpta Medica Foundation, International Congress ser. no. 132, p. 463.

Yates, F. E.: Physiological control of adrenal cortical hormone secretion. In Eisenstein, A. B., editor: The adrenal cortex, Boston, 1967, Little, Brown & Co., p. 133.

Chapter 13

Adrenocortical insufficiency

The eponym "Addison's disease" is generally restricted to atrophic or destructive lesions of the adrenal cortex. The broader term "adrenocortical hypofunction" or "insufficiency" (ACI) encompasses all varieties of adrenocortical failure (see outline below). There is a combined deficiency of cortisol and aldosterone, though rarely there may be an isolated deficiency of one or the other.

Etiology

ACI is caused by loss of adrenocortical tissue (see outline below, category 1, conditions a to c). A residuum of 10% of functional adrenal cortex is compatible with apparent eucortisolism in the unstressed subject. Idiopathic atrophy and tuberculosis account for fully 90% of cases; the other causes of ACI listed in the following outline are clinical curiosities:

1. Loss of adrenocortical tissue
   a. Idiopathic (cytotoxic, primary contracted) atrophy/necrosis (autoimmune?)
   b. Tuberculosis
   c. Infiltrative destruction or replacement by
      - granuloma
      - metastatic malignancy
      - lymphoblastoma, leukemia
      - amyloidosis
      - systemic fungus disease
        - histoplasmosis
        - blastomycosis
        - coccidioidomycosis
      - hemochromatosis

d. Adrenalectomy (bilateral)
e. Hemorrhage—fulminating infection (Waterhouse—Friderichsen), anticoagulants, trauma, metastatic malignancy, leukemia
f. Vascular occlusion

2. Adrenocortical atrophy secondary to anterior pituitary hypofunction and/or hypothalamic disorder
   Sheehan's syndrome, Simmonds' disease, pituitary tumor, monotropic loss of ACTH ("pituitary Addison's")

3. Defects of corticosteroid biosynthesis (enzymatic deficiency)
   Bilateral adrenocortical hyperplasia (adrenogenital syndrome)
   Drugs—triparanol, o,p'-DDD, amphenone, aminoglutethimide, Parnate, oral contraceptives
   Selective hypoaldosteronism

4. Transient inhibition of CRF-ACTH
   Withdrawal of corticosteroid therapy (iatrogenic)
   Cushing's syndrome (after removal of benign adenoma or carcinoma with contralateral adrenal atrophy)

In recent years there has been a decrease in cases due to tuberculosis and a proportionate increase in those due to idiopathic atrophy. Guttman, 1930, in his review of 403 autopsies performed from 1900 to 1929, reported the findings of tuberculosis in 70% and "primary atrophy" in 16%. Twenty years later O'Donnell, 1950, found tuberculosis in only 8 of 18 cases. At the U. S. Army Institute of Pathology, the number of tuberculosis/atrophy cases prior to 1940 was 21/6 and after 1940, 10/15 (Friedman, 1948). Systemic fungous diseases, particularly histoplasmosis, has been recognized more frequently. The majority emanate from the Central Mississippi Valley. A number of cases due to adrenal hemorrhage principally from anticoagulant therapy have been reported.

Autoimmune hypothesis. Autoimmunization may be an important mechanism to explain the destruction of the adrenal cortex. Circulating adrenal antibodies have been discovered in the sera of approximately 50% of patients with idiopathic atrophy. Examples of Addison's disease with hypothyroidism (Schmidt's syndrome), idiopathic hypoparathyroidism, Graves' disease, chronic thyroiditis, premature ovarian failure, and pernicious anemia in various combinations suggest polyglandular autoimmunization. The association of superficial moniliasis, hypoparathyroidism, and adrenal insufficiency has been observed principally in children and has a familial incidence. Eisenstein, 1968, summarized the following evidence that supports an autoimmune etiology: (1) the histology resembles that of other autoimmune processes; (2) specific antibodies are present; (3) antibodies to other tissues may be found; (4) the injection of adjuvant into animals produces similar adrenal changes; and (5) autoantibodies may be formed in experimental animals.

Pathophysiology

Bilateral adrenalectomy precipitates physiologic deterioration of the experimental animal and a fatal termination within 1 to 2 weeks. There is diminished activity, loss of aggressive behavior, anorexia, weight loss, inanition, diminished muscle tone and skin turgor, hypotension, hypothermia, and dehydration. Death follows from circulatory collapse and may be hastened by a supervening infection or hypoglycemic shock. Muscle work performance and the ability to withstand fasting or other forms of stress is obtunded. The effects of aldosterone loss leading to tissue anoxia and acidosis must exert

significant effects on protein, fat, and carbohydrate metabolism. The administration of a potent mineralocorticoid, desoxycorticosterone acetate (DCA), by correcting the water and salt deficiency, improves appetite and increases intestinal absorption of hexoses and thus indirectly replenishes liver glycogen stores and combats hypoglycemia. There will also be correction of extracellular fluid loss, partial restoration of blood pressure, renal plasma flow, and GFR. Azotemia is reduced, tissue anoxia is lessened, and acidosis diminishes. DCA, however, will not correct diminished muscle work performance, poor adaptation to stress, fasting hypoglycemia, inability to excrete a water load promptly, or hyperpigmentation. Muscular fatigue may be primarily a consequence of hypotension and reduced blood supply to the muscles. The ability of blood vessels to respond to pressor agents without developing refractoriness also requires an adequate milieu of corticosteroids. Melanosis is provoked by excessive MSH, which is ordinarily opposed by corticosteroids in normal subjects. Under certain circumstances, such as an MSH-secreting pituitary tumor, ACTH and MSH may be secreted independently.

Pathology

Tuberculosis. In tuberculosis (Fig. 13-1, A and B), both adrenals are enlarged, firm, and often nodular and on sectioning show a homogeneous yellow-white, yellow-gray, or grayish-red firm rubbery surface characteristic of Addison's disease and differing from caseation necrosis of other tissues. Calcification is found in 5% to 10% of cases. Both adrenals are almost totally replaced by either a necrotic lesion (massive necrosis surrounded by a fibrous capsule, few tubercles, small number of lymphocytes) or by a proliferative lesion (many tubercles, fibroblasts and connective tissue cells, only small areas of necrosis). Remnants of apparently viable tissue can usually be found by a meticulous search. Both healed and active lesions are found else-

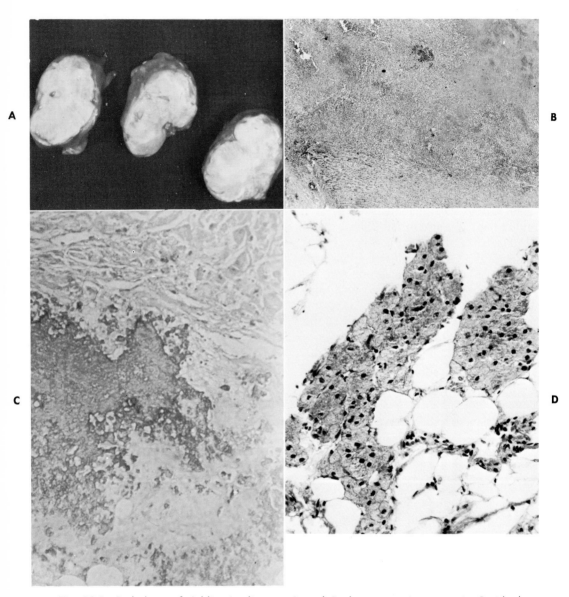

Fig. 13-1. Pathology of Addison's disease. **A** and **B** show caseation necrosis. Residual cells are shown in lower area of **B. C,** Idiopathic atrophy showing an area of calcification. **D,** Idiopathic atrophy with residual adrenocortical cells. (**A** courtesy Dr. Rachmiel Levine, New York, and Michael Reese Hospital, Chicago, Ill.; **B** to **D** from Department of Pathology, Hahnemann Medical College, Philadelphia, Pa.)

where, particularly in the lungs. Healed lesions are not found in the adrenals of tuberculous patients, the process being characteristically destructive. The peculiar susceptibility of the adrenal cortex to total necrosis in contrast to the resistance manifested by other tissues may be due to the local high concentration of corticosteroids in adrenocortical cells.

Idiopathic atrophy. The adrenals are small, misshapen, or so atrophic that they cannot be found. The microscopic picture (Fig. 13-1, *C* and *D*) varies from that of simple shrinkage of cortical tissue to a narrow rim with only the medulla remaining to that of nodular regeneration, often with central necrosis, that may obscure the underlying atrophy. There may also be connective tissue proliferation and a cellular reaction.

Hypopituitarism. The zona glomerulosa is preserved, but the zona fasciculata and zona reticularis undergo atrophy (Fig. 5-1, *D*).

Pathology of nonadrenal tissues. The thymus and lymph nodes are frequently hyperplastic. Cardiac weight is almost invariably subnormal. There is reduction in the number of basophils in the adenohypophysis. Significant involutional changes with lymphocyte and plasma cell infiltration are found in approximately 40% of thyroid glands. Thyroid abnormalities are usually associated with idiopathic atrophy of the adrenals.

Clinical features

Addison's disease is a rare disorder. Guttman, 1930, found 0.4 per 100,000 population, Forsham and Melmon, 1968, suggested a death rate of 4 per 100,000, and Soffer, 1961, reported 1 case per 4,500 hospital admissions. The most recent survey (Mason et al., 1968) identified 82 patients in a population of 3.2 million; in the age range 25 to 69 years the prevalence rate was 39 per million (12 tuberculous, 27 nontuberculous). Female predominate in nontuberculous cases. A genetic predisposition may exist.

Because the onset is gradual and the symptoms are not specific, the diagnosis is frequently overlooked until the patient becomes critically ill. The following discussion describes advanced ACI. Milder cases will present less clear-cut features.

Symptoms and signs

WEAKNESS AND FATIGUE. Muscle strength is impaired. Locomotion becomes slow and hesitant, and there is languor, a desire to sit or to remain in bed, and fatigability. The patient is sometimes refreshed after a night's sleep but tires in the morning or early afternoon. There is prolonged debility after an infection or a surgical procedure and even severe prostration. There is often a history of several episodes of collapse with recovery after intravenous glucose-saline solution.

WEIGHT LOSS. The diagnosis is in doubt if the patient has not lost weight. The loss is often minimal in the early stages but becomes progressively more severe because of anorexia, tissue wasting, and dehydration.

HYPERPIGMENTATION. Hyperpigmentation (melanosis) is often the first manifestation and may be associated with apparent good health for some time before other features appear. In such instances compensated adrenocortical failure with eucorticism because of hyperproduction of ACTH obtains, and the accompanying excess of ACTH-MSH induces early melanosis. Listed are varieties of hyperpigmentation in Addison's disease[*]:

Diffuse tan, especially of exposed areas
Multiple brown or black freckles
Extensor surfaces, pressure areas (belt line, shoulder straps, shoe pressure), palmar creases, scars
Mucous membranes and tongue
Areola, scrotum, perineum, perivaginal and perianal areas
Vitiligo
Hair darkening

Extreme hyperpigmentation with elevated circulating MSH may follow bilateral adre-

[*]Adapted from Thorn, G. W.: The diagnosis and treatment of adrenal insufficiency, Springfield, Ill., 1949, Charles C Thomas, Publisher, p. 29.

nalectomy for Cushing's syndrome. The pigmentation is less striking or even absent in blonds, redheads, and Northern Europeans. In the Negro natural melanosis is increased and becomes slate-gray or black. The gingivae may be heavily pigmented in normal Negroes (Plate I, *C*), but pigmentation of the tongue is usually abnormal. After adrenalectomy, melanosis is not found so consistently as in spontaneous Addison's disease. A search for hyperpigmentation should include an examination of the mouth, tongue, pharynx, and rectal and vaginal mucous membranes. The palmar creases are most frequently involved. Because hyperpigmentation is found in 95% of cases of ACI, its absence should suggest anterior pituitary insufficiency with loss of ACTH or normal adrenocortical function. Only scars that date after the onset of the disease become pigmented. Vitiligo may occasionally be the sole sign of pigmentary disturbance. Further skin darkening occurs with dehydration and may be a sign of impending crisis.

GASTROINTESTINAL SYMPTOMS. Symptoms of gastrointestinal origin suggest extensive disease. There is anorexia, a capricious appetite, a distaste for food, and nausea induced by the odor of food. Vomiting may herald crisis. Intermittent diarrhea, sensitivity to cathartics, and abdominal pain that can mimic intra-abdominal pathology are less common complaints. Salt craving is found in from 15% to 20% of patients. Hypochlorhydria is common but seems to play no role in producing symptoms.

HYPOTENSION, DIZZINESS, AND SYNCOPE. There is low blood pressure and a contracted pulse pressure causing faintness, syncope, and postural hypotension. Unless the patient has had hypertension, finding a normal blood pressure should raise doubts about the diagnosis. Profound hypotension leads to circulatory collapse and crisis. ACI is almost invariably associated with a small heart. Only a single case of congestive heart failure has been reported (Cushner et al., 1963).

CENTRAL NERVOUS SYSTEM. Apathy, withdrawal, irritability, confusion, drowsiness, and reduced mental acuity are symptoms of advanced disease, but minor personality alterations are frequent. The symptoms are a consequence of hypotension with impaired cerebral circulation, electrolyte disturbances, and hypoglycemia. Nonspecific EEG abnormalities have been described. Only 7 cases of flaccid muscle paralysis due to hyperkalemia have been reported (Bell et al., 1965).

HYPOGLYCEMIA. Hypoglycemic symptoms can occur at low-normal or mildly reduced blood sugar levels, since the threshold is reduced. Such symptoms tend to occur in the early morning or to follow a delay in mealtime, fasting, excessive ingestion of alcohol, or a heavy carbohydrate meal.

OTHER CLINICAL FINDINGS. Muscle cramps and intolerance to cold are frequent complaints. There is often loss of axillary hair and reduction of body hair. Poor mouth hygiene is associated with multiple dental caries. The pinnae may be sclerotic and calcified. Lymph nodes, tonsils, and the thymus may be enlarged. Costovertebral tenderness (Rogoff's sign) is unusual. Body temperature is often subnormal, but fever may be observed during or following a glucose infusion. If I.V. glucose is abruptly terminated, there is likely to be a severe hypoglycemic reaction. ACI is compatible with normal menstrual function and fertility. When there is weight loss, malnutrition, and debility, ovarian or testicular hypofunction ensues. Premature ovarian failure has been attributed to gonad-specific autoantibodies (Irvine et al., 1968).

Partial adrenocortical insufficiency. Addison's disease is not necessarily an all-or-none disorder but shows gradations of severity. Perhaps 5% to 10% of functional adrenal cortex can maintain life under nonstressful conditions. The remnant, already exerting its maximal secretory capacity under endogenous ACTH stimulation, is unable to augment its hormone output when the patient is subjected to stress, and adrenal insufficiency ensues.

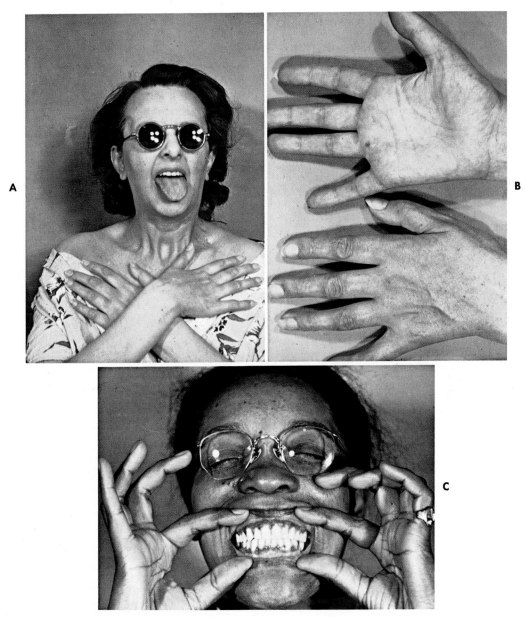

Plate I. Pigmentation in Addison's disease. **A,** Pigmentation of tongue, facies, neck, and hands. **B,** Pigmentation of knuckles, metacarpal and palmar creases, and melanotic spot on right palm. **C,** Heavy gingival pigmentation in a normal Negro woman. (**A** and **B** courtesy Dr. Rachmiel Levine, New York, and Michael Reese Hospital, Chicago, Ill.)

The patient may appear more or less healthy during basal conditions, though there may be hyperpigmentation because of elevated ACTH-MSH. The concentrations of plasma and urinary 17-OHCS may be normal or near normal but do not rise if stimulated by exogenous ACTH. The latent case may subsequently progress to the full-blown clinical state of complete ACI if the remnant is further ablated by a continuing disease process.

Isolated hypoaldosteronism (selective aldosterone deficiency). Seven cases of selective aldosterone deficiency with otherwise normal adrenal function have been reported (Vagnucci, 1969). The mechanism has been ascribed to an acquired impairment of the C^{18}-oxygenating enzyme. Hyperkalemia provoked cardiac arrhythmias, Stokes-Adams attacks, muscular weakness, and paralysis. Unless Na intake is severely restricted, Na conservation has been adequate.

Laboratory findings

The following are laboratory findings in Addison's disease (see also p. 215):

Plasma and urine 17-OHCS ↓; no response to ACTH

Plasma and urine cortisol ↓; no response to ACTH

Cortisol secretion rate ↓

Urine 17-KS and aldosterone ↓

Serum sodium and chloride ↓, serum potassium ↑, Na/K ratio less than 30

Urine and sweat sodium ↑, salivary Na/K ratio above 2

Delayed water excretion

Blood sugar—low fasting, hypoglycemia after prolonged fast, flat oral glucose tolerance, hypoglycemia after I.V. glucose, hypoglycemia unresponsiveness after I.V. insulin

Blood cells—normal to slightly elevated eosinophils and lymphocytes; hemoconcentration

Blood ACTH ↑, urinary MSH ↑

ECG and EEG—nonspecific abnormalities

X-ray findings—small heart, enlarged thymus, calcified pinnae, suprarenal calcification, evidence of pulmonary or vertebral tuberculosis, enlarged sella turcica (in pituitary insufficiency with tumor and secondary adrenocortical insufficiency)

Plasma and urinary 17-OHCS and urinary 17-KS are subnormal. Though finding normal values makes the diagnosis unlikely, this may rarely obtain in latent or partial adrenocortical failure or limited adrenocortical reserve (see discussion on partial adrenocortical insufficiency). The ACTH test is the best means of assessing the reserve capacity of the adrenal cortex. Failure to respond to ACTH can occur (1) when the adrenal cortex is completely destroyed or (2) when a remnant, already under continuous endogenous ACTH stimulation, can no longer respond to additional ACTH. The technique has been outlined on p. 49. Rarely, in a state of partial adrenal insufficiency with diminished reserves, some response may occur in the first 48 hours of the test; such a response may obscure a rapid exhaustion of adrenocortical reserve so that 17-OHCS production may not be sustained by day 3 or 4. A healthy adrenal will maintain and progressively increase its secretion of 17-OHCS for several days; so it is best to carry out at least 4 days of stimulation. Adrenal insufficiency in a patient on prolonged corticosteroid therapy may be a consequence of endogenous ACTH suppression or there may be underlying organic adrenocortical pathology. Prolonged ACTH stimulation, beyond the usual 4-day test, may be necessary to obtain a rise of plasma or urinary 17-OHCS with iatrogenic disease, whereas even prolonged stimulation will fail to evoke a response if the adrenal cortex is destroyed.

Reactions to ACTH can be avoided by giving the patient 0.5 mg. of dexamethasone twice daily during the test. The ACTH test is also used to differentiate Addison's disease from adrenocortical atrophy secondary to pituitary insufficiency. In the latter condition the adrenal cortex is responsive, and the plasma and urinary 17-OHCS will rise. This rise may not occur on the first day of stimulation with ACTH, but a stepwise increase will occur if a 4-day test is employed (Fig. 4-6).

In patients with severe ACI, adrenal crisis can develop precipitately, and the emergency situation does not permit elaborate testing. Blood can be drawn for total eosinophil count, BUN, and plasma Na and K immediately and a urine specimen obtained for Na content; I.V. cortisol therapy can then be started without delay. A portion of blood may be refrigerated for measurement of plasma 17-OHCS. ACI is likely if there is a normal or high eosinophil count, an elevated BUN, a reduced plasma Na and Na/K ratio (that is, below 30), and a urine Na greater than 20 mEq./L. The plasma 17-OHCS value can be determined later and will be low in adrenal insufficiency and high in other conditions causing shock. In salt-losing nephritis the urinary Na is high, but other tests will demonstrate a normal adrenal response to stress. At a later date, if the diagnosis is still in doubt, an ACTH test can be performed.

Even with ACTH testing the diagnosis may occasionally be equivocal, and the "indirect" tests are performed. The water excretion test (p. 221) may be helpful, though some patients with mild Addison's disease may excrete a water load as promptly as normal subjects. The plasma Na/K ratio is below 30, and the salivary Na/K ratio is above 2. Both the salt deprivation test, which can provoke severe adrenal insufficiency (crisis), and the insulin tolerance test, which can cause severe hypoglycemia, are hazardous procedures and are rarely employed. A 24-hour fast produces a progressive decline in blood sugar values in ACI (Thorn, 1949).

Blood. The total fasting eosinophil count is usually high-normal or elevated, so that the finding of a low count should cast doubt on the diagnosis. The total white count tends to be low-normal with elevated lymphocytes and reduced polymorphonuclears. A normocytic mild anemia is not infrequent but can be masked by hemoconcentration. Hypercalcemia parallels hyponatremia in adrenalectomized dogs (Walser et al., 1963) and may occur in patients with Addison's disease. Some reduction in serum total protein and albumin may be found.

X-ray findings. Adrenal calcification was found in 24 of 106 cases (23%) by Jarvis et al., 1954, but was also noted, albeit rarely, in normal individuals. The heart size was reduced, the average reduction being –13.5%. Inactive pulmonary tuberculosis was demonstrated in 38 of 116 patients and active tuberculosis in 9. Six patients had calcification of the pinnae, though this is not pathognomonic. Calcification of the costal cartilages was found in 93 of 104 patients.

Differential diagnosis

Difficulties in diagnosis can be encountered in the following situations.

Psychogenic disorders. Psychogenic disorders that are characterized by fatigue, weakness, and hypotension may mimic ACI. These disorders tend to remit spontaneously and to recur, whereas ACI usually follows a progressively downhill course. The response to corticosteroid therapy is vague and not the clear-cut rejuvenation that one observes in ACI. If pigmentation and weight loss are absent, Addison's disease is unlikely. The diagnosis may be rendered more obscure by the tendency for some patients with chronic asthenia to show a reduction in urinary 17-OHCS, a relative increase in the corticosterone/cortisol ratio, and a somewhat reduced response to ACTH stimulation (Albeaux-Fernet et al., 1957). Although anorexia nervosa and severe malnutrition occasionally exhibit hyperpigmentation, axillary hair is usually preserved, and although the basal secretion of adrenocortical steroids is often reduced, there is responsiveness to ACTH. Functional hypopituitarism due to a shunting of protein to meet caloric needs commonly occurs in prolonged starvation but rarely causes a significant ACTH deficiency.

Hyperpigmentation. Hyperpigmentation is observed in a host of other disorders, but in most instances there is no confusion with Addison's disease. The pigmentation of *hemochromatosis* resembles that of Addison's, and iron deposits in the pituitary and adrenals may lead to ACI, but in most cases there is a good response to ACTH and there is diabetes rather than hypoglycemia, and resistance rather than hypersensitivity to insulin. *Scleroderma* and *dermatomyositis* may be accompanied by melanin pigmentation, weight loss, weakness, and hypotension and, in scleroderma, by gastrointestinal complaints. Laboratory studies usually make the distinction. Rarely mistaken for Addison's disease is the pigmentation due to heavy metals (silver [in which case the condition is called argyria], bismuth, arsenic), hyperthyroidism and hypothyroidism, pellagra, polyostotic fibrous dysplasia, and von Recklinghausen's disease.

Tuberculosis. Patients with pulmonary tuberculosis may present features of Addison's disease and show evidence of adrenocortical depression that may be attributed to functional hypopituitarism. There is diminished response to ACTH in some patients. Low urinary adrenal steroid values and hyponatremia and hypochloremia are common findings. However, the patients are not pigmented, plasma 17-OHCS values are normal, and the serum potassium is not elevated.

Salt-losing nephritis. Excessive urinary Na loss in chronic renal disease due to failure of renal tubular responsiveness to adrenal steroids may be confused with ACI. Criteria for the diagnosis are (1) dehydration on a low sodium intake that is relieved by a high sodium intake, (2) persistent renal disease, (3) normal laboratory tests of adrenocortical function, and (4) failure to reduce urinary Na loss with DCA administration.

Treatment
Corticosteroid therapy

Replacement of the adrenal steroid deficiency is accomplished by the combined use of hydrocortisone (cortisol) or cortisone and 9α-fluorohydrocortisone (fludrocortisone), a potent synthetic mineralocorti-

coid. Cortisol is the naturally secreted hormone and is preferred for replacement therapy, though cortisone is satisfactory. Comparable doses are cortisol 20 mg., cortisone 25 mg. The daily production of cortisol in normal subjects varies from 15 to 30 mg. in the resting state and 150 to 250 mg. during stress so that replacement therapy must be guided by this knowledge.

Listed are preparations of corticosteroids for use in Addison's disease:

Corticosteroids
  Hydrocortisone, cortisol, U.S.P.
    Trade names: Hydrocortone, Cortef, Cortril, Cortifan
    Oral tablets: 5, 10, 20 mg.
    Parenteral preparations
      50% alcoholic solution
        50 mg./ml. in 5 ml. vials ⎫ For I.V. use, dilute in 500 to 1,000 ml. 5%
        5 mg./ml. in 20 ml. vials ⎭ glucose in normal saline solution
    Hydrocortisone 21-sodium succinate, U.S.P. (Solu-Cortef)—100, 250 mg. vials I.V. or I.M.
    Hydrocortisone 21-phosphate—50 mg./ml. I.V. or I.M.
    Hydrocortisone acetate—25 mg./ml. I.M.
  Cortisone acetate U.S.P.
    Trade names: Cortone, Cortogen
    Oral tablets: 5, 10, 25 mg.
    Parenteral preparation (suspension)
      25 mg./ml. in 10 and 20 ml. vials
      50 mg./ml. in 10 ml. vials
Mineralocorticoids
  9α-Fluorohydrocortisone, fludrocortisone 21-acetate
    Trade names: Florinef, F-Cortef, Aflorane
    Oral tablets: 0.1, 1 mg.
  Desoxycorticosterone acetate U.S.P.
    Trade names: Cortate, Percorten, Doca acetate, Decortin
    Buccal tablets: 2, 5 mg.
    Pellets: 75, 125 mg. for subcutaneous implantation
    Parenteral preparation:
      Oil solution: 5 mg./ml. in 1 and 10 ml. vials

If the patient is verging on crisis, ill from a complicating disorder, or unable to retain liquids by mouth, parenteral therapy is given initially as outlined below (Addisonian crisis) and oral therapy substituted later. If the situation is judged not to demand corticosteroids by I.V. infusion, I.M. hydrocortisone 21-sodium succinate U.S.P. (Solu-Cortef) powder (100 or 250 mg. vial) can be dissolved and given in a dose of 50 to 100 mg. every 6 hours or cortisone acetate in similar dosage for 24 hours or more as required. Oral hydrocortisone may then be tolerated in a dosage of 20 to 40 mg. every 6 hours with subsequent gradual reductions to a maintenance dosage. The daily maintenance dose is 20 to 40 mg. divided as follows:

Daily-dose cortisol	Schedule
20 mg.	10 mg. b.i.d. (q.12h.)
30 mg.	20 mg. on arising, 10 mg. 12 hours later
40 mg.	20 mg. on arising, 10 mg. 8 hours later, and 10 mg. at bedtime

The larger dose given in the morning simulates the normal diurnal variation. Because synthetic corticosteroids (Table 12-1) were designed to avoid sodium retention, they are not recommended for use in ACI.

Mineralocorticoid therapy

Although patients with mild ACI may require only 5 to 10 grams of supplementary NaCl daily, for optimum therapy all patients should receive 9α-fluorohydrocortisone. The dose is 0.05 to 0.1 mg. given once daily, since its effect lasts 24 hours. Aldosterone is not available. DCA in long-term treatment as long-acting injections (trimethylacetate, or acetate-in-oil), or as pellets, sublingual drops, or buccal tablets is rarely used since fludrocortisone became available.

Supplementary therapy

Very ill patients require I.V. fluids, NaCl, and glucose. DCA may be required and is given I.M. in 5 to 20 mg. doses (1 to 4 ml.) every 8 to 12 hours. There is no parenteral preparation of fludrocortisone. Antituberculosis therapy or antibiotics for infection may be necessary. A high calorie nutritious diet with supplemental vitamins is recommended until lost weight is regained. Some authorities advocate using androgens when there is extreme muscle weakness, muscle atrophy, or male sexual impotence. Adult, fetal, or hyperplastic adrenal transplants have been attempted but their effects are transient.

Response to therapy. The response is usually dramatic. Within 12 to 24 hours the bedfast or moribund patient may become euphoric from the surge of strength and the restoration of his sense of well-being. There is rapid rehydration, weight gain, rise of blood pressure, and return of appetite. If no complications arise, he is eager to leave the hospital within a few days. His appetite often becomes ravenous, and excessive weight gain must be guarded against. In severe and long-neglected cases, the response to therapy is less rapid or the patient may be beyond recovery.

Guides to subsequent therapy. Warning signs of decompensation are (1) weight loss, (2) fall of blood pressure, (3) loss of appetite or nausea, (4) onset of fatigue or weakness, and (5) muscle cramps. Addisonian patients are extremely sensitive to adrenal steroids, and overdosage, particularly from fludrocortisone, must be guarded against. There will be excess weight gain, hypertension, and edema. Headache may be a sign of hypertension, and muscle weakness may be caused by Na retention and K loss. ECG changes may occur, and there may rarely be cardiac arrhythmia or enlargement. The fludrocortisone is omitted for several days, and the patient is examined and serum electrolytes are measured daily until equilibrium is restored. K supplements may be necessary for hypokalemia. Diuretic therapy may be dangerous and is rarely necessary. An acute psychotic episode can occur, albeit rarely, during the first days of therapy, but recovery is usually rapid. Insomnia may be lessened by shifting the evening dose of cortisol to the late afternoon. Indigestion is combatted by taking cortisol immediately after meals or with an aluminum hydroxide gel or milk. Peptic ulcer, never seen in untreated cases, can be induced in susceptible subjects by the restoration of gastric secretion. The steroid is continued, together with a peptic ulcer regimen. Latent diabetes may become manifest.

Therapy and stress. In mild stress such as a respiratory infection, a tooth extraction, or a sprained ankle, the daily dose should be doubled for 2 or 3 days and then gradually tapered back to the maintenance dose. Severe stress requires a fourfold or greater increase, and the patient should consult his physician immediately. In patients far removed from medical assistance, parenteral corticosteroids should be available at home and a member of the family should be trained to give the injection. Surgical stress is discussed later. All patients should wear a medallion, anklet, or bracelet stating the diagnosis and therapy.* The patient must understand that he is unusually hypersensitive to narcotics, barbiturates, and antihistamines.

Prognosis

Prior to the cortisol era, the prognosis was poor. Guttman, 1930, reported that the tuberculous patient survived an average of 2.5 months and the nontuberculous 4.4 months. Today the outlook for prolonged survival is excellent under optimal conditions. Rowntree, 1955, described 8 patients who survived 15 years or more, and Thorn, 1968, observed 4 patients for 26 to 33 years. The patient must learn that he has a life-long illness and that, despite a sense of well-being, therapy does not restore complete health. Although only a minimum of medical supervision is usually necessary, he must guard against carelessness when subjected to stress. Hyperpigmentation rarely subsides completely, but any unexplained increase should be investigated.

Addisonian crisis
(acute adrenocortical insufficiency)

The causes of acute adrenocortical insufficiency are outlined:

Acute adrenocortical failure
    Classical Addisonian crisis or hypopituitary coma
    Withdrawal of long-term corticosteroid therapy

---

*Medic-Alert, Turlock, Calif.

    After bilateral adrenalectomy or after resection of benign adrenal adenoma in Cushing's syndrome
Acute adrenal hemorrhage
    Waterhouse-Friderichsen syndrome
    Complicating anticoagulant therapy
    Miscellaneous—adrenal vein thrombosis, tumor, trauma, blood dyscrasia
    In the newborn—complication of labor

The patient is usually brought to an emergency room in a shocklike state with profound hypotension, grayish cyanosis, sometimes fever and coma. If melanosis is obvious, the diagnosis is rarely missed. The history, if obtainable, is one of gradual onset of weakness, fatigue, weight loss, and anorexia, followed by a rapid exacerbation.

Treatment

Therapy is as follows:

1. Draw blood for total eosinophil count, plasma electrolytes, BUN, blood sugar, and 17-OHCS. Obtain urine, by catheter if patient is comatose, for Na concentration.

2. Start I.V. infusion through same needle containing:

  a. 5% glucose in normal saline solution, 2,500 to 3,000 ml./24 hr.

  b. 100 mg. hydrocortisone (see outline on p. 231, for preparations) per liter of fluid; approximately 200 to 300 mg. will be required in the first 24 hours. Infuse the first 100 mg. within 5 to 10 minutes.

  c. If systolic pressure is less than 70 mm. Hg, give metaraminol bitartrate (Aramine) in a separate I.V. so that the dose can be regulated quickly depending on the blood pressure. Available in 10 mg./ml. solutions; diluted in saline and infused at a rate depending on blood pressure response. Other vasopressors are *l*-arterenol (Levophed) and phenylephrine hydrochloride (Neo-Synephrine). Also inject an additional 100 mg. hydrocortisone rapidly through the I.V. tubing. The response to pressor agents can increase rapidly after hydrocortisone has been infused, so the blood pressure must be measured frequently.

3. DCA 4 ml. (20 mg.) I.M. immediately (2 ml. in 2 sites). The dose may be reduced to 5 to 10 mg. in elderly patients or those with cardiac disorders.

4. In severe shock use plasma, blood, or human albumin.

5. Antibiotic therapy is used empirically unless one obtains a clear-cut history of a stress agent other than infection or unless one learns that the patient omitted cortisol medication. Determine the precipitating cause of the crisis as soon as possible. If fever is present, antibiotics are always given.

Vital signs and fluid intake-output must be monitored frequently. Electrolytes and blood sugar should be measured again in 6 to 12 hours and thereafter as required. With recovery of consciousness and general improvement, I.M. cortisone acetate may be substituted for the I.V. cortisol in a dosage of 50 mg. every 6 hours and later 50 mg. every 8 hours. Oral cortisol therapy should be used as soon as feasible because it is absorbed more rapidly and provides a higher blood concentration than the I.M. steroid. A high carbohydrate liquid diet in small feedings every 4 hours may be tolerated within 6 to 12 hours, and by the second day the patient can be given a soft or even a full diet unless there is a complicating factor such as severe infection or toxemia. Maintenance levels of therapy are attained within the first week.

Adrenal hemorrhage ("apoplexy")

See outline on p. 233.

Waterhouse-Friderichsen syndrome. The Waterhouse-Friderichsen syndrome is a complication of cerebrospinal meningitis with meningococcemia but may occur in other fulminating infections. In earlier reports 90% of cases were found in children, but it has now been recognized more frequently in adults. The onset resembles a respiratory infection but there is rapid progression to a febrile toxemia with cyanosis, petechiae, purpura or coalescent ecchymoses of the skin resembling post-mortem lividity, shallow rapid respirations, circulatory collapse, and death. Cultures of the blood, the spinal fluid, and often the skin lesions yield meningococci. At autopsy there is bilateral adrenal hemorrhage varying from petechiae to large hemorrhages that can convert an adrenal into a bloody cyst. Although the adrenal hemorrhages were always viewed as the primary cause, a number of typical cases have been reported without hemorrhage. Rich, 1944, found adrenal cellular edema and necrosis in cases of circulatory collapse during acute infections. The solid cords of the zona fasciculata were transformed into tubular structures. Selye, 1951, described cortical cytolysis in acute intense stress with the formation of "lumina" resembling the tubular degeneration of Rich. Wilbur and Rich, 1953, produced adrenocortical necrosis, hemorrhage, and tubular degeneration by the administration of ACTH, and Greendyke, 1965, proposed a hypothesis that can be summarized as follows: stress → ACTH → adrenocortical necrosis → hemorrhage → adrenal vein thrombosis. The rapid downhill course has been ascribed to either acute adrenocortical insufficiency, overwhelming toxemia especially involving the central nervous system, or to the combination. To my knowledge there have been no reported studies of plasma or urinary 17-OHCS, but values obtained in patients with circulatory collapse due to sepsis have been normal. Treatment should be as outlined for Addisonian crisis together with measures to combat the specific type of infection.

Complicating anticoagulant therapy. McDonald et al., 1966, reviewed 41 cases. Seventy-five percent were found in patients 60 or more years of age. Heparin was the chief offender. The diagnosis is suggested by the onset, usually in the first 10 days of therapy, of anorexia, nausea, vomiting, steady abdominal or flank pain, fever, lethargy, disturbed sensorium, hypotension, upper abdominal or lumbar tenderness, and laboratory findings of ACI. The prompt administration of corticosteroids, stopping the anticoagulant, and the use of vitamin K, plasma, or blood transfusion may be life saving. Permanent ACI has been the usual sequela.

Miscellaneous causes. Greendyke, 1965, reviewed 33 cases of "idiopathic adrenal hemorrhage" and commented on the severity and wide diversity of the associated diseases. Shock was a prominent feature in 17 cases.

Newborn. Adrenal hemorrhage can occur after prolonged and difficult labor and may lead to neonatal death.

Adrenocortical insufficiency secondary to isolated deficiency of ACTH ("pituitary Addison's disease")

Odell, 1966, could find only 10 cases in the literature. The cause is unknown but could stem from an isolated deficiency of CRF. In the 2 patients who were autopsied, however, the hypothalamus appeared normal. In one case there was a decrease of pituitary basophils. The symptoms were those of adrenal insufficiency. The blood pressure was low. Axillary and pubic hair was normal in men but was absent or decreased in women. Hyperpigmentation was an unexpected finding in 3 patients and was ascribed to a hypothetical circulating polypeptide that was devoid of ACTH function but maintained MSH activity. Hyponatremia was found in 50% of patients. Plasma ACTH had not been measured in any patient, and the diagnosis of ACTH deficiency depended on indirect evidence. Therapy is the same as for primary ACI. ACTH has been used with success in patients with pituitary insufficiency, but for long-term therapy oral cortisol is recommended. If there are evidences of loss of other trophic hormones, therapy for pituitary insufficiency is carried out as outlined in Chapter 5.

Adrenocortical insufficiency following corticosteroid therapy (iatrogenic)

Corticosteroid therapy can cause ACTH inhibition, adrenocortical atrophy and reduction of the secretion of cortisol. The problem of whether the suppresison is due to a feedback inhibition of CRF, of ACTH, or of both or to direct inhibition of the adrenal cortex, which becomes unresponsive to ACTH, has not been established. Graber et al., 1965, studied several patients after prolonged suppression and found that in the first month after steroid withdrawal the adrenals were unresponsive to ACTH stimulation and plasma ACTH levels were low. During the second to the fifth month plasma ACTH values rose to even supernormal levels, but adrenal responses to ACTH remained subnormal. From the sixth to the ninth month plasma 17-OHCS finally returned to normal. Complete recovery was observed only after 9 months.

When corticosteroid therapy is discontinued, recovery of adequate adrenocortical secretion may be delayed, and the patient has adrenal insufficiency for an indefinite period of time. Even when therapy has not been interrupted, a stressful stimulus may unmask relative adrenal insufficiency unless the dosage of the corticosteroid is increased appropriately in relation to the severity and duration of the stress. Steroid withdrawal is often associated with painful aching joints and muscles, malaise, weakness, anorexia, nausea, mental depression, dizziness, and postural hypotension.

Robinson et al., 1962, Treadwell et al., 1963, and Danowski et al., 1964, showed that persistent adrenal suppression occurred only after continuous corticosteroid therapy for over 1 year in larger than physiologic doses, whereas small doses for up to 3 years, or interrupted therapy for longer periods, did not induce prolonged posttherapy ACI. When the unresponsive state of the adrenals is recognized, serious sequelae can be averted by supporting the patient through a stress by the administration of cortisol. The danger lies in the unrecognized case; the patient may not alert the physician to his previous steroid therapy, and a fatal outcome can be the result of anesthesia, surgery, or any other stress.

Posttherapy ACTH suppression or adrenal unresponsiveness can sometimes be averted (1) by slow stepwise reduction of steroid therapy rather than by precipitate withdrawal, (2) by using minimal effective doses, (3) by employing an intermittent dosage schedule, or (4) by the concomitant periodic administration of ACTH during or at least near the termination of corticosteroid administration. Data indicating the effectiveness of the above measures are limited.

Concurrent endocrine disorders in Addison's disease

Multiple endocrine deficiencies appear to be prevalent in the idiopathic variety of ACI.

Diabetes mellitus. Salomon et al., 1965, reviewed 113 cases and noted the prior onset of diabetes in 63%, of Addison's disease in 23%, and the simultaneous onset in 10%. Despite the susceptibility of diabetic patients to tuberculosis, adrenocortical failure was caused by tuberculosis in only 22%, whereas idiopathic atrophy was found in 74%. Tzagournis and Hamwi, 1967, found diabetes in 7 of 41 of their Addisonian patients. The diabetic patient who contracts Addison's disease shows diminishing insulin requirements and hypoglycemic reactions.

Hypoparathyroidism. An association has been observed with Addison's disease, superficial moniliasis, steatorrhea, posthepatitic cirrhosis, and a familial tendency.

Hypothyroidism. The combination has been called "Schmidt's syndrome" (Schmidt, 1926), and the hypothyroid state is usually attributed to lymphocytic thyroiditis. Diabetes mellitus is a frequent associated disorder. Autoimmune damage to the thyroid, adrenal cortex, and even the islets of Langerhans may be a causative factor. Gastineau and Arnold, 1963, reviewed 538 cases of Addison's disease from the Mayo Clinic and found only 11 cases of myxedema, an incidence of 2%, and concluded that this was a "slight but real increase above chance."

Hyperthyroidism. Approximately 3% to 4% of Addisonian patients have coexisting hyperthyroidism. The association may be more than fortuitous, but there is scant evidence to suggest a common etiology or a causative relationship. Occasionally hyperthyroid subjects show hyperpigmentation without definite signs of adrenal insufficiency.

Hypogonadism. The association with Addison's disease is unusual, but when it occurs, myxedema is often present.

Pregnancy and Addison's disease

Well-managed Addison's disease is compatible with fertility. Carefully supervised prenatal care is essential. The clinical course is usually uncomplicated but may become difficult should first trimester nausea or vomiting occur. Labor constitutes a stress stimulus that requires an increase of steroid dose and careful monitoring of vital signs and fluid and electrolyte balance. If cesarean section is done, the patient is prepared and maintained as described below in the discussion of surgery.

Addison's disease and surgery

Surgery imposes a major stress upon the human organism, which responds with an outpouring of adrenocortical secretions. The patient with Addison's disease lacks this protective mechanism. The following plan is recommended:

1. The day before surgery discontinue oral cortisol after the morning dose or after the noon dose (in patients on a thrice-daily schedule), and give a hydrocortisone preparation (see outline on p. 231) or cortisone acetate 50 mg. I.M. at 6 P.M., at midnight, and at 6:00 the next morning. If surgery is planned for the afternoon, another dose is given at 12 noon.

2. During surgery 100 mg. I.V. hydrocortisone is infused slowly. In case of a fall in blood pressure the dose is increased and vasopressor agents are added.

3. After surgery hydrocortisone or cortisone acetate 50 mg. I.M. is given every 6

hours for 24 hours, then given every 8 hours for the second day, and finally tapered gradually down to the patient's usual oral dosage.

4. In the event of unplanned emergency surgery, 100 mg. of hydrocortisone or cortisone acetate is given I.M. immediately, and 100 to 200 mg. hydrocortisone is infused I.V. during the operation. Thereafter the plan outlined in step 3 is followed.

5. In case of circulatory collapse, the plan outlined under the discussion on adrenal crisis is followed.

6. For minor surgery involving short anesthesia such as closed reduction of a fracture or a dilatation and curettage, 100 mg. of hydrocortisone or cortisone is given I.M. 1 or 2 hours before and 50 mg. 4 hours later. Thereafter oral medication can be resumed.

REFERENCES

Albeaux-Fernet, M., et al.: J. Clin. Endocr. **17:** 519, 1957.

Bell, H., et al.: Arch. Intern. Med. **115:**418, 1965.

Cushner, G. B., et al.: Ann. Intern. Med. **58:** 341, 1963.

Danowski, T. S., et al.: Ann. Intern. Med. **61:** 11, 1964.

Eisenstein, A. B.: Med. Clin. N. Amer. **52:**327, 1968.

*Forsham, P. H., and Melmon, K. L.: The adrenals. In Williams, R. H., editor: Textbook of Endocrinology, ed. 4, Philadelphia, 1968, W. B. Saunders Co., p. 322.

*Frawley, T. F.: Adrenal cortical insufficiency. In Eisenstein, A. B., editor: The adrenal cortex, Boston, 1967, Little, Brown & Co., p. 476.

*Friedman, N. B.: Endocrinology **42:**181, 1948.

Gastineau, C. E., and Arnold, J. W.: Proc. Mayo Clin. **38:**323, 1963.

Graber, A. L., et al.: J. Clin. Endocr. **25:**11, 1965.

*Greendyke, R. M.: Amer. J. Clin Path. **43:**210, 1965.

*Guttman, P. H.: Arch. Path. **10:**742, 895, 1930.

Irvine, W. J., et al.: Lancet **2:**883, 1968.

Jarvis, L., et al.: Radiology **62:**16, 1954.

Mason, A. S., et al.: Lancet **2:**744, 1968.

McDonald, F. D., et al.: J.A.M.A. **198:**1052, 1966.

*Odell, W. D.: J.A.M.A. **197:**1006, 1966.

O'Donnell, W. M.: Arch. Intern. Med. **86:**266, 1950.

Rich, A. R.: Bull. Johns Hopkins Hosp. **74:**1, 1944.

Robinson, B. M. B., et al.: Brit. Med. J. **1:** 1579, 1962.

Rowntree, L. G.: J.A.M.A. **159:**1527, 1955.

*Salomon, N., et al.: Diabetes **14:**300, 1965.

Schmidt, M. B.: Verh. Deutsch. Ges. Path. **21:** 212, 1926.

Selye, H.: The physiology and pathology of exposure to stress. Supplement: Annual report on stress, Acta, Montreal, 1951.

Soffer, L. J., et al.: The human adrenal gland, Philadelphia, 1961, Lea & Febiger, p. 257.

*Thorn, G. W.: The diagnosis and treatment of adrenal insufficiency, Springfield, Ill., 1949, Charles C Thomas, Publisher, p. 64.

Thorn, G. W.: Johns Hopkins Med. J. **123:**49, 1968.

Treadwell, G. L. J., et al.: Lancet **1:**355, 1963.

Tzagournis, M., and Hamwi, G. J.: Metabolism **16:**213, 1967.

Vagnucci, A. H.: J. Clin. Endocr. **29:**279, 1969.

Walser, M., et al.: J. Clin. Invest. **42:**456, 1963.

Wilbur, O. M., Jr., and Rich, A. R.: Bull. Johns Hopkins Hosp. **93:**321, 1953.

*Significant reviews.

Chapter 14

Cushing's syndrome

Cushing's syndrome is the clinical expression of the inappropriate hypersecretion of cortisol and, at times, of adrenocortical androgens. The excess cortisol arises from either hyperplastic or tumorous adrenal cortices. Almost identical clinical features can be reproduced in normal subjects by the administration of pharmacologic doses of corticosteroids or by sustained injections of ACTH (iatrogenic Cushing's syndrome). "Cushing's disease" refers to cases clearly of pituitary origin that usually exhibit a pituitary tumor. "Cushing's syndrome" refers to so-called nonpituitary cases. The distinction loses precision with the knowledge that bilateral adrenocortical hyperplasia is usually caused by excessive pituitary ACTH and should be called Cushing's disease, whereas it is generally included in the Cushing's syndrome category.

Etiology

An adrenocortical, adenohypophysial or ectopic (nonpituitary, nonadrenal) tumor serves as an obvious cause of the disorder. In the majority of cases, however, one finds only bilateral adrenocortical hyperplasia for which a satisfactory explanation is lacking. The following hypotheses have been offered.

Anterior pituitary pathology. Cushing, 1932, attributed the syndrome to the secretory activity of basophilic adenomas of the anterior pituitary and named the dis-

ease "pituitary basophilism." His hypothesis lost favor when identical tumors were found in up to 7% of routine autopsies. Crooke, 1935, described cytoplasmic hyalinization of the nontumorous basophils and suggested that they, rather than the basophilic adenoma, were responsible for the disease. Crooke's changes were relegated to a secondary role when it was found that they were reproducible by the administration of corticosteroids and occurred in patients with adrenocortical tumors.

More recent evidence indicating pituitary ACTH hypersecretion has been marshaled to substantiate a pituitary origin. Nelson and Meakin, 1959, first described an ACTH-producing anterior pituitary tumor that became manifest following bilateral adrenalectomy for Cushing's syndrome. Such tumors do not appear even in long-standing Addison's disease. The presence of extreme hyperpigmentation indicated hypersecretion of MSH as well as ACTH. A higher plasma ACTH concentration is found in patients with Cushing's syndrome than in Addison's disease or in normal subjects. An excessive response to the metyrapone test is characteristic of Cushing's syndrome from adrenal hyperplasia and is presumed to be the result of an excessively responsive endogenous ACTH-producing mechanism. Nugent et al., 1960, only slightly raised the plasma ACTH level of normal subjects for 4-day periods by means of constant I.V. infusions of small amounts of ACTH and produced an elevated plasma cortisol, abolished the normal diurnal plasma cortisol variation, and found hyperresponsiveness to ACTH, all characteristic phenomena of Cushing's syndrome. They suggested that the disease could be caused by a constant excessive secretion of ACTH so minimal that it escaped detection by currently available assay methods. Patients with Addison's disease have high circulating levels of ACTH that are easily suppressible with dexamethasone, whereas patients after subtotal adrenalectomy for Cushing's syndrome continue to demonstrate refractoriness, suggesting a continued abnormal pituitary regulating mechanism.

Hypothalamus. Heinbecker, 1944, described paraventricular nuclear atrophy in Cushing's syndrome and produced cushinggoid changes in dogs that had been subjected to complete denervation of the neural hypophysis or interruption of afferent nerve pathways to the supraoptic and paraventricular nuclei. The discovery of a corticotrophin-releasing factor (CRF) (Chapter 4) has suggested that the primary lesion may reside in the hypothalamus. There is also the possibility that disturbances of higher centers in the central nervous system may disturb the CRF → ACTH → cortisol pathway.

Intrinsic adrenocortical lesion. A non-ACTH dependent form of Cushing's without adrenocortical tumor but with extensive nodular hyperplasia has been described (Meador et al., 1967).

Pathophysiology

The common denominator, regardless of pathologic changes, is adrenocortical hyperfunction. The secretory rate of the adrenals and the total quantity of secreted cortisol are increased, but the cortisol content of tumors or of hyperplastic tissue has not been found to be elevated, nor is the in vitro production rate per gram of tissue increased, though because of a larger mass the total production per gland is greater.

The impact of persistent hypercortisolemia profoundly alters the physiology of all tissues. The mobilization of peripheral *fat* leads to a total increase with a truncal distribution and contributes to the development of arteriosclerosis. Protein antianabolism promotes a net loss of *protein*, muscle wasting, reduced muscular work performance, prepuberal growth retardation, cutaneous disruption and thinning with rubor and striae, impaired wound healing, and excessively fragile capillaries with ecchymoses. The rise of plasma growth hormone stimulated by insulin hypoglycemia in normal subjects is obtunded in Cushing's disease. Osteoporosis results from increased bone resorption, reduced osteoblastic activity and bone formation, and a contracted calcium pool. The diabetogenic action of cortisol leads to decreased *carbohydrate* tolerance in most cases, and frank diabetes in about 20% of cases. There is sodium retention, excessive urinary loss of potassium, some edema, occasionally hypochloremic hypokalemic alkalosis, and a susceptibilty to hypertension with its sequelae of cardiac, coronary, cerebral, and renovascular catastrophes. There is an increased susceptibility to infection and an attenuation of immune responsiveness. There may be excessive secretion of adrenal androgens, causing virilization of the female, that is, mixed Cushing's-adrenogenital syndrome. In bilateral hyperplasia the 17-ketosteroid (17-KS) excretion differs from the normal; there is an absolute and relative increase in the 11-oxy-KS, increased 11β-OH-androsterone, and a fourfold increase in the etiocholanolone/androsterone ratio. Dehydroepiandrosterone (DHEA) is usually greatly elevated in adrenocortical cancer. In the latter there is also a deficiency in the 11β-hydroxylating enzymes, resulting in an increased excretion of tetrahydro-S (Lipsett, 1963). Recurrent and metastatic adrenocortical carcinoma in Cushing's syndrome may be characterized by an increasing excretion of C_{19} compounds such as dehydroepiandrosterone, etiocholanone, and androsterone. Aldosterone production is usually within normal limits.

Pathology

Adrenal cortex. Adrenocortical hyperplasia is found in 60% to 74% and tumor in 25% to 28% of patients (Table 14-1). The hyperplasia may occasionally be of the nodular variety and resemble a benign adenoma, but a true adenoma usually, though not invariably, is associated with atrophy of the contralateral gland. In children, particularly before age 10 years, the prevalence of carcinoma is higher than in adults. In about 10% of patients the pathologist is unable to discern any abnormality.

Anterior pituitary. Pituitary tumors have been found in approximately half of all patients with adrenocortical hyperplasia in whom the pituitary was examined. In Table 14-2, Plotz's series included 45 tumors in 97 cases in which autopsy had been done, of which 31 were of the basophil variety, and Thompson and Eisenhardt, 1943, found 39 "pituitary adenomas" among 63 cases. Since the majority of adenohypophysial tumors are small basophil adenomas, they are discovered only if the pituitary is sectioned. The larger chromophobe adenoma is more likely to enlarge the sella turcica and constrict the visual fields. These tumors tend to become clinically evident particularly after bi-

Table 14-1. Pathologic anatomy of Cushing's syndrome*

	Plotz et al., 1952 (97 cases)*	O'Neal, 1964 (224 cases)	Soffer et al., 1961 (350 cases)	Riggs and Sprague, 1961 (203 cases)
Bilateral adrenocortical hyperplasia (ACTH-dependent)				
Idiopathic—excessive hypothalamic CRF (?) → ACTH	60%	40.2%	60%	74.4%
Pituitary tumor				
Benign—basophil, chromophobe, or eosinophilic adenoma	51%†	17.4%	—	—
Malignant—carcinoma (basophil or chromophobe origin)				
Ectopic tumor (nonadrenal, nonpituitary)	9.6%	14.7%		5.6% malignant 3.9% benign
Adrenocortical tumor‡	28%	27.7%	28%	25.6%
(Benign adenoma)	(11%)	(9.4%)	(16%)	(13.3%)
(Carcinoma)	(17%)	(18.3%)	(12%)	(12.3%)
Adrenals				
"normal"	9%	—	10%	—
Hypoplastic, or hemorrhage-infarct	3%	—	—	—

*The four series are literature reviews, so that there is probably considerable repetition; some cases are listed as showing both pituitary and adrenal pathology.
†Cases in which autopsy had been done (not included in totals).
‡Percentages in parentheses form the total percentages under the heading of adrenocortical tumor.

lateral adrenalectomy. Crooke's changes (1935) (p. 238) are the most pathognomonic histologic sign of Cushing's syndrome and have been found in 90% to 95% of cases. Malignant pituitary tumors are unusual.

Ectopic (nonendocrine) tumors. Tumors of neither adrenal nor pituitary origin may be associated with Cushing's syndrome. Most arise from the lung, thymus, or pancreas but they may originate from the prostate, parotid, ovary, testicle, kidney, breast, esophagus, colon, gallbladder, and brain, and even carcinoid tumors, pheochromocytoma, sympathicoblastoma, and ganglioma have been found. The thymic tumors are composed predominantly of epithelial cells, and the lung neoplasms are the oat cell or undifferentiated type. They produce a protein that resembles ACTH by bioassay and immunoassay, that suppresses endogenous ACTH, and that induces bilateral adrenocortical hyperplasia and excessive corticosteroid secretion. Even patients with bronchogenic carcinoma who lack the clinical features of Cushing's syndrome may exhibit adrenocortical hyperfunction, as evidenced by elevated plasma and urinary 17-OHCS, loss of the diurnal variation as the disease progresses, adrenocortical hyperplasia, and Crooke's cells in the anterior pituitary. The oat cell tumor of lung and mediastinum can elaborate not only ACTH but also vasopressin and serotonin. It has been suggested that bronchial carcinoid, oat cell carcinoma of the lung, and the anterior mediastinal malignant tumors associated with Cushing's syndrome are varieties of the same tumor and arise from similar tissue derived from the neural crest (O'Neal et al., 1968).

Miscellaneous. Rarely adrenocortical rest tumors of the ovaries or testes cause Cushing's syndrome. Other pathologic changes, not invariably present, are gonadal atrophy, atherosclerosis, nephrosclerosis, and cardiac hypertrophy. There is thinning of the corium and loss of subcutaneous fibrous supporting tissue with fat distention. Muscles are thin, flabby, and often grossly infiltrated with fat.

Table 14-2. The pituitary gland in Cushing's syndrome

	Plotz et al., 1952 ninety-seven cases with autopsy	*O'Neal, 1964 224 cases (25 tumors histologically verified, 14 clinically evident)*
Crooke's changes alone	33	7[*]
Basophil adenoma	31	9
Increased basophils	8	—
Chromophobe adenoma	7	10
Mixed chromophobe-eosinophil adenoma	3	—
Eosinophil adenoma	2	2
Mixed chromophobe-eosinophil adenoma	1	—
Increased eosinophils	1	—
Unspecified adenoma	1	—
Carcinoma		
Basophil	—	1
Chromophobe	—	3
Atrophy, fibrosis, or scar	2	—
Normal	6	—

[*]Seven of 8 nontumorous pituitary glands.

Clinical features

Cushing's syndrome is a rare disorder found more commonly in females than in males (3 or 4 to 1). In the latter it tends to be somewhat less florid and clear cut in its manifestations. Most cases occur in individuals between 20 and 45 years of age, but it has been reported in infants and in the aged. The onset is usually insidious, and the clinical manifestations progress slowly. Fully developed Cushing's syndrome is so striking that it is easy to recognize (Plate II), but symptoms and signs may be minimal and are often present for long periods before the diagnosis is made. Obesity and hypertension may be mistaken for the variety so commonly encountered in medical practice. With time the more typical manifestations appear, and atherosclerotic, cardiovascular-renal, or skeletal complications ensue. Intercurrent infections may be masked by the high levels of cortisol. Occasionally patients exhibit spontaneous, though usually transient, remissions. An accelerated clinical course is characteristic of adrenocortical carcinoma. Since the disease is usually curable, early diagnosis is essential.

Symptoms and signs

Obesity, weight gain. An increase in weight is the earliest and most characteristic physical change. Most, but not all, patients gain weight, though extreme obesity is rare. Occasionally though there may even be minor weight loss, the characteristic redistribution of fat to the trunk, shoulder, and pelvic girdles is manifest. There is thinning of the extremities as though fat were stripped from the arms and legs and deposited on the body, producing the characteristic buffalo adiposity, central or truncal obesity. Fat pads are found over the posterior cervical (cervicodorsal hump) and the supraclavicular areas. There is rounding of the face ("moon-face"—Plate II, A) caused by fat and fluid accumulation in the cheeks, periorbital area, and temples and plethora of the cheeks. The abdomen may become

pendulous, but more often resembles a distended pregnant belly because of thinning of the abdominal muscles and skin (Plate II, B). In the ectopic-ACTH syndromes the characteristic centripetal obesity may be lacking and weight loss is not unusual. The presence of a malignant ectopic lesion and consequent anorexia may be the explanation.

Hypertension. Hypertension is the second most common feature; its absence should render the diagnosis doubtful. It is usually quite fixed and moderate (160-170/115-105) but may attain high levels as the disorder progresses. Cardiovascular complications occur in long-standing cases.

Skin. The integument is thin and without resiliency. During venipuncture the needle penetrates without resistance, like a hot knife through butter. The underlying dilated blood vessels are visible, causing a reddening (rubor) particularly of the cheeks, producing a plethoric appearance. Veins are prominent especially over the lower abdomen and legs. Easy bruising and multiple ecchymoses are prominent features, and after several venipunctures the antecubital area becomes one large confluent ecchymosis. Liddle, 1967, describes the integument as being "so friable that it is denuded merely by removal of adhesive tape." Wounds often heal poorly, a phenomenon that is aggravated by frequent wound infection. Leg ulcers, skin pigmentation, rashes, and telangiectasia may be found. Striae form over the lateral and lower abdomen, flanks, anterior axillae and axillary portions of the breasts, and upper arms and thighs (Plate II, B). The striae are salmon red or purple, violaceous, flame shaped, long, and wide (more than 1 cm.), in contrast to the striae of obesity or pregnancy, which are short, thin, light pink, pale salmon color or white. Though striae are one of the most striking features of the disease, they are absent in one third of cases. *Fatigue, weakness,* and *asthenia* are prominent complaints. The patient appears ill and debilitated and is rarely spirited or cheerful. There is muscle

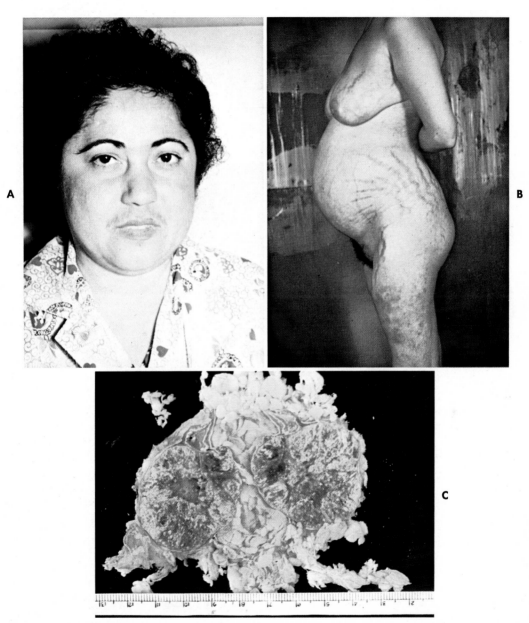

Plate II. Cushing's syndrome. **A,** Characteristic moon-face, mild hirsutism, and facial rubor.
B, The classical pregnant-belly lordosis and flame-shaped striae, cutaneous thinning with
prominent veins, and ecchymoses. **C,** Benign adenoma sectioned to show the color, areas
of necrosis, and uninvolved atrophic adrenal cortex. (**A** referred by Dr. Theodore H. Men-
dell, Philadelphia, Pa.; **B** and **C** courtesy Dr. Rachmiel Levine, New York, and Michael Reese
Hospital, Chicago.)

weakness, loss of tone, and wasting—findings that are likely to be more severe in older patients, in adrenal carcinoma, and in the ectopic-ACTH syndrome. The patient experiences great difficulty in rising from a squatting position.

Hirsutism and virilization. A scanty growth of hair on the upper lip, chin, and sideburns, together with mild acne is a frequent finding, but virilization is unusual. There may be a combination of the cushingoid (metabolic) changes because of excessive cortisol, and virilizing signs (adrenogenital syndrome) because of hypersecretion of both cortisol and adrenal androgens; in such cases adrenal tumors, especially carcinoma, are more prevalent than hyperplasia. Marked hirsutism, severe acne, temporal balding, and clitoromegaly may be striking in such patients.

Gonadal disorders. A menstrual disorder eventuating in amenorrhea occurs in the majority of cases. Maintenance of regular ovulatory menstruation is unusual, and fertility is rare. In the male there is reduced libido, partial-to-complete loss of sexual potency, and softening of the testes.

Osteoporosis. The reported incidence varies from 40% to 85%, probably because of differing criteria for diagnosis. The truncal skeleton is involved, whereas the extremities are often spared. The spine is kyphotic and lordotic. The commonest symptom is *backache,* but the patient may complain of rib pain, generalized bone pain, or nerve-root pain from a compression fracture of the dorsal or lumbar vertebrae. Backache can occur without demonstrable osteoporosis and is probably musculoligamentous in origin.

Renal calculi and even nephrocalcinosis are less frequent. Mental changes are common. There is no characteristic neuropsychiatric spectrum, but *depression* often associated with irritability predominates. Major psychoses and suicides have been

Table 14-3. Flow sheet for the laboratory diagnosis of Cushing's syndrome

Office screening procedures
1. Fasting eosinophil count, complete blood count
2. Postprandial blood sugar, or glucose tolerance test
3. Rapid (overnight) dexamethasone test (p. 221)

Hospital procedures
Day 1: a. Fasting plasma 17-OHCS, electrolytes, BUN, blood sugar, complete blood count, total eosinophil count, PBI, cholesterol
b. 4 P.M. plasma 17-OHCS, blood sugar 2 hours after oral glucose
c. Start collection of baseline 24-hour urine for 17-OHCS, 17-KS, and creatinine and save for future determination of 17-KGS, β-ketosteroids, tetrahydro-S, and DHEA if necessary
Day 2: a. Dexamethasone 0.5 mg. orally q.6h. for 2 days
b. X-ray chest, dorsolumbar spine and pelvis, skull and sella turcica
c. ECG
Day 3: 24-hour urine for 17-OHCS (first dose dexamethasone suppression test)
Day 4: Dexamethasone 2 mg. orally q.6h. for 2 days
Day 5: 24-hour urine for 17-OHCS (second dose dexamethasone suppression test)
Day 6: ACTH test
Day 8: Metyrapone test
Day 9, etc.: Radiologic studies to delineate tumor
In equivocal cases (if available)—cortisol secretion rate, urinary free cortisol, and items on Day 1, c.

reported. Paranoia, schizoid manifestations, irritability, hysteria, confusion, euphoria, hostility, or withdrawal and apathy have been observed. Neurologic changes have been reported and consist of tremors, visual changes, hemiplegia, paresthesias, and peripheral neuropathy.

Laboratory findings

The laboratory serves two purposes: (1) to establish the diagnosis by demonstrating adrenocortical hypersecretion of cortisol and (2) to differentiate adrenal hyperplasia from tumor. When both plasma and urinary 17-OHCS are elevated, one may immediately proceed to ascertain the nature of the adrenal lesion. Because a certain variability of hyperfunction is often exhibited by patients with adrenocortical hyperplasia, there may be fluctuations of cortisol secretion, of circulating blood levels, and of urinary excretion so that repeated testing and employment of multiple tests may be required. *The office screening procedures* (Table 14-3) are done in equivocal and suspected cases. When the diagnosis seems likely, the patient should be hospitalized for a complete study.

Studies to establish the diagnosis of Cushing's syndrome

Urinary 17-OHCS. Elevated values (above 15 mg./24 hr.) are found in 90% of patients with Cushing's syndrome if more than one 24-hour urine collection is examined. There is considerable variation in day-to-day steroid excretion, so that if one relies on a single determination, approximately 20% to 25% of values in Cushing's will fall within the normal range.

Very high values occur in adrenocortical carcinoma and in nonendocrine (ectopic) tumors. The urinary 17-ketogenic steroids (17-KGS) (p. 217) ordinarily correlate with the urinary 17-OHCS. Elevated 17-OHCS values may also occur in stress, hyperthyroidism, and simple obesity. Liddle, 1967, found that patients with Cushing's excreted more than 9 mg. 17-OHCS/gram creatinine, whereas normal subjects excreted 3 to 7 mg./gram creatinine.

URINARY FREE CORTISOL. Urinary free cortisol (p. 218) is more consistently elevated in Cushing's syndrome than the urinary 17-OHCS or 17-KGS. Nichols et al., 1968, after an extensive review of the literature, found free cortisol elevated in 90% of patients with Cushing's syndrome and in only 8% of those without Cushing's syndrome. Reported values are shown in Table 14-4. Values below 100 μg./24 hr. are rarely found. Free cortisol is usually normal in obese patients, whereas urinary 17-OHCS is often elevated.

PLASMA 17-OHCS. Fasting values of plasma 17-OHCS (p. 217) are usually above 20 μg./100 ml. and there is loss of the normal diurnal variation (Fig. 14-1), but occasionally they fall within the normal range. In such instances the late afternoon or evening value, normally about 50% of the morning, will usually, but not invariably, be elevated. The diurnal variation is occasionally preserved in Cushing's syndrome but is less distinct than in eucorticoid subjects. Ernest, 1966, published the values shown in Table 14-5 that demonstrate the overlap in morning and evening plasma 17-OHCS between normals and

Table 14-4. Elevation of urinary free cortisol in Cushing's syndrome (in μg./day)

Normal	Cushing's syndrome	Reference
Mean 15.4 (3-48)	58-710	Ross, 1960
Mean 71.4 (0-181)	297-3,605	Rosner et al., 1963
Mean 48 (0-108)	All above 120	Murphy, 1968

patients with Cushing's syndrome. Nichols et al., 1968, in their review, found that the fasting value was elevated in two thirds of patients with Cushing's and in 7% of patients without Cushing's.

CORTISOL SECRETION RATE (CSR). The CSR (p. 218) is grossly elevated, but the technical difficulties involved limit its availability. Then, too, somewhat elevated values have been found in obesity, hyperthyroidism, and late pregnancy and in 36% of patients without Cushing's syndrome in Nichols' review, 1968. The upper limit of normal is 30 mg./day, whereas in

Cushing's considerably higher values (40 to 400 mg.) are found.

DEXAMETHASONE SUPPRESSION TEST. The dexamethasone suppression test is described on p. 220. The overnight test can be used as a screening procedure to be followed by the 48 hour Liddle test when indicated. In obese subjects elevated urinary 17-OHCS, when present, are easily suppressed, in contrast to patients with Cushing's syndrome. Using Liddle's low dose (0.5 mg. every 6 hours for 48 hours), Nichols et al., 1968, found abnormal responses in 99% of patients with Cushing's

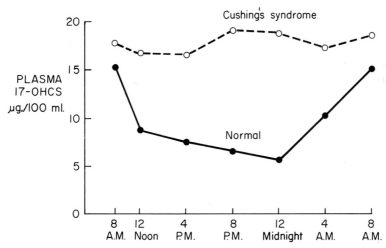

Fig. 14-1. Loss of the normal diurnal fluctuation of plasma 17-OHCS in Cushing's syndrome.

Table 14-5. Overlap of plasma 17-OHCS by case

	Plasma 17-OHCS μg./100 ml.			
	6-8 A.M.		11 P.M.-2 A.M.	
	Mean	Range	Mean	Range
23 Normal subjects	14.3 ± 4.3	8.6-27.8	3.5 ± 1.8	1- 6.6
46 Patients without Cushing's syndrome	11.3 ± 3.7	6.1-24.4	4.3 ± 3	0-15.2
36 Patients with Cushing's syndrome	20.7 ± 7.7	6-52.4	17.3 ± 4.7	2-30.1

syndrome and in 15% of patients without Cushing's syndrome. Thus *the dexamethasone test is the most reliable diagnostic laboratory study for the recognition of Cushing's syndrome.*

ACTH RESPONSIVENESS. Hyperresponsiveness in Cushing's syndrome is not found consistently enough to warrant using this test for the initial diagnosis, but it may be helpful to distinguish tumor from hyperplasia. Normally after an 8-hour infusion of 40 to 50 units of ACTH, there is a fourfold rise of urinary 17-OHCS to a range of 20 to 40 mg./24 hr. In patients with adrenal carcinoma and the majority with benign adenoma, little or no response occurs, though there have been rare notable exceptions. In bilateral hyperplasia there is usually a supernormal response to a range of 30 to 100 mg./24 hr. In benign adenoma one fourth to one third of patients will respond to ACTH.

METYRAPONE TEST. With the metyrapone test (p. 46) failure to respond is found in adrenocortical tumor, but considerable overlap of results in the various categories of Cushing's syndrome is found.

URINARY 17-KETOSTEROIDS (17-KS). In benign adrenocortical adenoma, normal or somewhat reduced values may be found. The height of the 17-KS tends to parallel the degree of virilism and is most elevated in adrenocortical carcinoma.

ROUTINE LABORATORY STUDIES. Approximately half of all patients have a neutrophilia above 80% and an eosinophilia below 40 cells/mm.[3]. One fourth show polycythemia. Finding a *fasting total eosinophil count above 100 cells/mm.[3]* should cast doubt on the diagnosis. Lymphopenia (below 20%) is common. Plasma electrolyte changes characteristic of Cushing's syndrome (decreased chloride and potassium) with alkalosis occur in 10% to 20% of cases and in almost 50% with ectopic tumor. Lowering of the serum potassium bears an inverse relationship to the degree of elevation of plasma 17-OHCS; there is usually no elevation of aldosterone. Diminished glucose tolerance is found in 80%

of cases and clinical diabetes mellitus in 20%.

For a review of laboratory tests see Nichols et al., 1968.

X-ray studies

The vertebrae, pelvis, ribs, and skull are often osteoporotic, whereas the long bones are not involved. *Spinal* osteoporosis may be severe, involving chiefly the lower dorsal and lumbar vertebrae with compression fractures and kyphosis. The changes closely resemble those of postmenopausal and senile osteoporosis, though Howland et al., 1958, believe that marginal condensation of the vertebral bodies with vertebral compression is more typical of Cushing's syndrome. Involvement of the *skull* may be diffuse or consist of irregularly decalcified areas particularly involving the frontal and parietal regions. Cranial osteoporosis is more common in Cushing's syndrome than in other osteoporotic disorders. Characteristically there are fractured osteoporotic ribs with heavy callus, often occurring spontaneously and frequently without pain.

Differential diagnosis

Obesity, particularly if associated with hypertension, diabetes, and/or mild hirsutism, is most likely to resemble Cushing's syndrome. The differentiation is outlined in Table 14-6. Steroid-induced (iatrogenic) Cushing's syndrome can be differentiated by the history. Although in the nephrotic syndrome there is facial and generalized edema, there is little resemblance to Cushing's. Myxedema is rarely mistaken for Cushing's syndrome.

Tumor versus hyperplasia

Clinical and laboratory differentiation. It is often impossible to distinguish between bilateral hyperplasia and tumor (Table 14-7) even when all available laboratory modalities are utilized. Ambiguous results are common; nevertheless, every effort must be made to define the responsible factor. Adrenal tumors are more frequent

Table 14-6. Differential diagnosis of obesity and Cushing's syndrome

	Obesity	*Cushing's syndrome*
Body weight increase	May be severe	Usually modest—rarely extreme
Truncal adiposity with thin extremities	Rare	Common
Duration of obesity	Usually lifelong	Definite onset
Moon-face	0	+
Mild hirsutism and acne	Rare	Common
Thin skin, rubor	0	+
Striae	White or pale pink, short, narrow	Salmon to purple, long, wide, flame shaped
Skin and muscles	Firm, good tone	Soft, atrophic, poor tone
Backache, osteoporosis	0	+
Cortisol secretory rate	May be elevated	Usually elevated
Urinary 17-OHCS	May be moderately elevated	Elevated
Urinary free cortisol	Normal	Elevated
Plasma 17-OHCS	Normal	Elevated
Diurnal variation	Present	Absent
Dexamethasone suppression (2 mg./day for 2 days)	Suppression	No suppression
WBC	Normal	Neutrophilia, lymphopenia, esoinopenia
RBC	Normal	Erythrocytosis

Table 14-7. Cushing's syndrome: hyperplasia, adenoma, or carcinoma?*

	Tumor		*Bilateral hyperplasia*
	Benign adenoma	*Carcinoma*	
Clinical observations			
Clinical course	Slow	Rapid	Slow
Clinical manifestations	Mild to moderate	Florid, severe	Mild to moderate
Virilization	Rare	Frequent	Rare
Palpable suprarenal mass	0	+	0
Signs of pituitary tumor	0	0	Occasionally
Laboratory tests			
Urine			
17-OHCS	++	++++	++
17-KS	Low-normal	Very high	Moderately elevated
β-Ketosteroid fraction	+	++++	0
Dehydroepiandrosterone	+	++++	0
Tetrahydro-S	0	+	0
Estrogens	+	++++	0
Dexamethasone suppression test (8 mg./day)	0	0	+
I.V. ACTH stimulation test	0 to +	0	++++
Metyrapone test	0	0	+
Plasma ACTH	0	0	Elevated
X-ray demonstration of tumor	+ or 0	Usually +	0

*0 = absent or normal.

in children than in adults; in the latter they are found in 25% of cases, and about half of these tumors are malignant. An abrupt onset with rapidly progressive full-blown clinical symptoms and signs, virilization, a palpable suprarenal mass, particularly if on the left side, very high urinary 17-KS and 17-OHCS, elevated urinary estrogens, and high values for tetrahydro-S and dehydroepiandrosterone (DHEA) (Lipsett et al., 1963) all suggest adrenocortical carcinoma. Urinary 17-KS's tend to be normal or low normal in adenoma (5 to 15 mg./24 hr.), markedly elevated in carcinoma (50 to 200 mg./24 hr.) and intermediate in hyperplasia (15 to 50 mg./24 hr.). The β-KS fraction is normally less than 15% of the total 17-KS, but is often 25% or greater in adrenal tumors and is most likely to be high in carcinoma. DHEA makes up a large part of the β-KS fraction; Lipsett et al. found increased DHEA in all 16 of their cases, but others have not found elevations as consistently.

The response to ACTH stimulation may aid in differentiating hyperplasia, adenoma, and carcinoma, but the results are often not sharply differentiated. Ordinarily there is overresponse in hyperplasia, no response in carcinoma, and a varying response in adenoma (none, mild, or moderate).

Plasma ACTH values tend to be elevated, or at least measurable, in bilateral hyperplasia and absent in tumor. Elevated values have been found in the nonendocrine (ectopic) tumor, presumably from an ACTH-like protein and not from ACTH of pituitary origin. When methods for measuring plasma ACTH become generally available, diagnostic precision will be greatly increased.

Radiologic diagnosis of adrenal tumor. Carcinomas, since they are usually bulky, are most likely to be demonstrated and can often be seen on the *flat-plate* or by body-section planigrams. A benign adenoma is smaller and more difficult to delineate. In Soffer's series (Iannoccone et al., 1960) 8 of 10 carcinomas and 6 of 9 adenomas were correctly diagnosed, indicating the optimum results by experienced workers. Downward displacement of a kidney on flat-plate or I.V. urography may be caused by tumor pressure. Retroperitoneal pneumography using the presacral approach and insufflating air, O_2, CO_2 or N_2O may outline a tumor that cannot be found by other means. The use of CO_2 or N_2O increases the safety of the procedure but requires rapid film exposure. Other techniques are selective adrenal arteriography or venography, aortography, inferior vena cavography, and nephrotomography.

All patients should routinely have an x-ray examination of the sella turcica to rule out the possibility of a pituitary tumor and a chest film to seek a lung tumor. Cushing's syndrome with an "ectopic" tumor is characterized by rapid onset, atypical clinical findings, frequent edema, a high incidence of hypokalemic alkalosis, a high cortisol secretion rate, greatly elevated 17-OHCS, elevated plasma ACTH, and failure to suppress the urinary 17-OHCS with dexamethasone or to rise with metyrapone. If the patient survives long enough, florid Cushing's syndrome develops.

Treatment

Benign adrenal tumor. If an adrenal tumor can be demonstrated or if the differential between hyperplasia and tumor is equivocal, both adrenals should be explored; if a tumor is found, it is resected. A functioning tumor almost invariably causes contralateral adrenocortical atrophy unless the syndrome is of brief duration. Thus finding hyperplasia of the contralateral gland suggests that an apparent tumor is simply a large adrenocortical nodule and the diagnosis is bilateral hyperplasia. I recommend unilateral adrenal resection if a tumor is not found, then followed by pituitary irradiation. Permanent adrenal insufficiency is avoided, and the rate of cure is about 70%. If pituitary irradiation is unsuccessful, the remaining adrenal can be resected at a later date.

The preoperative and postoperative management is outlined below. The surgical approach varies with the experience and preferences of the surgeon. The transabdominal, subpleural transdiaphragmatic, and bilateral simultaneous thoracolumbar approaches have their advocates. The transabdominal incision facilitates exposure of both adrenals. Some favor a two-stage exploration of one adrenal gland at a time. Preoperative and postoperative management of Cushing's syndrome is shown as follows:

Preparation for surgery

Treat intercurrent infections (antibiotics, etc.)

Control congestive heart failure (digitalize, use diuretics)

Correct potassium deficits with low Na diet and K supplements if required

Testosterone administration for protein depletion (except in virilized patients); (testosterone propionate 50 mg. I.M. every other day or thrice weekly)

Treat clinical diabetes, if present, with diet and insulin

For plasma volume deficit in polycythemia, give albumin or blood transfusion (Forsham, 1968)

Day before surgery

Cortisone acetate, 50 mg. I.M. 6 P.M. and midnight.

Day of surgery

1. Cortisone acetate, 100 mg. I.M. 6 A.M. and q.8h.
2. For shock and blood pressure decrease, use hydrocortisone (sodium phosphate or succinate), 100 mg. in normal saline solution I.V.; pressor agents (metaraminol bitartrate [Aramine bitartrate], levarterenol bitartrate [Levophed], or Neo-Synephrine hydrochloride)

Postoperative management

Days 1 and 2: Cortisone acetate, 100 mg. I.M. q.8h.

Days 3 and 4: Hydrocortisone (oral), 80 to 100 mg./day, divided doses

Days 5 and 6: Hydrocortisone (oral), 40 to 80 mg./day, divided doses

Days 7+: Taper hydrocortisone slowly to maintenance dosage, 20 to 40 mg./day

After resection of benign adenoma: Stimulate adrenals with ACTH-gel (see following paragraph in text)

After total bilateral adrenalectomy: Maintain hydrocortisone replacement therapy for life

The removal of a benign adenoma produces a complete cure. The atrophied contralateral adrenal cortex is restored to normal function only after several weeks or months so that corticosteroid supportive therapy is required. The patient must be treated similarly to one who has received pharmacologic doses of a corticosteroid for a prolonged period and will require increased doses during stress. Some authorities recommend the use of suboptimal cortisol replacement therapy to evoke a more rapid restoration of ACTH secretion. A dose of 10 mg. of hydrocortisone is given once daily in the morning. Intermittent ACTH therapy may hasten recovery of adrenocortical function. Various schedules have been advocated, such as 40 units of corticotrophin-gel I.M. every other day for 2 weeks, then twice weekly for another 2 weeks. However, ACTH is not universally employed because it may delay restoration of endogenous ACTH secretion.

Adrenocortical carcinoma. Complete resection can sometimes be accomplished. If metastasis has occurred, palliative removal of as much tumor tissue as possible is worthwhile. There are frequently retroperitoneal metastases that tend to produce large intra-abdominal masses. The most frequent sites of distant spread are the lung (53%) and the liver (44%) (Hutter and Kayhoe, 1966), whereas brain metastasis is unusual. Postsurgical radiation of the tumor site is usually without benefit because of the radioresistance of the lesion. Demonstrable skeletal or pulmonary metastases should be irradiated, however. An inhibitor of corticosteroid synthesis, 1,1-dichloro-2-(*o*-chlorophenyl)-2-(*p*-chlorophenyl)ethane (*ortho-para'*-DDD; *o,p'*-DDD) was introduced for the chemotherapy of adrenocortical carcinoma but is not available commercially. In a cooperative trial by the National Cancer Institute (Hutter and Kayhoe, 1966) in 138 patients, 58 of whom had Cushing's syndrome, 34% had objective tumor regression with a mean duration of 4.8 months. Toxic side effects were common and consisted chiefly of gastrointestinal disturbances, neuromuscular effects, and skin rash. Supplementary corticosteroid therapy may be necessary to combat adrenocortical insufficiency. Aminoglutethimide (Elipten) and metyrapone reduce cortisol secretion and may produce clinical improvement; Triparanol (MER-29) has a similar effect but is no longer available.

Bilateral adrenocortical hyperplasia. The most effective therapy is still a matter of controversy. The following methods are available.

Pituitary irradiation is employed to reduce excessive ACTH secretion, though it may also affect the hypothalamus and the production of CRF. Patients with relatively mild Cushing's syndrome of short duration in whom an adrenal tumor is unlikely after careful study should have pituitary irradiation as initial therapy. Cushingoid changes should regress within 6 months. After unilateral adrenalectomy a much higher percentage of cures (about 70%) may be expected. Conventional radiotherapy in the past was followed by relapse in 70% of patients. Dohan et al., 1957, suggested that more successful results might ensue if low total roentgen dosage was delivered in a more concentrated schedule (that is, 1,000 R in 5 days or 1,500 R in 10 days). A number of patients have experienced remission after implantation of radioactive seeds (^{90}Y, ^{198}Au) into the sella turcica. Teletherapy using a large accelerator to deliver alpha particles or proton beam to the pituitary has been used successfully by the Lawrence group at the University of California (Linfoot et al., 1963). Cobalt 60 irradiation delivers a therapeutic dose to the sella turcica with minimal soft tissue or brain damage.

Bilateral adrenalectomy is employed initially in severe progressive Cushing's syndrome and in patients who have failed to respond to, or relapsed after, pituitary radiotherapy. Bilateral total adrenalectomy is advocated as the most rapid and sure method of effecting a cure, but the patient thereafter has permanent adrenocortical insufficiency. Subtotal adrenalectomy is a less certain therapy; recurrences are common because the adrenal remnant is still subject to stimulation by excessive levels of ACTH, and hyperplasia of the hyperresponsive remnant is likely. If the remnant atrophies, the patient is in the same physiologic state as if a total adrenalectomy had been performed. Adrenal autotransplants have been attempted to avoid adrenal insufficiency, but the method is still experimental. Recurrent Cushing's syndrome after total bilateral adrenalectomy from persistent functioning ectopic foci of adrenal cortex tissue has been observed.

Pituitary tumor. Most clinically evident tumors are chromophobe adenomas; basophil tumors are quite small. Treatment of pituitary tumor has been discussed on p. 69. Irradiation is usually used initially, but hypophysectomy is indicated when the tumor is expanding rapidly, eroding the sella turcica, or encroaching upon vision. Even some aggressive tumors may be irradiated. In rapidly progressive severe Cushing's disease, immediate adrenalectomy has been advocated, although a trial of intensive radiotherapy with cobalt 60 or alpha particles may be considered in centers where these therapies are available. If the patient fails to respond to treatment directed to the pituitary, adrenalectomy is performed.

The appearance of an ACTH-MSH secreting pituitary tumor, usually a chromophobe adenoma, after bilateral total adrenalectomy (Nelson's syndrome) has been reported in 4% to 5% of cases (Nelson and Meakin, 1959). There is extreme cutaneous hyperpigmentation, visual field restriction, and other evidences of a pituitary tumor. Occasionally only hyperpigmentation in the absence of a demonstrable pituitary tumor occurs. Hypophysectomy has been the treatment of choice.

Nonendocrine "ectopic" tumors. Surgical removal of the primary lesion is desirable but is rarely possible because these tumors have usually metastasized at the time of diagnosis. The patient is usually too ill to survive adrenalectomy so that one must resort to various palliative measures such as local irradiation, cytotoxic chemotherapy to suppress the ectopic tumor, or the use of o, p'-DDD and metyrapone to inhibit cortisol production.

Prognosis

Plotz et al., 1952, reported that 17 of 32 of their patients died within an average of 5 years of the onset of symptoms. In regard to 114 cases collected from the literature in which autopsy had been done, the leading causes of death were bacterial infection (46.6%) and cardiovascular conditions (40%). There were 28 postoperative deaths. Since then the mortality rate has been substantially reduced with the availability of corticosteroids and antibiotics and more surgical experience. Notwithstanding, the patient with Cushing's syndrome is a delicate organism, and the risk and morbidity of surgery are still substantial. The postoperative course is likely to be stormy; there are the ever-present threats of complicating infections and wound dehiscence, and the convalescence can be prolonged.

Once the patient weathers the immediate postoperative period, the prognosis is best for benign adenoma. A complete cure is certain, and the contralateral gland after the first year can be depended on to function. Bilateral total adrenalectomy also ensures a complete cure, except in the very rare instance of ectopic adrenal tissue, and the prognosis thereafter is much the same as for a patient with Addison's disease. The onset of Nelson's syndrome alters the outlook but can usually be managed favorably. Carcinoma of the adrenal carries a poor prognosis. The outlook in the ectopic tumor syndrome depends on the primary tumor.

REFERENCES

Crooke, A. C.: J. Path. Bact. **41**:339, 1935.
Cushing, H.: Bull. Johns Hopkins Hosp. **50**:137, 1932.
Dohan, F. C., et al.: J. Clin. Endocr. **17**:8, 1957.
Ernest, I.: Acta Endocr. **51**:511, 1966.
Heinbecker, P.: Medicine **23**:225, 1944.
Howland, W. J., Jr., et al.: Radiology **71**:69, 1958.
*Hutter, A. M., Jr., and Kayhoe, D. E.: Amer. J. Med. **41**:572, 581, 1966.
Iannaccone, A., et al.: Arch. Intern. Med. **105**:257, 1960.
Liddle, G. W.: J. Clin. Endocr. **20**:1539, 1960.
*Liddle, G. W.: Cushing's syndrome. In Eisenstein, A. B., editor: The adrenal cortex, Boston, 1967, Little, Brown & Co.; a, p. 523; b, p. 543.
Linfoot, J. A., et al.: New Eng. J. Med. **269**:597, 1963.
Lipsett, M. B., et al.: Amer. J. Med. **35**:374, 1963.
Meador, C. K., et al.: J. Clin. Endocr. **27**:1255, 1967.
Murphy, B. E. P.: J. Clin. Endocr. **28**:343, 1968.
Nelson, D. H., and Meakin, J. W.: J. Clin. Invest. **38**:1028, 1959.
*Nichols, T., et al.: Amer. J. Med. **45**:116, 1968.
Nugent, C. A., et al.: J. Clin. Endocr. **20**:1259, 1960.
O'Neal, L. W.: Ann. Surg. **160**:860, 1964.
O'Neal, L. W., et al.: Cancer **21**:1219, 1968.
*Plotz, C. M., et al.: Amer. J. Med. **13**:597, 1952.
Riggs, B. L., and Sprague, R. G.: Arch. Intern. Med. **108**:85, 1961.
Rosner, J. M., et al.: J. Clin. Endocr. **23**:820, 1963.
Ross, E. J.: J. Clin. Endocr. **20**:1360, 1960.
*Soffer, L. J., Dorfman, R. I., and Gabrilove, J. L.: The human adrenal gland, Philadelphia, 1961, Lea & Febiger, p. 445.
Thompson, K. W., and Eisenhardt, L.: J. Clin. Endocrinol. **3**:445, 1943.

---

*Significant reviews.

Chapter 15

Adrenocortical androgenic hyperfunction (the adrenogenital syndrome) and hyperaldosteronism

ADRENOGENITAL SYNDROME

The adrenogenital syndrome is the clinical expression of the excessive elaboration of adrenocortical androgenic steroids. The androgens may arise from a benign or malignant adrenal tumor or from bilateral adrenocortical hyperplasia. The clinical manifestations depend to a large extent on whether the onset is before or after sexual maturity.

Congenital adrenal hyperplasia (CAH) (female pseudohermaphroditism)

CAH, an inherent disorder of adrenocortical biosynthesis originating in early fetal life, fosters the elaboration of androgenic steroids that distort the metamorphosis of the female external genital tract. Thus recognition of sexual gender at birth may be confused. The female appears virilized at or shortly after birth, the male shows sexual precocity, and there is accelerated somatic growth of both sexes. Fetal differentiation of the gonads is not affected.

The syndrome has been ascribed to a defective autosomal recessive mutant gene that is not sex linked and occurs clinically only in homozygous children (Childs et al., 1956). Only one type of CAH is ordinarily displayed in a single family; in the most prevalent form (21-hydroxylase deficiency), the simple virilizing or salt-wasting variety is rarely mixed in the same sibship (Bongiovanni et al., 1967).

Instances of CAH appearing in siblings, identical twins (Fig. 15-1), first cousins, and half sisters have been reported. Wilkins, 1965a, estimated an incidence of 1 person per 40,000 births and the heterozygous carrier 1 person per 100 population. There is an apparent predominance of females (104 females per 27 males, Wilkins, 1965b), but the diagnosis in males may be overlooked.

Pathology

The hyperplastic adrenals are largely composed of zona reticularis, the presumed source of excessive androgen production, though hyperplasia of the zona fasciculata has been implicated. In the hypertensive form there may be hyperplasia of the zona glomerulosa. The ovaries appear normal in infancy but become increasingly affected in older untreated children. In teen-aged females the ovaries contain developing primordial and atretic follicles, but there is no sign of previous ovulation. In males spermatogenesis is impaired.

Pathophysiology

The excessive secretion of adrogen commences in the fetus and results from an inherent defect of one of the adrenocortical enzymes responsible for the biosynthesis of cortisol. The most common defect involves the 21-hydroxylase enzymatic conversion of 17α-OH-progesterone to 11-desoxycortisol, but other enzymatic con-

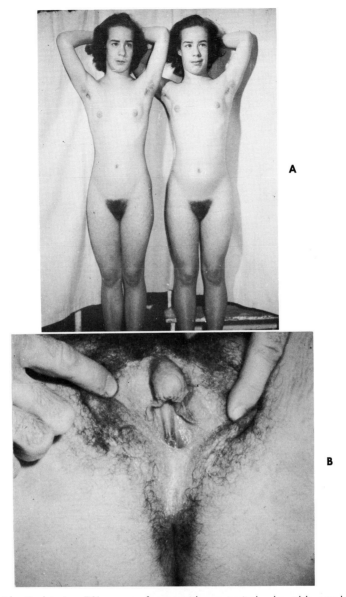

Fig. 15-1. A, Identical twins, 7½ years of age, with congenital adrenal hyperplasia. Early breast budding is the result of 2 months of corticosteroid therapy. Pretreatment photographs were technically unsuitable for reproduction. **B,** External genitalia showing separate urethra and vagina. (From Schneeberg et al.: J. Clin. Endocr. **203:**19, 1959.)

versions can be involved (Table 15-1). The blocked pathway is diverted from the synthesis of cortisol to the production of virilizing steroids that are excreted as 17-ketosteroids (androsterone, etiocholanolone, 11-OH-17-ketosteroids). The usual ratio of 11-desoxy- to 11-oxy-17-KS, being 3, becomes approximately 1 in CAH (Baulieu

et al., 1967), and the plasma androstenedione concentration is 4 to 18 times that of testosterone, whereas in normal males the concentration of testosterone is 6 times greater than that of androstenedione (Migeon, 1968). There is an accumulation of the cortisol precursors progesterone and 17α-hydroxyprogesterone and of 11β-hy-

Table 15-1. Varieties of congenital adrenal hyperplasia*

Clinical form	Biosynthetic defect	Urinary-compounds
Congenital lipoid adrenal hyperplasia	Cholesterol ↓ *Desmolase?* Pregnenolone	17-Ketosteroids ↓
3β-Hydroxysteroid dehydrogenase	| *3β-OH-dehydrogenase*	Δ⁵-3β-OH compounds 17-Ketosteroids (moderately) ↑
17-Hydroxylase	↓ Progesterone | *17-Hydroxylase*	Pregnanediol 17-Ketosteroids o Tetrahydro-B Tetrahydro-18-OH-dehydrocorticosterone
Simple and salt-losing	↓ 17α-OH-progesterone *21-Hydroxylase*	Tetrahydrocortisol ↓ Estrogens ↑ Pregnanetriol ↑, pregnanetriolene, 11-keto-pregnanetriol, 17-OH-pregnenolone, 11-keto-17-OH-pregnenolone, 17-ketosteroids ↑ (androsterone, etiocholanolone, 11-OH-17-ketosteroids) Testosterone ↑
Hypertensive	↓ 11-Desoxycortisol (Compound S) *11β-Hydroxylase* ↓ Cortisol	Tetrahydrocortisol ↓ Porter-Silber chromogens ↑ Tetrahydro-S ↑ Tetrahydrodesoxycorticosterone ↑ 17-Ketosteroids ↑ (especially etiocholanolone) Pregnanetriol ↑

*The enzymes involved are italicized; ↑ = increase, ↓ = decrease, o = no change.

droxyprogesterone, 11β,17α-hydroxyprogesterone, and Δ⁵-pregnenolone. Some 21 urinary metabolites of these compounds have been isolated; the most important are pregnanediol, pregnanetriol, 11-ketopregnanetriol, pregnenolone, 17-OH-pregnenolone, and pregnanetriolene. Abnormally large amounts of estrogens are secreted, but their effects may be blocked by the excessive androgen secretion. *The principal virilizing steroid is testosterone.* Degenhart et al., 1966, found an excretion of urinary testosterone glucuronide of 11 to 260 μg./day (normal < 5 μg.) and the production rate 0.34 to 11.4 μg./day (normal < 0.5 μg.). At least two pathways to testosterone exist in the adrenal cortex. The first is via 17α-OH-progesterone → androstenedione → testosterone, and the second is 17α-OH-pregnenolone → dehydroepiandrosterone ⎰ → Δ⁵-androstenediol or androsterone → ⎱ → androstenedione → → testosterone. Thus any enzyme block beyond 17α-OH-progesterone can generate the excessive production of testosterone as well as 17-KS. The resulting deficiency of cortisol, which may vary in degree, results in an elevated level of circulating ACTH. There follows adrenocortical hyperplasia, the continued elaboration of virilizing hormones, and some restoration of cortisol secretion often to near normal levels in the simple virilizing form but not in the salt-losing variety. There is considerable experimental evidence to substantiate this hypothesis:

1. Corticosteroid administration inhibits ACTH and causes a reduction of the urinary 17-KS, testosterone, pregnanetriol, and other progesterone derivatives and a regression of the clinical features.

2. There is a low or low-normal level of circulating cortisol and elevated circulating ACTH.

3. ACTH administration causes an increase of urinary 17-KS and pregnanetriol but little or no rise in cortisol metabolites, as one would expect in normal subjects.

4. The administration of 17-OH-progesterone normally evokes a rise of cortisol in normal subjects but not in CAH.

5. Large amounts of 17-OH-progesterone and deficient 21-hydroxylase enzymatic activity has been demonstrated in the adrenals.

Clinical features

More than 90% of cases of CAH are caused by a 21-hydroxylase deficiency. In Wilkins' series (1965b) of 131 cases, 123 were of this variety. The other forms will be discussed separately.

Simple virilizing ("compensated") form. The female external genitalia are more or less distorted at birth (that is, female pseudohermaphroditism). The clitoris resembles a male penis. There is labioscrotal fusion of varying degree that more or less obscures a persistent urogenital sinus so that there is a strong resemblance to that of a male infant with a hypospadic penis and bilateral cryptorchidism. Occasionally the onset of the disorder is later in fetal life (after the 162 mm. stage), and the

urogenital sinus has differentiated into urethra and vagina (Fig. 15-1). The effects probably commence between the 63 mm. and the 162 mm. stages of embryologic development. The external genitalia may even appear normal at birth, and the onset of the virilizing syndrome is delayed to later in childhood or adulthood. An adrenal tumor rather than CAH must be considered. Rarely there is a penile urethra, and the child may be reared as a male with cryptorchidism.

Rapid somatic growth occurs, but there is concomitant accelerated epiphysial maturation and closure so that the child is taller than his peers but becomes a short adult. The female acquires a deep voice, acne, seborrhea, a masculine habitus with broad shoulders and narrow hips, and excessive muscular development. Pubic hair may be present at birth or appear shortly thereafter, and axillary and coarse facial hair follow. In adolescence or early adult life, temporal and even apex scalp alopecia appears, particularly if there is a hereditary predisposition to baldness. At puberty there is primary amenorrhea and failure of breast development. The I.Q. tends to be above average.

In the *male* the disorder is not obvious at birth, and the first manifestation, excessive penile growth, is found in infancy. Virilization ensues, and a diagnosis of precocious puberty is entertained; the testes, however, do not enlarge as in most other varieties of premature puberty that are associated with gonadotrophin release but remain small and immature and lack spermatogenesis. Rarely the testes contain aberrant adrenal cortex tissue, and one or both enlarge but will regress during corticosteroid therapy.

Salt-losing variety. The enzyme deficit is 21-hydroxylase, as in the compensated or simple virilizing variety, but an excessive loss of urinary sodium predominates, resulting in clinical signs of adrenocortical insufficiency. In Wilkins' series (1965b) in which 123 cases were of the 21-hydroxylase deficiency, 45 were of the salt-wasting variety and 78 were of the simple virilizing type. This form of CAH usually becomes manifest in early infancy, with failure to thrive, anorexia, weight loss, vomiting, dehydration, lethargy, hypoglycemia, hypotension, hyponatremia, hyperkalemia, and metabolic acidosis and frequently terminates fatally unless treated promptly. There may be melanosis as in Addison's disease. An intercurrent infection can precipitate the syndrome, or circulatory collapse may occur without warning; many fatal terminations eluded diagnosis in the past until, at autopsy, bilaterally hyperplastic adrenal glands were found. The cause is still a subject for debate but may be due to (1) a salt-losing hormone, (2) a deficiency of aldosterone, or (3) a more complete loss of the 21-hydroxylase enzyme leading to a severe deficiency of cortisol. The first hypothesis has few adherents. A deficiency of aldosterone has been clearly demonstrated in several studies. A mechanism embodying both the second and third possibilities seems likely. The cortisol production rate in the simple form of CAH is normal, whereas it is diminished in the salt-losing variety. Bartter et al., 1968, have proposed the presence of two separate isozymes of the 21-hydroxylase enzyme to account for the aldosterone deficiency in the salt-losing variety and an intact pathway to aldosterone in the compensated form. The latter lacks 21-hydroxylation of 17-OH-progesterone alone, whereas the salt-losing patients lack 21-hydroxylation of both progesterone and 17-OH-progesterone. For a review see Bongiovanni et al., 1967.

Other varieties of CAH

HYPERTENSIVE FORM. The hypertensive form resembles the 21-hydroxylase defect with the addition of hypertension. There were 7 hypertensives among the 131 subjects with CAH in Wilkins' series (1965b). The defect resides in the 11β-hydroxylase enzyme (Table 15-1), resulting in a deficiency of cortisol and an accumulation of its immediate precursor, 11-desoxycortisol (Compound S) and the excretion of its tetrahydro-metabolite. Plasma and urinary Porter-Silber corticoids are elevated because of the rise of Compound S, and pregnanetriol is only modestly increased. Urinary 17-KS's are elevated, but 11-oxy-17KS's are not. A prepronderance of etiocholanolone has been demonstrated (Bongiovanni et al., 1967). The immediate cause of the hypertension is unknown but may be from an accumulation of desoxycorticosterone.

3β-HYDROXYSTEROID DEHYDROGENASE DEFICIENCY. A rare variety of CAH involves the transformation of pregnenolone to progesterone by the enzyme 3β-hydroxysteroid dehydrogenase. There is a lesser degree of female virilization, probably because testosterone is not produced, and incomplete differentiation of the male genitalia, suggesting a similar enzyme deficiency in the fetal testis. Salt loss, adrenocortical insufficiency, and a high fatality rate have characterized the few reported cases.

CONGENITAL LIPOID ADRENAL HYPERPLASIA. The adrenal cells are filled with lipoid material, and there is salt loss, adrenocortical insufficiency, and a high fatality rate. The enzyme deficiency may be similar to the 3β-OH-dehydrogenase variety or may involve the conversion of cholesterol to pregnenolone.

MISCELLANEOUS VARIETIES. A variety characterized by a deficiency of 17-hydroxylase has been reported (Biglieri, 1966). Hypoglycemia as a predominant symptom in 2 other cases and fever ascribed to etiocholanolone in 2 cases have been described (Baulieu et al., 1967). Two sisters reported by Mallin, 1969, showed hypertension, probably from excess secretion of desoxycorticosterone.

POSTPUBERAL CAH. See p. 259 for postpuberal CAH.

Laboratory diagnosis

Elevated urinary 17-ketosteroids (17-KS). Elevated urinary 17-KS is the *sine qua non* for the diagnosis. Normal values before 1 year of age are less than 0.5 mg./24 hr. except during the first postnatal month when up to 2.5 mg. are found. Normal values from 1 to 5 years are 0.5 to 2 mg., up to 9 years 1 to 3 mg., and 10 to 15 years 3 to 8 mg. Fractionation reveals a preponderance of androsterone and etiocholanolone and large amounts of 11-oxy-17-ketosteroids. In the hypertensive form (11-hydroxylase deficiency), etiocholanolone predominates and there are no 11-oxy-17-ketosteroids.

Elevated urinary pregnanetriol. Values above 0.5 mg./24 hr. are consistently found. However, elevated 11-ketopregnanetriol may be more specific for CAH since pregnanetriol has been elevated in adrenocortical tumor. In the hypertensive variety pregnanetriol is less markedly increased. Pregnanetriolene is elevated only in the 21-hydroxylase variety.

Suppression tests. The administration of dexamethasone in a daily dose of 3.75 mg./100 lb. body weight reduces the 17-KS and pregnanetriol to normal within 7 days in CAH but fails to do so in adrenal tumor, though a modest reduction occasionally is found. A 1-day test involving a 24-hour I.V. infusion containing 50 mg. of cortisol produces a fall of 17-KS within 2 to 6 hours.

Plasma and urinary 17-hydroxycorticosteroids. Values are normal or diminished. In the hypertensive variety, the 17-OHCS's are elevated from the accumulation of 11-desoxycortisol (Compound S), a compound measured as a Porter-Silber chromogen, or directly by chromatography.

Buccal smear and chromosome analysis. When there is ambiguity concerning the sexual gender of the newborn, genetic sex must be ascertained. The pattern in CAH conforms to the gonad of the individual. The buccal smear in affected females is chromatin-positive and the karyotype is XX.

Radiologic studies. If an adrenal tumor is suspected, intravenous urography, retroperitoneal air or gas insufflation, arteriography, or adrenal venography may be of value. The bone age is accelerated. Visualization of the urogenital structures can be accomplished by the injection of radiopaque dyes into the urogenital sinus or vagina.

Differential diagnosis

Adrenal tumor. Tumor rarely develops in fetal life or early enough in infancy to cause sexual ambiguity but is a common cause of the adrenogenital syndrome later in infancy. The urinary 17-KS is extremely high (above 50 mg./day) and is not suppressible. When fractionated, there are large amounts of DHEA. An elevated pregnanetriol is almost diagnostic of CAH rather than of tumor, though the presence of 11-ketopregnanetriol may be a more certain marker of CAH. Occasionally the 17-KS response to ACTH is used; theoretically the tumor should not respond and CAH should be hyperresponsive, but the results are not reliable. Attempts to visualize the tumor by radiologic studies may be helpful in diagnostic problems.

Intersexuality. The urinary 17-KS's are normal, and pregnanetriol is not elevated. Chromosome analysis is a critical study.

Sexual precocity. In the male one must differentiate an *interstitial cell tumor* from CAH. This lesion is ordinarily palpable, but so may be ectopic adrenal tissue in the testicle or along the spermatic cord. The elevated urinary 17-KS's are not suppressed by corticosteroids, and pregnanetriol is not found. *Constitutional sexual precocity* of the male produces testicular growth, modest elevation of the urinary 17-KS consistent with the sexual maturation of the patient, and no increase of pregnanetriol. Male sexual precocity may be associated with a hypothalamic or pineal tumor, hydrocephalus, hepatoma, or retroperitoneal sarcoma.

Female pseudohermaphroditism (nonadrenal). In female pseudohermaphroditism there may be a strong resemblance to CAH at birth, but virilization does not progress, the urinary 17-KS and pregnanetriol are not elevated, and pubertal maturation proceeds normally. In some cases the mother has received an androgen or a progestogenic compound during pregnancy because of threatened abortion, or there has been a maternal arrhenoblastoma. Occasionally there has been no apparent explanation for the presence of ambiguous external genitalia of the newborn.

Masculinizing ovarian tumors. Arrhenoblastoma is a rare, usually benign virilizing ovarian tumor that occurs in young women, and should not be mistaken for CAH. The urinary 17-KS may be elevated in one third of cases, but are not suppressible with dexamethasone or estrogens. *Adrenal rest tumors* exhibit elevations of urinary 17-KS that are suppressible with dexamethasone and often further suppressed with estrogens.

Treatment of CAH

Suppressive doses of a corticosteroid induce regression of the virilization and permit the underlying sexual gender of the patient to flower. Untreated patients become progressively more virilized, and function throughout life as males or as grotesque females. Adrenalectomy or estrogen therapy was unsuccessful before the cortisone era.

Cortisol (or cortisone), given in moderately large doses at first, suppresses androgen production within 5 to 14 days and is then tapered to a maintenance dosage. The goal is to ameliorate masculinization, to reduce the urinary 17-KS to values consistent with the age of the patient, and to provide steroid substitution for the frequently subnormal concentration of cortisol. All of these effects are accomplished when the excessive secretion of pituitary ACTH is blocked, thus permitting the hyperplastic adrenals to recede to normal. The average daily dose of I.M. cortisol or cortisone acetate advocated by Bongiovanni is 0 to 5 years 25 mg., 6 to 12 years 50 mg., and 13 years and above 75 to 100 mg.; the maintenance dosages, respectively, are 25, 35 to 50, and 50 to 100 mg. *every third day.* Oral cortisol may be used later in maintenance therapy

divided in 3 to 4 daily doses of 20 to 30 mg., 25 to 50 mg., and 50 to 100 mg., respectively, according to age. The daily oral dose is approximately double that of the I.M. dose. The principal guides to therapy are the clinical response and the urinary 17-KS. In infants a value of 1 to 2 mg./day and in older children less than 8 mg./day is desirable. If no cushingoid side effects appear, one should aim to restore normal urinary 17-KS. Overdosage with cortisol can impair growth. The dosage must be tailored to the patient, and variations of the above schedule may be necessary. As the child grows and matures, larger amounts of cortisol become necessary. If the child is subjected to stress, the dosage should be augmented, though not as markedly as in Addison's disease. Prednisone may be used, but other synthetic corticosteroids are not recommended because of their salt-wasting properties and their tendency to inhibit statural growth. The salt-wasting infant is a fragile person and requires water and NaCl replacement and I.M. desoxycorticosterone acetate in addition to cortisol. A regimen as described for Addisonian crisis (Chapter 13) may be necessary. Later oral fludrocortisol, 0.05 to 0.1 mg. daily, may be used. One may elect to implant DOCA pellets or to give long-acting DOC-trimethylacetate I.M. Despite good management, the mortality in later childhood is high.

Corticosteroid suppressive therapy must be maintained indefinitely. If treatment is omitted in the female, virilization gradually returns, accompanied by amenorrhea and anovulation; in the male, spermatogenesis regresses, though exceptions have been described. In both sexes excessive ACTH stimulation of the adrenal, a possible cause of neoplastic degeneration, is prevented.

Surgical correction of grossly distorted female external genitalia is usually performed, when necessary, in early childhood, preferably before the youngster recognizes the deformity. A grossly enlarged clitoris may require amputation. Consultation with a psychiatrist may be helpful.

Results of therapy and prognosis

Therapy started in infancy or early childhood promotes normal growth and development with few or no residual defects. If treatment is delayed, regression of virilization may be complete or somewhat incomplete, and there will be rapid breast development, menarche, and fertility. A number of treated patients have given birth to normal children. If epiphysial maturation is advanced, the patient will not attain his potential stature.

For reviews of CAH, see Baulieu et al., 1967, and Bongiovanni et al., 1967.

Virilizing adrenal tumors

Virilizing adrenal tumors are rare lesions occurring principally in young adult females. In infancy they have always been of postnatal origin, with a single exception (Kenny et al., 1968), and so are not a cause of sexual ambiguity at birth. Clinical differentiation of benign and malignant tumors is usually impossible, though a tumor in a young child, the appearance of cushingoid changes, or the finding of a very large tumor suggests cancer. Virilization is the principal physical sign in the adult female, and virilization and rapid statural growth with early epiphysial closure are the signs in the female child. Occasionally hirsutism is the sole manifestation. The onset is more abrupt, and progression is likely to be more accelerated in hyperplasia. In the prepubertal male there is macrogenitosomia praecox with small testes. The diagnosis is usually missed in the adult male unless there is gross testicular atrophy and hypospermatogenesis. The differential diagnosis from adrenocortical hyperplasia has been discussed (p. 257). The treatment is surgical resection. If there are preoperative manifestations or laboratory findings of concomitant Cushing's syndrome, the regimen outlined on p. 249 is recommended.

Adrenogenital syndrome (adult)

The adult adrenogenital syndrome may be generated by an adrenocortical tumor or bilateral hyperplasia. The clinical picture includes various degrees of defeminization (loss of female habitus, breast atrophy, genital atrophy, amenorrhea, and anovulation) and masculinization (male habitus, coarsened oily skin, acne, hirsutism, temporal recession of hair and cephalic balding, deep voice, clitoromegaly). More subtle varieties manifested only by infertility, menstrual disorders, and/or hirsutism may represent an adult counterpart of CAH. Studies of single cases or small groups have shown several of the following characteristics: menstrual disorder, failure to ovulate, hirsutism, clitoral enlargement, minimal elevation of urinary 17-KS, pregnanetriol and/or pregnanetriolene, suppression with corticosteroids, and overreaction to ACTH. Therapy with corticosteroids often induces ovulatory menstruation and fertility. Jefferies and Levy, 1959, reported successful results in 46 of 52 women with irregular menses, amenorrhea, or oligomenorrhea with the smallest dose of cortisone or hydrocortisone that would reduce the urinary 17-KS to 10 mg./day or less, that is, 2.5 to 5 mg. four times a day, or 5 mg. every 8 hours. Tyler, 1968, found that 13 of 15 patients ovulated while receiving human menopausal gonadotrophins. Several of these patients had ovulated during corticosteroid therapy but had not conceived. The distinguishing characteristics of tumor versus hyperplasia have been discussed under CAH (p. 257).

Feminizing adrenal tumors

The rare feminizing adrenal neoplasms cause gynecomastia, testicular atrophy, diminished libido and potency, and pain at the site of the tumor. In prepubertal boys there is, in addition, rapid growth and premature epiphysial maturation. The hypertension that frequently occurs has been attributed to an increased production of desoxycorticosterone from an 11β-hydroxylase deficiency (Solomon et al.,

1968). In Gabrilove's review of 52 cases (1965) 78% of the neoplasms were malignant and more than half were palpable. The urinary 17-KS or 17-OHCS tended to be elevated in cases of malignant tumor, and urinary estrogens were frequently high. Eighty percent of the patients were dead within 3 years of the diagnosis, and two thirds died within 1 year.

HYPERALDOSTERONISM
Primary aldosteronism
(Conn's syndrome) (PA)

A benign adrenal adenoma (aldosteronoma), inappropriately secreting aldosterone, induces potassium loss and hypertension. Its prevalence as a cause of chronic hypertension is probably considerably less than the hypothetical 20% once proposed by Conn (Fishman et al., 1968). Seventy-two percent of cases occur in the age range 30 to 50 years. Of 135 cases, 98 were women (Conn et al., 1964).

Pathology

Single adenomas have been found in 91% of cases and multiple adenomas in 9%. The majority spring from the left adrenal. A highly malignant form of carcinoma is a rare cause. Most of the tumors are small (Fig. 15-2), weighing less than 6 grams and measuring less than 3 cm. in diameter. They are canary yellow or yellow-orange in color. Atrophy of the contralateral adrenal is rare. Occasionally, particularly in young males, there is bilateral adrenocortical hyperplasia rather than an adenoma (congenital aldosteronism), or there may be nodular hyperplasia. Renal tubular epithelial degeneration results from hypokalemia. The histologic picture of an aldosteronoma is one of large cells with a clear vesicular cytoplasm and a small basophilic nucleus arranged in a glomerular-like pattern resembling the zona glomerulosa.

Pathophysiology

Hyperaldosteronemia probably initially induces Na retention, decreased Na excretion via urine, sweat, and saliva, and excessive urinary K loss. There ensues an increased blood and extracellular fluid volume, an increase in mean afferent renal arteriolar pressure, and suppression of the renin-angiotensin system. Histologic evidence consists of a reduced number of juxtaglomerular cells, together with almost complete absence of granularity. With continued K wasting, there is a decreased total exchangeable body K, increased exchangeable Na, and an elevated Na/K

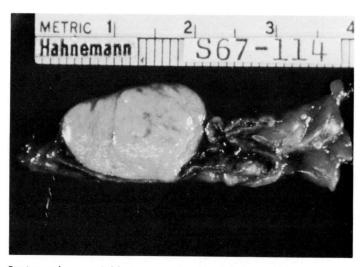

Fig. 15-2. Benign adenoma (aldosteronoma) excised from a patient with primary aldosteronism. (Courtesy Dr. Alexander Nedwich and Department of Pathology, Hahnemann Medical College, Philadelphia, Pa.)

ratio. The serum K eventually falls but may remain normal until near the end of the illness (Conn et al., 1969). The rise in blood pressure is generated by the elevated aldosterone. Renal and muscular symptoms probably depend on the profundity of K loss and the height of the blood pressure. An increased secretory rate of desoxycorticosterone and corticosterone has been found in 30% to 40% of patients (Biglieri et al., 1968).

Clinical features

The onset of clinical characteristics (Table 15-2) is insidious, probably with a prolonged asymptomatic phase marked solely by hypertension. The latter is usually moderate but may attain high levels, and the eyeground changes are minimal in relation to the blood pressure. Conn et al., 1964, classified the clinical features into three groups:

1. *Renal,* because of hypokalemic tubular damage, with polyuria, nocturia, and polydipsia; chronic pyelonephritis may intervene.

Table 15-2. Clinical features of primary hyperaldosteronism*

Major symptoms		Major signs	
Muscle weakness	(73%)	Hyper-tension	(100%)
Polyuria, nocturia	(72%)	Retinopathy	(50%)
Headache	(51%)	Cardio-megaly	(41%)
Polydipsia	(46%)		
Minor symptoms		*Minor signs*	
Paresthesias		Tetany	
Visual disturbances		Positive Trousseau sign	
Intermittent paralysis		Positive Chvostek sign	
Tetany		Paralysis	
Fatigue			
Muscle discomfort			

*Based on data from Conn et al.: Amer. J. Surg. 107:159, 1964.

2. *Muscular,* chiefly from hypokalemia, with episodic weakness and occasional flaccid paralysis. When there is metabolic alkalosis, tetany can develop or may be evident only on hyperventilation or be manifest by a positive Trousseau sign.

3. *Hypertensive* with severe frontal headache, retinopathy, and slight cardiomegaly. Abnormal sensitivity to the potassium-wasting properties of diuretic therapy may be the initial manifestation.

Laboratory findings

The following are laboratory findings in primary aldosteronism:

Urine
  Increased aldosterone (with normal 17-KS, 17-OHCS)
  Increased potassium (more than 30 mEq./24 hr.)
  Decreased concentrating ability; deficient response to vasopressin
  Neutral or alkaline dilute urine (reduced H^+, increased NH_4^+)
  Proteinuria
Electrolytes (with normal Na intake, that is, 80 to 165 mEq./day)
  Decreased serum potassium, chloride, and magnesium
  Increased CO_2, plasma pH, and sodium (above 140 mEq./L.)
  Increased total exchangeable sodium
  Decreased total exchangeable potassium
  Decreased sodium in sweat and saliva (Na/K $\downarrow$)
General
  Increased aldosterone secretory rate
  Impaired carbohydrate tolerance
  Increased extracellular fluid–plasma volume; low hematocrit
  EKG changes of hypokalemia
Stress tests
  Failure to raise plasma renin with low sodium diet (10 mEq./day), upright posture (suppressed plasma renin)
  Transient rise of serum potassium with potassium administration
  Restricted sodium intake { normal sodium retention, reduction of potassium loss, and rise of plasma K
  Saline infusion or DCA injection → failure to reduce aldosterone secretion rate or urinary levels
  Spironolactone administration → fall in urinary K, increased urine Na, rise in serum K, B.P. $\downarrow$

The diagnosis based on laboratory features, as in the preceding outline, is suggested by finding intermittent or persistent hypokalemia (K—2.5 mEq./L. or less) in a patient with hypertension. However, in 68 of Conn's patients (1969), 20 showed normal K levels. Estimations of plasma K must be repeated before labeling a patient normokalemic. Forearm exercise should be avoided before drawing the blood specimen, as this may lead to a marked increase of plasma K. Plasma rather than serum is preferred because K is released from platelets and blood cells when blood clots, thus tending to increase the K value. In occasional patients all electrolyte values are normal. The *urinary aldosterone* is almost always increased, but considerable day-to-day variation is found and single values may be within normal limits. Values above 22 μg./day are clearly elevated and values from 16 to 22 μg./day are borderline. The Na intake must be neither high nor low (about 100 mEq./day). In rare instances values have been persistently normal. Increased aldosterone may also be found in patients who are receiving diuretics, who are on a restricted salt intake, or who are receiving large amounts of potassium supplements; in malignant and renovascular hypertension; and in edema from liver cirrhosis, nephrosis, or congestive heart failure.

The *aldosterone secretion rate* (ASR) is a more reliable diagnostic index than is the excretion of aldosterone in the urine. An ASR above 160 to 170 μg./24 hr. on a normal Na intake is abnormal.

Stress tests. To confirm the diagnosis, tests have been devised to demonstrate a deficiency in the normal regulation of aldosterone and a tendency to K loss.

1. *Renin test.* The suppression of plasma renin activity (PRA) can be demonstrated by comparing a baseline PRA with the patient supine, to the PRA obtained after 3 to 5 days of restricted salt intake (about 10 mEq./day of Na) with the patient upright and ambulatory for 2 to 4 hours.

The lower limit of normal should be approximately 450 ng./100 ml. In normal subjects there is a significant rise of PRA, whereas in primary aldosteronism the response is suppressed. In one study (Jose and Kaplan, 1969) one fourth of 47 patients with essential hypertension had suppressed PRA. Thus the PRA test must be supplemented by finding increased aldosterone secretion before the diagnosis is confirmed. If measures to promote Na loss are too intense, such as the addition of a thiazide compound, a renin response can be stimulated that can mask evidence of suppressed PRA (Conn et al., 1969). The renin assay involves incubation of dialyzed plasma to promote angiotensin activity and then quantitation of the effect of incubated plasma on the blood pressure of rats.

2. *Demonstration of potassium deficiency.*

a. Administration of 100 mEq./day of K salts with an unrestricted diet causes retention of 200 mEq. or more of K and elevation of the plasma K (Luetscher, 1967). The effect is transient; when the K supplement is withdrawn, the plasma level falls.

b. Salt restriction results in normal Na retention, a reduction of K loss, and a rise of serum K. Thus *salt restriction can mask the electrolyte alterations of primary aldosteronism.*

c. Screening tests using chlorothiazide or furosemide with measurements of urinary electrolytes or PRA are not always reliable.

3. *Failure of Na administration or a high Na diet to reduce the ASR or urinary aldosterone.* Three methods can be utilized.

a. *High and low sodium diets.* Conn et al., 1969, compare urinary aldosterone excretion on the third day of a diet containing 120 mEq./day of Na and again on a diet of 10 mEq./day of Na. Normal subjects exhibit a significant increase after the low Na diet, whereas patients with primary aldosteronism do not, indicating that

PRA was not changed significantly. The test is particularly useful when renin assays are not available.

b. *Saline infusion* (Espiner et al., 1967). A diet of 10 mEq. Na and 100 mEq. K is given for 5 days. Two liters of 0.9% NaCl solution is infused I.V. from 10 A.M. to 2 P.M. on each of two successive days. The aldosterone secretion rate is reduced in normals but not in PA; the latter excrete more K and the serum K is lowered.

c. *Desoxycorticosterone acetate (DCA) administration* (Biglieri et al., 1967). DCA 10 mg. I.M. every 12 hours for 3 days after a 4- to 6-day period of metabolic control with a high Na intake of 120 mEq./day. Urinary aldosterone is reduced in normal subjects but not in PA.

4. *Spironolactone.* An aldosterone antagonist, spironolactone, causes increased urine Na and a reduction of K excretion, whereas normal subjects are not affected. A positive test denotes hyperaldosteronism but does not distinguish the primary and secondary forms. The drug is given orally in a dose of 50 to 100 mg. 3 or 4 times a day for 4 days. Serum K is measured before, on the fourth day, and 3 days after omitting the drug. The diet is moderate to high in Na (150 mEq./day) and average in K (60 to 90 mEq./day) (Leutscher, 1967).

Localization of these small tumors by air insufflation, tomography, or other techniques is rarely successful. In 73% of reported cases the tumors have been less than 3 cm. in diameter (Conn et al., 1964). Accurate localization has been accomplished by adrenal vein catheterization combined with assay of aldosterone in adrenal vein blood. Conn et al., 1969, recently reported good visualization of 9 of 12 tumors, utilizing a new technique of adrenal phlebography.

Congenital aldosteronism

Congenital aldosteronism is a rare nontumorous form of hyperaldosteronism associated with either bilateral adrenocortical hyperplasia or apparently normal adrenals that can be suppressed with corticosteroids. It affects young males predominantly and gives rise to severe or malignant hypertension, hypokalemic alkalosis, increased aldosterone secretion, and a long history of polyuria and polydipsia or tetany (Conn et al., 1964). A unique syndrome described by Bartter et al., 1962, consists of hyperaldosteronism, hypokalemic alkalosis, *normal blood pressure*, dilute urine, resistance to Pitressin, increased circulating angiotensin, and hypertrophy and hyperplasia of the juxtaglomerular cells. Liddle et al., 1963, reported a renal disorder simulating PA in a family. There was hypokalemic alkalosis and hypertension but no increase of aldosterone secretion and no response to spironolactone.

Secondary hyperaldosteronism (SA)

Excessive aldosterone secretion may occur with *malignant hypertension,* in *hypertension* from *renal artery stenosis,* and in some patients with renal functional impairment. The concurrence of hypokalemic alkalosis may render the differential diagnosis of SA from PA difficult. Hyperaldosteronism is often discovered in patients with *edema* from *hepatic cirrhosis, nephrosis,* and, to a lesser extent, *congestive heart failure.* There is reduction in effective blood volume from transudation of edema fluid, and the renin-angiotensin system is stimulated. The serum Na and K tend to be normal unless diuretic drugs have been administered or electrolyte intake has been curtailed for a long time. In *idiopathic edema* in females, often cyclic and frequently related to the menstrual cycle, aldosterone secretion may be increased to a limited degree, but the blood pressure and blood electrolytes are normal.

Differential diagnosis (Table 15-3)

The differential diagnosis revolves about the separation of primary (PA) from secondary (SA) aldosteronism and the elimination of other causes of hypokalemia, particularly in patients with hypertension. Hypokalemia is frequently induced by diuretic drug therapy, particularly when K supplementation has been inadequate. There is usually hyponatremia, some azotemia, and hyperuricemia. Potassium wastage ceases when the diuretic is omitted but persists in PA. In the face of lowered serum K, excretion in PA continues above 25 to 35 mEq./day, whereas in other hypokalemic states K excretion falls to less than 15 to 20 mEq./day. Potassium-losing renal disease (pyelonephritis, chronic nephritis, renal tubular acidosis, Fanconi syndrome) is accompanied by Na loss, by acidosis, and not infrequently by azotemia. Other possible, albeit rare, causes of hyperaldosteronism with hypokalemia are Cushing's syndrome, familial periodic paralysis, hyperthyroidism, and excessive licorice ingestion. Serum K may also be reduced by vomiting, or diarrhea, and from the administration of corticosteroids.

The presence of edema almost certainly, with very rare exceptions, eliminates PA. Since hypertension with hypokalemia is not a rare combination (20% essential hypertension, 40% malignant hypertension [Wrong, 1961]), the differential from PA commonly confronts the physician. Some of the differential criteria are shown in Table 15-3. Conn has emphasized the rarity of malignant hypertension in PA.

Hypervolemia and suppression of the renin-angiotensin system in the presence of supernormal aldosterone secretion strongly suggest PA. The renin test is

Table 15-3. Differential diagnosis of primary and hypertensive secondary aldosteronism

	Primary aldosteronism	*Essential hypertension with hypokalemia*	*Renal artery obstruction with hypertension*
Serum K	Markedly reduced Occasionally normal	Slightly reduced	Normal
Urinary K	High ($<$25 to 35 mEq./day)	Low ($>$15 to 20 mEq./day)	Normal or low
Serum Na	Normal or slightly elevated (140 to 150 mEq./L.)	Normal or slightly decreased	Normal or slightly decreased
Blood pressure elevation	Moderate to severe	Moderate to severe	Severe; rapid rise
Blood volume	Increased	Normal	Normal
Eyegrounds	Disproportionately mild in relation to blood pressure	Mild to severe	Mild to severe
Papilledema	None	None except in malignant phase	None or present
K repletion	Transient rise of serum K	Sustained rise serum K	Sustained rise serum K
Plasma renin activity on low Na intake, upright posture	Suppressed	Occasionally suppressed (20%)	Normal rise

probably the most accurate differential aid, and it is hoped that a simple technique for measuring renin will be forthcoming. Nevertheless, suppressed PRA has been found in about 20% of patients with essential hypertension, so that the determination of urinary aldosterone is not dispensable. The serum K reduction is more profound in PA and the serum Na tends to be somewhat elevated, whereas in SA it is normal or reduced. Studies to rule out renovascular hypertension (urography, angiograms, kidney biopsy, differential excretion studies) may aid in the diagnosis.

Treatment

Primary aldosteronism. The adrenocortical adenoma (aldosteronoma) is resected. The left side, the more frequent site, should be explored first, except in the rare instance where studies have successfully located the tumor on the right. However, because in 9% of cases more than one adenoma has been found (Conn et al., 1964), both adrenals must be inspected. If bilateral hyperplasia is found instead of a tumor, bilateral total adrenalectomy is necessary and the patient must be hormonally supported thereafter for permanent adrenocortical insufficiency. Hypertension has not always been ameliorated in patients with nodular hyperplasia of the adrenals. After operation, regression of symptoms and signs and restoration of normal electrolyte balance occur rapidly. Restoration of normotension may require weeks, depending on the previous duration of hypertension and the presence of renal damage. Only partial restitution of normal blood pressure may occur in 25% of patients. Patients who appear too ill for immediate surgery can be maintained on spironolactone 50 mg. four times daily, plus K supplements. This regimen can also be used preoperatively.

Secondary aldosteronism. The primary cause must be treated, and factors contributing to the disturbance should be eliminated. Again, spironolactone may be useful to antagonize the effects of excessive aldosterone.

REFERENCES

Bartter, F. C., et al.: Amer. J. Med. 33:811, 1962.

Bartter, F. C., et al.: J. Clin. Invest. 47:1742, 1968.

*Baulieu, E. E., et al.: Adrenogenital syndrome. In Eisenstein, A. B., editor: The adrenal cortex, Boston, 1967, Little, Brown & Co., p. 553.

Biglieri, E. G.: J. Clin. Invest. 45:987, 1966.

Biglieri, E. G., et al.: J.A.M.A. 201:510, 1967.

Biglieri, E. G., et al.: Amer. J. Med. 45:170, 1968.

*Bongiovanni, A. M., et al.: Recent Progr. Hormone Res. 23:375, 1967.

Childs, B., et al.: J. Clin. Invest. 35:213, 1956.

*Conn, J. W., et al.: Amer. J. Surg. 107:159, 1964.

Conn, J. W., et al.: J.A.M.A. 195:21, 1966.

Conn, J. W., et al.: Arch. Intern. Med. 123: 113, 1969.

Degenhart, H. J., et al.: Production and excretion of testosterone in children with congenital adrenal hyperplasia and precocious puberty. In Vermeulen, A., editor: Androgens in normal and abnormal conditions, Symposium on Steroid Hormones, Amsterdam, 1966, Excerpta Medica Foundation, International Congress Ser. no. 101, p. 81.

Espiner, E. A., et al.: New Eng. J. Med. 277: 1, 1967.

Fishman, L. M., et al.: J.A.M.A. 205:497, 1968.

*Gabrilove, J. L., et al.: Medicine 44:37, 1965.

Jefferies, W. McK., and Levy, R. P.: J. Clin. Endocr. 19:1069, 1959.

Jose, A., and Kaplan, N. M.: Arch. Intern. Med. 123:141, 1969.

Kenny, F. M., et al.: Amer. J. Dis. Child. 115: 445, 1968.

Liddle, G. W., et al.: Trans. Ass. Amer. Physicians 76:199, 1963.

*Luetscher, J. A.: Disorders associated with altered secretion of aldosterone. In Eisenstein, A. B., editor: The adrenal cortex, Boston, 1967, Little, Brown & Co., p. 639.

Mallin, J. C., et al.: Ann. Intern. Med. 70:69, 1969.

Migeon, C. J.: J. Pediat. 73:805, 1968.

Schneeberg, N. G., et al.: J. Clin. Endocr. 203:19, 1959.

Solomon, S. S., et al.: J. Clin. Endocr. 28:608, 1968.

Tyler, E. J.: J.A.M.A. 205:16, 1968.

*Wilkins, L.: The diagnosis and treatment of endocrine disorders in childhood and adolescence, ed. 3, Springfield, Ill., 1965, Charles C Thomas, Publisher; a, 407; b, 402.

Wrong, O.: Brit. Med. J. 2:419, 1961.

---

*Significant reviews.

Chapter 16

Adrenal medulla, pheochromocytoma, and the carcinoid syndrome

ADRENAL MEDULLA

The anatomy of the adrenal medulla is outlined in Chapter 12. The catecholamine compounds (epinephrine, norepinephrine, and dopamine) consist of an amine attached to a phenolic ring with two adjacent hydroxyl groups (Fig. 16-1). Epinephrine (E) originates in chromaffin cells in the adrenal medulla. Norepinephrine (NE) arises both from the adrenal medulla and from sympathetic postganglionic adrenergic neurons in many tissues (heart, brain, spleen). Thus NE is both a hormone and a neurotransmitter, whereas E is primarily a hormone. Approximately 15% of the total catecholamine content of the normal adrenal medulla is NE. The concentration of E in the urine is an approximate index of the secretion of the adrenal medulla, whereas NE reflects secretion from adrenergic nerves. Dopamine and its metabolites are excreted in increased amounts in neuroblastomas. Under the stress of hypotension, asphyxia, anoxia, acetylcholine, nicotine, or excitation of the splanchnic nerve of the dog, a preponderance of E secretion was found by Malmejac, 1958. No particular stress caused an obvious increase in NE secretion. Other studies have tended to show selective secretion of E from hypoglycemia and pilocarpine and NE from hemorrhagic shock and nicotine (Rubin and Miele, 1968).

Catecholamines are stored in subcellular membrane-lined granules that protect them from premature metabolic degradation by MAO and other enzymes; E resides in chromaffin granules and NE in granules within the adrenergic neuron. The granule contains the catecholamine, a small amount of a lipoprotein, and approximately 1 mol of ATP per 4 mols of E or NE (Crout, 1968). NE may exist in two equilibrated metabolic pools (Axelrod, 1962). The larger is bound within the granule, turns over slowly, and is metabolized within the nerve ending; the smaller pool is unbound, is free in cytoplasm, is susceptible to release by neural stimulation, and turns over rapidly. Granular NE is replenished both by synthesis and by reuptake of unused NE from the surrounding cytoplasm.

Biosynthesis of catecholamines

The biosynthetic pathways are shown in Fig. 16-1. L-Tyrosine is found in the circulation in a concentration of 10 to 15 mg./L. and is concentrated within cells of the adrenal medulla, sympathetic nerve endings, and brain. It is hydroxylated in mitochondria to form dopa probably by tyrosine hydroxylase, though albinos who lack this enzyme show no defect in catecholamine synthesis. Dopamine, the first catecholamine that is synthesized, can dif-

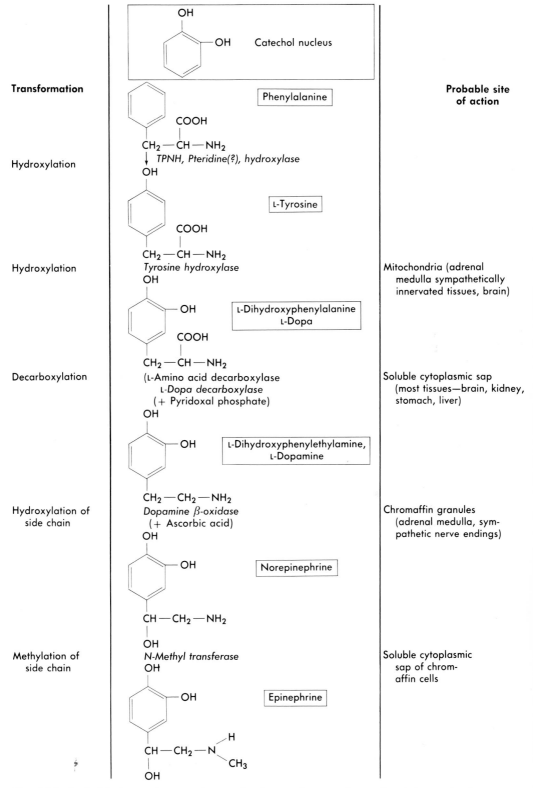

Fig. 16-1. Probable biosynthetic pathways for the production of norepinephrine and epinephrine. (Enzymes are italicized, and compounds are in rectangles.)

fuse into the circulation, can be excreted into the urine, can be metabolized, or can enter the granules in sympathetic nerve endings, chromaffin cells, and brain cells, and can be stored or hydroxylated by dopamine-β-oxidase to NE. This is probably the rate-limiting step in the synthesis of the catecholamines and is the final synthetic step in postganglionic adrenergic neurons and probably in the brain. Only the chromaffin cells largely in the adrenal medulla contain the necessary enzyme, n-methyl transferase, to methylate NE to E. NE diffuses from the storage granule and is methylated to E on the surface of the granule or in the cytoplasm of the adrenal medullary cells. Minute amounts of E are synthesized in the brain but are utilized in situ. The enzyme n-methyl transferase requires a considerable concentration of cortisol, which is supplied by the perfusion of the adrenal medulla by adrenal cortex blood (p. 196). Hypophysectomy lowers the level of circulating cortisol and thus the concentration of E; the level of NE rises from loss of conversion of NE to E. The reflex release of catecholamines from the adrenal is increased by cortisol (Harrison et al., 1968). Alternate biosynthetic pathways to E have been described and are under investigation, such as tyrosine → tyramine → octopamine → NE, and dopamine → epinine (n-methyldopamine) → E.

False neurotransmitters

The enzymes responsible for the synthesis of the catecholamines are not so specific that they may not act on other substrates and lead to the production of similar though less active compounds ("false neurochemical transmitters"). Thus β-oxidase dopamine can convert other phenylethylamines than dopamine to analogs of NE that are released by nerve stimulation. Monamine oxidase inhibitors can cause the accumulation of octopamine, a false transmitter that displaces NE and results in reduced sympathetic responsiveness. For a review see Cohen et al., 1966.

Circulating catecholamines

There is a continuous release of small amounts of catecholamines into the circulation and a sharp rise following a suitable stress signal. However, most secreted NE does not enter the circulation but is absorbed by the axonal membrane and is thus removed from the region of receptors. The half-life of infused isotopically labeled catecholamines is extremely short, that is, 10 to 30 seconds (Axelrod, et al., 1959) so that most of the E or NE utilized by an organ is accumulated during a single circulatory passage and the remainder is picked up by sympathetic nerve endings. Organs accumulating catecholamines store them in the granulated vesicles of sympathetic nerve endings rather than in the parenchyma, so that the extraction of catecholamines from the blood is proportional to the density of sympathetic nerve endings. The heart, being particularly rich in sympathetic nerve endings, contains a high concentration of NE. Since catecholamines do not diffuse readily across the brain-blood barrier, the rich content of brain catecholamine does not contribute to the circulating blood content.

Metabolism

Most metabolic transformations take place in the liver and kidneys (Fig. 16-2). Some E and NE is excreted unchanged or removed from the circulation and stored in sympathetic nerve endings. The major metabolic enzyme is catechol-O-methyl transferase, which methylates one hydroxyl to produce metanephrine (MN) from E and normetanephrine (NMN) from NE.

Three pathways are open to MN and NMN (Fig. 16-2): (1) a small amount is excreted unchanged, (2) a minor fraction is conjugated with glucuronic or sulfuric acid, and (3) the major portion is converted to vanillylmandelic acid (VMA) and a small fraction to methoxyhydroxyphenyl glycol (MHPG). The amount of urinary NE, E, and their metabolic products (particularly VMA) excreted per day is a rough estimate of the quantity of

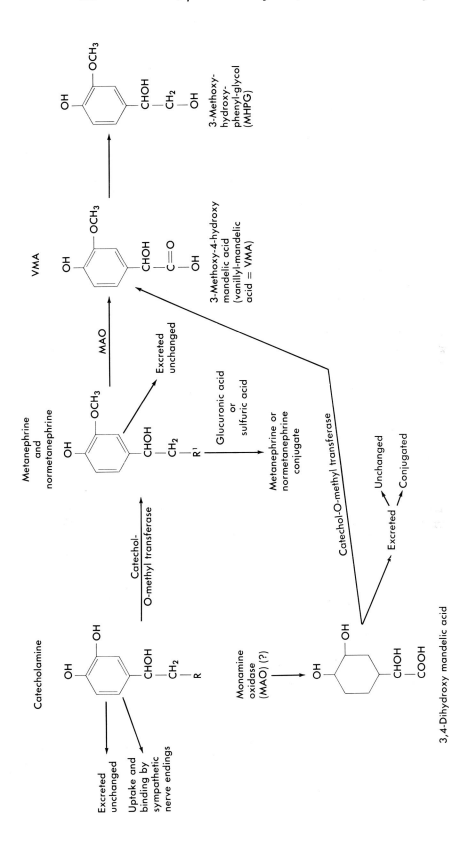

Fig. 16-2. Metabolic pathways of catecholamines. The chief product is VMA. The role of MAO has been questioned.

catecholamine synthesized daily. For a review see Wurtman, 1965.

Effects of drugs on catecholamines

Wurtman, 1965, has classified drug effects as follows: (1) interference with the uptake and binding of NE by sympathetic nerve endings, resulting in high catecholamine blood levels and enhanced physiologic responses (cocaine, imipramine, and chlorpromazine); (2) cause the release of bound NE (sympathomimetic agents such as ephedrine, amphetamine, and tyramine; reserpine depletes the brain and sympathetically innervated organs of most of their catecholamine by a destructive effect on the storage vesicle); (3) blockage of the release of tissue NE (guanethidine, ganglionic blockers, MAO inhibitors); and (4) false neurotransmitters.

Physiologic actions

Catecholamines are secreted in spurts to promote physiologic adaptation to emergency stimuli. There is also a lesser, more sustained secretion, particularly of NE, from sympathetic nerve endings. NE is released from granule binding as free NE, which diffuses from the neuron terminal to a receptor on the effector cell. A series of intracellular physiologic events are triggered within the effector cell, leading to the physiologic effect or to a particular response. Adrenergic receptors are cellular components located either on the cell membrane or within the effector cell that react or combine with E or NE. They are viewed as the primary site of action of the catecholamines and other adrenergic mediators, which produce adrenergic effects that are stimulating or inhibiting, depending on the effector organ. Ahlquist, 1948, proposed the existence of *alpha* and *beta* adrenergic receptors that can mediate the effects of E, NE, and sympathomimetic drugs. NE tends to preferentially stimulate alpha receptors, whereas E stimulates both alpha and beta. However, E is two to ten times more potent as an alpha stimulator

than is NE. In pharmacologic dosages both catecholamines can stimulate alpha and beta receptors depending on the dosage. Alpha receptor functions are chiefly excitatory and include vasoconstriction of certain vascular beds, iris dilator, nictitating membrane, pilomotor and splenic capsule contractions, and intestinal relaxation but little direct myocardial effect. Beta receptor functions are mainly inhibitory and include vasodilatation of certain vascular beds (Table 16-1); increased cardiac rate and output; myometrial, intestinal, and bronchial relaxation; and glycogenolysis. Both alpha and beta, however, show both excitatory and inhibitory actions. The principal physiologic and pharmacologic effects of the catecholamines are outlined in Table 16-1. Some of the responses have been observed in experimental animals and have not been completely verified in man, and in some the results have been contradictory. The hyperglycemic effects of E are the result of enhanced liver glycogenolysis from activation of hepatic glycogen phosphorylase. There is also a diminished rate of glucose utilization by peripheral tissues. E stimulates the release of ACTH probably via CRF and may also stimulate vasopressin secretion. For a review of adrenergic receptors see Abboud, 1968.

PHEOCHROMOCYTOMA (CHROMAFFINOMA)

Pheochromocytomas are chromaffin tumors of the adrenal medulla that store and secrete catecholamines in excessive amounts. Since they cause an unusual form of paroxysmal or sustained hypertension that can be fatal and their removal usually results in amelioration or cure, they have evoked medical attention disproportionate to their incidence as a cause of hypertension.

Pathology

The tumor is usually a small spherical, well-encapsulated mass that measures less than 10 cm. in diameter and weighs from

Table 16-1. Physiologic and pharmacologic effects of catecholamines*

System	Epinephrine		Norepinephrine	
	Small dose	*Large dose IV*	*Small dose*	*Large dose IV*
Cardiovascular responses				
Arteries and veins	Constriction		Constriction	
Vascular beds				
Skin	Constriction		Constriction (+)	
Mucosa	Constriction		Constriction (++)	
Striated muscle	Dilatation		Constriction	
Kidney	Constriction		Constriction (+)	
Splanchnic	Dilatation		Dilatation	
Lung	Constriction		Constriction	
Hepatic, mesenteric, uterine	Constriction		Constriction	
Coronary vessels	Dilatation		Dilatation	
Mean blood pressure		Increase (++)	Increase (+)	Increase (+++)
Systolic	Slight increase	Increase (+++)	Increase (+)	Increase (+++)
Diastolic	Slight decrease	Increase (+)	Increase (+)	Increase (+++)
Cardiac output	Increase (+)	Increase (++)	0	0 or decrease
Pulse rate	0 or increase (+)	Increase (++)	0	0 or decrease
Peripheral resistance	Decrease	Increase (++)	Increase (++)	Increase (++)
Eye—iris, orbital smooth muscle, nictitating membrane		Constriction (++++)		Constriction (±)
Bronchi		Relaxation (++++)		Relaxation (0 or ±)
G.I. sphincters, splenic capsule, urinary bladder, pilomotor apparatus		Contraction		Contraction
G.I. tract smooth muscle	Relaxation			Relaxation
Uterus	Relaxation			0?
Salivation	Decrease			?
Sweating	Increase			?
Calorigenic, BMR	Increase (++++)			Increase (++)
Liver glycogenolysis → hyperglycemia; muscle glycogenolysis → lactic acidemia and hyperkalemia	Increase (++++)			Increase (+)
Lipolysis, increase of plasma free fatty acids	Increase (++)			Increase (+++)
Central nervous stimulation	Increase (+++)			0

*Based on data from Levy, B., and Ahlquist, R. P.: Adrenergic drugs. In DiPalma, J. R., editor: Drill's pharmacology in medicine, ed. 3, New York, 1965, Blakiston Division, McGraw-Hill Book Co.

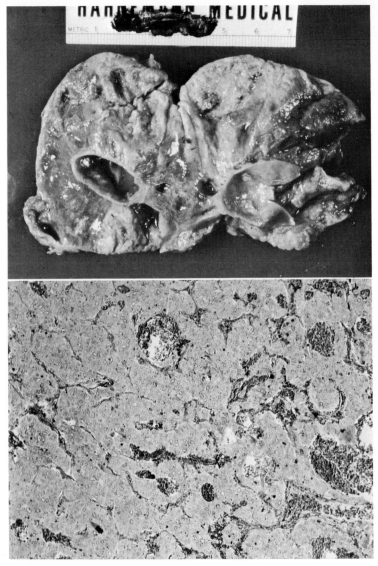

Fig. 16-3. A pheochromocytoma. The gross specimen has been sectioned and opened outward. The histologic section shows anastamosing cords of large polyhedral medullary cells with slightly pleomorphic nuclei. There is a rich vascular supply. (X20.) (Courtesy Dr. Alexander Nedwich and Department of Pathology, Hahnemann Medical College, Philadelphia, Pa.)

5 to 700 grams. The sectioned surface appears reddish or yellowish brown and often is cystic, necrotic, and hemorrhagic (Fig. 16-3). The microscopic appearance is that of cords of large polyhedral or irregular cells (Fig. 16-3), some of which stain brown after bichromate fixation. Groups of cells are surrounded by a vascular fine connective tissue stroma. Less than 10% are

malignant. Bilateral tumors have been found in 10% to 20% of reported series and up to 32% in children (Anderson and Cleveland, 1966) and are not infrequently associated with a familial occurrence and thyroid cancer. Ten percent of these tumors reside in extra-adrenal sites where chromaffin tissue can be normally present, that is, para-aortic sympathetic ganglia, organ of

Zuckerkandl on the ventral surface of the aorta, carotid body, and homologous structures in the thorax, brain, kidney, intestinal wall, urinary bladder, ovary, and testicle. Adrenal medullary hyperplasia rather than a tumor has been described in several patients.

Pathophysiology

Most tumors contain a higher concentration of catecholamines than normal medullary tissue. A rapid intravenous injection of E or NE produces clinical manifestations comparable to a paroxysm of pheochromocytoma. The symptoms and signs of the disease do not appear to be altered by differences in the ratio of NE to E, since large doses of E can induce overall vasoconstriction and large doses of NE will cause metabolic changes. Hypermetabolism and hyperglycemia result from much smaller doses of E than are needed to cause hypertension. Small tumors that contain 90% to 97% NE but not over 80 mg. tend to cause persistent blood pressure elevation resembling essential hypertension but without significant metabolic changes. If the content of NE were greater, metabolic changes become more striking even though NE is a less potent metabolic stimulator than E. Where E predominates, there is hypertension, tachycardia, hypermetabolism, and hyperglycemia. Occasionally tumors secreting large quantities of E produce a clinical state resembling essential hypertensive vascular disease without tachycardia, hyperglycemia, or hypermetabolism and show a negative or equivocal response to benzodioxane (Goldenberg, 1954).

Clinical features

An incidence of 1 case per 20,000 to 50,000 hospital admissions has been reported. It is a cause of less than 0.5% of hypertension, but it has been estimated that more than 1,000 cases occur annually in the United States. It may appear at any age, but the majority occur in the third to sixth decades.

Symptoms and signs

See outline below.

Major symptoms
  Headache (80)*
  Hyperhidrosis (71)
  Palpitation (64)
  Nausea and/or vomiting (42)
  Pallor (42)
  Tremor (31)
  Fatigue and weakness (28)
  Anxiety and nervous tension (22)
  Epigastric pain (22)
  Chest pain (19)

Miscellaneous symptoms
  Dyspnea, blurred vision, throat constriction, neck pain or throbbing, paresthesias or numbness, flushes, dizziness, faintness, convulsions, tinnitus, dysarthria, flank pain, psychic changes, weight loss

Physical signs
  Hypertension (sustained or intermittent)
  Cardiovascular changes secondary to hypertension (enlarged heart, congestive failure, retinopathy)
  Orthostatic hypotension
  Thin body build
  During a paroxysm—sweating, pallor, tremor, anxiety, tachycardia
  Related disorders—neurofibromatosis, thyroid carcinoma, Lindau-von Hippel disease, parathyroid adenoma

The symptoms tend to occur in spells or paroxysms and may become progressively more severe and frequent with time. Between attacks there is apparent health, except for persistent hypertension in some cases. Thomas et al., 1966, in a review of 100 cases from the Mayo Clinic, observed attacks as often as several times a day or as rarely as once every few months. Seventy-two percent of their patients had one or more attacks per week and 26% one or more per day. Paroxysms were nocturnal or appeared soon after arising. Precipitating factors are often reproducible and involve change of position or some mechanical stimulus to the tumor such as bending, turning over in bed, physical exertion,

*The numbers in parentheses are percent incidence from a review of 100 cases by Thomas, J. E., et al.: J.A.M.A. **197**:754, 1966.

excitement, or sudden marked change in environmental temperature (hot or cold shower). The major complaint is *headache.* It is usually sudden in onset, of brief duration usually lasting 15 to 60 minutes, of severe intensity, with throbbing, and often with nausea and vomiting. Brief drenching sweats and pallor or flushing of the upper half of the body accompany the paroxysm. There is a sense of impending death, chest or abdominal pain, and throat constriction. Personality changes and emotional disturbances may occur.

Gastrointestinal symptoms including nausea, vomiting, abdominal pain, diarrhea, melena, and severe constipation are not rare. Chronic peptic ulcer may be suspected. Occlusive endarteritis with intestinal infarction or hemorrhagic bowel lesions and deaths due to intestinal perforation have been reported (Greer et al., 1964). Other manifestations listed by Greer include "severe hypertension or unexplained hypotension during a routine administration of an anesthetic, a surgical procedure, or delivery; frequent miscarriage associated with hypertension, and hypertension developing or worsening in the last trimester of pregnancy."

In some patients there are no paroxysms, and symptoms are minimal or absent. The tumor may be unsuspected and encountered as an incidental finding at autopsy. Hypertension may exist alone with or without its complications (enlarged heart, congestive failure, retinopathy, cerebrovascular accidents). Orthostatic hypotension in a hypertensive patient is not unusual. Patients tend to be thin; obesity is uncommon. The presence of certain *related disorders* may suggest the diagnosis. Neurofibromatosis has been found in 2% to 8% of cases. Other neuroectodermal related disorders are Lindau-von Hippel disease (retinal, cerebellar, medullary, and spinal cord hemangioblastomas; lung, pancreas, kidney, liver, and epididymal cysts; hypernephroma), Sturge-Weber syndrome, and tuberous sclerosis. A triad of medullary carcinoma of the thyroid, hyperparathy-

roidism, and bilateral pheochromocytoma, with a familial occurrence, has been recognized (Sjoerdsma et al., 1966). Carman and Brashear, 1960, reviewed the familial cases and concluded that pheochromocytoma was probably inherited in a dominant genetic fashion with a high degree of penetrance.

Diagnostic studies
Urinary catecholamines and metabolites

The structure of the catecholamines and metabolites is shown in Figs. 16-1 and 16-2.

Urinary vanillylmandelic acid (VMA). VMA is the major metabolite of E and NE and serves as a good index of total catecholamine secretion. A 24-hour urine collection is required. Many laboratories use a commercial kit for the determination. These kits lack sensitivity, measure numerous phenols (coffee, vanilla, certain fruits and vegetables) and are not specific. It is important to reevaluate all positive tests obtained with these kits by more precise methods. Normal values range from 2 to 6 mg./day. False low values have been found in approximately 5% of cases; values from 6 to 10 mg. have been obtained in about 20%.

Urinary normetanephrine (NMN) and metanephrine (MN). The determination of the catecholamine metabolites NMN and MN is widely used because it is simpler to perform than the free catecholamine method or an accurate VMA determination and has indicated the correct diagnosis in 95% of patients. Normal values for NMN are 100 to 500 μg./day and for MN 50 to 200 μg./day, whereas in pheochromocytoma, values are usually above 250 μg./day for NMN + MN.

Urinary free total cathecholamine (NE + E). Determination of the free NE + E by the fluorometric trihydroxyindole method is probably the most accurate of the diagnostic tests. False high values will be produced by fluorescent compounds (tetracyclines, methyldopa, and quinidine). Normal values for NE range from 20 to 70 μg./day and for E from 0 to 15 μg./day, whereas in pheochromocytoma, values for NE + E exceed 100 μg./day. Stress, particularly heavy exercise, can produce elevated values. Free total catecholamines are occasionally elevated in cases of pheochromocytoma when the values for VMA and NMN + MN are normal. Catecholamines in nasal decongestants or antiasthma medications or α-methyldopa (Aldomet) can produce false elevated values. MN values may increase and VMA decrease in the presence of monamine oxidase inhibitors, but reserpine and guanethidine have caused no false elevations. For a review of an analysis of catecholamines see Crout, 1968.

Provocative pharmacologic tests

Provocative pharmacologic tests are adjunctive procedures to be used when the urinary catecholamine and/or metabolites are normal or equivocal.

Normotensive patient (or B.P. less than 170/100). Histamine, tyramine, and glucagon are three stimulating agents.

Histamine can provoke a hypertensive episode by inducing a reflex discharge of catecholamines from sympathetic nerve endings. In pheochromocytoma the concentration of catecholamines in sympathetic nerve endings is increased by continuous accumulation from the blood. It is probably these stores that are released by histamine rather than by any direct stimulation of the tumor. Histamine administration is preceded by a cold pressor test. When the blood pressure has returned to baseline values, histamine base in a dose of 25 to 50 μg. is rapidly injected I.V. through a previously established I.V. infusion of 5% glucose in water. An abrupt rise of blood pressure of 20/10 mm. or more above the maximum cold pressor values within 1 to 2 minutes is considered positive. Paroxysmal symptoms may be reproduced. Phentolamine (Regitine) should be available in case of a profound hypertensive response. Measurement of free urinary catecholamines (NE + E) before and after the his-

tamine injection adds further information. False positive tests are not rare; false negative tests are less likely. The injection of histamine is not without danger, causes flushing and throbbing headaches, and should not be used in patients with coronary heart disease or asthma.

Tyramine is a safer provocative agent with few side effects. It causes a direct release of excessive catecholamines stored in tissues and may inhibit their subsequent rebinding at the same sites. A positive test consists of a systolic rise of 20 mm. or greater after the rapid I.V. injection of 1 mg. of tyramine base. Occasionally doses up to 2 mg. are used. Engelman et al., 1968, reported positive results in 73% of patients with pheochromocytoma and 3 false positive tests in 88 patients with hypertension. Negative tests have been found in 10 of 14 patients with associated medullary thyroid carcinoma. Tyramine responses may be increased by methyldopa and MAO inhibitors to possibly fatal hypertensive levels. They may be inhibited by hydrochlorothiazide, reserpine, and α-methyl-*p*-tyrosine.

Glucagon (Lawrence, 1967) has been proposed as a safe provocative stimulus using 0.5 to 1 mg. I.V.

Hypertensive patient (B.P. above 170/110). Phentolamine (Regitine), an α-adrenergic blocking compound, neutralizes the pressor effects of catecholamines and promotes a sharp drop in blood pressure. With the patient supine and the blood pressure well stabilized, 1 to 5 mg. is flushed in about 1 minute through an already-established I.V. solution of 5% glucose in water. A positive test consists of a prompt fall of the B.P. of 35/25 mm. or more. The smaller dose should be tested first and then titrated upward until a positive response occurs or the maximum dose is attained. This precaution may prevent a serious hypotensive episode that can lead to coronary insufficiency or a cerebrovascular accident. False positive tests may occur in patients with uremia and in those taking antihypertensive drugs, sedatives, or narcotics. False negative tests are more likely to occur in patients with paroxysmal hypertension, since the depressor response will be obtained only if excessive circulating catecholamines are present at the time of injection. Other vasodepressor agents are piperoxan hydrochloride (Benodaine hydrochloride), Dibenamine hydrochloride, and tolazoline (Priscoline), but phentolamine has become the standard.

Routine laboratory studies

Finding diminished glucose tolerance and elevated blood sugar, free fatty acids, and BMR in a thin hypertensive patient warrants a search for pheochromocytoma. Most patients have a normal blood and plasma volume, but occasionally the hematocrit is increased and there is polycythemia.

X-ray studies

A flat plate of the abdomen will reveal a small percentage of tumors; occasionally the tumor is calcified. About half can be located by combined intravenous urography and planigrams. The kidney may be displaced downward. Presacral air or gas insufflation, selective arteriography, caval catheterization, or other measures are rarely used because they add little information and may provoke a hypertensive crisis. Rossi, 1968, however, recently described the value and safety of transfemoral retrograde arteriography. In 99% of patients this type of tumor is within the abdominal cavity, and in most of the remainder it is in the thorax. In the latter it presents as a posterior mediastinal paravertebral mass on anteroposterior or oblique chest x-ray plates.

Differential diagnosis

Patients with moderate or severe hypertension or with lability of blood pressure or patients with postural hypotension followed by hypertension should be studied for pheochromocytoma. Patients with any of the following manifestations should also be screened: (1) *anxiety states* in patients with an extremely labile pulse rate and blood pressure and with headache, sweating, tremor, palpitation, or hyperventilation; (2) *hyperthyroidism* suspected but with atypical manifestations and equivocal tests particularly if the BMR and blood sugar are elevated; (3) *thin, diabetic hypertensives;* (4) *obscure gastrointestinal complaints* associated with hypertension.

Treatment

Surgical removal is the treatment of choice, though pharmacologic control can be achieved if surgery is delayed or there is a metastatic malignant pheochromocytoma. A transabdominal approach permits exposure of both adrenals and examination of all areas of possible paragangliomas. Palpation and manipulation of all suspected areas while the blood pressure is continuously monitored may uncover hidden lesions. A definite, albeit small, blood pressure rise may indicate a functioning paraganglioma. The surgeon must maintain a high index of suspicion for a contralateral tumor even though one may have already been found in one adrenal gland; this fact is especially true in familial disease. A wide periadrenal resection is favored because of the possibility of adjacent tumors in the periadrenal fat.

Preoperative management

The danger of serious hypertensive crises during surgical manipulations can be avoided by the administration of the α-adrenergic blocking agents phentolamine (Regitine) and phenoxybenzamine (Dibenzyline). Because phentolamine is given on a 3- to 4-hour schedule for 10 to 14 days before surgery, because it may not control blood pressure smoothly, and because it frequently causes nausea and vomiting, phenoxybenzamine is favored. It is given in single or twice daily doses totaling 40 to 100 mg./day. The blood pressure is maintained at normal levels, and the patient is relieved of symptoms. If surgery must be delayed because of complicating illness, it can be continued for weeks or months. It is a useful agent for long-term therapy in patients with malignant pheochromocytoma. α-Methyl-*p*-tyrosine is an experimental compound that blocks the synthesis of catecholamines by inhibiting tyrosine hydroxylase and produces a clinical remission.

During surgery

Adequate replacement of blood loss is imperative to prevent the hypotension that so commonly follows resection of the tumor. In fact, the absence of significant hypotension should alert the surgeon to the possibility of residual tumor. The gallbladder should be carefully examined because of the prevalence of calculi. The operation may be attended by a hypertensive crisis, particularly if preoperative medical therapy has not been adequate. Cardiac arrhythmias, myocardial infarction, and cerebrovascular accidents are always potential threats.

Postoperative management

Removal of all tumor tissue cures the disorder. Follow-up examination and urine assays during the immediate postsurgical period and at regular intervals thereafter for several years are important to detect both cryptic disease that was overlooked by the surgeon and metastatic lesions from a malignancy. The thyroid gland should always be examined for an associated neoplasm. Family members who have hypertension should be studied.

SEROTONIN, KININS, AND THE CARCINOID SYNDROME

Serotonin (5-hydroxytryptamine, 5-HT) was named because of its vasopressor effects. It is found particularly in argentaffin (enterochromaffin) cells and is bound by platelets when it enters the circulation. The bound form is inactive and must be freed by platelet dissolution to exert physiologic activity. The concentration of 5-HT in a tissue is proportional to its content of the platelet-bound substance. The limbic system of the brain, the hypothalamus, the pineal, and the gastrointestinal tract (particularly the duodenum and jejunum) show the greatest concentrations. Serotonin is also found in bananas, tomatoes, certain mushrooms, insect venoms, and crustaceans. Tryptophan, an amino acid, is hydroxylated to 5-hydroxytryptophan (5-HTP) and thence, by decarboxylation, is converted to 5-HT. Decarboxylase deficiency with a resultant lack of serotonin may contribute to the syndrome of phenylketonuria. Monamine oxidase (MAO) converts 5-HT to 5-hydroxyindole acetic acid (5-HIAA), which is excreted in the urine.

The principal physiologic actions of 5-HT include stimulation of small-bowel contractility and tone, vasoconstriction, increased vascular permeability, increased cardiac output and pulmonary artery pressure, and bronchoconstriction. Its role in brain and CNS function is complex. Serotonin does not penetrate the blood-brain barrier but can be synthesized in central nervous tissue from 5-HTP. It is closely related to pineal, hypothalamic, and limbic function and is affected in various ways by numerous drugs.

Kinins (bradykinin, kallidin, etc.) are a group of vasodilator linear polypeptides found in mammalian plasma. The name "bradykinin" refers to the slow smooth muscle contraction that it generates in the isolated guinea pig ileum. The kinins are derived from a precursor alpha-2-globulin (kinogen) by the enzymatic action of kallikreins and are inactivated by kinases. One of the principal effects of kinins is to induce smooth muscle contraction, but this change varies with the organ studied and the species. Whether kinins play a role in the regulation of intestinal motility is unknown. The second important physiologic effect is vasodilator and hypotensive, though certain blood vessels are constricted (umbilical artery and vein, ductus arteriosus). This latter action has been proposed as the principal mechanism for the conversion of the fetal circulation to that of the adult (Melmon et al., 1968). Increased capillary permeability, catecholamine release, increased renal blood flow and GFR with diuresis, antidiuresis in some species, leukotaxis, and production of pain are other effects. Many of these responses to kinins resemble those of acute inflammation, and it has been proposed that they are the responsible agents for the changes of the inflammatory process.

For a review see Kellermeyer and Graham, 1968.

Carcinoid syndrome

The carcinoid syndrome (Lembeck, 1953, Thorson et al., 1954) is produced by the secretion of excessive amounts of serotonin and possibly kinins and histamine from a carcinoid tumor. The tumor arises from argentaffin cells and 80% to 95% of tumors are found near the ileocecal valve, particularly in the appendix and terminal ileum. Multiple tumors occur in 15% to 25% of cases. The tumor grows slowly and can metastasize to regional lymph nodes and liver and less commonly to ovaries, bones, and lungs. It can obstruct the small intestine.

Clinical features

The clinical manifestations are generated by liver metastases. Ordinarily serotonin, arising from the intestinal tract, enters the liver through the portal vein and is inactivated by MAO, but when secreted from the liver, it escapes the destructive action of MAO and directly enters the hepatic vein and the general circulation. The cardinal feature is the acute, brief, red, or cyanotic red cutaneous *flush* commencing in the face and often extending over the chest and extremities. There may be telangiectasia with chronic facial cyanosis. The flush may recur frequently and can be induced by exercise, emotional stimuli, eating, alcohol, or injection of catecholamines or histamine. It is probably caused by the vasodilator effects of serotonin and probably bradykinin, their interaction, and possibly the addition of other vasoactive substances. *Watery diarrhea* is

the second characteristic symptom and may be accompanied by colic and borborygmi. Late in the disease one finds signs of *right-heart disease*, principally *pulmonary stenosis*. The pulmonic and tricuspid valves become fibrotic, rigid, thick, and contracted. During the cutaneous flush, asthma may occur as a result of serotonin-induced bronchospasm. The liver may be enlarged from metastases. Edema, arthritides, pellagrous lesions, acute abdominal pain due to necrosis of liver lesions, and peptic ulcer are relatively rare additional clinical features. The bronchial carcinoid tumor exhibits certain distinctive characteristics. The cutaneous flush is severe and prolonged for 3 or 4 days and may be preceded by anxiety, disorientation, and hand tremors. There is facial and periobital edema, lacrimation, salivation, diaphoresis, fever, nausea, vomiting, explosive diarrhea, dyspnea and wheezing, sometimes profound hypotension, and oliguria. The endocardial lesions tend to involve the left heart and may cause pulmonary edema and death. The bronchial adenoma may itself, acting as an ectopic endocrine organ, produce 5-HTP and/or 5-HT. The prognosis is far worse than for the more common carcinoid syndrome. The diagnosis may be difficult because few patients present the entire clinical picture so that the existence of any one of the above symptoms or signs should arouse suspicion of a carcinoid tumor.

Laboratory findings

The cardinal finding is an elevated concentration of 5-HIAA in the urine. A simple qualitative test is used that becomes positive at a concentration of 40 mg. or more, whereas normal subjects rarely excrete more than 15 mg./24 hr. However, when the diagnosis appears likely and the qualitative test is negative, a quantitative determination of 5-HIAA should be done because some tumors do not produce enough serotonin to raise the level above a range of 9 to 25 mg. Minimal elevations can be caused by the ingestion of bananas, or the administration of reserpine, and are encountered in patients with sprue. False positive tests occur after the administration of mephenesin carbamate (Tolseram) or phenothiazines.

Treatment

Surgery is warranted even in the face of metastases because of the slow protracted natural history of the disease and because by reduction of the quantity of serotonin-elaborating tumor, amelioration of symptoms may ensue. Many patients live for 10 years or more after the diagnosis has been made. A large number of serotonin antagonists and antimetabolites have been tested, but most are without value. Vroom et al., 1962, tested eight compounds and found that chlorpromazine and cyproheptadine (Periactin) were effective. Antispasmodic and antidiarrheal drugs may be helpful in controlling gastrointestinal symptoms, and niacin is indicated if there is evidence of pellagra. The patient with a bronchial carcinoid tumor may respond dramatically to corticosteroid therapy, and some patients have remained asymptomatic for as long as 2 years. For a review see Melmon, 1968.

REFERENCES

Abboud, F. M.: Med. Clin. N. Amer. **52**:1009, 1968.

Ahlquist, R. P.: Amer. J. Physiol. **153**:586, 1948.

Anderson, W. A. D., and Cleveland, W. W.: Adrenal glands. In Anderson, W. A. D., editor: Pathology, vol. 2, St. Louis, 1966, The C. V. Mosby Co., p. 1125.

Armstrong, M. E., et al.: Biochem. Biophys. Acta **25**:422, 1957.

Axelrod, J., et al.: J. Pharmacol. Exp. Ther. **127**:251, 1959.

Axelrod, J.: J. Biol. Chem. **237**:1657, 1962.

Blaschko, H., and Welch, A. D.: Arch. Exp. Path. Pharmakol. **219**:17, 1953.

*Bridges, W. F.: Ann. Intern. Med. **56**:960, 1962.

*Carman, C. T., and Brashear, R. E.: New Eng. J. Med. **263**:419, 1960.

*Cohen, R. A., et al.: Ann. Intern. Med. **65**:347, 1966.

Crout, J. R., et al.: Amer. Heart J. **61**:375, 1961.

*Crout, J. R.: Anesthesiology **29**:661, 1968.

Elliot, T. R.: J. Physiol. **44**:374, 1912.

Engelman, K., et al.: New Eng. J. Med. **278**:705, 1968.

*Goldenberg, M., et al.: Amer. J. Med. **16**:310, 1954.

Greer, W. E. P., et al.: Amer. J. Surg. **107**:192, 1964.

Harrison, T. S., et al.: New Eng. J. Med. **279**:136, 1968.

Hillarp, N. A., et al.: Acta Physiol. Scand. **21**:155, 1954.

*Kellermeyer, R. W., and Graham, R. C., Jr.: New Eng. J. Med. **279**:754, 802, 859, 1968.

Lawrence, A. M.: Ann. Intern. Med. **66**:1091, 1967.

Lembeck, F.: Nature **172**:910, 1953.

Malmejac, J.: Bull. Acad. Roy. Med. Belg. **23**:50, 1958.

*Malmejac, J.: Physiol. Rev. **44**:186, 1964.

*Melmon, K. L.: The endocrinologic manifestations of the carcinoid tumor. In Williams, R. H., editor: Textbook of endocrinology, ed. 4, Philadelphia, 1968, W. B. Saunders Co., p. 1161.

Rossi, P., et al.: J.A.M.A. **205**:547, 1968.

Rubin, R. P., and Miele, E.: J. Pharmacol. Exp. Ther. **164**:115, 1968.

*Sjoerdsma, A., et al.: Ann. Intern. Med. **65**:1302, 1966.

*Thomas, J. E., et al.: J.A.M.A. **197**:754, 1967.

Thorson, A., et al.: Amer. Heart J. **47**:795, 1954.

von Euler, U. S., et al.: Acta Physiol. Scand. **59**:495, 1963.

Vroom, F. Q., et al.: Ann. Intern. Med. **56**:941, 1962.

*Wurtman, R. J.: New Eng. J. Med. **273**:637, 693, 746, 1965.

*Significant reviews.

Chapter 17

Parathyroid glands, calcium metabolism, and metabolic bone disease

PARATHYROID GLANDS
Anatomy

The parathyroids, usually four in number, are reddish or yellowish brown, thinly encapsulated, flat, ovoid structures each measuring 3 to 6 mm. by 2 to 4 mm. by 0.5 to 2 mm. and weighing 30 to 35 mg. They are located near the trachea and immediately posterior to the superior and inferior poles of the thyroid gland. Occasionally they reside within the thyroid capsule, may even be embedded in thyroid parenchyma, or may be found in the mediastinum. The blood supply is mainly from the inferior thyroid arteries. The nerve supply is chiefly vasomotor and arises from superior and recurrent laryngeal branches.

Histology and ultrastructure

The epithelial cells are arranged in cords separated by thin septa. Fat cells appear in the stroma during late childhood and puberty and increase steadily in number until by the fifth decade they occupy approximately 50% of the gland. The principal secretory cell is the *chief* cell, which measures 6 to 8 μ in diameter. It is believed to be the source of parathyroid hormone (PTH). There is a large central nucleus containing fine fibrillary or even pyknotic chromatin. The cytoplasm is usually slightly eosinophilic and often extensively vacuolated. The *oxyphil* cell is almost twice as large as the chief cell and contains pale acidophilic granules in the cytoplasm. It appears at puberty and increases in number with advancing age. The *water clear* cell, seen only in the adult gland, is large and polygonal and shows no visible cytoplasm. It is seen in states of pathologic hyperplasia. The ultrastructure has been described by Lever, 1965.

Calcium metabolism

Calcium (Ca) is essential for bone mineral, neuromuscular function, maintenance of cardiac rhythm, lactation, blood coagulation, acetylcholine synthesis and release, and maintenance of certain enzyme systems. The threshold of neuromuscular excitability is reduced by a deficiency of calcium ion (Ca^{++}), resulting in tetany. Excessive Ca^{++} causes reduced neuromuscular excitability, bradycardia, ventricular arrhythmias, reduced transport of urea, Na^+, and water across amphibian skin and urinary bladder, and reduced renal tubular reabsorption of Na. Membrane permeability is increased by a reduction of Ca^{++}.

Plasma Ca is maintained within narrow limits by a complex homeostatic mechanism comprising PTH, the kidney and small intestine, vitamin D, thyrocalcitonin (TCT), and bone (Fig. 17-1). Total body Ca is about 1 kg., of which 99% is in bone and 1% in extracellular fluids (ECF). Ca^{++} in ECF is constantly exchanged with available bone Ca and with the fluid of other cells and is excreted by intestinal mucosa and the kidney. Most blood Ca is

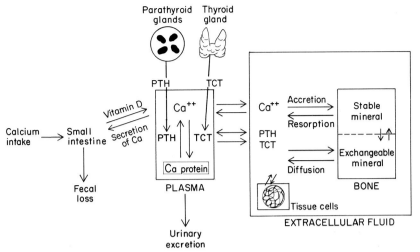

Fig. 17-1. Dynamics of calcium metabolism. **PTH,** parathyroid hormone; **TCT,** thyrocalcitonin.

in plasma, since the erythrocyte contains a negligible amount. Plasma Ca exists in three forms:

1. Ionized Ca++ (48%)
2. Complexed Ca—combined with citrate and phosphate (5%) } Diffusible
3. Protein-bound (Ca proteinate) (47%)— Nondiffusible

Albumin is the principal binding protein, 1 gram binding approximately 0.7 mg. of Ca. Alpha globulin binds little or no Ca, and gamma globulin binds only in multiple myeloma; beta globulin binds some Ca in normal subjects and in patients with hyperglobulinemia (except multiple myeloma). Ca++ is diffusible and biologically active, whereas the protein-bound form is neither ionized nor diffusible. Spinal-fluid Ca is almost protein free, and its concentration is almost identical with the diffusible fraction, but it is secreted by the choroid plexus and is therefore not a simple ultrafiltrate. The law of mass action governs the ionization of Ca. The equilibrium between Ca++ and protein is expressed by the formula (McLean and Hastings, 1935):

$$\frac{(Ca^{++})\ (Plasma\ protein^=)}{Ca\ proteinate} = K = 10^{-2.22(\pm0.07)}$$

Ca absorption is both an active and a passive process that occurs in the upper small intestine where the contents are acid and thus depends to an extent on normal gastric acidity. It is also enhanced by hypocalcemia, vitamin D, PTH, and reduced phosphate and is reduced by aging, an alkaline medium, vitamin D and/or PTH deficiency, excess phosphate–oxalates or sulfates, excessive fats that form insoluble Ca soaps, and cortisol. An average of 650 mg. of calcium is secreted into the gastrointestinal tract daily. This amount combined with unabsorbed ingested Ca provides 400 to 800 mg./day in the feces. Although urine rarely contains more than 200 mg. of Ca/day, Ca++ is filtrable, providing 5 mg./min. in the glomerular filtrate or about 7,200 mg./day. Thus fully 98% of Ca is reabsorbed by the renal tubule. The ability of the kidney to excrete Ca, even in the face of severe hypercalcemia, is limited. Calcium balance is positive in growing children, during pregnancy, in acromegaly, and after Ca deprivation and is negative in rickets, osteomalacia, sprue, osteoporosis, hyperparathyroidism, and hyperthyroidism and during calcium deprivation and lactation.

Inorganic phosphate metabolism (IP)

Phosphate ions form an essential part of the bone apatite crystal and participate in the formation of creatine phosphate, high-energy phosphates, phospholipids, hexose phospates of the carbohydrate cycle, and ribonucleic acids. The body contains approximately 700 grams of phosphate, of which 80% to 85% is in bones and teeth. The daily requirement is 1.2 grams or one and a half times that of Ca. The serum inorganic phosphate (SIP) comprises about one half the total blood phosphate. The normal blood level is 2.5 to 4.5 mg./100 ml. (1.45 to 2.7 mEq./L.) and is 1 to 2 mg. higher during growth and in active acromegaly and can be reduced by a restricted phosphate intake. Values tend to be low in the early morning and tend to rise to a late afternoon peak.

Free IP ion is freely excreted by the kidney; only 12% to 15% is protein bound. The tubular maximal reabsorption in humans is 139 to 148 μmole/min. (Longson et al., 1956). There is evidence that the human renal tubule secretes PO_4. The urinary excretion of IP increases progressively from 8 A.M. to 12 noon in normal subjects, and shows a negative correlation with plasma cortisol (Goldsmith et al., 1965). Ca and PO_4 tend to bear an inverse relationship in blood, which has been expressed by the "solubility product" Ca × PO_4 = K. The constant "K" remains relatively unchanged with minimal alterations of parathyroid activity, but K is not an absolute and does not necessarily reflect the effective plasma ionic concentrations of Ca and PO_4. The normal values for Ca × PO_4 are 40 to 55 for growing children, 30 to 40 for adults, and less than 40 for those with rickets.

Magnesium metabolism

Magnesium (Mg), a divalent ion, resembles Ca in its metabolism and has profound effects on many enzyme reactions and on Ca metabolism. The adult body contains about 24 grams, of which 70% is in the skeleton. Plasma contains 1.8 to 2.9 mg./100 ml. (1.5 to 2.4 mEq./L.), part of which is protein bound. Ca and Mg competitively share a common reabsorption system in the renal tubule and in the intestine, so that the absorption of either ion is increased at the expense of the other. Mg deficiency in animals causes hypercalcemia, hypocalciuria, and calcinosis.

Parathyroid hormone
Chemistry

Extracted pure bovine parathyroid hormone (PTH) is a single-chain polypeptide (molecular weight 8,500 to 10,000) composed of 74 to 81 amino acid residues (Potts et al., 1966). A tentative formula has been published. A 20-amino acid cleavage product representing one third of the molecule maintained typical PTH activity (Sherwood, 1968).

Assays

Biologic methods depend on the ability of the hormone (1) to restore the blood Ca level resulting from PTX (parathyroidectomy) or TPTX (thyroparathyroidectomy) in rats, (2) to produce phosphaturia, (3) to stimulate isolated liver or rat mitochondria in vitro, or (4) to stimulate the release of isotopically labeled Ca from cultured rat embryonic bone (Raisz, 1965). Radioimmunoassay depends on using purified bovine PTH and can detect as little as 10 $\mu\mu$g. in bovine plasma.

Regulation of secretion

Regulation of PTH secretion is accomplished by direct feedback control exerted by plasma Ca^{++}. Sherwood's group (Care et al., 1966) produced an 80% reduction of PTH secretion within 30 minutes by perfusing a goat parathyroid gland with blood containing 14 mg./100 ml. Ca, whereas perfusion with low Ca blood increased PTH secretion sevenfold. The rise of PTH is directly proportional to the fall of Ca. The parathyroid secretion is cut off at plasma Ca concentrations above 13 mg./100 ml. The half-life of PTH is approximately 18 minutes, and the volume of distribution is equivalent to 30% of body weight. The parathyroids store only small quantities of hormone; the secretion rate for a 500 kg. cow is 3 to 15 mg./day. Thus the parathyroid content of hormone would require replenishment 3 to 15 times per hour. The influence of PO_4 is indirect; hyperphosphatemia stimulates PTH secretion by lowering plasma Ca. PTH secretion may be inhibited by increased plasma Mg and stimulated by a decrease. The kidney has been shown to inactivate PTH.

Physiologic action

The principal function of PTH is to maintain circulating Ca^{++} within narrow limits and to conserve Ca by its action on bone and kidney and to a lesser extent on the intestine. The administration of PTH increases the concentration of plasma Ca and citrate and reduces the concentration of IP and Mg. It exerts important effects on mitochondria and on cellular membranes, particularly on the transport of divalent cations and anions.

Bone. The skeleton is a huge Ca reservoir made available to extracellular fluids by PTH. Even after PTX, if the blood Ca is lowered by EDTA (ethylenediaminetetraacetic acid), it slowly returns to its original level by release of bone Ca, but with intact parathyroids the restoration occurs far more rapidly. Bone mineral consists of a lattice structure of small apatite crystals whose aggregate surface area is huge, to which a surface layer of hydrated ions and a shell of water continuous with extracellular fluid is bound. A layer of hydrated Ca, PO_4, and OH ions is bound at the surface of the crystal and interchanges with similar ions in the surface layers of the lattice (Neuman and Neuman, 1957). Bone is directly resorbed by contact with parathyroid tissue. Bone formation and the protein biosynthetic capacity of osteoblasts is diminished. Bone resorption is an active process regulated by osteoclasts, osteocytes, or both. The resorptive process is probably enzymatic, involving dissolution of both mineral and protein matrix, and involves the release of both Ca and PO_4, but the mechanism remains obscure. An acid medium appears to be essential. Vitamin D promotes bone resorption and appears to be necessary for the action of PTH. Resorption is also favored by vitamin A, thyroxine, cortisol, heparin, and acidosis and inhibited by elevated plasma Ca, increased PO_4 intake, and TCT.

Kidney. PTE acts upon the mammalian proximal renal tubule and induces phosphaturia by reducing the tubular reabsorption of PO_4. There is also enhanced excretion of pyrophosphate, Na, K, Cl, and bicarbonate and reduced excretion of Ca, Mg, ammonia, and hydrogen ions.

Gastrointestinal system. PTE promotes Ca absorption from the small intestine in the presence of vitamin D. A decrease of Ca absorption occurs after PTX, and an increase is observed in hyperparathyroidism. Gastric secretory volume and total pepsin are increased, probably by a permissive effect through the influence of PTH on plasma Ca rather than by a direct action of the hormone. The action is probably one of inhibition of vagal activity. The administration of PTH, however, does not consistently influence gastric secretion in man. Numerous experiments have failed to reproduce a typical peptic ulcer in animals by the administration of PTH, Ca, or vitamin D, though large doses of PTH cause intramucosal hyperemia, petechiae, hemorrhages, and necrosis of the fundic glands in the stomach of dogs and rats. PTH generates an increase in active trypsin, pancreatic juice Ca, and pancreatic inflammation in experimental animals. Parathyroid hyperplasia can be produced in rabbits by the chronic administration of glucagon, and it has been postulated that the increased serum glucagon in acute pancreatitis may induce hypocalcemia and be responsible for PHP.

Mitochondria. The primary action of PTH is to alter the permeability of the inner mitochondrial membrane to Mg and K and to influence energy-dependent Ca and PO_4 mitochondrial transport (Arnaud et al., 1967). Ca is accumulated by mitochondria principally as $CaPO_4$ and is deposited as an amorphous precipitate in mitochondrial granules. The energy is provided by oxidative phosphorylation. In common with many other hormones, PTH action may be mediated via C-AMP.

Vitamin D

The provitamins can be transformed into vitamin D (Table 17-1) not only by ultraviolet irradiation but also by cathode rays, X rays, radium emanations, electric currents of high frequency, and electrons that open ring B in the ergosterol nucleus. The standard *assay*, or "line test," measures the capacity of the vitamin to calcify the epiphyses of the rachitic rat. The international unit is equivalent to a biologic activity of 0.025 mg. of pure crystalline cholecalciferol and equals 1 U.S.P. unit. Vitamin D is absorbed in the distal small intestine and stored principally in the liver but is also accumulated by skin, bone, brain, and spleen.

Physiologic actions. Certain of the physiologic actions of vitamin D and PTH are similar. Vitamin D promotes the intestinal absorption of Ca and PO_4 chiefly from the distal one third of the small bowel and from the large bowel. Vitamin D deficiency results in inadequate absorption of Ca and PO_4 and their excessive fecal loss. The rate of reabsorption of PO_4 by the renal tubule is increased. Vitamin D increases the free exchange between bone and ECF-Ca in young animals and is essential for bone resorption. The vitamin is necessary to promote normal bone growth and for calcification of rachitic bone. In rickets abnormal epiphysial ossification occurs and is characterized by a widened irregular plate with persisting cartilage cells and retarded ossification. The mechanism is unknown, but alkaline phosphatase must play some role because of its known function of converting organic phosphate to inorganic phosphate and because elevated serum alkaline phosphatase is found in rachitic children. Skeletal citrate and serum citrate levels are reduced in vitamin D deficiency as is mitochondrial citrate oxidation, whereas D stimulates citrate synthe-

sis in cartilage. Vitamin D tends to increase the $TmPO_4$, though the opposite effect is induced by excessive doses.

Dihydrotachysterol has less effect on Ca absorption from the intestine than does vitamin D but has a greater effect on bone resorption and thus a greater hypercalcemic action. It also increases renal PO_4 excretion far more than vitamin D by increasing the GFR. It therefore mimics the action of PTH more than does vitamin D.

Mechanism of action. A time lag has been observed between the administration of vitamin D to rachitic animals and the increased absorption of Ca across the intestinal wall. This interval is dose related and may reflect the period required for the synthesis of an intracellular protein that may be essential for Ca transport. Wasserman and Taylor, 1966, found a Ca-binding protein that might be identical with or related to an intracellular Ca carrier "operating in a facilitated diffusion or an active transport." DeLuca and Sallis, 1965, found that the Ca-release system in mitochondria was dependent on vitamin D but that the PO_4-uptake system was completely independent. Recently DeLuca et al. (Raisz, 1969) identified 25-hydroxycholecalciferol as the active metabolite of vitamin D_3.

Thyrocalcitonin (TCT) (calcitonin)

In 1961 Copp discovered thyrocalcitonin, a Ca-lowering hormone that he believed originated in the parathyroids. It has now been localized to subcellular vesicles of the parafollicular or "C" cells of the thyroid and the ultimobranchial glands of fowls and dogfish, and it is not detectable in thyroidectomized mammals. Electron-dense granular bodies found in some of these vesicles are released by Ca administration and are presumed to be the site of TCT. Extracts from the thyroid glands of humans and other mammals and from the ultimobranchial bodies of amphibians, teleost fish, and birds show TCT activity. Assays depend on Ca-lowering potency in the rat, and an assay of human plasma

Table 17-1. The D vitamins

Vitamin	Common name	Chemical structure	Precursor (provitamin D)	Source
Vitamin D₂	Calciferol (Ergocalciferol)		*Ergosterol (plant steroid; ergot, yeast)	Ultraviolet irradiation
Vitamin D₃	Cholecalciferol		Cholesterol → 7-dehydrocholesterol (provitamin D₃ in skin and duodenal mucosa)	Naturally occurring (butter, egg yolk, fish liver oil)
Dihydrotachysterol			Ergosterol	Ultraviolet irradiation

R—same as vitamin D₂ in rings A, B, and C.
X—same as vitamin D₂ in ring D and side chain.
*Same as calciferol, except for ring B.

showed levels of 60 to 120 mU./L. Recently a radioimmunologic method has been reported for the measurement of TCT in plasma (Deftos et al., 1968). The hormone is a polypeptide with a molecular weight of 3,700 and may exist in four separate active fractions designated alpha, beta, gamma, and delta calcitonin. The amino acid sequence has been characterized and the hormone has been synthesized (Rittel et al., 1968).

Physiologic actions. TCT lowers plasma Ca and SIP by inhibiting bone resorption. The hypocalcemic effect reaches its maximum within 1 to 2 hours of administration. Calcium accretion continues in bone when TCT prevents resorption and hypocalcemia ensues. An unsettled question is whether bone formation is enhanced. The urinary excretion of PO_4 and to a certain extent Ca and Na is increased as an indirect effect of the hypocalcemic stimulus to PTH secretion.

Regulation of secretion. The secretory signal is hypercalcemia and possibly glucagon, and the inhibitor is hypocalcemia. Whether TCT plays a physiologic role in regulating Ca metabolism remains to be established. It may well be that of fine adjustment of plasma Ca in conjunction with PTH, maintenance of Ca balance, and

regulation of bone resorption and growth. Mazzuoli et al., 1966, described a patient with hypocalcemia whose resected goiter showed a 100-fold increase of hypocalcemic activity. For reviews see Foster, 1968, and Tenenhouse et al., 1968.

DISEASES OF THE PARATHYROID GLANDS
Primary hyperparathyroidism (PHP)

PHP is generated by the autonomous hyperfunctioning of adenomatous or hyperplastic parathyroid tissue, resulting in the hypersecretion of PTH. The cause is unknown, but it is tempting to postulate a role for prolonged subtle hypocalcemia, perhaps from a mild excess of TCT. Patients with primary renal disease, secondary parathyroid hyperplasia, and subsequent adenoma formation have been described.

Pathology (Table 17-2)

Chief cell or water-clear cell hyperplasia was differentiated in only two reports in Table 17-2; Kyburz, 1966, found 10 chief cell hyperplasias and mentioned no water-clear cell cases, and Cope found 37 chief cell and 15 water-clear cell varieties of hyperplasia. Rarely there is no detectable histologic abnormality.

Adenoma. Most adenomas involve one

Table 17-2. Incidence of pathologic lesions in primary hyperparathyroidism

	Black and Zimmer, 1956	Ostrow et al., 1960	Wilder et al., 1961	Wilson et al., 1964	Kyburz et al., 1966	Cope, 1966	Goldsmith et al., 1966	Total
Number of cases	207	343*	50	51	55	343	44	1093
Benign adenoma	185	313	36	45	45	276	41	941 (86%)
Single	177	295	36	44	43	263	40	898 (82%)
Multiple	8	18	—	1	2	13	1	43 (4%)
Hyperplasia	15	24	12	5	10	52	2	120 (11%)
Hyperplasia + adenoma	—	—	1	—	—	—	—	—
Carcinoma	2	4	1	1	—	15	1	24 (2%)
Polyendocrine adenoma	5	2	—	—	—	—	—	7 (1%)

*Literature review.

of the inferior parathyroid glands. Over 90% are found behind the thyroid, but they may be intrathyroidal or may be in the thymus or other mediastinal sites. Tumor weight varies from 100 mg. to over 50 grams, and the shape varies from spherical to egg shaped or almost cylindrical. There is often a rough correlation between size and serum Ca concentration. The surface is usually smooth and tan to red or orange-brown or occasionally chocolate in color. The cut surface is darker, often largely hemorrhagic, or cystic with cyst spaces containing clear, colorless fluid. Calcification is rare. Distinguishing features are a distinct rim of normal parathyroid tissue outside the tumor capsule, the identification of another normal parathyroid gland, and the absence of fat in the tissue. Among the 941 cases in Table 17-2, 95% were single adenomas, and only 5% were multiple. More than two adenomas are very rarely found. Multiple adenomas or primary hyperplasia of all four parathyroids is found in hereditary hyperparathyroidism and may complete the multiple endocrine adenomatosis syndrome (MEAS). The light chief cell predominates, but all cell types (both light and dark chief cells, water-clear, oxyphil, and transitional forms) can be found (Fig. 17-2). The ultrastructure differs from that of normal tissue only by a loss of the reciprocal relationship between the amount of glycogen and the number of secretory granules.

Hyperplasia. The pathologist often experiences difficulty in distinguishing primary from secondary hyperplasia or adenoma. In the secondary variety fat is scanty or absent, more oxyphil cells are present than would be expected for the age of

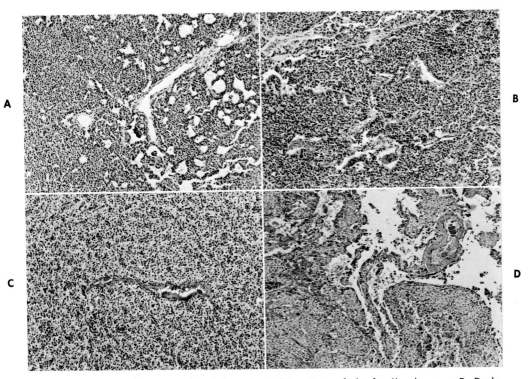

Fig. 17-2. Primary hyperparathyroidism. **A,** Light variety of chief cell adenoma. **B,** Dark variety of chief cell adenoma. **C,** Chief cell hyperplasia. **D,** Carcinoma (note tumor embolus in a blood vessel). (Courtesy Dr. Alexander Nedwich and Department of Pathology, Hahnemann Medical College, Philadelphia, Pa.)

the patient, and there is little variability from lobule to lobule. The chief cell variety was thought to be confined to secondary hyperparathyroidism until 1958, when Cope and his co-workers described *primary chief cell hyperplasia* (Fig. 17-2). In this variety all four glands are enlarged, are often nodular, and so closely resemble adenomas that some pathologists have maintained that they are indeed true tumors. The chief cell predominates, but oxyphil, water-clear, and transitional cells are found. In the *water-clear, or "wasserhelle," variety*, all four glands are enlarged, but the superior two are usually larger than the inferior two. They are quite irregular in shape and present large irregular projections or pseudopods from their surface. Masses of large water-clear cells with small pyknotic nuclei predominate.

Hyperplasia with adenoma. The presence of both lesions suggests a causal rather than a fortuitous relationship. One may project at least two possibilities: (1) primary renal disease → secondary parathyroid hyperplasia → autonomous adenoma formation, a sequence that has been called "tertiary hyperparathyroidism" and (2) primary parathyroid adenoma → renal insufficiency → secondary hyperplasia of remaining parathyroids.

Carcinoma. These rare, somewhat indurated, irregularly shaped, usually large tumors, firmly adhere to adjacent tissues. Although they show the usual histologic criteria of malignancy, rarely an apparently benign parathyroid adenoma will later metastasize, reflecting either a primary malignant potential or an acquired property. The cells are large, contain large nuclei, are arranged in sheets between fibrous bands, and often exhibit mitotic figures (Fig. 17-2, *D*).

Differential diagnosis by pathology (Roth, 1962)

Parathyroid tumor should be suspected if the gland is abnormally dark brown. The water-clear hyperplasia presents an irregular chocolate-colored gland with projecting pseudopods; on frozen section, sheets of large water-clear cells are evident, and the surgeon is alerted to the probable involvement of all four glands. Nevertheless, adenoma and primary or secondary chief cell hyperplasia cannot always be clearly differentiated by gross examination. Carcinoma is characteristically a large, somewhat indurated, adherent tumor. One cannot be certain of an adenoma unless one finds a true rim of normal tissue in the same gland, together with other normal parathyroid glands. When all glands are enlarged and particularly if they are nodular, hyperplasia is probable, though the enlargement may be so minimal as to be overlooked by the inexperienced surgeon. A gland larger than 5 mm. should be suspected as being abnormal. Multiple parathyroid gland involvement should be expected (1) if a well-defined adenoma is not found; (2) if one or more of the parathyroids appears enlarged, however minimally; (3) in MEAS particularly with islet cell pancreatic tumor; (4) in patients with minimal hypercalcemia; and (5) in the rare familial association of bilateral pheochromocytoma, medullary carcinoma of the thyroid, and multiple parathyroid adenoma (Sipple's syndrome). Seven patients with hyperparathyroidism from parathyroid adenoma and associated carcinoma of the thyroid have been reported (Ellenberg et al., 1962).

Pathophysiology

Excessive PTH secretion destroys bone matrix and mobilizes Ca and PO_4 from bone. The tubular reabsorption of Ca is increased and PO_4 is decreased, leading to a rising blood Ca and falling blood SIP. The renal loss of Na, K, and PO_4 is enhanced, whereas the excretion of Ca, Mg, and H is decreased. However, the rising concentration of blood Ca promotes hypercalciuria, nephrocalcinosis, and renal calculi. The urine tends to be alkaline, and there is some reduction of renal concentrating ability. There is enhancement of the intestinal absorption of Ca that may aggravate the hypercalcemia. The rise of gastric acid and pepsin secretion may favor peptic ulcer formation. The release of bone Ca, PO_4, citrate, hydroxyproline, and Mg results in osteoporosis and/or osteitis fibrosa cystica. There is thinning of cancellous spicules and marrow and even cortical replacement with fibrous tissue that may give rise to large and small degenerative fluid-filled cysts lined with fibrous tissue. The bones become soft and deformed. Fibrous tissue masses containing organized blood and pigment ("brown tumors") are formed. Microscopic examination of these tumors shows evidence of bone repair, numerous giant cells, and a reaction to hemorrhage. Studies of Ca kinetics have shown an increased accretion rate and often an increased bone turnover even in the absence of x-ray evidence of bone involvement.

Clinical features (Tables 17-3 and 17-4)

PHP is no longer classified as a rare endocrine disorder. The incidence appears to be directly proportional to the diligence with which it is sought. Boonstra and Jackson, 1965, for example, ordered serum Ca determinations on 26,000 consecutive patients attending a clinic in a small community and found 32 cases of PHP or 1 per 800; Keating found the incidence to be approximately 0.1% of the Mayo Clinic population. Vail and Coller, 1967, found 8 adenomas and 16 cases of hyperplasia among 200 unselected autopsies. Females predominate 2 to 1 in most series. PHP may appear at any age, but the majority of cases occur in the 30- to 60-year range. It is rare before puberty and uncommon but not so rare in old age.

PHP does not always exhibit the classic pattern of renal stones or bone disease but may be masked by a myriad of diverse and apparently unrelated symptoms often resembling a psychoneurosis. It may remain stable and occasionally remits for long periods of time or exacerbates to a severe toxic form. Occasionally it is symptomless and is revealed by the finding of

Table 17-3. Diagnostic features or presenting symptoms in primary hyperparathyroidism (in percent)

	380 cases, Keating, 1961	104 cases, Gordon, 1962	343 cases, Cope, 1966	Rasmussen, 1968
Bone symptoms	14	—	23	20
				3 (fracture)
				0.5 (local bone tumor)
Urologic signs	69	82	57	60
Symptomatic hypercalcemia	3	21	—	—
Asymptomatic hypercalcemia	—	7	—	3-8
Pancreatitis	1	1	3	—
Adenomatosis	1	—	1	—
Serendipity	12	—	—	—
Peptic ulcer	—	7	8	10*
Hypertension	—	29	2	1
Central nervous system signs	—	—	2	—
Mental disturbance	—	—	1	0.5
Fatigue	—	—	3	4

*Labeled "gastrointestinal."

Table 17-4. Clinical characteristics of hyperparathyroidism

	Symptoms	*Signs*
Kidney	Renal colic Polyuria, nocturia Polydipsia	Urolithiasis Nephrocalcinosis Hypertension Uremia
Hypercalcemia	Weakness, fatigue Malaise Myalgia Headache	Myopathy Hyperflexible extremities Band keratopathy Galvanic muscle stimulation—decreased excitability
1. CNS	Personality changes Depression, apathy Somnolence Epileptiform seizures Comatose episodes	Mental disturbance Hyporeflexia
2. G.I.	Dry mouth Anorexia, nausea dyspepsia, vomiting, weight loss, abdominal pain, "ulcer" pain, constipation	Peptic ulcer Pancreatitis, pancreatic calcification
3. Heart	Digitalis hypersensitivity	Bradycardia ECG—short Q-T interval
Bone	Pain Arthralgia	Tenderness to palpation or percussion Tender, stiff joints, limitation of motion, effusion Stubbing of ends of fingers Epulis of palate or mandible Fractures Skeletal x-ray changes

mild hypercalcemia, or by the fortuitous discovery of an adenoma during thyroidectomy or neck exploration. Only rarely is an adenoma palpable in the neck. One must consider PHP in such diverse disorders as pancreatitis, peptic ulcer, arthralgias and myopathies, renal failure, personality change, and depression. The diagnosis is made by a search for positive evidence of its presence and by the exclusion of other causes of hypercalcemia. Coexisting disorders or complicating conditions may be diagnostic signposts. Thyroid carcinoma has been found in 2% to 8% of cases. Florid PHP accompanied by a palpable mass in the neck, marked hypercalcemia, and bone lesions suggests parathyroid carcinoma. The disease may be familial and may be part of the multiple endocrine adenoma syndrome or may occur in concert with thyroid carcinoma and pheochromocytoma.

PHP tends to manifest itself in three clinical subgroups: (1) renal calculi, (2) overt bone disease, and (3) without calculi or bone disease. In general, patients with renal calculi rarely show overt bone disease, and patients with distinct bone disease usually do not show renal calculi. Moreover, there appears to be a lack of progression from one form to the other. There may be recurrent stone formation for years without bone disease and vice versa. Nephrocalcinosis, however, may occur in patients with bone disease.

Renal calculi. The majority of cases are encountered by studying patients with kidney stones or nephrocalcinosis; 5% to 12% of these individuals are found to have PHP. Repeated episodes of urolithiasis are typical. From 57% to 82% (Table 17-3) of patients with PHP show urologic pathology. Serious renal damage, probably accelerated by complicating pyelonephritis in patients with renal stones, can result from neglected long-standing disease. Mild polyuria, nocturia, and polydipsia, often attributed to the hypercalcemia, are more likely because of impairment of renal concentrating power. Uremia and hypertension are complications. Occasionally diabetes insipidus is suspected. The formation of renal stones probably depends not alone on hypercalciuria but also on a reduced excretion of H^+ ion and on the formation of an organic mucoprotein matrix released from bone by the action of PTH, and depolymerized, dissolved, and excreted by the kidney. PTH may also induce renal tubular binding of Ca salts. The typical parathyroid tumor in stone-formers is small, grows slowly, and is associated with minimal hypercalcemia.

Hypercalcemia. The symptoms are not specific for PHP and depend on the degree of plasma Ca elevation. They may vary from none, or so-called asymptomatic chemical hyperparathyroidism, to a profusion of often vague nondescript complaints. There may be motor weakness, increased flexibility of the extremities, fatigue, malaise, muscle and joint pains, headache, personality and mood changes, somnolence, dryness of the mouth and nose, anorexia, weight loss, constipation, bradycardia, and digitalis hypersensitivity. Rarely there is myopathy and muscle atrophy mimicking a primary polymyopathy. Neonatal tetany may alert the physician to search for PHP in the mother. Soaring plasma Ca concentrations cause hypercalcemic crisis (acute parathyrotoxicosis). Slit-lamp examination

may reveal band keratopathy—a deposit of $CaPO_4$ crystals usually in the palpebral fissure. Gray, hazy, granular, epithelial and subepithelial deposits concentric with the limbus are evident in the temporal and nasal areas, fading toward the center and often leaving a clear margin between the edge of the deposit and the limbus. They are occasionally visible with the naked eye. Bulbar conjunctival deposits resemble small crystal particles by slit lamp. Ocular irritation may result from a chalky white material in the palpebral conjunctiva. The eye changes are not specific for PHP but can be found in hypercalcemia of diverse origins. ECG tracings often reveal lengthening of the Q-T interval and bradycardia. Galvanic current stimulation of muscles shows decreased excitability.

Skeletal effects. Symptoms attributed to skeletal pathology occur in only about 20% of cases. However, histologic examination of bone reveals pathologic conditions in most patients even where the x-ray examination is negative. The incidence is especially high in children. Diffuse osteoporosis is more common and may be symptomless or may generate bone pain, backache, and some tenderness to palpation or percussion. A variety of articular and periarticular changes cause joint pains, stiffness, limitation of motion, and even effusions. A spontaneous fracture or one following minimal trauma may occur through a bone cyst or tumor. An epulis of the palate or mandible may be a "brown tumor." The dentist may be the first to suspect the disease by noting absence of the lamina dura or an isolated bone cyst of the mandible. Patients with overt bone disease usually have a large parathyroid adenoma and a higher plasma Ca than patients with kidney stones, and the history is relatively brief.

Peptic ulcer. PHP has been called "a disease of stones, bones, and abdominal groans" (St. Goar, 1957). Peptic ulcer is more common in patients with PHP than in the general population. Keating, 1961, found 59 patients with ulcer among 380 cases of PHP (15.5%), and Ostrow et al., 1960, reported an incidence of 9.1% in a composite series of 429 unselected patients. In the latter series a high incidence in males (14.9%) than in females (6.2%) was observed, though PHP is more common in females. The ratio of duodenal to gastric ulcer was 3.7 to 1. Symptoms of ulcer often could not be substantiated by x-ray examination. Multiple parathyroid adenomas and polyendocrine adenomas were more common in the ulcer group. Frame and Haubrich, 1960, studied 300 consecutive patients with peptic ulcer and discovered 4 cases (1.3%) of PHP. The significance of the relationship of peptic ulcer disease to PHP is obscure. The ulcer may long antedate PHP or vice versa. Cure of PHP may not always abolish ulcer disease. The serum Ca should always be measured in patients with peptic ulcer particularly if symptoms are persistent or aggravated by medical treatment, or if there is nausea or vomiting.

Pancreatitis. In various reports pancreatitis was found in from 1% to 12% of cases of PHP. Pancreatic calculi are common, and calcification of the pancreas may be found in the absence of renal calcification or bone changes. The pancreatic disease may be acute, chronic, postoperative, or recurrent. Acute pancreatitis can depress the serum Ca to normal values possibly by chelation of Ca by the products of fat digestion.

Familial occurrence and multiple endocrine adenomatosis (MEAS). Although PHP is usually a sporadic disease, a heritable factor has been compatible with an autosomal dominant mode (Jackson and Boonstra, 1967). The lesion usually consists of multiple parathyroid adenomas or primary chief cell hyperplasia. More than 80% of patients with MEAS have parathyroid adenomas. It has been suggested that familial PHP is a partial expression of MEAS and that MEAS may first arise in a single endocrine gland. Certain ectopic tumors may elaborate a PTH-like material. The resulting ectopic

PHP syndrome is more common in males and is characterized by a very high plasma Ca, anemia, weight loss, and a low incidence of renal calculi or bone involvement (Liddle, 1968).

Chemical or asymptomatic PHP

Chemical or asymptomatic PHP may prove to be the most common variety, so that the physician must consider adding a Ca determination to routine laboratory screening procedures. When the plasma Ca shows only minimal elevation, symptoms may be vague, mild, or lacking.

X-ray studies

Skeletal changes. Skeletal changes are detectable by x-ray examination in approximately 30% of cases. The pathognomonic finding is *subperiosteal cortical resorption of bone* (Fig. 17-3, *A* and *B*), most frequently found along the margins of the phalanges. The cortex is decalcified and appears as a peculiar lacelike or ragged spiculelike margin beneath the periosteum. In extreme cases the cortex may be completely absorbed (Fig. 17-3, *B*). When the distal phalanges are affected, the tufts tend to be absorbed (Fig. 17-3, *A*). The medial aspect of the upper third of the tibia is frequently involved. Erosions also involve the inferior aspect of the distal third of the clavicle and ulna, and the posterior or posterolateral portions of the ribs along their upper cortical margins especially affecting the third and fourth ribs. Loss of the *lamina dura,* seen in dental x-ray films, is another expression of subperiosteal resorption. Gordon et al., 1962, however, found the lamina dura to be intact in 39 of 42 dentulous patients with PHP. *Single* (Fig. 17-3, *D*) or *multiple bone cysts* and *brown tumors* (osteoclastomas) may be found in the mandible or long bones (Fig. 17-3, *C*). *Diffuse skeletal demineralization* (osteoporosis), since it is not evident in x-ray films until there is a loss of at least 25% of bone mineral, is seen in perhaps one third of cases. However, nonspecific bone abnor-

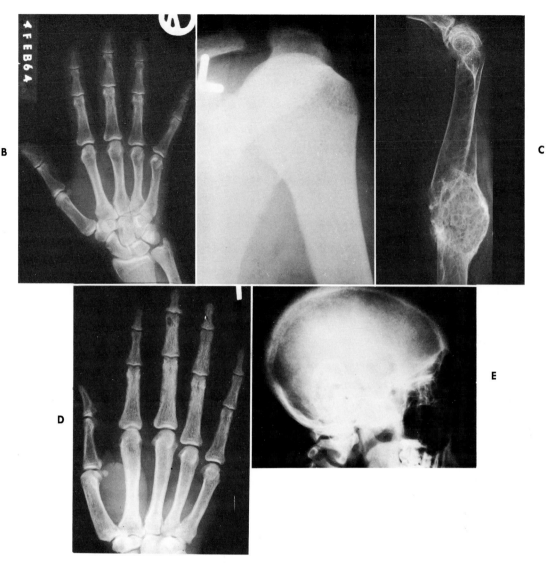

Fig. 17-3. Skeletal changes of primary hyperparathyroidism. **A,** Subperiosteal cortical resorption (note marked resorption of the middle phalanx of third finger and partial resorption of tufts of distal phalanges. **B,** Resorption of lateral end of clavicle. **C,** A "brown tumor." **D,** Single bone cyst of middle phalanx third finger and subcortical bone resorption of phalanges. **E,** Skull showing "ground glass" appearance. (Courtesy Dr. George Wohl, Department of Radiology, Philadelphia General Hospital, Philadelphia, Pa.)

malities, by a study of iliac-crest biopsies, have been found in some 90% of cases (Gordon et al., 1962), ^{125}I bone densitometry studies have shown low or distinctly abnormal values in 75% of cases (Forland et al., 1968), and microradiographic studies of iliac-crest biopsies revealed increased bone resorption in all of 26 cases of PHP (Riggs et al., 1965). The reason for the frequent absence of gross skeletal changes in PHP is unknown, but it has been suggested that it may depend on a compensatory hyperthyrocalcitonemia with some suppression of the bone-resorbing action of PTH. With advanced demineralization, a fine trabecular pattern appears later to become coarsened and even to disappear, leaving a ground-glass, moth-eaten, or wormwood appearance that is particularly striking in the skull (Fig. 17-3, *E*). There is also erosion of the inner and outer tables of the skull. Less commonly, owing to increased osteoblastic activity with increased bone deposition, *osteosclerosis* is evident. Diffuse osteitis fibrosa cystica (von Recklinghausen) is the most florid skeletal expression of PHP and displays multiple cystic disease, large and small brown tumors, and severe osteoporosis with extensive deformities and fractures.

Kidney. Renal calculi or nephrocalcinosis is found in 75% of patients, though the two seldom are found together. The latter is usually bilateral and is most prominent in the region of the renal papillae.

Ectopic calcification. Ectopic calcification is unusual in PHP and is manifested only in severe long-standing cases. There may be Ca deposits about the joints and in the articular cartilages, pancreas, and prostate.

For reviews of the radiologic findings see Bartlett and Cochran, 1964, and Gleason and Potchen, 1967.

Laboratory studies

Dependence on the laboratory for the diagnosis is a unique feature of PHP. One expects to find hypercalcemia, hypercalciuria, hypophosphatemia, and hyperphosphaturia.

Serum or plasma calcium. Persistent elevation of the blood Ca is the *sine qua non* for the diagnosis. It has been found in more than 95% of patients with PHP. Gordon and Roof, 1968, attribute "normocalcemic" PHP to the use of inappropriate normal standards, laboratory error, or coexistence of conditions that may lower the serum Ca. Nevertheless, rare examples have been reported. The usually accepted normal range of 9 to 11 mg./100 ml. (4.5 to 5.5 mEq./L.) has been reexamined by more precise techniques and found to be somewhat lower (Table 17-5). Any value above 10.5 mg./100 ml. (5.2 mEq./L.) obtained by EDTA titration, AutoAnalyzer or oxalate-permanganate methods, or above 11 (5.5 mEq./L.) by flame photometry should suggest PHP. Small deviations from the normal may be significant. Values between 10.5 and 11 mg./100 ml. are not uncommon in PHP. Factitial elevations of serum Ca can occur from prolonged venous stasis distal to a tourniquet or from the use of cork stoppers. Keating et al., 1969, reported a subtle but definite fall with aging in males but not in females. The ionizable or ultrafiltrable Ca may be elevated in hypoproteinemia (especially hypoalbuminemia) when the total Ca is normal. To avoid the technical difficulties of determining Ca^{++} ion, nomograms have been published (McLean and Hastings, 1935; Hanna et al., 1964) that offer

Table 17-5. Normal blood calcium

Method	Plasma Ca mg./100 ml.	Reference
EDTA titration	8.8 -10.4	Nordin and Smith, 1965
AutoAnalyzer	8.9 -10.5	Nordin and Smith, 1965
Flame photometry	9.5 -11.5	McIntyre, 1961
Flame photometry (McIntyre method)	9.6 -11.3	Gordon et al., 1962
Oxalate-permanganate	9.0 -10.8	Prunty et al., 1951
Various methods	8.93-10.05 (females) 9.04-10.3 (males)	Yendt and Gagne, 1968

an approximation of the Ca^{++} ion from knowledge of the serum protein and total Ca values. Acute pancreatitis, a high phosphate intake, renal failure with phosphate retention, or intestinal malabsorption may counteract the rise of serum Ca in PHP and mask the diagnosis. Other causes of hypercalcemia and hypophosphatemia are listed in the following outline*:

Hypercalcemia
  Nonparathyroid malignancies (117)
  Hyperparathyroidism (104)
  Vitamin D intoxication (37)
  Milk-alkali syndrome (12)
  Hyperthyroidism (12)
  Immobilization—Paget's disease,
    fracture, paraplegia (7)
  Idiopathic (infancy) (3)
  Sarcoidosis (3)
  Dysproteinemias
    (multiple myeloma, etc.) (2)
  Addison's disease (2)
  Leukemia
  Hodgkin's disease and lymphoma
  "Steroid withdrawal" syndrome
Hypophosphatemia
  Hyperparathyroidism
  Rickets and osteomalacia
  Low phosphate intake
  Renal tubular acidosis
  Renal failure (early)

Serum or plasma inorganic phosphate (SIP). Normal values range from 2.5 to 4.8 mg./100 ml. (1.45 to 2.8 mEq./L.) Keating et al., 1969, found a progressive decrease in males with aging; in females there is a decrease to age 40 followed by some increase. Though low values are thought to be the hallmark of the disease, Strott and Nugent, 1968, found that in 46% of 682 cases of PHP normal values were reported, and Gordon et al., 1962, discovered *normal values in 60%* of their cases. For investigation of the tendency for excessive renal PO_4 loss in PHP, a number of PO_4 excretion or clearance studies have been devised. None have been well standardized, and all are nonspecific in that a phosphaturic effect has been found in other disorders such as

*Modified in part from Gordon, G. S., et al.: Recent Progr. Hormone Res. 18:297, 1962; numbers in parentheses are from his publication.

SHP, osteomalacia, sarcoidosis, myeloma, Fanconi syndrome, urolithiasis, and gout and in patients receiving corticosteroids. The tests are of limited or no value in renal insufficiency. Phosphate excretion studies should be done after the discovery of hypercalcemia, because a high phosphate intake can mask hypercalcemia, whereas a low intake or the ingestion of aluminum hydroxide gels that bind PO_4 in the intestinal tract can mask phosphaturia.

PERCENT TUBULAR REABSORPTION OF PHOSPHATE (% TRP) TEST. The % TRP test measures the ratio of PO_4 to creatinine clearance, the latter being an estimate of glomerular filtration rate, from the following formula:

$$TRP = 1 - \frac{PO_4 \text{ clearance } (C_p)}{\text{Creatinine clearance } (C_{cr})}$$

or

$$\% \ TRP = \left[1 - \frac{U_p \times S_{cr}}{U_{cr} \times S_p} \right] 100$$

C_p is PO_4 clearance, C_{cr} is creatinine clearance, U_p is urine PO_4, U_{cr} is urine creatinine, S_{cr} is serum creatinine, and S_p is serum inorganic phosphate. Normal values are 78% to 90%. The test is performed in patients without renal insufficiency and on a normal PO_4 intake (1 to 1.5 grams/day) for at least 3 days. An inadequate PO_4 intake can produce a false normal value. To overcome PO_4 depletion, the patient is given 3,000 mg. of PO_4 daily for 3 days; this dosage can be accomplished by adding 1.2 grams neutral sodium phosphate and three 8 oz. glasses of milk daily. The TRP can fall as low as 67% in normal subjects, but in patients with PHP the fall is usually to below 60%. An overnight 12-hour urine is collected for creatinine and inorganic PO_4 and a fasting blood sample is obtained in the morning for SIP and creatinine. Chambers et al., 1956, simplified the procedure and reported normal values of $84.7 \pm 0.9\%$ (78% to 90%) in 13 normal subjects and $65 \pm 1.3\%$ (41% to 82%) in 10 cases of PHP. The % TRP test is viewed by many authorities as being the second most reliable test, though the overlap between normal subjects and patients with PHP is considerable, and values within the normal range are found in 20% or more of the latter. Becker et al., 1964, measured the percent TRP before and after the injection of parathyroid extract (PTE) and found that normal subjects or those with hypercalcemia from various causes showed a consistently decreased TRP whereas patients with PHP did not. Gershberg et al., 1966, reported that patients with primary kidney disease respond to PTE if the creatinine clearance was above 30 ml./min.

PHOSPHATE CLEARANCE. In mild renal failure the % TRP test is inaccurate but the phosphate clearance (C_p) is valid and is obtained from the formula:

$$C_p = \frac{U_p \times V}{S_p}$$

V is urine flow in milliliters per minute. Values above 15 ml./min. are found in PHP. Determination of the C_p depends on adequate hydration of the patient, accurate timing of urine collections, and complete collections. It varies with the SIP concentration. Creatinine need not be determined.

PHOSPHATE EXCRETION INDEX. PEI relates the clearance ratio of PO_4 to creatinine (C_p/C_{cr}) to the plasma PO_4 level and can be predicted as follows (Nordin and Smith, 1965):

$$C_p/C_{cr} = 0.055 \, (S_p - 0.07 \pm 0.09)$$

Deviation from the predicted normal mean is the PEI and normally falls within –0.09 to +0.09. It is calculated from the following formula:

$$PEI = C_p + C_c - 0.055 \, S_p + 0.07$$

Hyperparathyroidism is suspected if the PEI is above +0.12, whereas a PEI below –0.10 is found in hypoparathyroidism. The value of the test remains controversial.

MAXIMUM TUBULAR REABSORPTION OF PROSPHATE (TMP). TmP requires the I.V. infusion of a sodium phosphate solution until tubular reabsorption of PO_4 becomes constant. For details see Nordin and Smith, 1965. There is considerable overlap between normal subjects and patients with PHP, and the test is rarely employed. The "theoretical renal phosphorus threshold" (TRPT) is determined in a similar manner and has the same equivocal diagnostic value.

CALCIUM LOADING TEST. PTH secretion and urinary PO_4 excretion are inhibited in normal subjects by acutely raising the plasma Ca. In PHP the secretion of PTH is autonomous and cannot be reduced. As devised by Howard et al., 1953, urine is collected on 2 successive days from 9:30 A.M. to 9:30 A.M. On the second day Ca (calcium gluconate and calcium glucoheptonate, 15 mg./kg.) is infused I. V. at a steady rate for 4 hours; the plasma Ca must be elevated to at least 11 mg./100 ml. Blood for Ca, PO_4, and serum proteins is obtained before the test, at 2 hours, and at 4 hours. Several modifications of Howard's original technique have been proposed. There is a rise of serum Ca and PO_4 and a fall of at least 20% in the 24-hour PO_4 excretion in normal subjects. In PHP there is little or no change in SIP or urinary PO_4. According to Pronove and Bartter, 1961, the sensitivity of the test may be enhanced by additionally measuring the urinary PO_4 the day after the Ca infusion. The diagnostic value of Ca loading remains in doubt. Strott and Nugent, 1968, reviewed the literature and found considerable overlap between patients with PHP and renal stones and normal subjects.

PHOSPHATE DEPRIVATION (Pronove et al., 1961). The patient is given a low PO_4 diet (less than 450 mg./day) and aluminum hydroxide gel before and after each meal for 3 to 6 days. The expected reduction of SIP should cause a greater rise of plasma Ca and calciuria in patients with PHP than in euparathyroid subjects, as a result of enhanced PTH secretion.

Urinary calcium. Patients with PHP and good renal function are expected to excrete more Ca than do normal subjects, but so do patients with other conditions causing hypercalcemia, as well as those with renal stones and idiopathic hypercalciuria. If the 24-hour urinary Ca is greater than 250 mg. on an unrestricted diet, the patient is given a low Ca diet for 5 to 7 days (less than 150 mg./day). The urinary calcium-creatinine ratio can be measured on a random sample, though two consecutive 24-hour collections are preferred. Persistent hypercalciuria warrants suspicion of PHP. However, 24% of 650 patients reviewed by Strott and Nugent, 1968, and 28% of 54 patients of Yendt and Gagne, 1968, all with proven PHP, excreted normal quantities of Ca. The most common cause of hypercalciuria in patients with calcium-containing renal stones is idiopathic hypercalciuria, a disorder almost entirely confined to males. Yendt investigated 600 patients with renal calculi and found that the hypercalciuric male had only a 12% chance of having PHP, whereas the female had a 65% chance.

Suppression of hypercalcemia by corticosteroids. Hypercalcemia caused by sarcoidosis, certain malignancies, or vitamin D intoxication is usually reduced by corticosteroid administration, whereas in PHP a reduction is unusual. A malignant tumor that secretes a PTH-like substance will usually not respond to corticosteroids. The patient is given 150 to 200 mg. of cortisone, or 30 to 40 mg. prednisone, daily for 10 to 14 days, and the plasma Ca is measured daily. The test is useful in evaluating equivocal cases.

Urinary hydroxyproline. Normal values are 36.6 ± (S.E.) 1.96 mg./24 hr. (range 19 to 65 mg./24 hr.) (Johnston et al., 1966) and become elevated in PHP in proportion to the degree of bone involvement. After an I.V. infusion of calcium, hydroxyprolinuria is reduced in normal subjects but not in patients with PHP (Klein, 1963).

Radioimmunoassay of plasma PTH concentration. Methods are being evaluated for application to problems of human parathyroid disease. It is discouraging to note that Berson and Yalow, 1966, found normal plasma levels in 15 of 29 cases of PHP. Present methods lack sufficient sensitivity to be of diagnostic value. Reiss and Canterbury, 1968, have developed a more sensitive assay using chicken antibody and have noted a rise in plasma PTH after massaging over an adenoma.

Localization of a parathyroid adenoma

PARATHYROID SCANNING. Selenomethionine labeled with ^{75}Se, concentrates in a parathyroid adenoma and may prove to be a diagnostic aid when the technique is improved. If a goiter is present, a "cold" nodule delineated by ^{131}I thyroid scanning in a suspected case of PHP serves to heighten suspicion of a parathyroid adenoma. Toluidine blue, a phenothiazine dye, visibly stains the parathyroids in vivo and is being investigated as a means of identifying the glands at surgery (Hurwitz et al., 1967).

BARIUM-SWALLOW ROENTGENOGRAPHY OR CINEROENTGENOGRAPHY. Occasionally indentation or deviation of the cervical esophagus may help to localize the tumor.

ANGIOGRAPHY. Bilateral subclavian arteriography may aid in the location of the tumor. Recognition depends on distortion and displacement of the inferior thyroid artery.

PNEUMOMEDIASTINOGRAPHY. The method involves the introduction of CO_2 into the anterior mediastinum to delineate a mediastinal adenoma.

VENOUS CATHETERIZATION. Selective venous catheterization of the major veins draining the neck and thorax and measurement of an increased local PTH concentration was reported by Reitz et al., 1969.

Bone biopsy. Iliac-crest biopsies may show nonspecific bone pathology in patients with PHP in whom skeletal x-ray films appear normal and the serum alkaline phosphatase is not elevated.

Miscellaneous studies. Wills and Mc-Gowan, 1964, found a *serum chloride above 102 mEq./L.* in all of 32 cases of PHP, whereas levels of 102 mEq./L. or lower were the rule in 28 cases of nonparathyroid hypercalcemia. Lafferty, 1966, stated that a serum chloride below 102 mEq./L. in the absence of vomiting or respiratory acidosis is definite evidence against the presence of a parathyroid adenoma. The serum alkaline phosphatase may or may not be increased in the presence of bone disease. Hypomagnesemia and hypokalemia are nonspecific and inconsistent findings. Hypertonic NaCl administered I.V. may stimulate calciuria in patients with PHP and has been proposed as a diagnostic test (Axelrod, 1966). Measurement of the rate of bone formation with strontium or various isotopes is experimental. The finding of increased urinary cyclic AMP in hyperparathyroidism in contrast to suppressed excretion in other hypercalcemic states may prove to be a useful test in the future (Chase and Aurbach, 1967). For a review of laboratory studies see Goldsmith, 1969.

Differential diagnosis

One must distinguish PHP from other causes of hypercalcemia (see outline on p. 295), from other bone disorders, and from other varieties of urolithiasis. PHP must be suspected when there is associated MEAS, medullary carcinoma of the thyroid, pheochromocytoma, Zollinger-Ellison syndrome, or intractable peptic ulcer, and especially when there is a positive family history for PHP or one of the associated disorders. PHP may coexist with other causes of hypercalcemia in 15% of cases.

Malignancy. The principal cause of hypercalcemia is malignancy even in the absence of demonstrable bone metastases. Some tumors secrete a PTH-like hypercalcemic polypeptide (pseudohyperparathyroidism). In the absence of obvious skeletal metastases, the differential from PHP can be perplexing, particularly when the biochemical picture mimics that of PHP. The hypercalcemia associated with breast cancer may be from the elaboration of a nonphosphaturic osteolytic sterol (Gordon et al., 1966), is associated with a normal or elevated SIP, and responds to corticosteroids, whereas hypercalcemia associated with bronchogenic carcinoma may show low SIP and resistance to corticosteroids. Lafferty, 1966, reviewed 50 cases of pseudohyperparathyroidism and found that hypernephroma and bronchiogenic carcinoma accounted for 60%. Seventy-five percent of patients were males, and the duration of symptoms was briefer than in PHP; significant weight loss and anemia were common, renal calculus and peptic ulcer were unusual, the serum Ca was above 14 mg./100 ml. in over 75%, and the serum alkaline phosphatase was elevated without bone disease in 20 of 42 cases, a probable indication of liver metastases.

Vitamin D intoxication. Individuals who ingest toxic quantities of vitamin D may be infants, food faddists, arthritic victims seeking relief of pain, or overtreated patients with hypoparathyroidism. The SIP is more likely to be high than low. Withdrawal of vitamin D is followed by a slow regression of the plasma Ca to normal.

Milk-alkali syndrome. The prolonged excessive ingestion of milk and alkali can induce a hypercalcemic syndrome that can mimic PHP without bone disease but with renal failure and peptic ulcer. There is no hypercalciuria, SIP is normal or elevated, serum alkaline phosphatase is normal, and there is mild alkalosis, frequently an alkaline urine, and metastatic calcification in the more severe cases. However, there have been patients who did have hypercalciuria, hypophosphatemia, and elevated alkaline phosphatase. Osteosclerosis has been found in some 20%. In the early stages the syndrome is usually reversible when milk and alkali are omitted, though the hypercalcemia may persist for long periods of time, whereas in PHP the syndrome persists. In the more advanced cases with metastatic calcification, renal damage is irreversible and there is a fatal outcome.

Sarcoidosis. There may be hypercalcemia, hypercalciuria, increased serum alkaline phosphatase, low % TRP, band keratopathy, conjunctival calcification, bone lesions, renal damage, and urolithiasis. The SIP, however, is usually normal, and the serum globulins show a distinctive rise. The hypercalcemia is attributed to enhanced intestinal absorption of Ca, and both are suppressed by corticosteroids. A positive diagnosis of sarcoidosis can usually be verified by well-known methods, but the differential from PHP is occasionally difficult.

Renal lithiasis. In patients with renal lithiasis or nephrocalcinosis, PHP must be eliminated as a cause, particularly when hypercalciuria is found. In idiopathic hypercalciuria, serum Ca is normal, SIP may be normal or reduced, % TRP is usually normal, and the excretion of Ca does not fall with a low Ca intake, whereas in PHP it may or may not. When this condition is found in females, PHP is more likely even if there is normocalcemia.

Multiple myeloma. There may be hypercalcemia but usually normal SIP and serum alkaline phosphatase. The diagnosis can usually be verified by typical findings. The elevated serum Ca is reduced by corticosteroid administration.

Miscellaneous findings. Secondary hyperparathyroidism (SHP) is discussed in Table 17-6 and on p. 301. Hypercalcemia is occasionally found in hyperthyroidism and Addison's disease. The bone lesions of Albright's syndrome (polyostotic fibrous dysplasia) may resemble PHP but are focal rather than diffuse, and the biochemical changes of PHP are lacking. In Paget's disease (osteitis deformans), hypercalcemia can occur if the patient is immobilized, but the other biochemical findings of PHP are not found, and the serum alkaline phosphatase is markedly elevated. In the differential diagnosis one's suspicions of PHP should be heightened where adequate therapy for a hypercalcemic disorder is not effective. For a review of the diagnostic spectrum of hypercalcemia, see David et al., 1962.

Acute hyperparathyroidism (acute parathyrotoxicosis, hyperparathyroid crisis)

There is a sudden major elevation of the blood Ca (usually about 17 mg./100 ml.)

Table 17-6. Differential diagnosis of primary from secondary hyperparathyroidism

	Primary	Secondary (renal osteodystrophy)
Age (years)	30-60	Often below 30
Clinical features	Protean	Renal failure (long duration)
Metastatic calcification	Rare	Common
Serum Ca	Elevated	Normal or low
Serum inorganic phosphate	Low or normal	Elevated
Ca × PO₄ product	Normal	Elevated
BUN	Normal*	Elevated
Urine Ca	Often increased	Decreased
Alkaline phosphatase	Often normal	Elevated
Renal biopsy	Interstitial inflammatory changes, peritubular calcification	Diffuse parenchymal destruction (far-advanced pyelonephritis)

*Except in chronic cases with renal damage.

and the patient will die if untreated. Anglem, 1966, could find only 82 recorded cases prior to 1966. The disorder is associated with progressive renal failure, hyperphosphatemia, azotemia, dehydration, hypochloremic alkalosis, oliguria, and metastatic calcification. The clinical manifestations are protean and many encompass the gastrointestinal, renal, skeletal, nervous, and neuromuscular systems, with particular emphasis on the first. Anorexia, nausea, vomiting, abdominal pain, and diarrhea or constipation predominate, but there is often dehydration, thirst, and polyuria from renal involvement. The hypercalcemia provokes myalgia, motor weakness, headache, irritability, confusion, depression, lethargy, obtunded mentation, and eventual coma. The ECG may first suggest the diagnosis by the characteristic shortening of the Q-T interval. Acute parathyrotoxicosis should be considered in any acutely ill patient with bizarre manifestations, disturbed behavior, or coma. Attempts to lower the serum Ca and to provide hydration and replacement of electrolyte losses are all a prelude to *mandatory emergency surgery*. These measures are outlined on p. 301.

Therapy of PHP

The most important preoperative measure is a frank exposition of all the surgical problems involved so that the patient will be prepared to accept a second or even third exploration should it become necessary. The surgeon identifies all parathyroid tissue and decides, with the aid of a frozen section, whether he is dealing with a single adenoma, multiple adenomas, or hyperplasia. If hyperplasia is found, he usually removes three glands and spares a portion of the most accessible gland (Cope, 1966). If the parathyroid glands appear normal and no adenoma is found, the surgeon must remove the thymus gland and perform a subtotal thyroidectomy, since the adenoma may be buried within these organs. Mediastinal exploration should always follow, rather than precede, these operations. Large fixed tumors are completely resected with care to preserve the capsule so as to prevent local seeding if there is parathyroid carcinoma. When the disorder persists after surgery, a second neck or mediastinal exploration may be required to locate an elusive tumor. Special preoperative measures are necessary only in the face of severe hypercalcemia when a low Ca–high PO_4 diet and increased fluid intake precede surgery. Renal insufficiency is not a contraindication to immediate surgery except when there is severe azotemia. Transient improvement sufficient to permit surgery may follow hemodialysis or the use of sodium ethylenediaminetetraacetate (EDTA), sodium sulfate, or sodium phosphate.

After surgery the serum Ca returns to normal within 24 to 48 hours, but the SIP requires 2 to 10 days. Rarely Ca values may later rise to high values in patients who do not appear to have persistent disease. A significant fall was observed in 7 hypercalcemic patients of Goldsmith et al., 1966, following negative neck exploration, and a nonspecific fall has been observed after surgery not involving the neck. Excessive phosphaturia disappears within 12 to 18 hours and may be a more reliable indication of the accuracy of the preoperative diagnosis than the fall of the serum Ca. Transient latent tetany despite normocalcemia in the immediate postoperative period is not unusual and is self-limited. Clinical tetany is found in patients with diffuse osteoporosis and often with an elevated serum alkaline phosphatase and has been attributed to cessation of bone resorption coupled with rapid calcification of the calcium-hungry bone matrix. It does not respond to vitamin D, A.T. 10, or PTH administration in the immediate postoperative interval but can be managed with a high Ca intake combined with intravenous Ca infusions as required. Hypomagnesemia should be treated with Mg supplements. Tetany disappears after several months or even a year and may first appear after a prolonged latent period. Permanent hypoparathyroidism may result from atrophy of residual parathyroid tissue.

Medical palliation may be necessary in patients too ill to withstand surgery and in metastatic parathyroid carcinoma. A high PO_4 intake combined with oral PO_4 supplements may raise the SIP, promote phosphaturia, and reduce hypercalcemia and hypercalciuria. Oral orthophosphates, neutral or alkaline phosphates, or other preparations in dosages of 2 to 4 grams/day may be used. Occasionally diarrhea can be an annoying side effect. Testosterone, estrogens, and growth hormone have been used for their anabolic effects and tend to reduce the hypercalcemia and hypercalciuria. More heroic measures to counteract severe hypercalcemia may be required, as the following:

1. *Saline infusions*, the safest measure for initial therapy, promote urinary Ca excretion and correct dehydration.

2. *I.V. isotonic sodium sulfate* prevents renal tubular reabsorption of Ca and augments calciuria. Magnesium supplements are required because sulfate increases magnesium excretion and may aggravate the hypomagnesemia found in many patients with PHP.

3. *I.V. phosphate salts* are potent, rapidly acting hypocalcemic agents but are thought to be a cause of hypotension, cardiac complications, metastatic calcification, and acute renal failure. Goldsmith and Ingbar, 1966, gave a solution of 0.1M disodium and monopotassium phosphate to 20 patients with hypercalcemia from diverse causes, without deleterious effects. If PO_4 infusion is reserved for the seriously ill patient and the minimal effective dose is employed with frequent monitoring of the blood Ca, adverse effects can be avoided. It may lower Ca by a simple physico-chemical precipitation of dibasic calcium phosphate as its solubility is exceeded.

4. Ethylenediaminetetraacetic acid disodium salt (EDTA) chelates Ca and lowers the plasma level but has nephrotoxic properties that have limited its use. It is available for parenteral administration as disodium edetate injection U.S.P. (1 Gm. in 5 ml. and 3 Gm. in 20 ml. of distilled water).

5. *Hemodialysis* or *peritoneal dialysis* has been effective in a few patients.

6. *Corticosteroids* are rarely effective in PHP. TCT may become available in the future and will undoubtedly be evaluated for its therapeutic efficacy.

Clinical course and prognosis

The natural history of untreated PHP remains undocumented. The relatively recent recognition of asymptomatic "chemical PHP" prompts the question of the duration of the disease prior to diagnosis and suggests the possibility that this variety may remain asymptomatic and need not progress inexorably to symptomatic hypercalcemia with ultimate renal and skeletal pathology. Whether such patients require surgery or can be kept under medical supervision for months or years cannot be answered at this time. Permanent spontaneous remissions have been rare and in several instances have been the result of infarction and necrosis of an adenoma. An increased incidence of complications of pregnancy and of fetal morbidity and mortality has been observed.

The long-term prognosis after surgery has not been well documented. Goldsmith et al., 1966, reported that 22 of 43 patients operated on were enjoying a state of health consistent with their age, 5 patients had low-grade hypertension, and 6 showed progression of their original renal problem. Of 14 patients with peptic ulcer, 1 patient had a gastric ulcer 2 years after healing of a prior gastric lesion and the remaining 13 were well. Parathyroid carcinoma exhibits local recurrences, cervical lymph node metastases, and often uncontrollable hypercalcemia. Survival for more than 5 years is rare.

Secondary hyperparathyroidism (SHP)

Chronic hypocalcemia promotes parathyroid hyperplasia and increased PTH secretion, that is, secondary hyperparathyroidism (SHP). The plasma concentration of PTH measured by radioimmunoassay is considerably higher than in PHP (Berson and Yalow, 1967). The principal cause is chronic renal failure (renal or azotemic osteodystrophy).

Renal osteodystrophy. Chronic renal disease can be associated with osteomalacia, osteoporosis, osteosclerosis, and osteitis fibrosa. The radiologic picture cannot be distinguished from that of PHP. The pathogenesis is not clear, but impaired Ca absorption, acquired vitamin D resistance, the decalcifying effects of PTH, and reduced bone responsiveness to the calcium-mobilizing effects of endogenous PTH have all been implicated. A continuum of bony changes has been noted with rickets or osteomalacia at one extreme and normally mineralized bone with generalized osteitis fibrosa indistinguishable from PHP at the other. The patient with SHP and defective mineralization is likely to have a low plasma Ca with a normal Ca $\times$ PO$_4$ product, whereas SHP with osteitis fibrosa shows a normal or near-normal Ca, a high Ca $\times$ PO$_4$ product, and more advanced renal damage. Thus Stanbury and Lamb, 1966, reported that in 79 cases with defective mineralization the mean plasma Ca was 7.63 mg./100 ml., PO$_4$ 6.03, Ca $\times$ PO$_4$ 45.7, and BUN 77.6, whereas the values in 55 cases of generalized osteitis fibrosa were 10.05, 8.79, 86.5, and 130.7, respectively. In general, the serum total Ca in SHP is normal or slightly depressed, and the SIP is always elevated. The renal lesion is more likely to be far-advanced pyelonephritis and only occasionally uncomplicated glomerulonephritis.

Rickets and osteomalacia. There is normocalcemia (or Ca is slightly subnormal), hypophosphatemia, and an elevated alkaline phosphatase. Mild SHP as evidenced pathologically by parathyroid gland hyperplasia may result.

Primary versus secondary hyperparathyroidism. In SHP, prolonged renal disease predominates. In some instances it is difficult to distinguish prolonged PHP with secondary renal damage from primary renal disease leading to SHP (Table 17-6). Renal biopsy may be of value; in PHP, chronic inflammatory cells and fibrosis are found predominantly in interstitial tissue and Ca deposits tend to be adjacent to or in the tubular basement membrane. In SHP the lesion is one of far-advanced pyelonephritis. However, in late cases of PHP the histologic picture may be considerably modified.

Therapy. Vitamin D stimulates mineralization of bone, heals subperiosteal erosions, and relieves skeletal symptoms. The initial dosage of calciferol is 50,000 units daily with subsequent increases as required. In resistant patients 250,000 units or more daily may be necessary. Because hypercalcemia and metastatic calcification can occur quite rapidly, a diet with a Ca to PO$_4$ ratio of 1:1 is recommended, and treatment should be stopped as soon as improvement becomes evident and the serum Ca or the alkaline phosphatase return to normal. Vitamin D has a cumulative effect that may last as long as 6 months. Where vitamin D therapy has failed to promote involution of the hyperplastic parathyroid glands, subtotal or even total parathyroidectomy may be effective in producing a fall of plasma Ca and the Ca $\times$ PO$_4$ product, absorption of metastatic calcifications, and remineralization of bone. Vitamin D therapy is then resumed, though it may be dispensable once the skeletal lesions have regressed. Experience with parathyroidectomy in SHP is limited to some dozen cases.

Tertiary hyperparathyroidism. The term was coined to designate patients with SHP in whom parathyroid hyperplasia had become autonomous or where one or more parathyroid adenomas appeared. This situation may develop after prolonged hemodialysis or after renal homotransplantation.

Hypoparathyroidism (HypoP)

The principal cause of HypoP is inadvertent parathyroidectomy or damage to the parathyroids or their blood supply during thyroidectomy. After subtotal thyroidectomy 0% to 3.6% of patients develop permanent HypoP, and after one-stage total thyroidectomy for thyroid cancer approximately 30% do the same. Transient hypocalcemia followed by recovery is not uncommon. Fourman et al., 1963, however, found that a fourth of the patients they investigated after thyroidectomy had partial parathyroid insufficiency and about half of these had symptoms of tension and anxiety, occasionally with attacks of panic, often with depression and lassitude. [131]I therapy directed to the thyroid gland is a rare cause of HypoP; the impairment of Ca mobilization may be principally from RAI-induced hypothyroidism. *Idiopathic HypoP* (IdHypoP) occurs without apparent cause, although an autoimmune mechanism has been implicated. A number of cases associated with varying combinations of Addison's disease, superficial moniliasis, Hashimoto's thyroiditis, or pernicious anemia and exhibiting the appropriate autoimmune antibodies have been reported in children. The suggestion of a polyglandular autoimmunity bears further investigation. A famial tendency has been observed.

Pathology of IdHypoP

The parathyroid glands may be absent, hyperplastic, or grossly normal. Histologic examination usually reveals replacement of parathyroid tissue by fat. Adrenocortical atrophy may be an associated finding. In the few cases in which autopsy and brain examination have been done, there has been calcareous replacement of the basal ganglia and deposition of a homogenous material in and about the media and adventitia of small blood vessels, together with areas of tissue calcification.

Pathogenesis

After parathyroidectomy (PTX) in a dog there is a rapid decline of the plasma Ca from an average of 10 mg. to 5 to 6 mg./100 ml. and a rise of SIP from 4 to 5 mg. to 8 to 10 mg./100 ml., together with a decrease of urinary Ca and PO_4. Within 24 to 48 hours there are fibrillary twitchings of muscles followed by clonic and tonic muscle contractions. Hyperpyrexia, hyperpnea, and respiratory alkalosis appear, and death ensues from laryngeal stridor and respiratory muscle tetany. Convulsive seizures may occur at any time. Bone resorption decreases when PTH is lacking, but bone formation may be normal or slightly decreased; the net effect may increase bone density. Neuromuscular excitability is increased. Cataract formation after PTX has been attributed to hypocalcemia in blood and aqueous humor, with subsequent metabolic alterations of the lens. There is experimental evidence for a relationship between plasma Ca concentration and cataract formation, but the mechanism is obscure. The cause of intracerebral calcifications is unknown.

Clinical features

Surgical HypoP. The onset after surgery is within the first 10 days in 90% of cases. However, the diagnosis is sometimes delayed for several years. Hypothyroidism is a frequent companion in postsurgical cases.

IdHypoP. Denko and Kaelbling, 1962, reviewed most of the world literature to 1962 and found only 151 cases (80 females, 71 males). The onset is more gradual and insidious than in surgical HypoP.

Symptoms

Tetany. Paresthesias (numbness and tingling) of the extremities precede the onset of tetany. Carpopedal spasm is the first sign manifested by the classic "accoucheur's hand" (spastic adduction of the thumb with the wrist, metacarpophalangeal joints hyperflexed, and the carpal joint hyperextended). There may follow other muscle spasms, laryngeal stridor, and convulsions. Rarely asphyxia may cause death. Convulsive seizures, occurring in about 75% of cases, may recur for years sometime in patients without tetany and be mistaken for grand mal. There may be syncopal attacks without convulsions or episodes resembling petit mal. The administration of diphenylhydantoin and phenobarbital may mask the hypocalcemia by elminating tetany, tetanic equivalents, or the Chvostek and Trousseau signs. Tetany may appear only during or after the stress of surgery, infection, the menses, pregnancy, parturition, or lactation. Tetanic episodes may be infrequent, minor, and nonprogressive in some cases.

Central nervous system symptoms. The disease may manifest itself by psychiatric changes as a well-defined organic brain syndrome, a less specific psychosis, intellectual impairment, or a heterogeneous group of ill defined symptoms. There may be personality change, anxiety, agitation, irritability, hysteria, depression, hypochondriasis, bizarre behavior, syncopal attacks, delirium, frank psychoses, or late mental retardation. Transient choreiform movements may occur in children.

Signs

Chvostek and Trousseau's signs. The following two signs may be elicited in any hypocalcemic condition as evidence of latent tetany. *Chvostek's sign* is produced by tapping sharply over the preauricular region, site of the facial nerve, resulting in a quick contraction of the facial muscles, particularly those of the corner of the mouth, the upper lip, and sometimes the alae nasi and eyelids. A contraction confined to the corners of the mouth can be provoked in some normal subjects, but the more marked contractions occur only with hypocalcemia. *Trousseau's sign* is carpopedal spasm produced within 3 minutes of compression of the upper arm with a sphygmomanometer holding the pressure above systolic.

Erb's sign. Increased motor nerve excitability is elicited by galvanic current.

Cataracts. Lenticular abnormalities are common in long-standing cases but may develop rapidly in untreated or inadequately treated postthyroidectomy cases. There may be advanced bilateral cataracts, small punctate opacities, or other lens changes.

The incidence of cataracts is 36% to 50% in IdHypoP and 5% to 28% in postoperative HypoP (Dimich et al., 1967). Once established, lens changes are permanent despite elimination of hypocalcemia. *Papilledema* and other signs of *increased intracranial pressure* have been described.

Radiologic changes. Bilateral, usually symmetrical, focal calcifications of the basal ganglia occur chiefly in IdHypoP and are rare in postsurgical cases. Cerebellar and sometimes vascular, bursal, or tendinous calcifications have been observed. Calcification, however, of the choroid plexus, falx cerebri, habenula, and pineal gland is a physiologic change observed in some normal adults. Pathologic cerebral calcifications may also be encountered in tuberculosis, trichinosis, toxoplasmosis, cysticercosis, brain tumor and abscess, hematoma, and vascular lesions. Some increased density of bones, particularly of the skull, or rarely demineralization, is found, but usually the skeletal architecture appears normal.

ECG and EEG. Hypocalcemia causes prolongation of the Q-T interval and sometimes inverted T-waves. Nonspecific diffuse and focal EEG abnormalities may be confused with true epilepsy in patients with convulsive seizures. The EEG pattern may or may not correlate with the presence of hypocalcemia.

Ectodermal lesions. Ectodermal lesions are unusual changes found in IdHypoP and consist of dry, coarse, scaly skin; pigmentation; thinning of the hair with patchy alopecia and loss of axillary and pubic hair, eyelashes, and eyebrows; and atrophy, deformity, and fragility of fingernails and toenails. IdHypoP can cause aplasia or hypoplasia of the teeth during the years of dental development. With onset before age 10, blunting of the roots of the molar teeth occurs. Widespread chronic moniliasis may be associated with IdHypoP.

Laboratory studies

The diagnosis depends on finding a low plasma Ca and elevated SIP. Calcium values range from 4 to 8 mg./100 ml. and

SIP from 5 to 10 mg./100 ml. However, in mild postsurgical cases normal values can be found. The serum protein should be measured because a high protein value can mask hypocalcemia or a low value can produce an apparent hypocalcemia that does not exist. Ca values obtained before thyroid surgery are helpful for comparison with postoperative determinations. In equivocal cases provocative measures to reveal hypocalcemia such as a high PO$_4$– low Ca diet, physical exercise, or the use of chelating agents may be necessary. Fujita et al., 1966, gave calcium-disodium EDTA 70 mg./kg. I.V. in 20 minutes and measured serum Ca for 3 hours by a special stepwise titration with disodium EDTA. A markedly delayed recovery from hypocalcemia characterized the cases of HypoP and permitted a clear separation from normal individuals. Side effects were less than with disodium or trisodium EDTA preparations.

Other biochemical changes include a normal or reduced alkaline phosphatase, low serum citrate, a reduced urine Ca and hydroxyproline, a reduced PO$_4$ clearance, and an increased % TRP. Mg values are usually normal. The urine is negative for Ca with Sulkowitch's reagent, a solution that precipitates urine Ca as calcium oxalate.[*]

Differential diagnosis

HypoP must be distinguished from other causes of tetany and /or hypocalcemia. The most common nonparathyroid stimulus for tetany is *hyperventilation,* an emotionally induced disorder usually seen in young anxious females. Hysterical gasping and hyperventilation produce alkalosis and carpopedal spasm, positive Chvostek and Trousseau signs, vertigo, faintness, and occasionally syncope. Recovery is rapid when respiration becomes normal and can be hastened by breath holding or rebreathing into a paper bag. The plasma and urinary Ca and SIP are normal, but the arterial CO$_2$ is low. Alkalosis from excessive ingestion of alkali or vomiting can also induce tetany. Hypocalcemia in rickets, osteomalacia, renal failure, or acute pancreatitis is rarely severe enough to cause tetany, and

---

[*]Sulkowitch solution contains 2.5 grams each of oxalic acid and ammonium oxalate, 5 ml. of glacial acetic acid, and water q.s. to make 150 ml.

Table 17-7. Clinical features that may distinguish idiopathic hypoparathyroidism from pseudohypoparathyroidism

	Idiopathic hypoparathyroidism	*Pseudohypoparathyroidism*
Familial and hereditary effects	Rare	Common
Sex—M:F	Approximately equal	F2:M1
Average age of onset	17 years	8½ years (usually before age 20)
Ectodermal changes	More common	Less common
Monilial infections	Present	Absent
Addison's disease	Occasional	Absent
Subcutaneous calcifications	Rare	Common
Brachydactyly	Absent	Frequent
Round face	Rare	Common
Thickset, stocky build	Rare	Common
Mental retardation	Occasional (18%)	Common (63%)
Calcification of basal ganglia	Common	Rare
Cataracts	Common	Rare

the biochemical differences from HypoP are distinctive. Tetany may develop in patients with azotemia if the acidosis is treated. Rare causes of tetany are hypomagnesemia and primary aldosteronism. Pseudohypoparathyroidism is discussed on p. 307 and in Table 17-7.

Treatment

Tetany is relieved promptly by I.V. injection of 10 to 20 ml. of a 10% solution of calcium gluconate. Frequent repetition may be necessary, or a continuous I.V. infusion may be more efficacious. If tetany is difficult to control, *parathyroid extract**[*] 50 to 200 U.S.P. units is administered I.M. until other measures become effective. To avoid the pain of the injection, which can be considerable, the extract can be infused I.V. in a glucose solution (5% in water). Sedation with barbiturates may be necessary.

Vitamin D_2 (ergocalciferol) is the standard therapeutic agent. It is available in 50,000-unit (1.25 mg.) gelatin capsules. The initial dose varies from 100,000 to 300,000 units, although occasionally up to 500,000 units can be required. The maintenance dose is 50,000 to 100,000 units daily. Oral Ca is usually essential early in therapy because the effects of vitamin D can be delayed for 6 to 10 days. Numerous preparations are available, but one of the most effective and cheapest is calcium lactate powder dissolved in hot water and taken in a dosage, of 2 to 4 Gm. thrice daily. The plasma Ca should be measured frequently in the early weeks of treatment to ensure restoration of normal values (9 to 10 mg./100 ml.). It is important to avoid mild hypocalcemia with its complications of latent tetany, cataracts, and mental deterioration, as well as hypercalcemia with attendant nephrocalcinosis and renal damage. Because vitamin D has a prolonged half-life, the dangers of hypercalcemia can persist for several weeks. The SIP is restored more slowly. As con-

trol of blood Ca is achieved, oral Ca supplements can be gradually withdrawn, the diet is unrestricted, and normocalcemia is maintained in most patients with vitamin D_2 alone.

In *postthyroidectomy hypoparathyroidism*, if the hypocalcemia is minimal (7.5 to 9 mg./100 ml.), there is no tetany and only paresthesias are experienced by the patient; therapy can be restricted to oral Ca until it becomes evident that permanent, rather than transient, HypoP has been established. In patients receiving vitamin D as long-term therapy, at least once an attempt should be made to cautiously withdraw medication to be certain that there is no functioning parathyroid tissue. Most postsurgical cases suffer concomitant hypothyroidism and require thyroid hormone replacement.

An occasional patient is *resistant* to the usual therapeutic measures, and other agents must be added or substituted. *A.T. 10 (Hytakerol)* is an isomer of dihydrotachysterol, consisting principally of dihydrovitamin D_2. It has fallen into disfavor because considerable variation in potency from one preparation to another has been found. It is available in capsules containing 0.625 mg./0.5 ml. or in an oily solution containing 1.25 mg./ml. The initial dose is 2 to 10 capsules or 3 to 5 ml. and the maintenance dosage is 1 capsule or 1 ml. daily or every other day. *Crystalline dihydrotachysterol* has recently become available for general use[*]. It is marketed in 0.2 mg. tablets and the recommended initial dosage is 0.8 to 2.4 mg. daily. Harrison et al., 1967, reported that it exhibited three times the potency of vitamin D_2. It is probable that this agent will become the treatment of choice in patients resistant to vitamin D. Rasmussen, 1968, found that magnesium, in a dose of 4 mEq./kg., enhanced the response to vitamin D. Other measures to increase Ca absorption have been advocated, such as the ingestion of aluminum hydroxide gel

---

*Lilly & Co., Indianapolis, Ind.

*Philips Roxane Labs, Inc., Columbus, Ohio.

5 to 10 ml. thrice daily with meals to reduce phosphate absorption, or the administration of probenecid, 0.5 to 1 Gm. once
or twice daily, to inhibit the tubular resorption of phosphate. A high Ca–low PO_4
diet is usually advocated, though doing so
would require the elimination of meat, fish,
seafood, and fowl, as well as milk and
dairy products, beans, corn, whole wheat,
and liver.

Clinical course and prognosis

In the majority of patients, control is
easily achieved and maintained. The complications encountered in untreated cases
such as cataracts, psychiatric symptoms,
mental deficiency, and ectodermal changes
should not occur. Cataracts, once formed,
do not regress. Psychiatric symptoms, if
related exclusively to the hypocalcemia,
usually subside after weeks or months of
treatment, but mental retardation may be
permanent. The patient is promptly re-
warded for any lapse of treatment by a
recurrence of symptoms, although occasionally this may be delayed for weeks or even
months.

Pseudohypoparathyroidism (SH) (Albright's hereditary osteodystrophy)

Pseudohypoparathyroidism is a rare disorder characterized by the same biochemical phenomena as IdHypoP but exhibiting
resistance to the effects of PTH in contradistinction to the sensitivity shown by patients with IdHypoP. The parathyroid
glands may be normal or hyperplastic,
whereas in IdHypoP they are absent or
atrophic. In addition, there are certain
pathognomonic stigmas, as short stature,
thickset figure, facial rounding, blank expression, subcutaneous calcinosis and/or
ossification, brachydactyly, thickened calvarium, and mental retardation. There is
shortening of one or more metacarpals
(Fig. 17-4) and metatarsals involving, in
order of decreasing incidence, I, V, IV,
and III metacarpals, with II rarely affected
(Mann et al., 1962). The short fourth
metacarpal is responsible for the "meta-

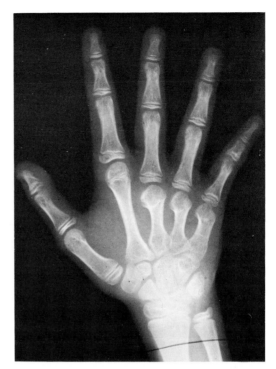

Fig. 17-4. Pseudohypoparathyroidism. The third, fourth, and fifth metacarpals are shortened.

carpal sign"—a dimple replaces the knuck-
le when a fist is made and a line drawn
through the heads of the fifth and fourth
metacarpals passes through the head of the
third instead of clearing it. Other less
constant features include radius curvus,
exostoses, abnormally short and wide fingernails, palmar creases resembling a simian fold, signs of hypometabolism with a
normal PBI, hypercholesterolemia, carbohydrate intolerance, or frank diabetes, and
coincident Turner's syndrome.

Pseudo-pseudohypoparathyroidism (SSH)

An even rarer variant that is identical in
all features, except that the serum Ca and
SIP are normal and tetany or other consequences of hypocalcemia are absent, is
pseudo-pseudohypoparathyroidism (SSH).
SSH and SH undoubtedly represent modified expressions of a single genetic disorder of which SH is the more complete
form. In some patients SH becomes transformed to SSH with a spontaneous rever-

sion of the plasma Ca and SIP to normal. Mothers with SSH have had children with SH (Fromm, 1965). The hereditary mode may be a dominant sex-linked transmission with an abnormal gene on the x-chromosome or an autosomal transmission. A positive family history has been elicited in one third of the cases. Todd et al., 1961, include SSH with progressive myositis ossificans, multiple hereditary exostosis, hereditary brachydactyly, multiple epiphysial dysplasia, and Turner's syndrome, though the mode of inheritance is different.

Etiology and pathogenesis of SH

The Albright hypothesis (1948) of renal tubular end-organ refractoriness to PTH is supported by the finding of normal or hyperplastic parathyroid glands on biopsy and the finding of Tashjian et al., 1966, of a PTH-concentration in thyroid vein blood that was elevated sevenfold. The mechanism is unknown but does not appear to be related to disturbances of vitamin D metabolism or of hyperthyrocalcitoninemia, nor has it been proven that an abnormal PTH is secreted or a normal hormone is blocked by some hypothetical inhibitor. Insensitivity to PTH may be limited to the renal tubule, and bone may respond normally, as shown by an elevated serum alkaline phosphatase and the occasional finding of osteitis fibrosa cystica. However,

the finding of thick osteosclerotic bones in some cases suggests an additional bone resistance to the resorptive effects of PTH. Resistance to PTH may not be absolute, as shown by the production of phosphaturia after large doses of a highly purified extract.

Features that may aid in distinguishing IdHypoP from SH are listed in Table 17-7. In many instances it may be impossible to make a differentiation by physical examination alone. On the average the serum Ca reduction and SIP increase tend to be less marked than in IdHypoP. Resistance to the phosphaturic effect of PTH (Ellsworth and Howard, 1934) has been the principal laboratory evidence of SH. The test is performed as follows: after an overnight fast, 3-hour urines are collected before and after the intravenous infusion of 200 units of parathyroid extract (PTE), and the PO_4 and creatinine concentrations are measured; it is essential to perform the test on a normal subject using the same batch of extract to be certain of its potency. In normal subjects and in patients with IdHypoP, the PO_4 excretion rises by at least 100% and the SIP may fall by 1 to 2 mg./100 ml., whereas in SH there is little or no change (Table 17-8). In renal failure, steatorrhea, or rickets, there may be a poor response. The test is often unreliable. Assuming that the extract is active, its

Table 17-8. Ellsworth-Howard test*

Diagnosis	Number of patients	Urinary phosphate (mg./hr.)		
		Before	Maximum rise after PTH	Increase (%)
Normal subjects	19	22 (4-53)	50 (19-89)	230 (90-150)
Idiopathic hypoparathyroidism	26	18 (5-42)	78 (23-209)	450 (120-320)
Pseudohypoparathyroidism	19	18 (3-50)	16 (2-43)	90 (20-350)

*From Bronsky, D., et al.: Medicine **37:**317, 1958

potency may vary from batch to batch. Some normal subjects may fail to respond, whereas an occasional patient with SH may exhibit considerable phosphaturia. The latter phenomenon may be caused by an increased renal plasma flow and GFR. In order to improve the accuracy of the test, Arnstein, 1966, recommends giving at least 600 to 800 units I.M. daily for 5 to 7 days. Normal subjects given large doses of PTH (500 units or more daily for 3 or more days) show a rise of serum Ca of 2.5 to 5.5 mg./100 ml. and a marked increase in urinary hydroxyproline, whereas patients with SH fail to show any increase of Ca concentration. Though the plasma PO₄ in SSH is usually normal, it can occasionally be elevated. A high Ca–low PO₄ diet may raise the serum Ca and the SIP toward normal in some patients with SH but not in those with IdHypoP. The urinary hydroxyproline is expected to be normal, or increased in SH and low in IdHypoP.

Therapy is the same as for IdHypoP, though the requirement for vitamin D is often less. For reviews of SH and SSH, see Mann et al., 1962, and Bartter, 1966.

METABOLIC BONE DISEASE (OSTEOPOROSIS AND OSTEOMALACIA)*
Osteoporosis

Osteoporosis is a metabolic disease in which bone of normal chemical composition is reduced in mass and density. It is the most prevalent generalized bone disorder, occurring predominantly in postmenopausal and elderly females and may indeed be a physiologic concomitant of aging.

Pathogenesis

Recent studies have shown that there is excessive bone resorption rather than decreased bone synthesis and osteoblastic activity. The diminution of bone mass is the net effect, therefore, of bone resorption continuously outstripping bone formation, whereas in normal bone these pro-

---

*Written with the assistance of Dr. Harry Banghart.

cesses tend to remain in balance. In corticosteroid-induced osteoporosis, however, bone synthesis is impaired by the antianabolic action of the steroid and resorption may remain normal. The parathyroids regulate bone resorption, and they probably respond to the negative Ca balance by increasing their secretion (SHP). The reduction of bone mass is a physiologic process that commences between 30 and 40 years of age and continues throughout the life of the individual. There is a linear loss of bone mass in both sexes approximating 5% to 10% per decade or 15 to 30 μg. of calcium per day (Whedon, 1968).

Although osteoporosis is associated with a variety of clinical disorders (see outline below), its etiology and pathogenesis remain speculative.

Endocrine
  Postmenopausal occurrence—spontaneous or artificial (by surgery or X rays)
  Senescence
  Cushing's syndrome (or corticosteroid administration)
  Hyperthyroidism
  Acromegaly
  Diabetes mellitus
  Eunuchoidism
  Gonadal dysgenesis and ovarian agenesis
Nutritional
  Malnutrition, calcium deficiency
  Chronic diseases—collagen disease, malignant tumors
  Avitaminosis C
Inactivity (local or generalized osteoporosis)
  Prolonged immobilization
  Paralyses
Miscellaneous
  Excessive doses of ultrasonic waves
  Excessive doses of roentgen rays
  Heparin administration
Idiopathic

Osteoporosis has been attributed to several factors.

Hormonal factors. Current evidence suggests that lack of estrogen serves as a modifying rather than causative factor that accelerates the natural osteoporotic tendency accompanying aging. Evidence both favoring and negating the effect of the menopause on osteoporosis has been presented. The disorder is far more prevalent in females, and the process appears to be accelerated particularly in the first 5 postmenopausal years. Estrogen therapy inhibits bone resorption and promotes mineral retention, but there is no evidence of increased bone density. Testosterone insufficiency in the male may play a similar though less important role. An increased corticosteroid–gonadal hormone ratio that evolves with aging favors the production of osteoporosis, an imbalance that Urist and Vincent, 1960, found to be more severe in patients with osteoporosis than in nonaffected subjects.

Calcium deficiency. Nordin, 1961, proposed that a deficient intake of Ca played an important role and demonstrated significant improvement in patients treated with Ca supplements and vitamin D. Though many individuals adapt to a low Ca intake by increasing intestinal absorption and decreasing urinary loss of Ca, some remain in negative balance. Dietary surveys have both confirmed and denied the role of Ca deficiency, but it probably is a contributing factor. Poor intestinal absorption of Ca, as in steatorrhea, may result in bone demineralization. Clinical steatorrhea has been reported in 15% of patients with osteoporosis (Riggs et al., 1968). However, several independent investigations have demonstrated that the intestinal absorption of Ca varies inversely with age in both osteoporotic and nonosteoporotic female populations, so it probably does not play a primary role in causing bone demineralization. Idiopathic hypercalciuria, a source of chronic Ca loss, has been found in 20% of osteoporotic patients. The administration of Ca supplements has been found, in Nordin's studies, to increase vertebral density.

Racial factors. Autopsy data have demonstrated the greatest bone mass in Negro males, less in Caucasian males and Negro females, and least in Caucasian females. Clinical osteoporosis is much less common in Negroes, probably because of a higher initial bone mass.

Immobilization. Skeletal homeostasis is favored by physical activity, whereas inactivity, and particularly immobilization, promotes bone resorption and loss of bone mass. Local osteoporosis occurs in an extremity immobilized in a plaster cast or by paralysis.

Heaney, 1965, proposed a unified concept that centered upon the integrating force of Ca homeostasis, such that "osteoporosis is a multifactoral disease, in its homeostatic varieties produced whenever bone is forced to provide Ca that the organism fails to obtain from its environment." Thus if Ca balance is maintained, bone resorption tends to equal bone formation and bone density remains constant. If the balance shifts to the negative, the parathyroid glands increase their secretion, Ca is mobilized from the skeleton to maintain homeostasis, and bone mass decreases.

Secondary osteoporosis

Cushing's syndrome or corticosteroid administration in pharmacologic doses interferes with the synthesis of the bony matrix, antagonizes the action of vitamin D, and enhances calciuria.

Hyperthyroidism promotes negative protein and Ca balance, minimal hypercalcemia in some cases, and an increased turnover of Ca. The summation of these changes generates osteoporosis.

Scurvy can promote osteoporosis by interfering with the formation of collagen fibrils and thus reducing mineral deposition.

Prolonged *heparin* therapy appears to cause or accelerate osteoporosis, and the effect is dose related.

Clinical osteoporosis

Incidence. Osteoporosis is the most prevalent generalized bone disorder in man. Since a linear loss of bone mass is a physiologic accompaniment of the aging process, the disease is probably extremely common but becomes manifest only when there are symptoms or physical signs. Radiologic studies of inmates in a home for the aged showed a prevalence of asymptomatic vertebral fractures in osteoporotic spines of 20% in males and 29% in females (Gershon-Cohen et al., 1953). An epidemiologic survey conducted in Puerto Rico and Michigan (Smith and Rizek, 1966) showed a prevalence rate of 50% in women over 45 years of age and 80% over 65 years of age, though only 5% showed vertebral fractures. Necropsy studies of lumbar vertebrae showed a prevalence rate of 59% of females and 36% of males. The onset of osteoporosis in young adults and during pregnancy is rare.

Symptoms and signs. Symptoms are lacking until mechanical strain or a fracture ensues. Vague, dull, lower-back pain may be present for months or years. The pain is sharply increased by spontaneous compression fracture of a vertebral body and is aggravated by change of position or physical activity. Occasionally the compression may be the presenting symptom, and at times fractures occur in patients who have few complaints. Radicular pain results from vertebral wedging and affects the pelvis, lower extremity, or chest. Fractures of ribs or the femoral neck can occur from minor trauma.

Physical signs of osteoporosis include local tenderness of the vertebrae on deep palpation or punching, paravertebral muscle spasm and tenderness, and gradually developing kyphosis and loss of stature. Serial measurements of height provide an objective appraisal of the progress of the disorder. Progression is rapid in the early phases and slower in the later phases.

Laboratory studies. The plasma Ca, PO_4, and alkaline phosphatase remain normal. In immobilization osteoporosis and in a small percentage of elderly patients, there is hypercalciuria.

X-ray studies. In x-ray studies (Fig. 17-5) demineralized bone is found particularly in the spine and pelvis. In mild cases the diagnosis is difficult because it depends on an assessment of the probable mineral content of bone by judging its translucency. Attempts to establish bone-

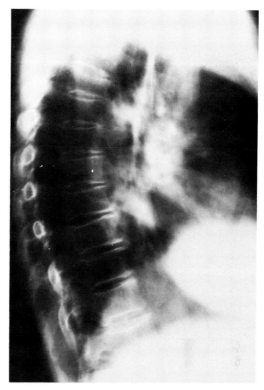

Fig. 17-5. Senile osteoporosis. Note the increased translucency, biconcave compression, wedge-shaped collapse of the third dorsal vertebra, and apparent increased density of end plates. (Courtesy Dr. Marvin E. Haskin, Department of Radiology, Hahnemann Medical College, Philadelphia, Pa.)

density standards have been made by comparison with aluminum step-wedges, by measurement of the thickness of bone cortex or the concavity of lumbar vertebrae, and by measurement with various types of bone densitometers, but there is no uniform method. Criteria for diagnosis include (1) increased bone translucency, (2) collapse of vertebrae, (3) decreased number and thickness of horizontal trabeculae and prominence of vertical trabeculae, (4) thinning of cortical plates, (5) biconcave compression (fish-mouth vertebrae), (6) expansion of intervertebral disks, and (7) absence of evidences of degenerative arthritis of spine (spurring, etc.) consistent with the age of the patient.

Differential diagnosis

MULTIPLE MYELOMA. Multiple myeloma causes bone pain and produces x-ray findings that can resemble osteoporosis. The pain of myeloma is usually more intense. In the absence of typical punched-out areas of bone, the differential diagnosis by x-ray study may be difficult. Hypercalcemia and hypercalciuria occur in about half of all cases, and anemia and thrombocytopenia are common.

OSTEOMALACIA. The disease is the adult counterpart of rickets and is rare in the United States.

HYPERPARATHYROIDISM. The x-ray and laboratory findings are usually diagnostic.

Treatment

GENERAL MEASURES. Maximum physical activity consistent with comfort should be maintained, depending on symptoms, the presence or absence of fractures, and the need for traction or for a back brace. A firm mattress and/or bedboard is recommended. Analgesic, tranquilizer (muscle-relaxant) or narcotic drugs are employed as necessary. Correction of an associated disorder such as Cushing's syndrome or thyrotoxicosis or maximum control of diabetes mellitus may arrest further demineralization.

SEX HORMONES. Estrogens alone or combined with androgens reduce bone resorption, promote positive Ca balance and arrest the progress of demineralization in postmenopausal and senile osteoporosis. Henneman and Wallach, 1957, reported on the effects of estrogen treatment of 200 women for 1 to 20 years. Progress of the osteoporosis was arrested, as judged by serial x-ray studies and measurements of height. However, not "a single instance of increase of bone density" was found. This result may be attributed to a reduction in bone formation and hence in skeletal turnover that occurs after a few months of treatment. The following regimen is proposed: stilbestrol 1 to 3 mg., ethinyl estradiol 0.1 to 0.2 mg., or conjugated estrogens (Premarin) 1.25 to 2.5 mg. orally, daily for 4 weeks, omitted for 1 week, and continued indefinitely in this cyclic order. Withdrawal bleeding may or may not occur and, if not tolerated by the patient, may sometimes be avoided by reducing the dosage. Androgen therapy does not prevent bleeding and may be attended by undesirable virilizing effects. Some authorities advocate its routine use, whereas others recommend androgen only when there is malnutrition and in severely debilitated patients. Patients receiving estrogens should have breast and pelvic examinations and Papanicolaou smears at intervals.

CALCIUM SUPPLEMENTS. Despite the controversy concerning the role of Ca deficiency, treatment with Ca supplements and vitamin D has become an integral part of therapy. Though 1 quart of milk provides approximately 1 Gm. of Ca, many elderly patients cannot tolerate more than one or two glassfuls daily. Fortified skim milk may be preferred to whole milk because of its low fat content. Calcium lactate provides a satisfactory supplement in dosages of 1 to 4 Gm./day, to which vitamin D 1,000 to 5,000 units per day or a single dose of 50,000 units every second week is added.

EXPERIMENTAL AGENTS. Sodium fluoride in small doses augments bone formation and decreases bone resorption. It has been used experimentally for several years but has not received FDA approval. High PO_4 supplements may induce positive Ca balance in osteoporotic subjects. TCT is being investigated because it inhibits bone resorption.

Osteomalacia

In osteomalacia, a rare generalized bone disease that is the adult counterpart of rickets, the decrease of bone density is from inadequate mineralization of bone matrix. There is softening and loss of the structural strength of bone with the production of bending, deformities, and cortical fractures.

Etiology

Most, but not all, cases can be attributed to a deficiency of vitamin D from inadequate intake, excessive loss from the bowel, or vitamin D resistance but may also derive from conditions causing Ca and protein deficiency. Ca deficiency alone is probably not a cause of osteomalacia. The etiology of osteomalacia is presented below:

Vitamin D deficiency or resistance
Idiopathic renal hypercalciuria
Renal tubular acidosis
Fanconi syndrome
Malnutrition
   Inadequate intake of Ca and vitamin D
   After gastrectomy
   Intestinal malabsorption
Pancreatic steatorrhea
Tropical sprue
Nontropical sprue

Pathogenesis

Vitamin D deficiency leads to the following sequence of events: reduced intestinal absorption of Ca and PO_4 → reduced plasma Ca and PO_4 → excessive PTH secretion → bone resorption → restoration of a low normal plasma Ca + phosphaturia → further reduction of plasma PO_4 → inadequate bone mineralization (uncalcified osteoid seams). The uncalcified soft bones bend, become deformed, or form multiple symmetrical ribbonlike zones of focal decalcification that resemble incomplete fractures (Milkman's syndrome with "pseudofractures").

Clinical features

There is pain in the lower back and lower extremities accentuated by physical activity and especially by rising from a bed or chair, pelvic and pectoral muscle weakness, and later a clumsy waddling gait, bone tenderness, and skeletal deformities (Edeiken and Schneeberg, 1943). If one of the conditions listed above is present, there may be additional symptoms and signs from renal disease, sprue, steatorrhea, or malnutrition.

Laboratory findings

The serum Ca is low or low normal, the SIP is reduced, and the product of Ca × PO_4 (normal 30 to 40) is below 30.

Alkaline phosphatase is increased and urinary Ca is low.

X-ray findings

There are translucent transverse bands, irregular pseudofractures, or circular areas of demineralization. The lesions tend to be symmetrical and bilateral and show no callus. In late cases osseous deformities occur (coxa vera, abnormal angulations, separation or overlapping, settling of vertebral column, heart-shaped pelvis).

Treatment

Calciferol (vitamin D_2) 2,000 to 4,000 units daily for several months until there is x-ray evidence of cure except in vitamin D–resistant osteomalacia, where 50,000 to 500,000 or even 1 million units daily may be required. The diet should be nutritionally optimal; additional Ca (calcium lactate 1 Gm. four times a day) is usually added. Other measures directed to an underlying disorder (see list above) may be required.

REFERENCES

*Albright, F., and Reifenstein, E. C.: The parathyroid glands and metabolic bone disease, Baltimore, 1948, The Williams & Wilkins Co., p. 40.

Anglem, T. J.: Surg. Clin. N. Amer. **46:**727, 1966.

*Arnaud, C. D., Jr., et al.: Ann. Rev. Physiol. **29:**349, 1967.

Arnstein, A. R.: Ann. Intern. Med. **64:**996, 1966.

Axelrod, D. R.: J. Clin. Endocr. **26:**207, 1966.

Bartlett, N. L., and Cochran, D. Q.: Radiol. Clin. N. Amer. **2:**261, 1964.

Becker, K. L., et al.: J. Clin. Endocr. **24:**347, 1964.

Berson, S. A., and Yalow, R. S.: Science **154:**907, 1966.

Berson, S. A., and Yalow, R. S.: New Eng. J. Med. **277:**640, 1967.

Black, M. B., and Zimmer, J. F.: Arch. Surg. **72:**830, 1956.

Boonstra, C. E., and Jackson, C. E.: Ann. Intern. Med. **63:**468, 1965.

*Bronsky, D., et al.: Medicine **37:**317, 1958.

Care, A. D., et al.: Nature **209:**55, 1966.

Chambers, E. L., Jr., et al.: J. Clin. Endocr. **16:**1507, 1956.

---

*Significant reviews.

Chase, L. R., and Aurbach, G. D.: Proc. Nat. Acad. Sci. USA **58**:518, 1967.

Cope, O., et al.: Ann. Surg. **148**:375, 1958.

Cope, O.: New Eng. J. Med. **274**:174, 1966.

Copp, D. H., et al.: Proc. Canad. Fed. Biol. Soc. **4**:17, 1961.

°David, N. J., et al.: Amer. J. Med. **33**:88, 1962.

Deftos, L. J., et al.: Proc. Nat. Acad. Sci. USA **60**:293, 1968.

DeLuca, H. F., and Sallis, J. D.: Parathyroid hormone: Its subcellular actions and its relationship to vitamin D. In Gaillard, P. J., Talmage, R. V., and Budy, A. M., editors: The parathyroid glands, ultrastructure, secretion, and function, Chicago, 1965, University of Chicago Press, p. 181.

°Denko, J. D., and Kaelbling, R.: Acta Psychiat. Scand. **38**(suppl. 164):1, 1962.

Dimich, A., et al.: Arch. Intern. Med. **120**:449, 1967.

Edeiken, L., and Schneeberg, N. G.: J.A.M.A. **122**:865, 1943.

Ellenberg, A. H., et al.: Surgery **51**:708, 1962.

Ellsworth, R., and Howard, J. W.: Bull. Johns Hopkins Hosp. **55**:296, 1934.

Forland, M., et al.: Arch. Intern. Med. **122**:236, 1968.

°Foster, B. V.: New Eng. J. Med. **279**:349, 1968.

Fourman, P., et al.: Brit. J. Surg. **50**:608, 1963.

Frame, B., and Haubrich, W. S.: Arch. Intern. Med. **105**:536, 1960.

Fromm, G. A.: Clinical and humoral evaluation of pseudo-pseudohypoparathyroidism. In Gual, C.: Proceedings of Sixth Pan-American Congress of Endocrinology, Mexico City, Oct. 10-15, 1965, Amsterdam, 1966, Excerpta Medica Foundation, International Congress Ser. no. 112, p. 197.

Fujita, T., et al.: Endocr. Jap. **13**:338, 1966.

Gershberg, H., et al.: Metabolism **15**:206, 1966.

Gershon-Cohen, J., et al.: J.A.M.A. **153**:625, 1953.

Gleason, D. C., and Potchen, E. J.: Radiol. Clin. N. Amer. **5**:277, 1967.

Goldsmith, R. E., et al.: Acta Endocr. **52**:221, 1966.

Goldsmith, R. S., et al.: J. Clin. Endocr. **25**:1649, 1965.

Goldsmith, R. S., and Ingbar, S. H.: New Eng. J. Med. **274**:1, 1966.

°Goldsmith, R. S.: New Eng. J. Med. **281**:367, 1969.

°Gordon, G. S., et al.: Recent Progr. Hormone Res. **18**:297, 1962.

°Gordon, G. S., and Roof, B. S.: J.A.M.A. **206**:2729, 1968.

Gordon, G. S., et al.: Science **151**:1226, 1966.

Hanna, E. A., et al.: Clin. Chem. **10**:235, 1964.

Harrison, H. E., et al.: New Eng. J. Med. **276**:894, 1967.

Heaney, R. P.: Amer. J. Med. **39**:877, 1965.

Henneman, P. H., and Wallach, S.: Arch. Intern. Med. **100**:715, 1957.

Howard, J. E., et al.: J. Clin. Endocr. **13**:1, 1953.

Hurvitz, R. J., et al.: Arch. Surg. **95**:274, 1967.

Jackson, C. E., and Boonstra, C. E.: Amer. J. Med. **43**:727, 1967.

Johnston, N. G., et al.: Metabolism **15**:1084, 1966.

°Keating, F. R., Jr.: J.A.M.A. **178**:547, 1961.

Keating, F. R., Jr., et al.: J. Lab. Clin. Med. **74**:507, 1969.

Klein, L.: Clin. Res. **11**:298, 1963 (abstract).

Kyburz, B. A., et al.: Southern Med. J. **59**:273, 1966.

°Lafferty, F. W.: Medicine **45**:247, 1966.

°Lever, J. D.: Fine structural organization of the human and rat parathyroid glands. In Gaillard, P. J., Talmage, R. V., and Budy, A. M., editors: The parathyroid glands, ultrastructure, secretion, and function, Chicago, 1965, University of Chicago Press, p. 11.

Liddle, G. W.: Ectopic hormones. In Astwood, E., editor: Clinical endocrinology, New York, 1968, Grune & Stratton, Inc., p. 767.

Longson, D., et al.: J. Physiol. **131**:555, 1956.

°Mann, J. B., et al.: Ann. Intern. Med. **56**:315, 1962.

Mazzuoli, G. F., et al.: Lancet **2**:1192, 1966.

McIntyre, I.: Advances Clin. Chem. **4**:1, 1961.

McLean, F. C., and Hastings, A. B.: J. Biol. Chem. **108**:285, 1935.

°Neuman, W. F., and Neuman, M. W.: Amer. J. Med. **22**:123, 1957.

Nordin, B. E. C.: Lancet **1**:1011, 1961.

Nordin, B. E. C., and Smith, D. A.: Diagnostic procedures in disorders of calcium metabolism, Boston, 1965, Little, Brown & Co., pp. 35-42.

°Ostrow, J. D., et al.: Amer. J. Med. **29**:769, 1960.

°Potts, J. T., Jr., et al.: Recent Progr. Hormone Res. **22**:101, 1966.

Pronove, P., and Bartter, F. C.: Metabolism **10**:349, 1961.

Prunty, F. T. G., et al.: A laboratory manual of chemical pathology, Elmsford, N. Y., 1951, Pergamon Press, Inc.

Raisz, L. G.: New Eng. J. Med. **281**:616, 1969.

°Raisz, L. G., et al.: Regulation of parathyroid activity. In Gaillard, P. J., Talmage, R. V., and Budy, A. M., editors: The parathyroid glands, ultrastructure, secretion, and function, Chicago, 1965, University of Chicago Press, p. 37.

°Rasmussen, H.: The parathyroids. In Williams, R. H., editor: Textbook of endocrinology, ed.

4, Philadelphia, 1968, W. B. Saunders Co., pp. 853, 918, 921-922.

Reiss, E., and Canterbury, J. M.: Proc. Soc. Exper. Biol. Med. **128**:501, 1968.

Reitz, R. E., et al.: New Eng. J. Med. **281**:348, 1969.

Riggs, B. L., et al.: J. Clin. Endocr. **25**:777, 1965.

Riggs, B. L., et al.: J. Bone Joint Surg. (in press) (quoted by Whedon, 1968).

Rittel, W., et al.: Helvet. Chim. Acta **51**:924, 1968.

Roth, S. I.: Arch. Path. **73**:75, 1962.

St. Goar, W. T.: Ann. Intern. Med. **46**:102, 1957.

*Sherwood, L. M.: New Eng. J. Med. **278**:663, 1968.

Smith, R. W., Jr., and Rizek, J.: Clin. Orthop. **45**:31, 1966.

Stanbury, S. W., and Lamb, G. A.: Quart. J. Med. **35**:1, 1966.

*Strott, C. A., and Nugent, C. A.: Ann. Intern. Med. **68**:188, 1968.

Tashjian, A. H., et al.: Proc. Nat. Acad. Sci. USA **56**:1138, 1966.

*Tenenhouse, A., et al.: Ann. Rev. Pharmacol. **8**: 319, 1968.

Todd, J. N., et al.: Amer. J. Med. **30**:289, 1961.

Urist, M. R., and Vincent, P. J.: Clin. Orthop. **18**:199, 1960.

Vail, A. D., and Coller, F. C.: Missouri Med. **64**:234, 1967.

Wasserman, R. H., and Taylor, A. N.: Science **152**:791, 1966.

*Whedon, G. D.: Osteoporosis. In Astwood, E. B., and Cassidy, C. E., editors: Clinical endocrinology, vol. 2, New York, 1968, Grune & Stratton, Inc., p. 349.

Wilder, W. T., et al.: Ann. Intern. Med. **55**: 885, 1961.

Wills, M. R., and McGowan, G. K.: Brit. Med. J. **1**:1153, 1964.

*Wilson, R. E., et al.: Ann. Surg. **159**:79, 1964.

Yendt, E. R., and Gagne, R. J. A.: Canad. Med. Ass. J. **98**:331, 1968.

Chapter 18

Carbohydrate metabolism

Ralph A. Shaw, M.D., Ph.D.

The metabolism of carbohydrates provides energy and materials for synthetic purposes. Energy derived from the oxidation of carbohydrates (primarily glucose) is referred to as free energy, and the reaction is called exergonic. In contrast, a reaction that requires energy is termed endergonic. In biologic systems free energy is used (1) for coupled reactions in which an exergonic reaction is coupled to an endergonic reaction to provide energy for the latter reaction to proceed, and (2) for the synthesis of materials that can subsequently catabolize and release energy. Energy-rich compounds are, in general, either hydrogenated materials such as reduced nicotinamide adenine dinucleotide (NAD) or phosphorylated compounds such as creatine phosphate and adenosine triphosphate (ATP). The metabolism of carbohydrates can provide both immediate and stored energy for a cell.

A cell may derive, in addition to energy, certain materials from the metabolism of carbohydrates that are not provided in sufficient quantities by the diet or that may not be provided at all. For example, glucose may be metabolized to oxalacetate, which by transamination becomes the amino acid aspartate that can be incorporated into a protein. Conversely, proteins can be metabolized to provide amino acids, which can be converted into carbohydrates. The same can be said for some of the fatty acids and lipids. Thus, carbohydrate, protein, and fat can all contribute to, or be derived from, a metabolic pool.

ENTRY OF GLUCOSE INTO THE CELL

Glucose enters cells by an active metabolic process rather than by simple diffusion. The latter process can be effective at high blood sugar levels, but insulin permits cellular penetration of the cell membrane at normal concentrations of blood glucose. The insulin effect on permeability is dependent on the chemical configuration of the sugar since D-galactose may enter a cell rapidly while L-galactose is almost totally excluded. Furthermore, insulin acts prior to phosphorylation since it increases the entrance of glucose even when hexokinase has been inactivated by cooling. Insulin acts probably by altering the permeability of the cell membrane.

METABOLIC PATHWAYS OF GLUCOSE

Intracellular glucose may enter any of several metabolic pathways and is phosphorylated to glucose-6-phosphate (G6P). The factors that dictate the particular pathway depend on the presence and concentration of key enzymes and may vary from one organ system to another. In certain tissues, such as brain and skeletal muscle, enzymes favor the glycolytic pathway.

In the liver, adipose tissue, and red blood cells, enzymes of alternative pathways are more prominent. The liver is the primary site of gluconeogenesis and the principal source of free glucose released from intracellular precursors because glucose-6-phosphatase is present almost exclusively in the liver.

Embden-Meyerhof pathway

The Embden-Meyerhof pathway is the major route of glucose metabolism. Glycolysis is the breakdown of glucose into other metabolites (catabolism). Gluconeogenesis is the formation of glucose from metabolites of the pathway. The ratio between glycolysis and gluconeogenesis is the glycolytic flux. The glycolytic pathway is shown in Fig. 18-1. The two separate arrows in reactions 1, 3, and 10 indicate that one enzyme catalyzes the reaction in one direction and a different enzyme is required to reverse the reaction. For example, in reaction 1, hexokinase catalyzes the conversion of glucose into G6P, whereas the enzyme glucose-6-phosphatase catalyzes the opposite reaction. Such enzyme systems are rate limiting and are thought to be the sites where factors that influence the metabolic activity of a pathway exert their maximum effect. In glycolysis there are three rate-limiting enzymes: hexokinase, phosphofructokinase, and pyruvic kinase, which catalyze reactions 1, 3, and 10, respectively. In gluconeogenesis there are two rate-limiting enzymes: glucose-6-

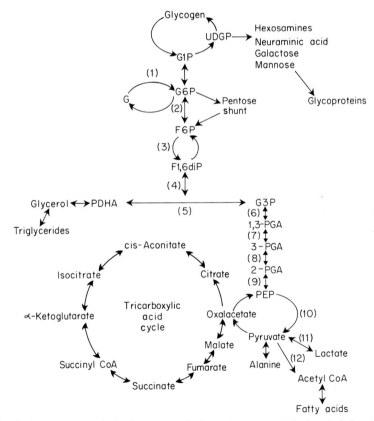

Fig. 18-1. Pathways in carbohydrate metabolism. Reactions of the Embden-Meyerhof pathway are numbered (1) through (12), respectively. *G*, glucose; *G6P*, glucose-6-phosphate; *G1P*, glucose-1-phosphate; *UDPG*, uridinediphosphoglucose; *F6P*, fructose-6-phosphate; *F1,6diP*, fructose-1,6-diphosphate; *PDHA*, phosphodihydroxyacetone; *G3P*, glyceraldehyde-3-phosphate; *1,3-PGA*, 1,3-diphosphoglyceric acid; *3-PGA*, 3-phosphoglyceric acid; *2-PGA*, 2-phosphoglyceric acid; and *PEP*, phosphoenolpyruvic acid.

phosphatase and fructose diphosphatase, which catalyze reactions 1 and 3, respectively. Reaction 10 is more complicated, since the conversion of pyruvate to phosphoenolpyruvate does not appear to occur in the living cell. In fasting, some 90% of the pyruvate in the liver going to form glycogen does so by an alternate pathway involving part of the Krebs cycle and the malic enzyme.

In the glycolytic pathway the conversion of glucose to fructose diphosphate requires an energy input, since a compound with a higher energy level has been made. One mol of ATP is required for both reactions 1 and 3 to convert 1 mol of glucose to fructose diphosphate. However, when fructose diphosphate is split into two three-carbon sugars by aldolase, each three-carbon sugar is then oxidized to pyruvic acid and this series of oxidations yields 4 mols of ATP and 2 mols of reduced nicotinamide

adenine dinucleotide (NAD) for each mol of glucose metabolized. Thus, glycolysis provides energy for the cell in the form of ATP and reduced NAD, which can then be used for other reactions. Fig. 18-1 reveals that two compounds serve as significant branch points in the glycolytic pathway, that is, G6P and pyruvate. G6P can enter the pentose shunt, be converted to free glucose, or enter the nucleotide pathway, in addition to proceeding through glycolysis.

Pentose shunt

The pentose shunt (Fig. 18-2) is thought to be the major source of reduced NADP, which is necessary for the synthesis of fatty acids, steroids, and amino acids. G6P is oxidized to 6-phosphogluconolactone by a reaction catalyzed by G6P dehydrogenase. This enzyme appears to be important in influencing the activity of the pentose pathway in carbohydrate metabolism, since the concentration may be influenced by drugs or race. After enzymatic hydrolysis of the lactone, 6-phosphogluconate is oxidized to the five-carbon sugar, ribulose-5-phosphate. These reactions require 2 mols of oxidized NADP and produce 2 mols of reduced NADP for each mol of G6P metabolized. CO_2 is formed from the first carbon of glucose. Ribulose-5-phosphate may be converted to either xylulose-5-phosphate or ribose-5-phosphate. These two five-carbon sugars may then be converted to fructose-6-phosphate through either a seven-carbon sugar, sedoheptulose-7-phosphate, or the four-carbon sugar, erythrose-4-phosphate. The major functions of the pentose shunt pathway for the cell appear to be for synthesis. Ribose is needed for such important compounds as nucleic acids, nucleotides, ATP, NAD, and NADP.

Enzymes of the pentose-shunt pathway, like those for glycolysis, are present in many different tissues and are particularly active in adipose tissue and in lactating mammary gland, less active in liver, and almost absent in skeletal muscle. Studies of the pentose shunt have been stimulated by reports of reduced amounts of G6P de-

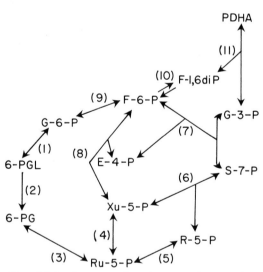

Fig. 18-2. Pentose phosphate pathway. The reactions of this pathway are numbered (1) through (11) sequentially. *G-6-P,* glucose-6-phosphate; *6-PGL,* 6-phosphogluconolactone; *6-PG,* 6-phosphogluconate; *Ru-5-P,* ribulose-5-phosphate; *R-5-P,* ribose-5-phosphate; *Xu-5-P,* xylulose-5-phosphate; *S-7-P,* sedoheptulose-7-phosphate; *E-4-P,* erythrose-4-phosphate; *G-3-P,* glyceraldehyde-3-phosphate; *F-6-P,* fructose-6-phosphate; *F-1,6diP,* fructose-1,6-diphosphate; and *PDHA,* phosphodihydroxyacetone.

hydrogenase and 6-phosphogluconic dehydrogenase in alloxan-diabetic rats. Since reduced NADP is important in the synthesis of fatty acids, this pathway might contribute to hyperlipemias.

NUCLEOTIDE PATHWAY

Carbohydrates are stored in mammalian tissue as glycogen. However, the glycogen store is small in comparison with the deposits of lipid, will furnish only about 50% of the daily caloric requirement of an adult, and must be conserved. As is true for glucose, the route of synthesis of glycogen (glycogenesis) and the pathway of its degradation (glycogenolysis) are different. Again, when two entirely different enzymes are necessary to promote a reaction in different directions, a more delicate control can be effected. Such reactions can also be expected to be influenced by hormones or other factors.

G6P is converted to glucose-1-phosphate (G1P) by the reaction catalyzed by phosphoglucomutase. G1P is added to the nucleotide uridine triphosphorylase to produce uridine diphosphoglucose (UDPG). The UDPG thus formed may donate its glucose to a molecule of preformed glycogen in the presence of glycogen synthetase or the glucose may be converted to other sugars while still regulated by the nucleotide. Since nucleotides other than uridine triphosphate are known to accept glucose molecules (in the presence of other enzymes), the pathways have been lumped into the general category of the nucleotide pathway. Although the nucleotide pathway has not yet received much attention, hexosamines and other carbohydrates present in glycoproteins (Stadtman, 1966) may be synthesized by this pathway. Glycoproteins may constitute the major portion of PAS-staining material found in the small-vessel disease of diabetics.

In contrast to the stepwise conversion of G1P into glycogen, the latter is broken down into G1P by a single reaction catalyzed by phosphorylase. This enzyme exists principally in an inactive form that can be activated by epinephrine and glucagon. The ability of these hormones to quickly elevate blood glucose stems from the rapid breakdown of glycogen stores.

PYRUVATE METABOLISM

Pyruvate serves as a significant branch point in the glycolytic pathway. It may be converted into lactate, transaminated to alanine, be converted into glucose or glycogen, can enter the tricarboxylic acid cycle either as acetyl coenzyme A (or as malate or oxalacetate), or be converted to a lipid. Pasteur noted that yeast cells supplied with oxygen would rapidly stop producing alcohol but would vigorously produce CO_2. This "Pasteur effect" is a general property of animal tissues, with several notable exceptions such as brain and neoplastic and embryonic tissues. In mammalian tissues pyruvate is not converted to alcohol, as in yeast, but rather to lactate when the supply of oxygen is diminished.

Liver tissue from fasted rats converts pyruvate to tricarboxylic acid intermediaries at a rate ten times that of liver tissue from fed rats (Kaeppe, 1959). In fasting conditions, if pyruvate is used to provide free energy by the tricarboxylic acid cycle, then fatty acids must be used to a greater extent than pyruvate to form acetyl coenzyme A (Fig. 18-1). As the pyruvate and fatty acids are further utilized for energy, glycogen stores are depleted and proteins are also catabolized to supply the need for energy. Eventually, as fatty acid utilization increases, the enzyme systems for fatty acid metabolism are overwhelmed and ketone bodies accumulate (starvation ketosis). A check of the plasma or urine will reveal strongly positive ketones with a relatively low sugar level. If glucose cannot be utilized by the cells because of insulin deficiency, the lipids and proteins are similarly used for energy and there is diabetic ketoacidosis.

TRICARBOXYLIC ACID CYCLE (KREBS CYCLE)

The Krebs cycle provides most of the high-energy phosphate and is the final pathway for most energy-yielding reactions of fat, protein, and carbohydrate metabolism. Two different substrates are required for its operation: (1) a dicarboxylic acid obtained as a product of the previous turn of the cycle, from glucogenic amino acids, or directly from pyruvate via the malic enzyme, and (2) acetyl coenzyme A, which can be obtained from fatty acids, pyruvate, or ketogenic amino acids. The products of the cycle are CO_2, reduced NAD and NADP, and the amino acids aspartate and glutamate.

INSULIN

Insulin is a protein with a molecular weight of approximately 6,000 (Fig. 18-3). It is composed of 48 amino acids of 17 different varieties arranged in two straight chains (A and B) linked by two disulfide bridges. The A chain contains an internal disulfide bridge. The amino acids 3, 29, and 30 of the B chain and 4, 8, 9, and 10 of the A chain distinguish the insulins of various species and explain the altered antigenicity and serum binding observed between insulins from different species. In the United States commercial insulin is derived mainly from beef, pork, and sheep.

Insulin has a direct effect on both lipid and glucose metabolism. It inhibits the breakdown of lipids into fatty acids (lipol-

ysis), so that an excess of insulin favors lipogenesis whereas a deficiency of insulin promotes lipolysis. Since insulin is a major factor for the entry of glucose into the cell, insulin deficiency causes a rise of blood glucose. As the deficiency persists, the cells must utilize glycogen, lipids, and proteins for both free energy and materials required for synthetic reactions. Because the glycogen stores are limited, lipids and proteins become the principal catabolic targets in insulin deficiency. As hyperglycemia increases, the kidney continues to filter and excrete glucose (glycosuria) until its capacity is exceeded. As lipolysis proceeds more rapidly, the capacity of the enzyme systems for lipid metabolism is exceeded and ketone bodies are formed. The kidney excretes ketone bodies until its capacity is exceeded, whereupon ketonemia and metabolic acidosis ensue.

Not all diabetics lack insulin. In fact, some diabetics have marked elevations in the levels of plasma insulin when compared to normal subjects (Yalow and Berson, 1960). To explain hyperglycemia in the presence of an insulin excess, there must be something wrong with either the insulin or the cells. Many theories to explain a defective insulin have come forth. Recently, a proinsulin or heavy insulin,

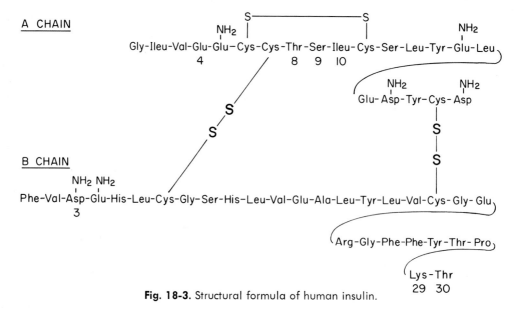

Fig. 18-3. Structural formula of human insulin.

which has a greater molecular weight than insulin, has been characterized (Steiner et al., 1968). If a peptide is split off this heavy insulin, insulin is formed. Since heavy insulin is similar to insulin, some investigators think that both are measured by radioimmunoassay methods. If heavy insulin is not biologically active, then the presence of hyperglycemia in a state of "insulin" excess could be explained. It has been suggested that insulin might be bound to some factor and become active when freed (Antoniades, 1961). Antagonists to insulin such as lipids and synalbumin have been sought to explain a defective action of insulin. Excess lipids and particularly fatty acids impair carbohydrate metabolism. Since hyperlipemias are common in diabetics, it may be that defective fatty acid metabolism is a primary factor in the etiology of diabetes. Plasma from diabetics and even prediabetics (Vallance-Owen, 1965) contains greater amounts of the synalbumin antagonists than does the plasma of nondiabetics. The nature of the antagonist remains unknown. The liver contains an enzyme that can split the alpha and beta insulin chains. Circulating plasma levels of both the alpha and beta chains may be determined by radioimmunoassays (Meek, 1968). In diabetics there does appear to be an increased titer of chains, especially the alpha chain, when compared to nondiabetics. It has been suggested that a reduced beta chain might be combined with albumin to form the synalbumin antagonist (Vallance-Owen, 1965). Epinephrine and growth hormone are also known to antagonize insulin. The major role of these hormones seems to be glycogenolysis through activation of phosphorylase. Similarly, ACTH and corticoids probably do not directly antagonize insulin, but do stimulate gluconeogenesis.

Some investigators favor a cellular defect in the pathogenesis of diabetes. Recently, insulin has been shown to increase the *de novo* synthesis of rate-controlling glycolytic enzymes (hexokinase, phosphofructokinase, and pyruvic kinase). The production of pyruvic kinase by liver homogenates was increased by addition of insulin. When actinomycin (which inhibits protein synthesis) was added, no increase in pyruvate kinase production was found. Thus the stimulating action of insulin on pyruvate kinase production must occur through synthesis of new enzyme rather than through release of stored enzyme (Gevers, 1967). Evidence is also available that the genes for the production of hexokinase, phosphofructokinase, and pyruvic kinase are present on the same genome (Weber, 1966). It is not surprising then that these enzymes seem to act in unison. In another study (Lowenstein, 1966), pyruvic kinase was found to be deficient in the white blood cells of diabetics. It has been suggested that defective glycolysis in diabetes might result from deficiencies of glycolytic enzymes as well as from a lack of glucose entry into cells.

HORMONAL INFLUENCES ON CARBOHYDRATE METABOLISM

Many drugs and hormones increase the insulin requirements of diabetics or reveal a latent diabetic state. Cortisone is known to increase gluconeogenesis, to promote the catabolism of protein, and to increase the synthesis of glucose-6-phosphatase and fructose diphosphatase. The importance of these rate-limiting enzymes for gluconeogenesis now becomes apparent. If cells are induced to produce glucose by cortisone, chemical diabetes can ensue. A rise in glucose would also stimulate insulin secretion by negative feedback. The excess insulin might inhibit lipolysis to promote deposition of fat. One might even speculate that the nucleotide pathway would become more active with an increase in glycogen stores and glycoproteins for deposition into blood vessels.

Glucagon and epinephrine activate phosphorylase, which catalyzes the breakdown of glycogen to G1P. The G1P can be converted to glucose via gluconeogenesis, and such a mechanism may explain the hyperglycemic effect of these hormones. Thyroid hormones appear to regulate the actions of epinephrine and also potentiate the effects of insulin on glucose utilization and glycogen synthesis. Some of the effects of thyroid hormones are dose dependent. For example, in rats, small doses enhance the glycogenolytic effect of epinephrine, whereas large doses depress this response. Large doses of thyroid hormones enhance gluconeogenesis by increasing the availability of precursors derived from protein and fat. Thyroid hormones enhance the rate of intestinal absorption of glucose and appear to increase insulin degradation. Such actions may explain the diminished sensitivity to exogenous insulin that is sometimes seen in thyrotoxicosis. Thyroid hormones affect nearly all aspects of carbohydrate metabolism, and many of these influences are dependent on or modified by other hormones. The mechanisms remain poorly understood. The inhibitory effects of growth hormone (GH) on carbohydrate metabolism occur mainly by antagonism of insulin action. Prolactin acts similarly to GH. Large doses of estrogen and progesterone have caused diabetes in experimental animals, but whether or not these findings can occur in clinical situations is a subject of debate.

REFERENCES

Antoniades, H. N., et al.: Endocrinology **69**:46, 1961.

Gevers, W.: Biochem. J. **103**:141, 1967.

Kaeppe, R. E., et al.: Biochem. J. **234**:2219, 1959.

Lowenstein, B. E.: Med. World News, March 25, 1966, p. 79.

Meek, J. C., et al.: Diabetes **17**:61, 1968.

Stadtman, E. R.: Advances Enzym. **28**:41, 1966.

Steiner, D. R., et al.: Diabetes **17**:725,1968.

Vallance-Owen, J.: Insulin antagonists. In Leibel, B. S., and Wrenshall, G. A., editors: On the nature and treatment of diabetes, Amsterdam, 1965, Excepta Medica Foundation, International Congress ser. no. 84, p. 351.

Weber, F., et al.: Advances Enzym. Regul. **4**: 59, 1966.

Yalow, R., and Berson, S.: Diabetes **9**:254, 1960.

Chapter 19

Diabetes mellitus

Gordon Bendersky, M.D.

Definition

Diabetes mellitus may appear in stages. *Prediabetes* occurs prior to a discernible disorder of glucose metabolism. *Latent (chemical, "subclinical") diabetes* is an asymptomatic stage associated with an elevated postprandial blood sugar and impaired glucose tolerance. "Early" latent diabetes shows only reactive hypoglycemia. *Clinical (overt) diabetes* manifests fasting hyperglycemia. Ketoacidotic diabetes is the most extreme form.

Etiology and classification

Primary diabetes mellitus (essential diabetes, familial diabetes)

Primary diabetes mellitus with an inherited predisposition includes both the relatively stable adult-onset diabetes not prone to ketoacidosis as well as the unstable, ketosis-prone juvenile diabetes. The cause is unknown but several theories have been proposed:

1. There may be a circulating insulin antagonist such as a small polypeptide, the albumin-bound B chain (phenylalanyl-NH_2) component of insulin representing the synalbumin of Vallance-Owen (Jervell and Vallance-Owen, 1967). This component exhibits insulin antagonism on perfused rat muscle, but its activity regarding in vivo studies has yet to be confirmed and in fact may be artifactual. To explain the observed elevation of circulating insulin levels in diabetics given a glucose load, other antagonists have been proposed such as binding substances, alpha globulin or β-lipoprotein.

2. There may be an inherited deficiency of the enzyme pyruvate kinase (Lowenstein, 1968). Being a significant rate-limiting catalyst in glycolysis, deficiencies of this enzyme lead to a bottleneck in the metabolism of sugar. Since this kinase deficiency can be compensated for in many cases by an excess of endogenous insulin, the observation that most diabetics have too much circulating insulin is not incompatible.

3. There may be an impairment of insulin by excesses of free fatty acids (FFA). A genetically influenced defect in adipose lipase activity would allow excesses of serum FFA in the serum and at the same time permit dietary carbohydrate to be diverted (instead of adipose tissue) toward direct stimulation of greater insulin release. The FFA act to antagonize the insulin, allowing chronic elevations in circulating insulin that would not be wholly active.

4. There is depletion of the enteric hormones, gastrin, secretin, pancreozymin, and enteroglucagon, which are said to be agents stimulating the islets of Langerhans to release insulin.

5. A possible explanation is that there is an enzymatic defect in the islet cell synthesis of insulin with compensatory overproduction of an abnormal insulin-like chemical that is biochemically less active in glucose transport but normal in regard to lipogenesis. The discovery of *proinsulin* (Steiner et al., 1968) helps to account for an active and inactive form of insulin, similar to "big" and "little" insulin (Gordon and Roth, 1969). In the prediabetic state, the beta cell would be deficient in the enzyme breaking down proinsulin to insulin.

6. Diabetes is a syndrome involving many different genetic diseases similar to the different species of rat hyperglycemia, implying that hyperglycemia is caused by a variety of genetic etiologies.

7. The pancreatic hyposecretion theory states that the intrinsic defect in the beta cell is that a slow insulin release occurs in response to glucose and can even occur in the prediabetic person as a result of a genetically induced substance interfering with beta cell release. However, the prediabetic's slow insulin response cannot be consistently demonstrated.

8. Other concepts include autoimmune destruction of islet cells (applicable but unproved for juvenile diabetes), disorder of Krebs cycle preventing lactate incorporation (and resulting in diminished ATP required for glucose transport), viral infection (as mumps), and peripheral tissue as the source of insulin resistance (the hypertrophic adipose cell is insensitive to insulin).

Secondary diabetes mellitus

The following evident *endocrinologic causes* are Cushing's syndrome (see steroid diabetes on p. 212), acromegaly (see Chapter 5), hyperthyroidism (the incidence of diabetes ranges from 3% to 10%), pheochromocytoma (see epinephrine hyperglycemia on this page), and primary hyperaldosteronism; the hyperglycemia may be caused by potassium depletion. Some authorities predict that a large percentage of diabetics will be found to have primary hyperaldosteronism as the cause of their hyperglycemia.

Pancreatic disorders (islet cell deficiency) compose the following: hemochromatosis and the other diseases of iron storage, pancreatitis (including mumps virus as a cause), cystic fibrosis especially in those surviving to adult stage, pancreatectomy and cysts and neoplasms of the pancreas.

Other types of diabetes mellitus

Neonatal diabetes. Neonatal diabetes is a rare occurrence in the first 30 days of postpartum life.

Diabetes-like states

Starvation diabetes refers to the impairment of glucose tolerance and glucosuria occurring after either fasting or carbohydrate deprivation and is characterized by a normal or low fasting blood sugar and an excessive postabsorptive rise and delayed return of blood sugar. It has been attributed to a form of disuse atrophy with a temporary delay, or failure of insulin secretion, in response to hyperglycemia. Peripheral glucose uptake is impaired. Starvation can induce other diabetes-like conditions such as ketosis and hyperuricemia.

Epinephrine hyperglycemia, as in pheochromocytoma, manifests both fasting and postprandial hyperglycemia. Epinephrine inhibits peripheral glucose assimilation, inhibits secretion of insulin, and may destroy beta cells. It induces glycogenolysis by influencing phosphorylase activity and enhances lipolysis with the release of FFA, which may act as an insulin antagonist. Epinephrine hyperglycemia explains the means by which infection and stress can aggravate diabetes. Catecholamine activates cyclic adenosine-3',5'-monophosphate (AMP), which enhances phosphorylase and lipolytic activity.

Steroid diabetes. The action of corticosteroids on carbohydrate metabolism is discussed in Chapter 12.

Glucagon diabetes. Glucagon diabetes

occurs when repeated injections of glucagon are given, resulting in a condition similar to starvation diabetes.

Hepatogenous diabetes. Patients having liver cirrhosis exhibit a 50% incidence of impaired glucose tolerance and a 12% to 25% incidence of fasting hyperglycemia. Other liver diseases with a higher incidence of abnormal glucose tolerance include hepatitis and obstructive jaundice because of stones.

Syndromes in which diabetes is known to occur

Werner's syndrome. See Chapter 25.

Lipo-atrophic diabetes. Lipo-atrophic diabetes is characterized by the complete absence of body fat, hyperlipemia, hepatomegaly, and a high BMR. The diabetes is usually insulin resistant but free from ketosis.

Congenital lipodystrophic diabetes. Congenital lipodystrophic diabetes with acanthosis nigricans can appear.

Leprechaunism. Leprechaunism is a more severe form of congenital Seip-Lawrence syndrome (than either lipo-atrophic diabetes or congenital lipodystrophic diabetes).

In addition to enlarged genitals, hirsutism, and neurologic abnormalities, they have retarded bone growth and increased sensitivity to insulin.

Pseudophlorhizin diabetes. Pseudophlorhizin diabetes occurs in dwarfed children who have reddened cheeks, protruding stomachs, massively enlarged livers, and bone disease. Although there is impaired glucose tolerance, the extreme glycosuria is more impressive, suggesting a similarity to the experimental induction of renal glycosuria with phlorhizin.

Uric acid diabetes. Under certain experimental conditions, uric acid (whose chemical structure resembles that of alloxan) is diabetogenic. Gouty patients have a high incidence of impaired carbohydrate tolerance (20% to 50%). Moreover, hyperuricemia, hypercholesterolemia, hypertriglyceridemia, and early coronary artery disease may be associated with hypertension and diabetes.

Refsum's syndrome. Refsum's syndrome consists of peripheral neuropathy, ataxia, progressive nerve deafness, retinitis pigmentosa, and diabetes.

Schmidt's syndrome. Schmidt's syndrome consists of Addison's disease and thyroid insufficiency. Diabetes is frequently associated.

Mauriac's syndrome. Mauriac's syndrome consists of diabetes occurring in infancy and adolescence with dwarfism, hepatomegaly, osteoporosis, "moon-face," and delayed sex maturation.

Prader-Willi syndrome. Prader-Willi syndrome consists of mental deficiency, short stature, a peculiar type of obesity, muscle hypotonia, undescended testes, and diabetes.

Other causes of hyperglycemia or abnormal glucose tolerance

Burns (blood glucose levels greater than 1,000 mg./100 ml.).

Hypothermia (glucose rising above 600 mg./100 ml. in some cases).

During dialysis when hyperglycemic fluids are employed in the treatment of edema.

Postgastrectomy patients (even in the absence of the dumping syndrome).

Chronic uremia (due to diminished pancreatic release of insulin, decreased pancreatic reserve, and/or paradoxically low total body potassium).

Head injuries, cerebral vascular disorders, and myocardial infarction.

Drug-induced (stress) hyperglycemia: impaired carbohydrate tolerance occurring during treatment with various pharmacologic agents, such as nicotinic acid, thiazide drugs (by potassium depletion and/or depression of insulin secretion), corticosteroids, thyroid hormone, epinephrine, and nonthiazide diuretics; under unusual circumstances, human growth hormone, testosterone (and other anabolic agents), large doses of Dilantin sodium, prostaglandin, morphine, cyclic AMP, and I.V. arginine are known to cause hyperglycemia.

Hyperlipoproteinemia.

Malnutrition and carbohydrate deprivation.

Advanced age, race (Pima and Cherokee), obesity (because of elevated FFA or increased gluconeogenesis), sex (female), and parity.

Islet cell tumors (the impaired glucose tolerance is probably related to persistant elevations of plasma growth hormone arising from chronic hypoglycemia or beta cell suppression in the remnant after surgery).

Alpha cell tumors (glucagon secreting).

High-sucrose diet.

Pathophysiology

Beta cell "inertia" is a characteristic feature of diabetes, that is, the sluggish release of insulin after a glucose load. The peak of insulin output during an oral glucose tolerance test (OGTT) is from 90 to 120 minutes, whereas in normal subjects it is from 30 to 45 minutes. In addition, there is a reduced increment in insulin release, causing hyperglycemia. The hyperglycemia, in turn, stimulates a more persistent insulin release, thus accounting for the *late high peak of insulin* output in the OGTT. When a *continuous* intravenous glucose infusion is given, diabetic patients display an absence or marked reduction of and delay in the *initial* insulin peak. In normal subjects there is a biphasic insulin curve during glucose infusion. Prediabetic and early diabetic patients also manifest this decreased insulin response, which has been considered the genetic factor and the earliest insulin abnormality in the pathogenesis of diabetes. Other stimuli for insulin release are ketone bodies and amino acids.

Diabetic patients may have decreased, normal, or elevated levels of serum insulin. The paradoxically *elevated* insulin levels have been proposed as a cause for obesity as well as for the deposition of lipids in

atherogenesis. Exposure of the arterial tunica intima to elevated levels of insulin and/or lipids (or enhanced endogenous synthesis of lipid in the vessel wall) may promote the development of atheromatous plaques. There is an increased incidence of hypercholesterolemia, high levels of FFA, phospholipids, chylomicrons (similar to type I hyperlipoproteinemia) and triglycerides. There is also a higher incidence of type III hyperlipoproteinemia (low-density β-lipoprotein), type IV (sucrose- and starch-induced hyperglyceridemia) and type V, a mixed group (Levy and Glueck, 1969). The triglycerides may rise higher than 2,000 mg./100 ml. in diabetic lipemia, and range between 300 to 2,000 in carbohydrate-induced hyperlipemia (upper limit of normal, 150 mg.). The FFA in nonketotic diabetics may reach 1,000 or more μEq./L. and in those with ketosis 1,700 μEq./L. (normal of 300 to 800). The cholesterol level usually ranges from 300 to 400 mg./100 ml. in hypercholesterolemic diabetics and rises further if there is nephrosis. Recent surveys indicate that 40% to 70% of nonketoacidotic diabetics have hyperlipidemia in association with decreased lipoprotein lipase activity. There is a 5% to 10% incidence of hyperlipidemia even in the mild well-controlled diabetic subject. These and other biochemical disorders of diabetes mellitus are listed in the following outline:

Serum abnormalities
    Elevations in glucose, glycerol, and phosphate
    Elevations in FFA,* cholesterol, phospholipids,* triglycerides,* and lipoprotein
    Low, normal, or elevated plasma insulin levels
    Elevations in lactic,* amino, uric,* ascorbic, and citric acids
    Acidosis* and hyperosmolarity
    Elevations in acetyl coenzyme A,* acetoacetyl coenzyme A,* β-hydroxybutyryl coenzyme A,* and acetone*
    Elevations in glycoprotein and L-xylulose
    Elevations in epinephrine,* adrenocortical-,* and growth-hormone* levels

---

*Particularly in the very uncontrolled diabetic; see section on diabetic coma for additional abnormalities.

High β-glucuronidase activity

Functional hypoglycemia in early course of diabetes

Intracellular abnormalities

High glucose-6-phosphatase and fructose-1, 6-diphosphatase activity

Low glucose-6-phosphate dehydrogenase activity (suppressed pentose pathway)

Low pyruvate dehydrogenase, pyruvatekinase, glucokinase and phosphofructokinase activity

Decreased oxidation in the Krebs cycle

Suppression of fatty acid synthesis arising from inhibition of coA-carboxylase by acyl coA–thioesters and from deficient TPNH

Low lipoprotein lipase activity

High cardiac, renal, and pancreatic glycogen (fatty acid utilization suppresses glycolysis)

Low hepatic glycogen* (from relative deficiency in insulin)

Enhanced glucose utilization by glucuronic acid pathway

Enhanced sorbital synthesis

The classic pathologic finding in the pancreas of the juvenile diabetic is a marked decrease in the number and mass of islets and number of beta cells. In maturity onset diabetes there is a relatively normal complement of islets with beta cells containing normal or decreased amounts of secretory granules. Other pathologic changes include hyalinization, glycogen infiltration, and leukocytic infiltration.

Diagnosis

The diagnosis depends on finding an elevation of blood glucose. The typical complaints are polyuria, polydipsia, polyphagia, pruritus, fatigue, and drowsiness. Some patients have undetected asymptomatic diabetes for years. "Prediabetes" defines the genetic disorder before an alteration in carbohydrate metabolism is demonstrable.

Listed are the characteristics of prediabetes:

Clinical characteristics

Women whose pregnancies are complicated by:

Macrosomia of newborns (weight of 9 lb. or greater)

Renal glycosuria

Repeated miscarriages, unexplained stillbirths

Hydramnios, premature labor, toxemia, excessive lactation

Cushingoid appearance of the fetus

Neuropathy, retinopathy, cataracts, parotid gland enlargement, xanthelasma, necrobiosis lipoidica, etc. (occurring before any carbohydrate abnormalities)

Pathologic characteristics

Thickened capillary basement membrane, for example, nodular glomerulosclerosis

Increased conjunctival venous/arteriolar diameters

PAS–positive endothelial proliferation in arterioles

Chemical characteristics

Phenformin lowers the serum level of triglycerides in those subjects who have hypertriglyceridemia

Abnormally high insulin levels after a glucose meal

High β-glucuronidase activity

Carbohydrate-induced hyperlipemia

Physical examination is usually of little help in making the diagnosis of diabetes but there may be diabetic retinopathy, juvenile cataracts, hepatomegaly in children, dermopathy, parotid gland enlargement, or hemochromatosis.

The two commonly used "true" blood glucose methods most closely conforming to values obtained with glucose oxidase are the ferricyanide AutoAnalyzer and the Somogyi-Nelson procedures.

The red blood cell contains less glucose than plasma, so that tests using plasma will be 15% higher than those using blood. Diagnostic conclusions should be based on at least two blood samples because in normal individuals there may be a slight elevation of blood glucose in a single sample. At least one third of diabetic subjects show a normal fasting blood glucose (FBG). When other causes of hyperglycemia have been eliminated, a *definite* diagnosis of diabetes can be made when the blood glucose is 120 mg./100 ml. or higher on two or more samples of blood. A value between 100 and 120 mg. is borderline, though some authorities accept a value of over 110 mg. as diagnostic. An elevated value 1 to 2 hours after a meal is the earliest manifestation of diabetes and will detect about 90% of cases. The most sensitive screening test for this postprandial elevation utilizes the 100-gram load of glucose. However, since the 2-hour postprandial blood glucose (PPBG) is not standardized and varies between eating an unspecified meal and taking a 75-gram glucose drink, criteria vary with different authorities. A 2-hour PPBG of 190 or above indicates definite diabetes, 170 to 190 diabetes suspect, 150 to 170 suggestive of diabetes, and 120 to 150 borderline. Levels below 120 are nondiabetic. If the 2-hour PPBG is elevated, retest with FBG and if negative do a GTT.

All adults in the population are recommended to obtain an annual screening test. When there are clues suggesting the presence of prediabetes, or if there is a positive family history, acromegaly, Cushing's syndrome, signs and symptoms of diabetes, and hypoglycemia, or when diabetogenic drugs are used, a more careful evaluation is indicated.

Despite its drawbacks, the *oral glucose test* (OGTT), is the most widely employed procedure for the diagnosis of *early* diabetes. The criteria are a FBG of 110, 1-hour level of 170, and 2-hour level of 120. Obtaining two or more elevations indicates definite diabetes; one elevation would be *probable diabetes.* Some believe that in a person 50 years of age or over the 1- and 2-hour levels are normally increased by 10 mg./100 ml. for each decade. The OGTT is done after an overnight fast and the subject should have had an adequate carbohydrate intake for the 3 prior days. A *5-hour* GTT is often preferred because the early detection of diabetes may be enhanced by finding reactive hypoglycemia at the fourth or fifth hour. The OGTT is indicated in the following situations: (1) when the 2-hour PPBG is normal but diabetes is still suspected; (2) when the blood glucose is only mildly elevated; (3) when glucosuria occurs with a normal FBG; (4) in the presence of unexplained neuropathy or angiopathy; (5) and as an aid in the diagnosis of prediabetes. The *intra-*

venous GTT has greater reproducibility, takes only 1 hour to complete and is not affected by changes in gastrointestinal absorption. However, it has the disadvantages of lack of sensitivity (poor detection of early diabetes), lack of uniform criteria, and occasional phlebitis. The *tolbutamide test* (both I.V. and oral) is based on the failure of the blood glucose in diabetics to fall to 80% or less of the FBG at 20 minutes and 78% at 30 minutes after 2 Gm. of tolbutamide and indicates ineffective insulin. It is not as sensitive as the OGTT but has the advantage of brevity.

The *corticosteroid* glucose tolerance test (CGTT) is based on the observation that subjects with a normal OGTT but with a positive CGTT had a likelihood of becoming diabetic or were already early diabetics. Yet there is considerable question as to its reliability in detecting prediabetics, and false negative test results have appeared too often (normal CGTT but a diabetic GTT). *Afternoon diabetes* refers to the occasional patient whose morning OGTT is normal but the GTT is positive when done in the afternoon. Also, in the afternoon reactive hypoglycemia is more frequently elicited. For *factors raising the blood glucose level* and thus influencing the diagnosis by laboratory means, see the section on insulin hypoglycemia on p. 335.

Urine testing for glucose when used for screening tests and to establish the adequacy of therapy is frequently done with Clinitest tablets, which utilize the copper sulfate technique (as in the Benedict's solution). This technique detects not only glucose but also other sugars, such as fructose, lactose, maltose, galactose, and the pentoses, such as in persons eating large amounts of fruit, inborn errors of metabolism like galactosemia, congenital pentosuria, lactating women, and avocado eaters (mannoheptulosuria). Other "reducing substances" include uric acid, ascorbic acid (when in huge quantities), and homogentisic acid. *Clinistix* or *Test-Tape* specifically detect glucose, but the color transition for grading degrees of glucosuria is not sharp and the test may detect normal amounts of glucose. Although glycosuria is most commonly due to diabetes, it is still a nonspecific finding. Glycosuria (as determined by the glucose oxidase method) may be caused by nondiabetic renal disturbances (de Toni-Fanconi syndrome, pregnancy, nephritis) and alimentary glycosuria.

Other laboratory tests include the finding of yeast in a voided specimen of urine; mucormycosis infection (usually in sinuses); radiographic evidence of calcification of the prostate, vas deferens, and pelvic arteries; cystitis emphysematosa; or a neuropathic joint.

Therapy

The objectives of therapy are (1) prevention of ketoacidosis, (2) avoidance of hypoglycemia, (3) prevention of the hyperosmolar state and attainment of normal blood glucose and absence of glycosuria, (4) relief of symptoms (polyuria, pruritis vulvae, polydipsia, etc.), (5) avoidance of obesity, and (6) control of hyperlipemia. Classification of control is sometimes oversimplified by analysis of the blood glucose (Table 19-1). Ideally, the major objective should be the prevention of the disorders of glucose, protein, and lipid metabolism and the prevention of the microangiopathies and macroangiopathies. Treatment consists of giving the patient an appropriate diet, permitting regular exercise, embarking on a program of patient education, and prescribing oral antidiabetic drugs or insulin when required.

Diet

The diet for the adult is designed to avoid or treat obesity, restrict intake of sucrose, favor frequent small meals, and keep the daily intake isocaloric (especially if insulin is used), while at the same time providing adequate vitamins and appetite-controlling bulk. Most of the fat in the diet should consist of unsaturated fatty acids so as to reduce serum cholesterol and triglycerides and to inhibit atherogenesis. The polyunsaturated vegetable oils include corn, cotton seed, safflower, and soybean. Obesity does not cause diabetes, but it may uncover a predisposition and can further aggravate carbohydrate intolerance in the known diabetic. Erratically eating different quantities of calories (or carbohydrate) from day to day may lead to wide swings of blood sugar. Little or no sucrose is permitted because sugar absorption is rapid, the blood glucose elevation is steep and erratic, and hypertriglyceridemia is promoted. Multiple small feedings are known to promote improved carbohydrate tolerance and to stabilize the blood glucose. The diet is calculated by first ordering the proper total daily caloric intake (as predicted by using standard ideal height and weights) based on 20 to 40 calories/kg. of ideal weight, depending on whether the patient is sedentary or engages in laborious work. The daily protein allowance is 1.5 grams/kg. for hard-working men (and patients with infection, ketosis, or protein loss), 1 gram/kg. for sedentary adults, and 2 gram/kg. for growing children. The number of grams of protein multiplied by 4 gives the total daily calories from protein.

Table 19-1. Criteria for deciding adequacy of diabetic treatment when all other criteria are met (blood glucose in mg./100 ml.)*

	2-Hour postprandial	Preprandial
Excellent	130-150	100
Good	150-170	130
Fair	170-200	160

*For the very *mild*, stable diabetic patient, these figures should be lowered by about 10% to obtain the best possible control. For the *labile* patient, these figures should be raised by 10% to 20% to avoid hypoglycemia.

To calculate the carbohydrate and fat content, substract the protein calories from the total daily caloric allowance. Probably no less than 30% of the daily calories should be carbohydrate, less than 125 grams being conducive to ketogenesis. Ordinarily, the diet would be apportioned as follows: 2/7 of the daily requirement should be allowed for breakfast, 2/7 for lunch, and 2/7 for dinner, with an additional 1/7 for a snack or prebedtime feeding. By having the patient prepare a list of foods consumed as to type, quantity, and the time of day, his personal likes and dislikes can be taken into consideration.

An occasional patient will fail to cooperate and the directions must be adjusted to his eating pattern. Since diet alone can be effective in about 50% of patients, it is justified to advise strict adherence, even to the extent of initially weighing the foods. Instead of calculating the diet, one of nine standard American Diabetic Association diets can be ordered. Successful weight reduction in the obese has achieved remissions in gouty subjects, in hyperglycemia, and in starch-induced hyperlipemia. Marked weight reduction usually promotes improvement in carbohydrate tolerance whereas the use of insulin may increase obesity. As a method of rapidly losing weight, complete starvation

for obese diabetics is not recommended; there can be precipitation of gout, ketosis, marked negative nitrogen balance, and orthostatic dizziness. Although "diabetic" foods are marketed to provide sweets without sugar (low-calorie ice cream, carbonated beverages, etc.), some have considerable caloric value that must be taken into account. Alcohol consumed in occasional small quantities is harmless; however, it potentially can cause hypoglycemia (with irreversible neurologic changes), acetonuria, hyperglyceridemia, beer-drinker's cardiomyopathy, and intoxication simulating an insulin reaction. It may also lead to fatty infiltration of the liver to which diabetics are already prone, and it may cause incompatibility with sulfonylurea drugs.

In the office management of the adult diabetic, the physician observes the effects of diet alone by obtaining blood glucose levels and occasionally 24-hour urinary glucose determinations every 3 to 7 days in the moderately severe group and every 2 to 8 weeks in the mild group (many of whom have only chemical diabetes). If the hyperglycemia persists, oral antidiabetic agents are then tried. Even if the patient does not attain an ideal weight, if the 2-hour postprandial blood glucose remains at 200 mg.% or less and the pa-

Table 19-2. Oral drugs for diabetes

Generic name	Trade name	Size tablet available	Minimum dose	Maximum dose	Half-life (hours)
Sulfonylureas					
Tolbutamide	Orinase	500 mg.	250 mg.	3 Gm.	5
Chlorpropamide	Diabinese	100 and 250 mg.	50 mg.	750 mg.	36
Acetohexamide	Dymelor	250 and 500 mg.	125 mg.	1.5 Gm.	8
Tolazamide	Tolinase	100 and 250 mg.	100 mg.	1.0 Gm.	7
Biguanide					
Phenformin	DBI	25 mg.	50 mg.	200 mg.	3
Phenformin hydrochloride		50 mg.			
(long-acting)	DBI-TD	(capsule)	50 mg.	200 mg.	6

tient is free of symptoms, the use of the oral agents may be deferred. Diet alone can effectively control about 50% of diabetic patients; 25% to 35% of cases are controlled by insulin and 24% to 35% by oral antidiabetic agents.

Oral hypoglycemic agents

Oral hypoglycemic agents (Table 19-2) are not effective in preventing ketoacidotic complications, controlling the unstable diabetic patient, or managing diabetes in the presence of acute stress. They should not generally be used in the juvenile diabetic, in the severely ill patient, and in acidosis. They are still not recommended in pregnancy. When used with insulin they occasionally produce a more stable course than with insulin alone. It is interesting to note that a placebo can cause a temporary fall in fasting blood glucose in about one fourth of the cases.

Sulfonylureas. Sulfonylurea drugs promote stimulation of an increase in plasma insulin-like activity, decrease of beta cell granules and assayable insulin in the pancreas, decrease in hepatic gluconeogenesis, slight inhibition of ketogenesis in the absence of insulin, and a 10% reduction in serum cholesterol if elevated but no reduction of triglycerides. The incidence of primary failures is 20% to 30%. A variable number of apparent secondary failures are of dietary failure; the average incidence is 10% to 20%. This failure may occur at any time over a matter of years but is most common in the first 3 years. There is a leveling off after the fifth year. Secondary failure to one sulfonylurea does not mean that another will fail to work. Large loading doses are no longer used and, in fact, may induce hypoglycemia. Primary failures occur in underweight patients, in patients less than 45 years of age, in those requiring large doses of insulin, and in patients having a record of acetonuria; however, there are many exceptions. In substituting a sulfonylurea agent for insulin one should not reduce the insulin stepwise over several days while the

oral agent is being increased, because the risk and harmful effects of hypoglycemia outweigh any dangers from transient hyperglycemia. The insulin is omitted completely when the oral agent is started. Determining responsiveness to sulfonylureas with an I.V. tolbutamide test is no longer practiced. During surgery or in the presence of necrosis or infection, it is best to substitute insulin. Some patients (30% to 60%) who are not responsive to either a sulfonylurea or a biguanide alone may be responsive to a combination; this fact is not true for the patient under 40 years of age. Only 5% of secondary failures respond to a different sulfonylurea. In some cases combined therapy merely postpones insulin therapy for a short time. The success of combined therapy is not dependent on the previous duration of the diabetes. Side effects occur in about 5% of patients and include nausea, vomiting, diarrhea, epigastric distress, headache, constipation, nervousness, insomnia, paresthesias, lethargy, pruritus, leukepenia, anemia, hemolysis, thrombocytopenia, cholestatic jaundice, fever, vertigo, and photosensitivity. Severe unexpected and occasionally prolonged hypoglycemia occurs particularly with renal failure, hepatic disease, and congestive failure, or in those patients taking salicylates, Dicoumarol, sulfonamides, and phenylbutazone, but in general hypoglycemia with oral agents is less frequent than with insulin. Cutaneous reactions include urticaria, maculopapular, and morbilliform eruptions; purpura, erythema multiforme; and exfoliative dermatitis. Despite the evidence that some patients develop hypothyroidism, diminished ^{131}I uptake and goiters, there is no general agreement that this is due to the sulfonylurea. Patients taking sulfonylurea drugs may exhibit a sensitivity to alcohol, resulting within 5 to 20 minutes in flushing, headache, dyspnea, tachycardia, and nausea.

INDIVIDUAL CHARACTERISTICS. *Tolbutamide,* although the most expensive compound, causes fewer and milder side effects. It is the most rapidly metabolized sulfonylurea.

Some patients respond to a single daily dose despite its short duration of action (6 to 10 hours). *Chlorpropamide* can induce more side effects unless one uses the lower doses recently advocated. Its action is more prolonged (up to 60 hours), and it is therefore effective in a single daily dose. It is more likely to be effective in severe diabetes. *Tolazamide* is effective in single doses.

Phenylbiguanide. With phenylbiguanide, there is increased anaerobiosis with suppression of oxidative phosphorylation, enhanced peripheral glucose uptake, and probably increased oxidation of glucose to CO_2; there is decreased blood glucose in the absence of the pancreas, but in the usual doses phenylbiguanide requires the presence of insulin (endogenous or exogenous), does not ordinarily lower blood glucose in normals, lowers plasma insulin after a glucose load (particularly in the obese), causes weight loss in diabetic patients (70%) because it is anorexigenic and inhibits lipogenesis (by lowering insulin levels), decreases hepatic gluconeogenesis (via suppression of ATP formation), and decreases cholesterol and triglyceride levels in some hyperglyceridemic diabetics.

Side effects (2%) include anorexia, nausea, metallic taste, diarrhea, dizziness, and weakness. Hypoglycemia is unusual. The reported predisposition to lactic acidosis is not proved; most of the reported cases were associated with circulatory collapse, hypoxia, bleeding, myocardial infarctions, alcoholism, hepatic disease, infection, pancreatitis, and other factors known to induce lactic acidosis even in nondiabetics. However, when a diabetic on phenformin develops any serious intercurrent illness, it is wise to change to insulin.

Phenformin (DBI) is the drug of choice particularly in obese patients who do not respond to dietary management. Used in conjunction with insulin, DBI decreases the oscillations from hypoglycemia to hyperglycemia more efficiently than is observed with insulin-sulfonylurea combinations. Occasionally DBI is usefully combined with a sulfonylurea. This combination may reduce the incidence of secondary failures. In juvenile diabetic patients it sometimes eliminates the need for a small evening dose of insulin, for example, 12.5 mg. of the rapid-acting DBI tablet given with the evening meal.

Insulin

Insulin therapy prolongs the life of the juvenile diabetic, but does not correct all metabolic derangements. It is indicated for almost all children, often for the lean diabetic, in pregnancy, ketoacidosis, surgery, and infection, and when sulfonylurea-biguanide combinations fail. The various forms of insulin are listed in Table 19-3. Insulin is available in 10 ml. vials; a vial of U-80 contains 800 units (80 units per milliliter), and one of U-40 contains 400 units (40 units per milliliter).

Regular insulin is unmodified quick-acting crystalline insulin in a clear solution that can be injected subcutaneously or intravenously. It is available in U-40, U-80, U-100, and U-500 concentrations. Indications for its use are (1) urgent situations such as ketoacidosis, infections, and surgical complications and (2) as an aid in conjunction with more prolonged-acting insulins for controlling labile cases.

Protamine zinc insulin (PZI) was designed to prolong insulin action in a depot form. When used alone it may have the disadvantage of permitting excessively high blood glucose during the day, with hypoglycemia during sleeping hours. For this reason a bedtime feeding is required. To overcome daytime hyperglycemia, regular insulin can be mixed with PZI in the same syringe. Since PZI has an excess of protamine, which combines with added insulin, it is necessary to exceed a 1:1 ratio of regular insulin to PZI before the added regular insulin will be free to act. In the stable diabetic patient who requires less than 30 units, PZI may promote satisfactory control. Giving more than 40 units of PZI is not safe because of the danger of early-morning hypoglycemia.

NPH insulin (neutral protamine Hage-

Table 19-3. Classification of insulin

	Appearance	Added protein	Average timing in hours (quite variable)		
			Onset	Peak	Duration
Rapid					
Regular (crystalline)	Clear	None	1	3	7
Semilente	Turbid	None	1.5	5	9
Intermediate					
Globin	Clear	Globin	4	9	16
NPH	Turbid	Protamine	3	14	24
Lente	Turbid	None	3	15	26
Slow					
PZI	Turbid	Protamine	10	22	36
Ultralente	Turbid	None	10	23	36

dorn or isophane insulin) has an intermediate action. It allows mixing with regular insulin without saturating extra protamine. When more than 50 units is needed, giving two injections (before breakfast and dinner) is preferable in order to avoid hypoglycemia. When a single injection is used, a midafternoon snack is necessary. If the FBG remains high when a single dose is employed, a small dose of NPH insulin is added at supper.

Globin insulin is a modified insulin that has an onset and peak of action earlier than that of NPH insulin or Lente. It is used principally in the elderly in whom nocturnal hypoglycemia is likely and who have been refractory to oral agents.

Lente insulin is a mixture of 3:7 amorphous Semilente and the crystalline form, Ultralente. Lente is similar in action to NPH insulin. Do not mix PZI or NPH insulin with Lente because the Lente crystal solubility will be disrupted. The advantage of the Lente series is the absence of added protein, though this does not necessarily prevent sensitivity reactions.

Semilente is similar to regular insulin but is not as rapid acting.

Ultralente is long acting like PZI. To Ultralente or Lente, any amount of Semilente can be added to speed its effect.

The choice of a particular insulin depends on the time of the day when hyperglycemia occurs. In most cases a single dose of NPH insulin or Lente before breakfast suffices. Nocturnal hyperglycemia requires either a long-acting preparation or an evening dose. Midmorning hyperglycemia is controlled with regular insulin; in case of daytime hyperglycemia, that is, morning and early evening, an intermediate insulin can be added to the regular insulin. Patients exhibiting early afternoon hyperglycemia are best treated with globin insulin.

Patients with labile blood sugars may need a morning dose and a before-supper dose of insulin, each consisting of a mixture of fast-acting and intermediate types. PZI and Ultralente are indicated when there is hyperglycemia through the night and before breakfast. A 2:1 mixture of regular insulin and PZI is slightly more active in the first 4 hours than the equivalent amount of NPH insulin.

Method of using insulin. A single-scale syringe is preferable (U-40 syringe for U-40 insulin). It is best to start with 10 units and measure the blood glucose and/or the 24-hour urine glucose value. The insulin dosage can then be increased in increments of 5 units if the 2-hour postprandial blood sugar or urine sugar is too high. The same dose can be given for a few days to allow the effects to stabilize. U-80 insulin is used when the patient requires more than 40 units to achieve control.

If more than 40 to 50 units is required, the insulin dosage can be increased by 10-unit increments. In the patient with labile diabetes, hypoglycemia can be prevented by not attempting to lower the blood glucose below 150 mg. A blood sugar of 200 mg. or higher may have to be tolerated.

In the hospital, precision in choosing the appropriate type and dosage of insulin will be aided by (1) measuring urine glucose concentrations in four aliquots to determine the time of day of the peak glycosuria and the day-to-day total 24-hour urine sugar and by (2) obtaining renal threshold determinations (that is, a blood sugar just before a second voided "fresh" specimen). Regulation involves trial and error based on repeated blood and urine determinations. If, with an intermediate insulin, there is glycosuria or hyperglycemia before breakfast, two injections are usually more effective than changing to one long-acting preparation. When shifting from a single dose to two injections, the total dose is often reduced by one fourth; then three fourths the remaining insulin is given before breakfast and one fourth before supper. If postprandial hyperglycemia or glycosuria persists with the two-injection regimen, regular insulin can be mixed with the intermediate insulin in the same syringe.

The potency of regular insulin is preserved for 3 years when refrigerated, but deteriorates more rapidly at room temperature. All modified insulins (NPH insulin, PZI, etc.) maintain their original potency for 3 years at room temperature and longer when refrigerated. At 122° F. there is a 50% reduction in potency of all insulins every few months.

Special forms of insulin. Dalanated (or desalinated) pork insulin closely resembles human insulin and with sulfated insulin shares the characteristic of being less antigenic and binds less readily with antibodies. Other insulins infrequently used are Actrapid and Rapitard and insulins from specific animal sources.

Problems in therapy

INSULIN ALLERGY. Up to 50% of patients beginning insulin therapy may experience swelling or itching at the site of injection; rarely there is eosinophilia, respiratory symptoms, urticaria, thrombocytopenia, serum sickness, or anaphylactic shock. With continued administration, the symptoms usually disappear spontaneously. Antihistamines may be helpful. If reactions continue, species-specific insulin can be used, such as pure-beef or pure-pork insulins. Patients can also be desensitized, using regular insulin greatly diluted with saline in increasing doses starting with a 1:1,000 dilution. Boiling insulin sometimes abolishes the cutaneous reacting factors without significantly altering potency. Occasionally epinephrine or corticosteroids are required. Hypersensitivity is caused by IgA, and probably IgM and IgG, antibodies.

INSULIN RESISTANCE

Definition. Arbitrarily a daily insulin requirement exceeding 200 units per day is considered to be insulin resistance.

Causes. The causes of resistance (usually unknown) include stopping insulin for 2 weeks or more and then resuming it, cyclic change with menses, emotional stress, necrosis, infection, hyperglyceridemia, Cushing's syndrome, pheochromocytoma, the transient resistance of diabetic ketoacidosis, excessive doses of insulin (reactive hyperglycemia), and excess circulating antibodies binding insulin.

Characteristics. At the site of insulin injections there can be local tissue reactions (painful swelling, lymphadenopathy, or allergic reactions). Spontaneous remission occurs in a few weeks or months. Extreme examples involve "peripheral end-organ unresponsiveness" with as much as 38,000 units of insulin required in 24 hours.

Therapy. U-500 crystalline insulin is a useful preparation that acts over a prolonged period of time. One injection per day may suffice. The site of insulin injection should be changed. The rapid-acting insulins should be used intravenously in ketoacidosis accompanying resistance. Switch to insulins of different origins. Change from beef to pork NPH insulin. Dalanated pork or sulfated insulin may be effective. Phenformin alone or occasionally the sulfonylureas may suffice. ACTH and steroids may cause an initial increase in hyperglycemia followed in a few days by a remission (due to interference with antigen-antibody reaction and perhaps to a decrease in binding capacity of the antibodies). Close observation is necessary because hypoglycemia may follow a remission of insulin resistance.

INSULIN HYPOGLYCEMIA. Characteristic symptoms of insulin hypoglycemia occur when the blood glucose is less than 50 mg./100 ml. but can rarely occur at normal glucose levels. Symptoms may depend on the rapidity of the blood glucose fall, the type of insulin, and the age of the patient. Frequently occurring mild symptoms suggesting hypoglycemia should not be accepted unquestioningly; blood glucose confirmation is necessary. The manifestations have a variable onset and multitudinous expression, may be difficult to diagnose, and may exhibit no necessary relationship between the degree of hypoglycemia and the severity of symptoms. Some patients develop severe hypoglycemia without warning, for example, sudden frank coma or convulsions. Although there may be great variation in symptoms and signs from one patient to another, in any one individual the pattern of insulin reactions is consistent.

Causes. The causes are overdosage (failure to recognize rebound hyperglycemia and errors in technique of administration) and decreased insulin requirements due to unaccustomed exercise, decreased caloric intake, termination of pregnancy (postpartum), uremia causing a more prolonged insulin half-life, coexistence of conditions and drugs causing hypoglycemia (see hypoglycemia, p. 353), cure of conditions that had elevated the insulin requirement, and hypoglycemia from sulfonylurea drugs.

Symptoms. The symptoms are syncopal feeling, hunger, nervousness, anxiety, trembling, weakness, sweating, restlessness, crying spells, mental depression, somnolence, frequent yawning, tingling, numbness, headache, double vision, poor judgment, confusion, hostility, abusiveness, convulsions, and occasionally hallucinations.

Signs. The signs are pallor, early tachycardia, coolness, clammy skin, hyperventilation, tonic and clonic spasms, hypothermia, hyporeflexia, acetonuria (and acetonemia, which could be confused with ketoacidosis), aphasia, pyramidal-tract abnormalities (Babinski sign), late bradycardia, miosis, amnesia, coma, hypotensive shock, temporary blindness, and catatonia.

Treatment

1. Correct a *mild* reaction by oral ingestion of candy, 10 grams of sugar, or orange juice; if the patient is using a long-acting insulin, a meal (fat and protein) should follow to prevent recurrences.

2. In more severe reactions give 20 to 30 grams or more of sugar.

3. If the patient is *unconscious,* the parenteral route is used.

4. A relative at home may be prepared to give glucagon, 1 mg. (1 vial) or more I.M., I.V., or subcutaneously.

5. Give I.V. 30 to 50 ml. of 50% glucose, followed by 500 to 1,000 ml. of 20% glucose, if a long-acting insulin was the cause.

6. Epinephrine, 0.3 to 0.5 ml. of a 1:1,000 solution subcutaneously is effective, but is less desirable than glucagon because of cardiovascular effects.

7. Glucocorticoids.

8. When doubt exists in differentiating hypoglycemia from ketoacidotic coma, glucose is given, since it will not aggravate ketoacidotic coma; very rarely glucose ingestion aggravates a state of hyperosmolar nonketotic coma.

9. General management of the *unconscious* patient: Check airway, arterial bleeding, shock, and injury to the spine; catheterize and test for acetone and glucose; draw blood for glucose, acetone, BUN, alcohol, and barbiturates; type and crossmatch; examine patient each day for skin ulcers, thrombophlebitis, or gangrene; keep patient warm.

Complications. Although mild, brief reactions are not harmful even if recurrent, too frequent or more severe episodes are detrimental. There can be various degrees of cerebral damage, reductions in intelligence, personality changes (including schizophrenia), hemiparesis or hemiplegia, angina, myocardial infarction, prolonged and irreversible coma, decerebrate rigidity, and sometimes death.

The vicious cycle of rebound hyperglycemia may occur, whereby hypoglycemia causes hyperglycemia; the defense mechanism of hepatic glycogenolysis overcompensates for the hypoglycemia. The result may also be hyperlability.

MANAGEMENT OF LABILE (BRITTLE) DIABETES. Hyperlability is most frequent in the lean, juvenile diabetic; it may be transient or permanent. It is characterized by frequent ketoacidosis, labile blood sugar, and a high incidence of infection and vascular complications. Curiously, nondiabetic oscillations in blood glucose can occur as frequently as every 30 seconds with an amplitude of 10 to 30 mg. The hyperlabile patient's glucose level swings from one hour to another through a 100 mg. amplitude; from day to day the blood sugar may vary from a level of 50 mg./100 ml. to 500 mg./100 ml. The cause is unknown but may occasionally be caused by faulty administration or poor absorption of insulin, underlying infection, alcoholism, or other factors. The therapy is as follows:

1. Search for an underlying cause (as above) before designating the lability as a natural characteristic.

2. Use multiple feedings.

3. Daily adjustments in the dosage of insulin may be necessary to accommodate variations in caloric intake and exercise.

4. Use divided doses of intermediate insulin rather than single morning mixtures. It may be necessary to take a breakfast and supper mixture of regular and intermediate insulin.

5. The patient whose blood glucose varies from 50 to 400 every day may need three or more injections of regular insulin each day, even a small dose at 2 A.M.

6. Weighing the food may be necessary to control the dietary variable.

7. Phenformin in combination with a long-acting insulin (for example, given in the evening as a substitute for a second insulin injection) may aid in achieving smoother control with less danger of hypoglycemia than when regular insulin is used. Combinations of insulin and oral agents, however, are not often helpful.

ERRORS IN MANAGEMENT OF THE DIABETIC. The sliding-scale method of ordering insulin on hospital order sheets with the dosage depending on the amount of glycosuria (for example, 20 units for 4+) is erroneous because it gives the wrong dose at the wrong time and assumes that insulin works retroactively and stoichiometrically. It also ignores any threshold disorders and promotes repeating the same inadequate dose.

MANAGEMENT OF DIABETICS DURING SURGERY. Elective surgery is postponed if acidosis is present. Any kind of anesthetic can be used, although chloroform, ether, and tribromoethanol are to be discouraged. About 1,000 calories derived from carbohydrate should be administered daily to avoid ketoacidosis and depletion of hepatic glycogen. Only half the usual requirement of insulin should be given on the morning of surgery, with supplements of regular insulin if the blood glucose rises too high or if ketoacidosis develops. Oral antidiabetic agents can be continued if surgery does not preclude the oral route; however, if surgery or its complications are prolonged or if the parenteral route is necessary, insulin must be employed. A postoperative blood glucose and acetone determination should be obtained. In the juvenile or labile diabetic undergoing any prolonged procedure, these determinations should be measured during the operation.

Juvenile diabetes
Characteristics

The major characteristics that differentiate juvenile from adult diabetes are the following:

1. There is a state of absolute insulin deficiency usually after the initial 2 years in contrast to maturity onset diabetes where there may be compensatory hypersecretion of insulin.

2. Ketoacidosis occurs readily.

3. Unstable blood sugars not readily explainable on the basis of variations in calories, activity, or insulin dosage occur frequently; some children, however, have the adult-obesity type of stable diabetes.

4. There is short stature, usually manifested after 5 years' duration of diabetes and associated with obesity, infantilism, delayed bone development, and hepatomegaly (due to fat infiltration).

5. There are microangiopathy and gross vascular complications.

6. Other features include the onset of ketoacidosis in a matter of hours or days if insulin is stopped, markedly accelerated increase in insulin requirements accompanying puberty, equal incidence among boys and girls in contrast to the predominance among female adults, and a high incidence of insulin lipodystrophy and hypertrophy at sites of insulin injection.

Diagnosis

More than one third of juvenile diabetic patients are first recognized in acidosis or coma. Failure to gain weight in spite of a good appetite is a classic symptom. Other symptoms suggesting the diagnosis include enuresis, cataracts, irritability, weight loss, fatigue, and abdominal pain.

Therapy

Diet. In the juvenile patient, diet alone is ineffective but is still important. Enough calories should be provided to satisfy hunger and attain growth measurements within the 90 percentile on anthropometric charts. The diet should be isocaloric from day to day. A rule of thumb is 1,000 calories plus 100 calories per year of age over one. Restrict disaccharides to avoid sucrose-induced hyperlipemia. Prescribe a diet low in animal fat and high in polyunsaturated fats and containing adequate protein (1 to 3 grams/kg.) to promote growth. Patients on an unmeasured diet must eat at regular times and have extra food at bedtime and midafternoon; measurement of the food at the first interview is still advisable to give the patient an approximate idea of quantity.

The main objections to a "normal" diet are that it is too high in fat and is not isocaloric. In the uncooperative patient, one should not hesitate to modify the above principles toward the free diet; otherwise patients may resist all the other suggestions. The "free" diet is not an unlimited diet; as it is generally used, this term signifies permission to eat one's fill, including sugar and sweets, but obesity is avoided.

Insulin therapy in the juvenile. The commonest regime is a combination of short- and long-acting insulins. As age progresses, the insulin requirements increase. In the first few days of therapy use 0.25 unit/lb. of body weight. Subsequent doses should be based on 24-hour urinary glucose testing. The urine is collected in separate fractionated containers to aid in the selection of the proper type of insulin. Because of the lability of blood sugar levels from hour to hour, they are of limited use in the routine management of the juvenile diabetic patient. Insulin dosage varies from day to day because of a multiplicity of factors and is often a trial-and-error process. Because children are quite sensitive to insulin, only 2-unit adjustments are used, in comparison to the 5- to 10-unit adjustments used for adults. If excessive postprandial glycosuria occurs, add regular insulin to the intermediate insulin in the same syringe. Supplement the daily insulin program with regular insulin at the slightest appearance of acetonuria or increase in glycosuria. Urine for acetone should be tested at least once daily. Competitive sports are permitted with the understanding that exercise has an insulin-sparing effect.

Miscellaneous. Some children develop hepatomegaly and edema after initiating therapy. The oral hypoglycemic agents have not been effective, except for the occasional case in which phenformin improves stabilization in combination with insulin and the unusual circumstance of responsiveness to sulfonylurea (for example, cases of recent onset of diabetes).

Criteria for control in the juvenile diabetic

In the very labile patient, normoglycemia and aglycosuria are usually unattainable without precipitating insulin shock. In view of the detrimental effects of hypoglycemia, slight hyperglycemia is permitted as long as ketoacidosis is avoided. In most cases, an average of 75% of the pre–evening meal specimens may be negative or trace; the remaining 25% are permitted to range from 1 to 4+ and blood sugars of 250 to 500 mg./100 ml. may have to be tolerated if an attempt to achieve better control induces hypoglycemia. An attempt should be made to restrict the urinary glucose to less than 10% of ingested carbohydrate (as long as hypoglycemia can be avoided).

Prognosis

The mortality is 24% after 20 years of diabetes; the life expectancy is shortened by 20 to 25 years. There is not unanimous agreement regarding the relationship between the state of control and the incidence of diabetic complications. Duration of disease may be of greater importance than degree of control. Prior to the availability of insulin, the average life expectancy of the diabetic child was 2 years

after the onset of the disease. Those patients exhibiting recurring coma have a death rate of approximately 60% in 20 years. Those who are characterized initially by hyperglycemia and acetonuria may rarely develop a normal glucose tolerance after losing weight. Diabetic ketoacidosis may occur at any time, not necessarily as a result of an obvious precipitating factor.

Pregnancy and diabetes

The principal goal in the care of the pregnant diabetic patient is the prevention of fetal mortality.

Influence of pregnancy on diabetes

1. Pregnancy is a diabetogenic stimulus that unmasks the disease. Insulin requirements often increase. Increasing parity leads to greater risk of permanency of diabetes. The placenta itself exerts antagonism to insulin. The half-life of human insulin in (nondiabetic) pregnancy is 20 minutes versus 35 minutes for pregnancy in diabetic patients (Gitlin et al., 1965). Placental lactogen or a proteolytic enzyme may be responsible.

2. Pregnancy predisposes to ketoacidosis (by vomiting and dehydration) and to acetonuria, which may be confused with or superimposed on diabetic ketonuria. The incidence of acetonuria among pregnant nondiabetics is 10% to 50%; pregnancy accelerates starvation metabolism.

3. Pregnancy predisposes to hypoglycemia because of glycosuria due to diminished tubular reabsorption. The course of the diabetes may be more labile.

4. It may induce an exacerbation of retinopathy and pyelonephritis. Three percent of cases have an aggravation of preexisting vascular disease.

5. There may be confusion in diagnosis because of nondiabetic galactosuria, lactosuria (particularly in the last 6 weeks of pregnancy), and renal glycosuria. In addition, among known diabetic patients, urine testing for glycosuria often has to be abandoned because of its unreliability, unless the renal threshold is known ap-

proximately and is consistent from week to week. Although the degree of carbohydrate intolerance and insulin requirement is unpredictable, there is a tendency about the tenth week for the diabetes to improve for 2 to 3 months (with an occasional insulin reaction if not anticipated). About the twenty-fourth to twenty-eighth week, there is a worsening associated with ketoacidosis that may subside at the thirty-seventh to thirty-ninth week. Following delivery, an abrupt drop in insulin requirement occurs. Lactation further promotes glucose tolerance (Pederson, 1967).

Influence of diabetes on pregnancy

Diabetes increases the risk of toxemia, hydramnios, gigantism, abortion, congenital anomalies in the fetus (5% to 10% versus 2% in nondiabetic subjects), stillbirths, and placental infarcts. The incidence of perinatal mortality in prediabetic patients is about 10% to 30% in contrast to 2% to 3% for all pregnancies in the United States. The untreated pregnant diabetic individual has a 50% perinatal mortality; under optimal circumstances this can be reduced to 10% to 15%. The risk of intrauterine death of the fetus is greater in the last 4 weeks and increases near term. In contrast, the earlier the fetus is delivered, the greater the risk of death from prematurity. The curve of increasing hazard of intrauterine death and the curve of decreasing danger of prematurity cross at approximately the thirty-seventh week. Maternal mortality in the pregnant diabetic is no longer higher than in nondiabetics. The presence of ketoacidosis imparts a 50% increase in the incidence of intrauterine deaths. Antepartum pituitary necrosis is rare but is peculiar to diabetic individuals.

Management of the pregnant diabetic patient

1. Preconception advice includes warning of fetal risks and reassurance as to the general outcome. The menses should be accurately recorded so as to time the

length of pregnancy. The need for hospitalization, the expense, and the need to terminate pregnancy early should be discussed.

2. Diagnosis: Every pregnant woman deserves a 2-hour postprandial blood sugar test at the first office visit and in the last trimester. However, if there is any evidence of prediabetes or a family history of diabetes, these tests are mandatory; and when the blood sugar is borderline or normal in a case of suspected diabetes, a glucose tolerance test should be performed.

3. Frequent visits are needed to observe and educate, check weight, teach the action of medications and the technique of urine acetone testing and insulin injection, and perform a complete history and physical examination.

4. Hospitalize the newly diagnosed pregnant diabetic at the time of the diagnosis.

5. Diet control alone is sufficient in about 10% of patients who show only a positive glucose tolerance test result and no overt diabetes. Some authorities use insulin in addition to diet even when there is only a positive GTT.

6. Insulin is preferred to the oral hypoglycemic agents. It shows a correlation with reduced fetal morbidity and mortality. Then, too, the juvenile form of diabetes is prevalent in this age group. Generally those pregnancies in patients with stable diabetes cause few difficulties, except for adjustment of diet and insulin and the birth of immature large babies. Those mothers with the brittle juvenile pattern have a greater likelihood of complications and intrauterine deaths and need combinations of insulin and the strict avoidance of acidosis.

7. The early observations of possible teratogenic effects of oral hypoglycemic agents was not subsequently substantiated.

8. Some believe that insulin should be given even in latent diabetes and in cases with a normal fasting and slightly elevated postprandial blood sugar.

9. Urine cultures should be done at

least once near the end of the first trimester.

10. Twice-weekly urinary-estriol determinations are performed if the course of diabetes is complicated. In normal pregnancy, the estriol excretion rises slowly from the seventh to the twentieth week of gestation, after which it accelerates. Values above 12 mg./24 hr. obtained within 2 days of delivery usually foretell a healthy infant. Fetal jeopardy is likely when values are below 12 mg.; fetal mortality correlates with levels below 4 mg.

11. Immediate hospitalization is necessary for ketoacidosis, infection, excess weight gain, albuminuria, abrupt fall in insulin requirement, onset of hypertension, and inappropriate drop in estriol levels. Sex-steroid therapy is probably ineffective.

12. Indications for termination of pregnancy earlier than the thirty-seventh week are as follows:
   a. Onset of albuminuria, hypertension, and retinopathy
   b. Rapid progression of retinal lesions or cardiovascular-renal pathology
   c. Uncontrollable ketoacidosis
   d. Drop in urinary estriol below 4 mg./day for 48 hours
   e. Disorder of fetal movements or disturbance in heart tones

13. Generally the time selected for delivery is the thirty-seventh week; the baby has the best chance of survival if the mother can be delivered 14 to 21 days before term. However, if the pregnancy passes the thirty-sixth week without significant complications, continue it to full term.

14. Management at delivery is performed as follows:
   a. Hospitalize the patient several days before the anticipated delivery.
   b. Vaginal delivery is attempted (often even in the primigravida) unless there are obstetric indications for a cesarean section. It has been popular to deliver the primigravida by cesarean section, particularly when the cervix is not favorable for induction of labor or the attempted oxytocic induction fails. Section is indicated particularly for toxemia, severe hydramnios, an oversized baby, in the elderly, a history of previous cesarean section, decreasing fetal movements, change in fetal heart sounds, fetal halo, and decreasing insulin requirements.
   c. Delivery is preferably performed under caudal or other regional anesthesia.
   d. Intravenous 10% dextrose or fructose 1,000 ml. is given every 8 hours.
   e. Insulin: discontinue long-acting insulin at the time of the first stage of labor or 12 to 24 hours before induction. Proceed with fractions of the total anticipated dose using regular insulin, which may be less than the usual daily dose. There occasionally is an abrupt reduction in the insulin requirement in the first stage of labor, which justifies maintaining some hyperglycemia to avoid insulin reactions. In fact, it is usually best to withhold insulin during labor until the blood sugar and/or urine sugar rises, unless there is ketoacidosis.

Diabetic coma
Ketoacidotic coma

Ketoacidosis is characterized by ketonemia, acidosis, hyperosmolarity, usually hyperglycemia, dehydration, and eventually coma. The morbidity and mortality of diabetic coma correlate more closely with the concentration of plasma acetone than with the presence or depth of the coma. Many patients with profound dehydration, Kussmaul breathing, and 4+ plasma acetone are alert or, at the most, slightly confused. The ketone bodies are β-hydroxybutyric acid, acetoacetate, and acetone. Ketoacidosis can occur prior to a significant rise in blood glucose. Also, persisting hyperketonemia after therapy may occur when the blood glucose is normal or below. The principal proton donors are β-hydroxybutyric acid and acetoacetic acid.

Pathogenesis. See Fig. 19-1.

KETOGENESIS. In ketoacidosis the production of ketones exceeds the physiologic limits, leading to the accumulation of ketones beyond the normal concentration of approximately 100 μM./L. The blood level may reach 5,000 μM./L. When plasma acetone reaches 4+ with the Acetest tablet or powder, the acetone is about 200 mg./ 100 ml. In uncontrolled diabetes, lipolysis occurs, releasing excessive fatty acids. With reduction in glycolysis, glycerol phosphate is unavailable for at least one of the pathways of fatty acid utilization, that is, the formation of triglycerides. Fatty acids promote the shift of accumulating acetyl coA toward increased acetoacetate formation by facilitating the appropriate oxidation-reduction potential (fatty acid oxidation enhances DPNH accumulation) and also by inhibiting the condensation of acetyl

coA with oxaloacetate (in the entrance of acetyl coA into the citric acid cycle). In addition, fatty acid synthesis is suppressed in diabetes, promoting the reversal of another pathway of acetyl coA utilization (at the acetyl carboxylase point, the rate-limiting step of lipid synthesis, and perhaps also TPNH-dependent steps, crotonyl coA and malonyl coA involving acetoacetyl coA reductase).

At the center of intermediary metabolism is acetyl coA, the common intermediate in the breakdown of fatty acids, glucose, and amino acids. The three main pathways for its disposal are (1) condensation with oxaloacetate to form citrate for oxidative metabolism, (2) fatty acid synthesis via malonyl coA, and (3) condensation of acetyl coA to form acetoacetate, which in turn can be reduced to β-hydroxybutyrate or decarboxylated to

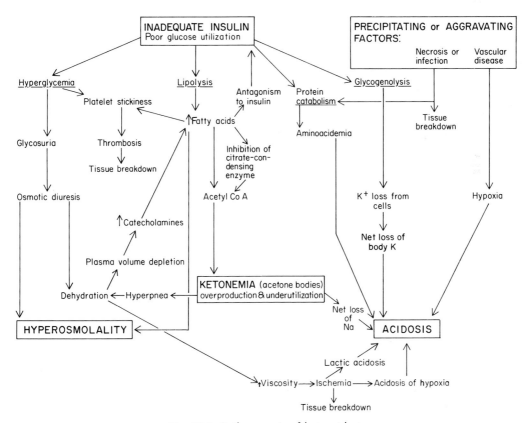

Fig. 19-1. Pathogenesis of ketoacidosis.

acetone. With the failure of the first two pathways, the third path proceeds as the major route in ketogenesis.

A vicious cycle is produced when the anorexia of ketosis and the anorexia associated with precipitating factors of ketoacidosis induces a starvation state, which itself promotes ketosis. Hypoglycemia and the depletion of hepatic glycogen also cause ketosis.

OSMOTIC DIURESIS. Hyperglycemia leads to dehydration by the mechanism of solute diuresis, a phenomenon that is further enhanced by breakdown products from tissue destruction as well as gluconeogenesis, amino acids, fatty acids, and the release of intracellular potassium. Furthermore, the increased viscosity of dehydration contributes to ischemia, leading to further tissue destruction and lactic acidosis. In the process of diuresis, electrolyte and water losses amount to the following deficits in milliequivalents per kilogram of body weight: Na 5 to 13, K 4 to 6, Cl 2.5 to 9.5, Mg 0.6 to 0.8, inorganic P 0.5 to 1.3, and water 100 ml./kg.

ACIDOSIS. Ketoacids produce 1,000 to 2,000 mM./day of hydrogen ions. With the excretion of ketoacetate and β-hydroxybutyrate in the form of Na and K salts, the loss of alkali predisposes to further acidosis. The frequent coexistence of renal disease and the associated loss of buffer mechanisms particularly in the presence of dehydration further compounds the injurious acidosis to the extent that the pH of arterial blood may fall to 7.1 (normal 7.4). Hypoxic acidosis, renal acidosis, lactic acidosis, the ketoglutaric acid of hepatic failure, and coincidental acidosis of unrelated causation may enter this sequence.

Precipitating factors. Precipitating factors may be the omission of insulin, or the presence of infection, diarrhea, emotional upset, alcoholism, anesthesia, shock, pregnancy, or necrosis. Other factors include the use of oral hypoglycemic agents, insulin resistance, thyrotoxicosis, fever, steroid therapy, and diuretic therapy. Ketoacidosis may be spontaneous in new cases.

Manifestations. Except for marked ketonemia, there is no specific diagnostic feature, and even 4+ plasma acetone has been known to occur in nondiabetic starvation ketosis. However, any illness occurring in a known juvenile diabetic patient may be due to ketoacidosis. Vomiting and abdominal pain are typical manifestations; the vomitus may be blood tinged. Tachypnea and more characteristically Kussmaul breathing occur and there is also the occurrence of weakness, intensification of polyuria and polydipsia, dryness of mucosa and skin, headache, drowsiness, stupor and coma with dilated pupils, florid face, hyporeflexia, acetone odor on the breath, and soft eyeballs. With reduction of plasma pH below 7.2, cyanosis and hypotension occur. Kussmaul breathing or hyperventilation may continue after the CO_2 combining power is normal, perhaps because of persisting acidosis in the cells of the respiratory center. Cerebral edema may occur during otherwise successful therapy. Other complications include acute renal tubular necrosis, bacteremia, gangrene, stroke, coronary occlusion, pancreatic arterial thrombosis, and myoglobinuria. Tachycardia may persist for several days after proper therapy and may be caused by pulmonary emboli or myocardial necrosis. Similarly polyuria may continue (hypokalemic nephropathy?, recovery phase of tubular necrosis?).

The serum CO_2 combining power is usually below 10 mEq./L. when Kussmaul breathing is present and is 15 to 20 mEq./L. with milder ketonemia. Although glycosuria and ketonuria are almost invariably present, the urine does not accurately reflect the degree of hyperglycemia or ketonemia. In fact, rarely as a result of a high renal threshold, acetonuria may be absent. Usually, the relationship between ketonuria and ketonemia is such that when there is a slight amount of ketone over equal production, all the excess appears in the urine and remains normal in the plasma (for example, negative plasma Acetest). Only when the maximum renal excretory capacity is exceeded do ketones accumulate in the blood (hyperketonemia). Therefore, once ketonemia disappears, urine testing is utilized to follow milder degrees of ketoacidosis. However, when urine acetone is 4+, then plasma testing is indicated to quantitate the adequacy of therapy. The blood glucose ranges between 150 mg. and 2,000 mg. There is no necessary relationship between the glucose and acetone levels, the latter being more closely related to the severity of the condition. A polymorphonuclear leukocytosis is common even in the absence of infection from dehydration and increased adrenocortical activity. Azotemia is common, usually resulting from a combination of prerenal deprivation (dehydration) and protein catabolism, as well as renal insufficiency. There is commonly hyperlipemia, with elevations of FFA, cholesterol, phospholipids, and triglycerides. Occasionally the serum is lactescent. Hyperuricemia, hypomagnesemia, and elevated serum amylase and lactic acid may occur. Although in coma patients there is a loss of 300 to 700 mEq./L. of sodium and 200 to 700 of potassium, serum values may be normal or high.

Hyperpotassemia appears before treatment and during the first few hours of therapy. Thereafter there is a tendency to hypopotassemia. This sequence is unpredictable, however. Rarely an ECG demonstrates the effects of hyperpotassemia when the serum level is normal or low. Some patients have no signs or symptoms despite a serum K as low as 2 mEq./L.

Differential diagnosis. Other conditions causing acetonuria are starvation states, uncomplicated pregnancy, fever, salicylate overdosage, cold weather, intestinal obstruction, hyperventilation, excessive fat intake, dehydration, acromegaly, Cushing's syndrome, thyrotoxicosis, hypoglycemia, Fanconi syndrome, anesthesia, severe exercise, and hepatic necrosis. Other conditions causing acidosis are renal failure, renal tubular acidosis, methyl acohol intoxication, overdosage of paraldehyde, salicylates, lactic acidosis, hypoxia, gastrointestinal fistula, tremetol (snake root) and ethylene glycol poisoning, hyperbaric oxygen, open-heart surgery, excessive boric acid absorption, hepatic failure (ketoglutaric acid), and excessive intake of ammonium chloride.

In an attempt to differentiate diabetic ketoacidosis from starvation ketosis, one can infuse intravenous 10% glucose in water or one to two small doses of oral or parenteral corticosteroids, both of which correct the ketosis of starvation.

Causes of death. The causes of death are myocardial and cerebral infarction, unrecognized lactic acidosis, hypopotassemia, bacteremia, acute renal insufficiency, acute pancreatitis, and lateral sinus thrombosis. Overzealous fluid therapy may induce acute pulmonary edema in the elderly. Approximately one third the deaths are unexplained (apparently uncomplicated). The overall mortality from diabetic coma, using the criterion of 4+ plasma acetone or CO_2 of 10 mEq./L., is 10%.

Therapy

1. In one venipuncture, draw the necessary blood specimens, give 25 to 50 units of *regular insulin* (intravenously), and start an I.V. infusion (at a rapid flow) of *isotonic saline* (see p. 344). The blood specimens should include plasma acetone, blood sugar, CO_2 combining power, BUN, hematocrit, serum osmolarity, and occasionally serum potasium, sodium, and chloride.

2. If the patient is in shock, type and crossmatch the blood and perform a cutdown, or consider central venous pressure. Upon completion of the plasma acetone, supplement the intravenous insulin with regular insulin given subcutaneously as follows: 50 to 100 units if plasma acetone on the undiluted specimen is 4+; 100 to 200 units if the first one-to-one dilution is 4+; 150 to 300 units if on the second dilution it is 4+; acetone determinations correlate better with morbidity and mortality than do glucose and CO_2 levels. Depending on the severity of diabetic acidosis in the initial evaluation, the above total initial dose (or an integral fraction

thereof) of regular insulin may have to be repeated hourly or every 2 hours until acidosis is relieved or modified, depending on the degree of improvement. If the patient remains in peripheral vascular collapse, most of the insulin should be given I.V.

3. Examine the patient for signs of trauma and consider doing a pelvic examination to search for inflammatory disease that may have precipitated the coma. Incise, drain, and culture the pustule or boil and check the urine smear for the organism that may be the cause of pyelonephritis, etc. Whenever the factor precipitating diabetic coma is unknown or in case of any suspicion of a complicating infection, draw a blood culture. Administer parenteral antibiotics appropriately. Persistent acetonuria and delayed resolution of the diabetic coma may be due to failure to treat an underlying infection.

4. Although the ideal *fluids* are hypotonic (for example, 0.45% saline solution, or one can add 100 ml. of sterile distilled water to 900 ml. of isotonic sodium chloride) usually the immediately available unmodified isotonic saline solution is adequate. Isotonic saline as the sole replacement therapy is theoretically a poor choice; the body requires free water in view of the priority of the total body deficit for water. This water is required for the replenishing of the intracellular stores and for utilization in the excretion of acetone bodies and glucose. Secondly, sodium chloride itself in any concentration is a poor choice because the body is more depleted of sodium and bicarbonate than of chloride. However, saline solution is more acidic than is blood (blood is alkaline normally, whereas saline solution is neutral). Hence, one is placed in the position of giving an acid solution to a patient in acidosis. One can add sodium bicarbonate so that the ratio of chloride to bicarbonate is the same as that in the blood (100 mEq. of chloride, 30 mEq. of bicarbonate). Up to as much as 10 L. of fluid may be necessary in the first 24

hours in severe cases. As a rough guide, follow the fluid balance to ensure that the patient is receiving at least 1 liter of fluid every hour (in the first 2 to 4 hours) more than his urinary volume output. Thirty grams of sodium chloride probably is the maximum that should be given in the first 24 hours. Glucose solutions need not be given in the first 4 hours (it may increase dehydration, electrolyte loss, and hypopotassemia and can interfere with blood sugar determinations), except in mild cases when the serum glucose drops rapidly. Consider using sodium bicarbonate when an extremely low CO_2 is associated with Kussmaul breathing. In the presence of oliguria, in cardiac decompensation, or in the elderly, fluids must be limited as judged by the venous pressure determinations, the hematocrit, serum osmolalities, and the response in urine output.

5. Catheterization of the bladder for urinalysis, culture, and urine volume determinations is not recommended; half-hour urine, sugar, and acetone determinations (which may be done at hourly or two-hourly intervals, once a definite improvement is evident) do not necessarily require catheterization.

6. As soon as possible, an initial ECG should be obtained; this is to be repeated at the time of anticipated hypopotassemia.

7. *Gastric lavage* is sometimes carried out, particularly if there is abdominal distention, vomiting, and abdominal pain. Aspirate completely and wash the stomach with warm water. Some advise leaving sodium bicarbonate in the stomach.

8. Repeat the blood sugar, CO_2 combining power, and plasma acetone between the second and fourth hours. Adjust the hourly or two-hourly dose of insulin accordingly. If the blood sugar has significantly increased and the plasma acetone remains unchanged, sufficient insulin has not been given. If the blood sugar is at normoglycemic levels while plasma acetone persists, infuse 5% to 20% glucose solution I.V., while continuing to provide insulin. At this stage, glucose solutions have

the further advantage of enhancing glycogen repletion and of providing a hypoosmolar solution.

9. Once the patient is alert and can swallow, give fluids by mouth as tolerated, limiting them at the beginning to 100 to 150 ml. hourly. Give broths, dilute juices, or milk, which also provide potassium 10 to 15 mEq./glass. Hypopotassemia does not usually occur until 6 to 18 hours after therapy. Potassium by mouth at this time may be given prophylactically. It is preferable, however, to repeat the serum potassium and the ECG at the anticipated time. Oliguria and particularly anuria are contraindications to potassium therapy. One gram of potassium every 3 to 4 hours is provided in the oral liquids. Potassium chloride is a gastric irritant and should not be used. If the patient is unable to swallow at the time that the hypopotassemia has been confirmed, parenteral potassium therapy is justified; in such instances, 20 to 30 mEq. of potassium may be given every 2 to 4 hours if the urine output is more than 50 ml./hr. Rarely, hypopotassemia develops during the first hour of therapy. Correct any fecal impaction and consider giving an enema for relieving abdominal distention. If oral fluids are well tolerated, parenteral fluids may be gradually decreased. If anuria occurs and the BUN rises progressively despite adequate fluid replacement, peritoneal or blood dialysis may be necessary. More complete reliance on the urine, sugar, and acetone may now be made in adjusting the insulin dosage. Optimally, the patient should be free of acidosis at about the sixth to tenth hour, at which time insulin may be given according to the urine tests every 2 to 4 hours. Obtain an occasional blood sugar to verify the renal threshold. Oral feedings can be substituted.

Hyperosmolar nonketotic diabetic coma

The patients may or may not have an increase in ketones or lactic acid or show acidosis. Their disturbed consciousness is ascribable to cellular dehydration resulting from hyperglycemic osmolar diuresis. They are usually elderly, often are obese, and have mild diabetes, severe dehydration, frequent seizures, and a predisposition to hypernatremia and to potassium depletion. Few of them are known diabetic patients. The WBC tends to be high. Those who recover often respond to oral antidiabetic agents. The osmolarity ranges from 350 to 465 mOsm./L. and blood glucose from 500 to 2,200 mg./ml. The CO_2 combining power and pH may be normal to low. The serum potassium is usually normal or high and the BUN is frequently elevated (60 mg. or greater). Some patients have hypotension that can lead to lactic acidosis; the breath is nonacidotic and has an acetone-free odor. Typically there is failure of large amounts of I.V. fluids to induce a diuresis. The diagnosis is suggested by finding a blood glucose above 700 mg./100 ml. and a CO_2 above 18 mEq./L. (patients with CO_2 below 18 are diagnosed as lactic acidosis if there is no ketonemia). Complications include hemiparesis, convulsions, hemianopia, nuchal rigidity, acute renal tubular necrosis, hepatic necrosis, acute pancreatitis, venous thrombosis, gangrene, stupor, and coma. Mortality is about 40% in the more than 150 reported cases. Precipitating factors have included pancreatitis, glucocorticoid therapy, burns, or high carbohydrate therapy. The treatment is insulin and 0.5N saline solution I.V. in large amounts.

Lactic acidosis

Lactic acidosis is suspected when a low plasma bicarbonate level occurs without ketonemia or when acidosis develops during phenformin therapy, especially in the presence of decreased renal function. Characteristically there is an anion gap (acidosis without ketosis) of sudden onset with no other obvious preexisting cause. Levels of pH as low as 6.96 have been reported. There is a frequent incidence of high levels of sodium glutamic oxaloacetic transaminase (SGOT) and lactic acid dehydrogenase (LDH) (possibly arising from hepatic impairment) and high serum phosphorus. The rise in blood lactate is out of proportion to the rise in pyruvate. Normally the fasting blood lactate level ranges from 0.4 to 1.4 mM. or a mean of 12 mg./100 ml. (pyruvate 0.7 to 0.14 mM./L.). Lactic acidosis is diagnosed when the level rises above 7 mM./L. or the lactate to pyruvate ratio is 10:1 or greater. Other conditions besides diabetes that can be associated with increased lactic acid levels include cardiovascular disorders with ischemia, bleeding peptic ulcer, shock, pneumonia, pulmonary infarction, subacute bacterial endocarditis, leukemia, high alcohol intake, pyelonephritis, cirrhosis, hepatitis, acute pancreatitis, and starvation states.

Signs and symptoms consist of tachypnea, cyanosis, weakness, fatigue, Kussmaul respiration, stupor, and death. The mortality is about 75%.

Treatment is directed toward correcting the acidosis with fluids and alkali, bicarbonate being given at a rate of 40 mEq. every 15 minutes. Since excess lactate is an index of the gravity of any possible underlying pathologies, their correction and relief of anoxia are essential. Promising results using large doses of regular insulin with 20% glucose infusions even when blood glucose levels were not significantly elevated, have been described. Methylene blue therapy is no longer recommended and peritoneal dialysis has not been effective. When patients on biguanide therapy develop any serious intercurrent illness or renal failure, insulin should be substituted despite adequate control of the blood glucose.

Hypernatremia

Although hypernatremia most frequently coexists with hyperosmolar coma when it occurs in diabetics, it may occur alone, in association with other complications, and of course in nondiabetic patients (as hypothalamic lesions, salt intoxication in infants, derangement of thirst center, plus high "setting" for ADH secretion). The serum level may reach 200 mEq./L. Clinical signs include hyperirritability, stupor, convulsions, and decerebrate rigidity. Treatment is the same as for hyperosmolar coma.

Chronic manifestations of diabetes
Vascular disease

Microangiopathy. The vessel walls and basement membrane of arterioles, capillaries, and venules are thickened by endothelial proliferation with a deposition of lipid, and the PAS layer is 10 times thicker than in nondiabetic patients. The pathology is not specific. The cause of small-vessel pathology is unknown, and though it appears to vary directly with the degree of diabetic control, vascular and carbohydrate changes are separate but concomitant defects. The former is not a complication but rather an integral part of the disease. Basement membrane hypertrophy may be the initial lesion of diabetes. It is present in more than 50% of prediabetic subjects and in 97% of patients with clinical diabetes.

Doubt has been cast on the statistical significance of the angiopathic prediabetic concept, especially in view of the failure to demonstrate basement membrane thickening in glomeruli with early diabetic lesions (Kimmelstiel et al., 1966); in fact, the changes in the renal basement membrane most likely result from, rather than precede, those in the glomerular mesangium (Fisher et al., 1967). Also, this membrane thickening may occur in the nondiabetic subject; its high incidence in diabetic patients has not been consistent. In addition, the endothelial proliferation occurs in about 20% to 35% of nondiabetic individuals. Furthermore, whereas diabetic retinopathy is essentially a venous disease initially, diabetic nephropathy is an arterial lesion.

Retinopathy

Diabetic retinopathy is characterized by angiopathy (microaneurysms, retinal hemorrhage, retinal edema, and venous dilation), exudates, proliferative processes, and vitreous hemorrhages. Its presence is almost pathognomonic of diabetes. In the juvenile diabetic patient, of all the clinically expressed vascular complications, retinopathy is the commonest and the first to appear. Although the microaneurysms alone are not pathognomonic and do not represent a *sine qua non* feature, multiple microaneurysms are characteristic and are the earliest clinically recognizable sign of diabetes; using retinal photographs, one may observe venous dilation before microaneurysms occur. Other causes of retinal microaneurysms are central vein thrombosis, sickle cell anemia, glaucoma, malignant hypertension, Takayasu's disease, carotid arterial occlusion, macroglobinemia, and uveitis.

Pathology. The initial lesion has been described as degeneration of the pericyte (mural cell), but hyalinization of the endothelial basement membrane probably precedes this degeneration. Characteristic features include capillary sheathing (the basement membrane is stained by PAS) with A-V shunt or microaneurysms of the arteriolar-venular capillaries that develop when the pericytes disappear. Exudates represent leaking serum from ruptured blood vessels. Stagnant anoxia of the retina leads to neovascularization. *Retinitis proliferans* refers to the white fibrous bands carrying blood vessels in a membrane across the retina or floating into the vitreous. Vasoproliferation produces friable new blood vessels and recurrent vitreous hemorrhage. Connective tissue proliferation produces traction on the retina, distortion of the macula, and subsequent retinal detachment. Once glomerulosclerosis occurs, the ophthalmoscopic picture may be complicated by hypertensive changes.

Natural history. Half of all patients with retinopathy will exhibit spontaneous improvement (Davis, 1968). Regression with disappearance of all hemorrhages and exudates, leaving either microaneurysms alone or a normal fundus, occurs in 45% of diabetic patients 29 years of age or younger (Burditt et al., 1968). Of the 50% of diabetic patients who develop retinopathy in the tenth to fifteenth year of their disease, those with a change in visual acuity have a 50% chance of becoming blind within 5 years. The presence of engorged retinal veins suggest a poor prognosis. Although vision deteriorates in the vast majority of all patients with "malignant" retinopathy (new vessel formation, glial proliferation, or vitreous hemorrhage), 15% retain good vision for at least 5 years. Once a diabetic patient becomes blind, the average survival is only 5 years. When the patient exhibits retinopathy, there is an almost two-thirds probability of coexisting nephropathy, whereas almost all patients with glomerulosclerosis develop retinopathy.

Therapy. Low fat and rice diets, heparin, anabolic agents, Atromid-S, and salivary gland removal have been ineffective. Pituitary ablation and photocoagulation are controversial therapies. The intelligent and cooperative patient who is under 40 years of age and is free of clinically overt arteriosclerosis and renal insufficiency is a candidate for pituitary ablation when at least one fairly healthy macula remains, but the mortality is 0% to 10%, and the results sometimes are equivocal. Those who favor pituitary ablation cite 50% to 75% improvement (including arrested cases), benefit sustained for long periods, and the absence of other therapy yielding similar benefits; whereas untreated patients in the younger age groups have about a 45% chance of spontaneous improvement (including arrested cases). Using radio-frequency thermal-coagulation techniques, more than 80% exhibited arrest of the retinopathy (Zervas, 1969). Pituitary ablation has no effect on nephropathy, neuropathy, peripheral vascular disease, and most cases of retinal detachment. Laser photocoagulation seals off leakage from microaneurysms and from sites of small hemorrhages and prevents the sequence of events leading to vitreous change. It obliterates neovascular tufts, thus preventing hemorrhage, and produces adhesions under the retina to prevent retinal tears and detachment.

Neuropathies

Diabetic neuropathy may be the initial clinical manifestation of diabetes, even in the absence of hyperglycemia, and occurs eventually in at least one half of all adult diabetic patients. It may appear abruptly when diabetes is brought under control. Transient symptoms may coincide with severe hyperglycemia. When adults eventually exhibit all three components of the "triopathy," the usual sequence is for the neuropathy to develop first, then retinopathy, and finally the nephropathy.

Pathogenesis. There is either myelin sheath degeneration (segmental demyelination) and/or angiopathy of the vasa nervorum. Small infarcts can occur within nerve trunks (ischemic mononeuropathy multiplex). The Schwann cells possess not only a thickened basement membrane but also the means for an inordinate turnover of the sorbitol pathway (polymeric fructose accumulation); the adlose reductase enzyme, which converts glucose to sorbitol, is localized to the Schwann cell.

Manifestations

CRANIAL NEUROPATHY. There may be an isolated palsy, complete or partial paralysis, and, uncommonly, bilateral involvement. The ophthalmoplegia of diabetes is benign, self-limited, and unassociated with pupillary changes. Symptoms include diplopia, orbital pain, and ipsilateral headache. Optic neuritis, transient unilateral papilledema, anisocoria, and changes resembling Argyll Robertson pupils have been described but usually do not occur with ophthalmoplegia. It is characteristic for third, fourth, sixth, and seventh nerve involvement to recover in less than 2½ months, but there may be recurrences. All cranial nerves have been involved in diabetes, except the first and twelfth nerves. Up to 40% of diabetic patients exhibiting ophthalmoplegia have a nondiabetic cause such as myasthenia gravis, Graves' disease, aneurysm, demyelinating disease, and tumor. Cerebral aneurysms frequently manifest pupillary changes with ophthalmoplegia, where as diabetic cranial neuropathy usually shows no pupillary involvement.

PERIPHERAL NEUROPATHY. *Sensory involvement* is usually symmetric and is more common in the lower extremities. Pain is the most outstanding symptom. It is usually of a shooting, sharp, boring, or crampy quality, usually improves partially, is characteristically worse at night, is aggravated by cold, and is alleviated by activity. One of the earliest findings is impairment of vibratory sense, often with diminished or absent deep tendon reflexes. Probably the most frequent peripheral nerve involved is the femoral, with pain, paresthesias, and tenderness along its pathway; stretching by extension of the thigh from the hip is painful.

Motor involvement is unilateral, appears early, and can be controlled with treatment of the diabetes. There is almost always a recovery in patients with pure foot drop. Motor changes can improve even in poorly controlled patients. In the upper extremity the most frequent manifestation of neuropathy is hand-muscle atrophy; in fact, unexplained interosseus atrophy should suggest the presence of diabetes. Isolated absence of the Achilles reflex is more common than subjective symptoms and is present in half of all patients with diabetes; patella areflexia is less common. Tenderness in the calves and thighs has been noted frequently. Sometimes mononeuropathies begin acutely and may cause muscle weakness and wasting, again usually asymmetrically. Improvement or recovery occurs in a few months to several years.

SPINAL INVOLVEMENT. Although cord changes are less pronounced than changes in peripheral nerves, occasionally the changes are severe even in the young patient. The process is diffuse, usually symmetric, and affects gray as well as white matter, resulting in atrophy of the cord, necrosis of the posterior columns, and fibrosis of the leptomeninges. Neurogenic atrophy of muscles may occur as can ataxia, spasticity, and sensory symptoms.

ENCEPHALOPATHY. Young patients with long-term diabetes develop degenerative diffuse cerebral disease that is often accompanied by angiopathies, pseudocalcinosis, and brain softening. Manifestations include mental impairment, sudden neurologic deficits (brain hemorrhage), vertigo, hemiparesis, slurred speech, and cerebellar ataxia.

VISCERAL (OR AUTONOMIC) NEUROPATHY. Diabetic enteropathy causes intermittent diarrhea productive of brown, watery stools. It is commonly accentuated postprandially and nocturnally and is often accompanied by fecal incontinence. Patients may have malabsorption and less commonly steatorrhea. Constipation may alternate with diarrhea. Frequently, but not necessarily, other autonomic and peripheral neuropathies are present. X-ray studies show a deficiency pattern of the small bowel, segmentation, and partial obliteration of folds; either slow or rapid transit may occur. Gastric atony with delayed emptying, reduced peristalsis, nausea, heartburn, vomiting, "bloating," and gastric dilatation may resemble the postvagotomy syndrome. Atony (paralysis) of the bladder and neurogenic vesicle obstruction may cause abnormal cystometrograms without abnormal residual urine. With advanced bladder neuropathy, pyuria and azotemia become associated with residual urine and occasionally with a marked increase in bladder capacity. The increased frequency of renal infection in diabetic patients may be caused by progressive decompensation of the neurologically involved bladder. There may be impaired vasomotor and pilomotor control (anhidrosis or drenching night sweats), disturbed heat regulation, dependent edema, orthostatic hypotension, tachycardia, retrograde ejaculation, and impotence. Impotence may affect the whole coital act or may be partial and limited to one or more components (libido, erection, orgasm, ejaculation).

TROPHIC CHANGES. The Charcot joint in diabetes primarily affects the tarsal, or ankle, joint and produces an edematous, deformed foot. Fragmentation and obliteration of the joint spaces is followed by marked destruction of joints and bones. Occasionally the changes resemble chronic osteomyelitis. Advanced osteoporosis of tarsal and metatarsal bones has been described as a complication of diabetic neuropathy. Neuropathic painless fractures occur in the tibia and fibula (minimal trauma plus bone changes). Trophic ulcers (mal perforans) are recurrent, persistent, frequently spontaneous, sharply demarcated, deep, and painless. Occasionally the earliest lesion is a bleb easily mistaken for a burn. Ulcers usually occur under the metatarsal and other pressure points of the plantar surface. If they are not traumatized, the prognosis for healing is excellent.

Laboratory findings. The cerebrospinal fluid protein is elevated in more than 80% of cases. Finding reduced motor nerve conduction velocity by electromyography may aid in making the diagnosis.

Differential diagnosis. Old people normally have progressive impairment of vibratory sense. The association of sensory symptoms, symmetric areflexia of the lower extremities, autonomic involvement, and high CSF protein strongly suggest diabetes. Psychotherapy and hypnosis can often relieve psychogenic impotence. Metastatic tumor, pernicious anemia, collagen vascular disease, cervical spondylosis, alcoholism, cerebral aneurysm, tabes, syringomyelia, herniated disk, myasthenia gravis, and Grave's disease must be ruled out.

Treatment. Treatment includes analgesics, local surgery, physiotherapy, antidiarrheal agents, antibiotics and steroids for diarrhea, orthopedic devices for Charcot joints, resection of internal vesical sphincter in some cases of neurogenic bladder, and avoidance of weight bearing and elimination of pressure points for neuropathic ulcers. In some cases strict diabetic control will be effective. Dilantin is sometimes used for the pain of neuropathy. The effectiveness of vitamin therapy and vitamin B_{12} by injection remains unproved but is frequently employed.

Nephropathy (glomerular)

Nodular glomerulosclerosis. The Kimmelstiel-Wilson lesion is probably specific for diabetes. It consists of spherical deposits of variable size of glycoprotein-laden PAS material in the mesangial region (intercapillary space) of the glomerulus. This lesion has been found occasionally by means of renal biopsy of prediabetic subjects but is less common than the diffuse form.

Diffuse glomerulosclerosis. The *diffuse* form of *glomerulosclerosis* is nonspecific, is seen in 50% to 90% of patients with diabetes, and refers to the increased deposition of PAS-positive material throughout the mesangium. It consists of a diffuse enlargement of the glomerular structure and a thickening of the capillary membrane. The basement membrane thickening parallels or follows, rather than precedes, mesangial deposition. This lesion, rather than the nodular type, is said to cause the nephrotic syndrome, although the diffuse and nodular often coexist.

Exudative glomerulosclerosis. Exudative glomerulosclerosis or "capsular drop" consists of characteristic localized deposits of acidophilic fibrinoid material into Bowman's space. It is a late finding mainly in the uremic stage.

Fibrin cap. The *fibrin cap* (lipohyalin lesion) is a nonspecific crescent in a capillary and is not as common as intercapillary glomerulosclerosis. The lesions may be spherical and resemble fibrinoid material. Diabetic glomerulosclerosis is the cause of death in over half of juvenile diabetic patients. Edema or albuminuria appearing in a patient with known diabetes should suggest the presence of glomerulosclerosis. Numerous other renal diseases occur in diabetes (see discussion on renal disorders).

Natural history. The average survival is 5 years after the onset of proteinuria; death occurs about 50 to 55 years of age. Only about 10% of patients with proteinuria and glomerulosclerosis manifest the nephrotic syndrome. Other causes of proteinuria are the nephrosclerosis of hypertension and pyelonephritis. Similarly edema in diabetic individuals is usually not nephrotic (and probably nonrenal). Besides edema, hypoproteinemia, 4+ proteinuria (4 to 5 grams of protein per day), doubly refractible "fat bodies" in urine, and hypercholesterolemia of the nephrotic syndrome, there is hypertension, azotemia, retinopathy, and rarely microscopic hematuria. Incomplete forms occur with milder consequences; occasionally slight proteinuria of many years' duration may not impair renal function. The serum cholesterol may be normal. The apparent amelioration of diabetes with onset of nephropathy consists only of a reduction in insulin requirement (prolongation of half-life of circulating insulin). The vascular disease does not improve. There is ordinarily no quantitative relationship between the severity of glomerulosclerosis and the insulin requirement. Glomerulosclerosis is found in nondiabetic siblings and in patients whose diabetes springs from hemochromatosis or pancreatitis.

Therapy. Therapy is symptomatic and usually ineffective. It includes diuretics, antihypertensives, transfusions for anemia, therapy for hypocalcemia, low protein diet, dialysis, autotransplantation, and prevention of infection and ketosis.

Arteriosclerosis

Premature, rapidly progressive arteriosclerosis is more prevalent in a diabetic than in a nondiabetic population. The incidence of intimal fibrosis, with medial hypertrophy and hyalinization of intramural vessels, is double that of nondiabetic subjects, but atherosclerosis (plaque formation) may be increased only in the obese and/or hypertensive diabetic patient. Hyperlipemia and diabetic microangiopathy (of vasa vasorum) may be important factors. There is a predilection for involvement of peripheral vessels (anterior and posterior tibial arteries) whereas in nondiabetic subjects the large vesels (femoral, popliteal) are more extensively affected. Arteriolosclerosis involves larger vessels than those involved with microangiopathy and shows intimal concentric fibrosis, PAS-negative material, and medial hypertrophy and hyalinization.

Coronary artery disease. Ischemic heart disease is the leading cause of death in adult diabetic patients and the male to female ratio is equal. In coronary heart disease fully 65% of cases show abnormalities of carbohydrate metabolism, and many are unrecognized cases of diabetes.

Peripheral vascular disease. Diabetic patients frequently suffer vascular occlusion of the popliteal and tibial arteries, and gangrene is far more prevalent than in the nondiabetic population. The dorsalis pedis pulse is palpable in 20% of cases of gangrene, attesting to the contribution of microangiopathy. Features of the diabetic foot include the following:

1. Diabetic neuropathy favors unrecognized local infection from painless trauma.

2. Traumatic and infectious lesions are more likely to occur than when vascular occlusion affects the nondiabetic subject.

3. Females are as prone to gangrene as males.

4. Arterial calcification is frequent in cases with gangrene.

5. Corns, calluses, and paronychia are frequent sources of infection and lead to cellulitis and gangrene.

6. Juxta-articular osteolysis, loss of tips of distal phalanges, and osteomyelitis can occur. Osteoporosis indicates sufficient arterial supply to permit bone resorption, whereas opacification suggests ischemic necrosis.

7. Associated pathology (gout, Charcot joint, neurotrophic ulcer) and complications (thrombophlebitis, pulmonary emboli, osteomyelitis). In cases involving amputation for gangrene the 5-year mortality exceeds 50%. Gangrene occurs in the other leg in almost half of all cases.

Renal disorders

1. Necrotizing papillitis occurs in obstructive uropathy, phenacetin abuse, and diabetes. The lesion, frequently associated with pyelonephritis, is often bilateral. Localized to the medulla, it is a rapid process resulting in separation of the necrotic tissue with sloughing off into the urine. Symptoms are similar to pyelonephritis except that they are more sudden in onset and involve more hematuria, more severe renal colic, fever, vomiting, chills, and azotemia. An early radiologic sign is raggedness of the calyx. Treatment is the same as that for pyelonephritis. Occasionally it is necessary to surgically remove the necrotic papilla when it obstructs the lower ureter.

2. Pyelonephritis and urinary tract infection are further renal disorders. About 30% of diabetic patients have asymptomatic bacilluria. Females and patients confined to bed are particularly susceptible. Factors predisposing to urinary infection include catheterization, incomplete emptying of the bladder (neuropathy), and the vulvovaginitis associated with glycosuria. Bacteriuria can usually, in time, be equated with pyelonephritis. The incidence of significant bacteriuria following a single bladder catheterization in nondiabetic females is about 8%. During pregnancy the incidence of bacteriuria is 15% to 35%; many of the episodes are acute pyelonephritis.

3. Multiple renal abscesses (cortical as well as medullary) and perinephric abscesses.

4. Glycogen nephrosis (Armanni-Ebstein nephropathy) consists of vacuolization of the epithelial cells of the proximal convoluted tubule, unassociated with any clinical manifestations.

5. Efferent arteriosclerosis is almost specific for diabetes.

6. Fibrinoid necrosis is found in the small vessels (without malignant hypertension or collagen disease).

7. Among hypertensive subjects with renal arterial stenosis, 40% have diabetes.

Skin disorders

1. Furuncles, carbuncles, and staphylococcus infection.

2. Necrobiosis lipoidica diabeticorum is more common in females. There is a predilection for the shins. The lesions show an ivory-yellow center with red or violet periphery laced with telangiectasis. One half the patients have diabetes that may precede or follow the lesions. Histologically both the collagen and small blood vessels are involved.

3. Diabetic dermopathy (shin spots, "spotted leg" syndrome) refers to multiple, atrophied, circumscribed, usually brownish lesions of the lower extremity. There is a predilection for males. It is a characteristic but not specific lesion in diabetes.

4. Scleredema diabeticorcum is a persistent hardening of the skin, usually of the back, due to excess dermal collagen and acid mucopolysaccharide.

5. Rubeosis (flushed face) occurs in almost 50% of all long-term diabetic patients.

6. Xanthelasma.

7. Acute eruptive xanthomatosis is a rare but well-recognized complication.

8. Dermatitis gangrenosa.

9. Dupuytren's contracture.

10. Hirsutism in diabetic individuals of Mediterranean origin has been called Achard-Thiers syndrome.

11. Werner's syndrome.

12. Dermatophytosis. Fungus infections include onychomycosis (*Candida albicans*), genital mycosis, and erythrasma (involving groins, axillae, and trunk).

13. Generalized pruritus.

14. Insulin lipodystrophy, atrophy, and hypertrophy. The atrophy of subcutaneous fat may occur at sites *distant* from areas of injection and may symmetrically follow the cutaneous nerve supply.

15. The lipodystrophy of Seip-Lawrence.

16. Carotinosis is yellow discoloration of the skin due to impaired conversion of carotene to vitamin A (xanthochromia).

17. One out of 4 patients with porphyria cutanea tarda has diabetes.

Eye disorders

There are transitory refractive changes, cataracts in 50% to 75% of patients, night blindness, lipemia retinalis, glaucoma, wrinkling of the posterior surface of the cornea, and weakness of accommodation. The onset of a relative myopia with blood glucose increase and a relative hyperopia with a glucose reduction is caused by osmolar changes. Senile cataracts resemble those found in subjects without diabetes but occur earlier and with greater frequency. The metabolic cataract occurs in juvenile diabetic patients, develops rapidly, is subcapsular (rather than central), appears as a snowflake-like flocculation, and may disappear spontaneously.

Mouth

There are periodontal infections, gingivitis with pocket formation, and alveolar destruction with mobility of teeth.

Parotid gland

Asymptomatic bilateral enlargement occurs rarely and often precedes the recognition of the diabetes.

Gastrointestinal system (other than the visceral neuropathies)

There is a higher incidence of cholecystitis and cholecystitis emphysematosa (usually nonclostridial), cholelithiasis, and pancreatitis. Other complications include gallbladder hypotony, fatty infiltration of the liver, glycogen-laden liver (hepatomegaly), and megasigmoid.

Bones

Almost 50% of patients with infected leg ulcers have at least radiologic evidence of osteomyelitis underlying the skin infections.

Genitourinary system

There may be cystitis emphysematosa, calcification of the vas deferens, pneumaturia, and vulvovaginitis.

Miscellaneous

Hypertension is prevalent among patients with diabetes because both are mutual manifestations of such diseases as pheochromocytoma, Cushing's syndrome, and primary aldosteronism and because diabetes predisposes to numerous renal diseases (glomerulosclerosis, renal arteriosclerosis, pyelonephritis), which then cause hypertension. Then too, widespread microangiopathy increases peripheral resistance. There is a heightened susceptibility to many infections, particularly when the blood sugar level is not stabilized. Idiopathic intermittent edema in females may be a sign of early diabetes.

HYPOGLYCEMIA

Hypoglycemia is a clinical syndrome elicited by a reduced blood sugar concentration. In adults the level is usually below 50 mg./100 ml., whereas in the newborn it may be below 30 mg./100 ml.; in low birth weight, often premature, infant values may be less than 20 mg./100 ml. The causative factors of hypoglycemia are outlined below .

Organic
  Neoplasms
    Pancreatic islet cell adenoma and rarely beta cell hyperplasia
    Pancreatic islet cell carcinoma
    Extrapancreatic tumors
  Hepatic diseases
    Hepatitis (only in severe cases and rarely)
    Cirrhosis
    Hereditary enzyme defects (Table 19-4)
    Chronic venous congestion (rarely)
    Fatty infiltration
      "White liver disease" (usually infants with metabolic acidosis, uremia, and cerebral edema of unknown cause)
      Kwashiorkor
    Primary malignancy—it is controversial that secondary metastatic malignancy to the liver causes hypoglycemia
    Biliary disease (rarely and not particularly in severe cases)
    Hepatotoxins: urethane, phosphorus, chloroform, neoarsphenamine, mushrooms, cinchophen, hypoglycin (from the unripened akee plant used as a "bush tea," see under the miscellaneous part of this outline) and alcohol
  Hypopituitarism, including isolated growth hormone deficiency
  Hypoadrenocortical function
  Congenital adrenal hyperplasia (defective synthesis of cortisol)
  Adrenomedullary deficiency (rare cases of diminished release of epinephrine)
  Central nervous system lesions, for example, cerebral damage in childhood, but the evidence is not convincing
  Starvation (fasting hypoglycemia but without a pathologic lesion)
  Pancreatic disease—acute or chronic pancreatitis, atresia of the pancreatic duct
  Hypothyroidism
  Alpha cell deficiency (hypoglucagonosis)
  Sudden diarrhea
Functional (no histopathologic lesion)
  Idiopathic reactive hypoglycemia
  Early diabetes mellitus
  Alimentary (postgastrectomy, dumping syndrome)
  Reactive hypoglycemia in asthma, intestinal helminthiasis, multiple sclerosis, renal glycosuria, mental depression, epilepsy, narcolepsy, cyclic edema, and tobacco toxicity (Marks and Rose, 1965)
  Neonatal and childhood hypoglycemias—infants of diabetic mothers, ketotic hypoglycemia, leucine sensitivity, etc.
  Strenuous muscular work—not convincing as a cause of hypoglycemia (in fact, slight hyperglycemia has been known to occur)
Chemically induced hypoglycemia
  Insulin, for example, factitious hypoglycemia
  Salicylates
  Alcohol (ethyl and methyl)
  Potentiation of oral sulfonylurea drugs by Dicumarol and phenylbutazone
  Ganglion-blocking agents, for example, propranolol
  Monamine-oxidase inhibitors
    Hydrazines—phenelzine, pheniprazine, isocarboxazid, mebanazine, iproniazid, nialamide
    Nonhydrazine—tranylcypromine
  Miscellaneous—methandienone, phentolamine (Regitine), human growth hormone (early), ethacrynic acid, intravenous potassium in the treatment of familial periodic paralysis and hypoglycin (α-aminomethylenecyclopropanepropionic acid) from unripened fruit causing Jamaican vomiting sickness
Artifactual—in leukemia as a result of the glycolytic WBC

The symptoms depend to a large extent on the speed of the blood sugar fall, the degree of hypoglycemia, and the age of the individual. In most cases of spontane-

Table 19-4. Hereditary enzyme diseases

Name	Enzyme involved	Organ	Comments
Galactosemia	Galactose-1-phosphate-uridyl transferase	Liver	Hypoglycemia follows ingestion of galactose
Hereditary fructose intolerance	1-Phosphofructaldolase	Liver	Hypoglycemia follows ingestion of fructose and is not connected with glucagon
Familial fructose and galactose intolerance (Dormandy's syndrome)	Not known		Hypoglycemia follows ingestion of either hexose
Types of glycogen storage diseases			
Von Gierke's disease	Glucose-6-phosphatase	Liver and kidney	Fasting hypoglycemia; diminished hyperglycemic response to catecholamine or glucagon
Pompe's disease	α-Glucosidase	Generalized	Usually no hypoglycemia
Forbes' disease (limit dextrinosis)	Amylo-1,6-glycosidase (debrancher enzyme)	Liver, heart muscle, and WBC	Fasting hypoglycemia
Andersen's disease (amylopectinosis)	Amylo-4,6-transglucosidase (brancher)	Liver	Fasting hypoglycemia is mild or infrequent
McCardle's syndrome	Muscle phosphorylase	Muscle	No hypoglycemia
Hers' disease	Liver phosphorylase	Liver and WBC	Occasional hypoglycemia; hypoglycemia follows use of catecholamines or glucagon
Glycogen synthetase deficiency	Glycogen synthetase	Liver	Fasting hypoglycemia

ous hypoglycemia the glucose concentration is 30 mg. or less per 100 ml. The symptoms include loss of consciousness, confusion, weakness, sweating, fever, amnesia, abdominal pain, hypothermia, localizing neurologic abnormalities (hemiplegia, paraplegia), mental depression, apathy, and hysteria. Tetany and psychosis may be simulated. Prolonged hypoglycemia may produce neuronal damage. Prolonged and often irreversible coma may result. Bilateral and complete necrosis of the cerebral cortex has been described. Hypoglycemia can also, albeit rarely, precipitate angina or myocardial infarction.

Diagnosis

The diagnosis must be verified by finding a low blood glucose concentration. The glucose tolerance test will not distinguish organic from functional hypoglycemia and only occasionally provokes hypoglycemia. A prolonged fast may cause hypoglycemia in insulinoma, whereas a high carbohydrate meal or the administration of glucose may provoke mild hypoglycemia. The intravenous tolbutamide test uses Orinase Diagnostic (1 Gm.), and plasma insulin is measured. Values show an initially higher level and a characteristically more delayed rise with a sustained elevation in functioning islet cell tumors than either in normal subjects or in patients with reactive hypoglycemia; however, finding normal plasma insulin levels after I.V. tolbutamide does not rule out insulinoma. Also, patients with an islet cell tumor have glucose values below 35 mg./ 100 ml. after tolbutamide that are maintained for three hours, but the glucose pattern is nonspecific compared to the insulin results. Using the glucose determinations alone, false positives can occur in the presence of severe liver disease, sarcomas, undernutrition, and alcoholism. Glucagon and leucine provocative tests are less sensitive and less specific than the tolbutamide test, although the leucine test is less likely to induce severe hypoglycemia. The glucagon test may in fact cause a paradoxical

hypoglycemia in patients with islet cell tumors. In adults a marked drop in blood glucose (more than 25 mg./100 ml.) and a large rise in insulin levels (over 25 μU./ ml.) after leucine strongly suggests insulinoma, but a negative response does not rule out insulinoma.

Pancreatic islet cell tumors

A few well-documented cases of diffuse islet cell hyperplasia have been reported, but the majority are caused by benign adenomas, 32% of which are in the tail of the pancreas and 27% in the head. Multiple adenomas are found in 13%. Ectopic adenomas occur in 2% in such locations as the duodenum, hilus of the spleen, or posterior aspect of the pancreas. Adenomas of other endocrine organs, such as parathyroids, adrenal, or anterior pituitary may accompany insulinomas and are frequently familial. In addition, the Zollinger-Ellison syndrome may occur. Some islet cell tumors rarely are accompanied by severe diarrhea and hypokalemia. The non–beta cell pancreatic tumors contain gastrin.

The symptoms provoked by functioning islet cell tumors are protean. Attacks are usually unrelated to meals. The demonstration of Whipple's triad (fasting hypoglycemia, symptoms associated with low blood glucose, relief by glucose administration) is no longer considered diagnostic since hepatic disease, pituitary and adrenal insufficiency, alcohol ingestion, and nonendocrine tumors can produce a similar triad. Although the GTT is not a reliable test, a flat hypoglycemic curve at approximately the third to the fifth hour is characteristic. A diabetic curve may be seen before and after surgery; rarely, proved cases of adenomas have exhibited no fasting hypoglycemia, a flat curve or a curve similar to hepatogenous hypoglycemia, and hypoglycemia occurring several hours after a test meal. Although a high fasting plasma insulin may aid in differentiating a functioning islet cell adenoma from a fibrosarcoma, the insulin level may be normal in about one third of cases of pancreatic adenoma. Preoperative angiography of the celiac axis sometimes localizes the tumor, but this procedure is not without risk.

Although numerous drugs are available for raising the blood sugar, surgical removal is the treatment of choice. If at operation a careful search does not reveal the tumor, partial pancreatic resection is carried out. Temporary hyperglycemia may follow removal of the adenoma.

Malignant insulinomas comprise 20% of all secreting islet cell tumors and are usually slow growing; survival with known metastasis for 25 years has been observed. Antimitotic agents may be effective and diazoxide, ACTH, steroids, human growth hormone, and glucagon are used for palliation. However, even in the presence of metastasis it may be helpful to remove insulin-producing tissue to minimize the hypoglycemia.

Extrapancreatic tumors

About 250 cases of hypoglycemia caused by nonendocrine tumors have been reported. The theoretical mechanisms of the hypoglycemia include overuse of glucose by the neoplasm, deficient liver gluconeogenesis (impaired glucose-6-phosphatase and fructose-1,6-diphosphatase), insulin-like material secreted by the tumor, and suppression of physiologic insulin antagonists. The tumors are usually large, slow-growing mesothelial lesions (fibromas, sarcomas, fibrosarcomas) that arise in the thoracic or retroperitoneal area. Generally they do not produce high fasting insulin levels, and there is little response to oral glucose or intravenous tolbutamide. The differential diagnosis includes a coexisting insulinoma, a large epithelial tumor in the abdomen metastasizing to the liver, and a malignant insulinoma.

Hepatic disease

Almost all forms of liver disease (Table 19-4) have caused hypoglycemia. However, there may be only laboratory evidence of hepatic dysfunction. Typically, the GTT shows a low fasting glucose followed by a hyperglycemic curve with a fall to hypoglycemia 4 to 7 hours later. Occasionally, patients are erroneously diagnosed as having hepatic coma rather than hypoglycemia. Patients with liver cirrhosis may give a false-positive result because the tolbutamide test (probably because of prolongation of the half-life of tolbutamide) can induce hypoglycemia almost as severe as in insulinomas. The hypoglycemia in the glycogen storage diseases is ascribable to the unavailability of glucose from glycogen. Thereapy includes treatment of the underlying liver disease and a high protein–high carbohydrate diet. Diazoxide has been helpful.

Idiopathic reactive hypoglycemia (functional hyperinsulinism)

There is hypoglycemia 2 to 4 hours after a meal and postprandial hyperinsulinism. Convulsions or loss of consciousness is rare.

The disorder does not become progressively worse as in insulinoma and may spontaneously disappear. The mechanism is one of an excessive response to the normal stimulus for insulin secretion by hypersensitive, histologicaly normal islet cells. Although the etiology is unknown, most patients are hyperkinetic, tense, and anxious. Occasionally repeated 5-hour GTT is necessary to document the hypoglycemia in otherwise characteristic cases. The response to 1 Gm. I.V. tolbutamide is recovery to nearly normal glucose within 90 minutes after the initial fall in glucose.

Therapy includes a high protein–low carbohydrate diet preferably divided into 6 feedings. Occasionally this aggravates the condition, apparently because the protein induces further attacks; however, leucine or arginine sensitivity is not responsible. The sulfonylurea drugs are paradoxically effective, probably because they stimulate a more smooth insulin release. Anticholinergic drugs may be helpful. Coffee, alcohol, tobacco, and stress should be avoided.

Hypoglycemia of early diabetes

Hypoglycemia is now well established as a feature of early diabetes. The hyperinsulinism contributes to obesity by promoting an increased appetite and by its lipogenic mechanisms. The implication is that the obesity therefore may be a manifestation of the diabetes (Faludi et al., 1968). Since this variety of hypoglycemia may not appear until the fourth to fifth hour of the GTT, a 5-hour test should be done. Although the hypoglycemia is typically postprandial, rarely there may be a fasting component even late in the course of diabetes. The impaired initial insulin response to a glucose meal in early diabetes results in a prolonged hyperglycemic stress on the beta cell; this burden precipitates an exaggerated, albeit delayed, insulin response at a time when the blood sugar is starting to fall, resulting in a precipitous drop in glucose. Plasma insulin determinations during the GTT are helpful because there is a delayed peak of plasma insulin in early diabetic hypoglycemia.

Hypoglycemia in infants and children

Neonatal hypoglycemia. The majority of cases in the newborn have transient idiopathic hypoglycemia. The oral GTT is of little value.

1. Persistent or recurrent neonatal hypoglycemia—liver glycogenoses, fructose intolerance, galactosemia, lactose-induced hypoglycemia, inherited disorders of amino acid metabolism, hormonal abnormalities, leucine sensitivity, the "infant giant," and mesothelial tumors.

2. Transient neonatal hypoglycemia

a. Infants of diabetic mothers: The majority are asymptomatic and the blood glucose rises to normal by 4 to 8 hours after birth. The mechanism is probably hyperinsulinism, but the hypoglycemia occurs while fasting. Hypoglycemic agents given to the mother occasionally cause neonatal hypoglycemia. Treatment is I.V. 10% fructose given to the mother 2 to 3 hours before delivery (0.25 to 0.5 Gm./kg./hr.).

b. Idiopathic neonatal hypoglycemia (transient): This form is among the commonest causes of hypoglycemia.

The majority of infants have low birth weight and manifestations occur 12 to 72 hours after parturition while fasting. They have a reduced store of glycogen and a relatively large brain.

c. Miscellaneous—maternal hyperthyroidism, CNS hemorrhage or injury, adrenal hemorrhage, and cold injury.

Idiopathic hypoglycemia of childhood.

1. Ketotic hypoglycemia is the commonest type of idiopathic hypoglycemia in the age group 1 to 5 years and is characterized by acetonuria, hypoglycemia and convulsions (especially while fasting), spontaneous improvement or complete remission, and some degree of mental deficiency. There is a diminished quantity of subcutaneous fat. Diazoxide is used with the occasional need of other benzothiadiazine drugs for enhancement of the hyperglycemia.

2. Leucine sensitivity (McQuarrie's syndrome, idiopathic familial hypoglycemia) occurs usually at the age of 6 to 12 months, when infants are switched to cow's milk. There results increasingly severe attacks of clouding of consciousness leading eventually to convulsions. When it occurs after 4 years of age and particularly in adults, the possibility of an underlying islet cell adenoma arises. Symptoms may occur during fasting or after leucine or arginine ingestion. The disorder usually regresses by the age of 6 to 10 years. There is commonly a family history of diabetes. Early recognition of leucine sensitivity is important since two thirds of the infants have subsequent mental retardation and neurologic deficits. Leucine increases insulin secretion and is known to decrease hepatic gluconeogenesis.

Therapy includes humanized milk, long-acting zinc glucagon, diazoxide, or sodium glutamate. High carbohydrate supplements are given 20 to 30 minutes after meals and at bed time.

Other causes of childhood hypoglycemia.

1. Poisonings—salicylate, phosphorus, insecticides, alcohol.

2. Severe malnutrition, for example,

kwashiorkor, restrictive diets in phenyl-ketonuria, "white liver disease" (that is, the wet-brain, fatty liver syndrome).

Alimentary hypoglycemia (tachyalimentation)

Postgastrectomy hypoglycemia occurs usually 1 to 3 hours after eating. Initially there is an elevated blood glucose level of 200 to 300 mg./100 ml. that stimulates a prompt release of insulin. The high glucose levels arise from the rapid delivery of ingested carbohydrate into the small intestine, followed by rapid absorption.

Therapy includes oral hypoglycemic agents and a diet similar to that recommended for idiopathic reactive hypoglycemia. Anticholinergic agents occasionally are helpful.

Alcohol hypoglycemia

Hypoglycemia can be induced by ethanol ingestion after a 2- to 3-day preliminary fast, but in susceptible people hypoglycemic coma commonly appears within 12 hours. It is not corrected by glucagon. There may be an increased formation of α-glycerophosphate and long-chain fatty acids; the resulting formation of triglyceride accounts for the fatty infiltration of the liver in alcoholism. There is metabolic acidosis and lacticemia. The tolbutamide test results simulate islet cell tumor, causing confusion in diagnosis. There is no increase in immunoreactive insulin. Signs of liver damage are only occasionally present.

Diazoxide therapy

Diazoxide has been useful in the dosage range of 50 to 600 mg./day in controlling the hypoglycemia in islet cell adenoma, pancreatic carcinoma and hyperplasia, ex-trapancreatic neoplasma, hepatic hypoglycemia (including the glycogen storage diseases and hepatotoxic disorders), leucine sensitivity, hypopituitarism, and insulin shock. It has been utilized particularly when hypoglycemia is not satisfactorily controlled by diet, glucagon, and glucocorticoids. The mechanisms by which diazoxide induces hyperglycemia are not fully understood. Side effects include hirsutism, which usually disappears several weeks after termination of the drug, gastric symptoms (anorexia, nausea, vomiting), edema, tachycardia, hyperuricemia, dermatitis (pruritus and erythematous eruption), drug-induced fever, decreased plasma immunoglobulins, and ketoacidosis.

REFERENCES

Davis, M. D.: In Kimura, S. J., and Caygill, W. M., editors: Vascular complications of diabetes mellitus, St. Louis, 1967, The C. V. Mosby Co., p. 139.

Faludi, G., et al.: Ann. N. Y. Acad. Sci. **148:** 868, 1968.

Gitlin, L., et al.: Pediatrics, **35:**65, 1965.

Gordon, P., and Roth, J.: Arch. Intern. Med. **123:**237, 1969.

Jervell, I., and Vallance-Owen, J.: Lancet **2:**21, 1967.

Kimmelstiel, P., et al.: Amer. J. Clin. Path. **45:**21, 1966.

Levy, R. I., and Glueck, C. J.: Arch. Intern. Med. **123:**220, 1969.

*Marks, V., and Rose, F. C.: Hypoglycemia, Philadelphia, 1965, F. A. Davis Co.

Pedersen, J.: The pregnant diabetic and her newborn, Baltimore, 1967, The Williams and Wilkins Co., p. 146.

Randle, P. J., et al.: The glucose-fatty acid cycle. In Leibel, B. S., and Wrenshall, G. A., editors: On the nature and treatment of diabetes, Amsterdam, 1965, Excerpta Medica Foundation, International Congress Ser. no. 84, p. 361.

Steiner, D. F., et al.: Diabetes **17:**725, 1968.

*Significant reviews.

Chapter 20

Female endocrinology—the ovary and menstrual disorders

Bernard A. Eskin, M.D.*

PHYSIOLOGY OF THE MENSTRUAL CYCLE

The menstrual cycle comprises three interrelated sequences: (1) hypothalamic-pituitary-ovarian, (2) ovarian-endometrial, and (3) ovarian–secondary sexual tissue.

Hypothalamic-pituitary-ovarian cycle

Luteinizing hormone releasing factor (LRF) and follicle-stimulating hormone releasing factor (FRF) of hypothalamic origin reach the adenohypophysis via the hypophysial portal circulation and provoke the release of FSH and LH. The cycle starts when FSH (p. 43) is released and stimulates follicular maturation. LH probably acts in concert with FSH to release estrogen. When the ratio of FSH to LH becomes optimal, the mature ovum is released from the ovary. LH then acts on the residual cells in the erupted graafian follicle to form a corpus luteum that secretes both progesterone and estrogen. If the ovum is not fertilized, nidation in the uterus does not follow. Progesterone feedback to the hypothalamus and estrogen effect on both hypothalamus and pituitary cause a falling gonadotrophin level, with a subsequent sharp drop in estrogen and progesterone resulting in menstruation.

*Grateful acknowledgment is made to Dr. S. Leon Israel for his advice and criticism of the manuscript.

Ovary

Ovaries are paired ovoid bodies, each consisting of a cortex that contains follicles in various stages surrounded by a stroma. Internally, there is a medulla of loose connective tissue, elastin and smooth muscle fibers, and one hilar area composed of blood vessels, lymphatics, and nerves. The principle functions of the ovaries are the cyclic release of ova and the production of estrogen and progesterone. Embryologically, the human ovum (oocyte) is thought to migrate by ameboid motion to the mesenchyme of the mesenephric coelomic folds where mitotic division of the oocyte ceases. There follows encirclement by cells of the area, creating the primordial follicles. The lifetime supply of oocytes is approximately 500,000 cells and is present at birth.

At puberty, the hypothalamus matures and FRF stimulates the anterior pituitary to produce FSH. Although most of the follicles become atretic, a dominant follicle grows by the multiplication of its granulosa and theca layers, with an enlargement of the ovum, and by the accumulation of an estrogen-rich fluid. This fluid results from the degeneration of some granulosa cells. The ovum assumes an eccentric position in the follicle and becomes completely ensconced by a mass of proliferating granulosa cells, the discus proligerus. The inner cells of the discus

359

are so arranged that the long axis of each is radially directed, forming the corona radiata. At the same time, stromal cells condense about the growing follicle, where they acquire a capillary plexus and multiply to form the theca interna. All such theca cells, whether from the follicle destined to ovulate or from the follicles that become atretic, secrete estrogen. Estrogen causes further proliferation of the follicle and stimulates the release of increasing quantities of LH; this shift in the FSH:LH ratio accounts for ovulation.

Histologically, the theca interna consists of loosely arranged polygonal cells with vacuolated cytoplasm and vesicular nuclei, rich in lymphatics and capillaries. There are also smaller cells with small hypochromatic nuclei and eosinophilic cytoplasm called K cells because of a presumed high content of ketosteroids. Their exact origin and purpose is unknown, although it has been suggested that they secrete progesterone. They appear in the theca interna near the time of ovulation and invade the granulosa layer during luteinization. The theca externa, the outermost and probably nonsecretory portion of the condensed stromal cells, melds gradually into the surrounding stroma, although it is more prominent as the follicle enlarges.

After ovulation, the group of maturing follicles become atretic and eventually disappear. The liberated oocyte directly enters the fimbriated opening of the fallopian tube. Approximately midway down the tube fertilization may occur. The sperm coursing through the cervix and uterus is probably assisted both mechanically and enzymatically to its final rendezvous with the ovum. Following ovulation, the walls of the ruptured follicle collapse with an insignificant diapedesis of erythrocytes into the newly formed corpus luteum. This small gray structure begins its growth when the granulosa cells rapidly proliferate to form an orderly layer of large carotin-containing epitheloid cells, the luteum cells. The latter is quickly invaded by V-shaped capillary-laden extensions from the theca interna, the cells of which are also luteinized, constituting the paralutein cells. Within a few days, the well-vascularized corpus luteum, consisting for the most part of fat-laden polyhedral cells that secrete both estrogen and progesterone, is completed.

If the ovum is not fertilized, there is no trophoblast to produce very high levels of chorionic gonadotrophin, most of which is LH. Without the luteotrophic activity of LH, the corpus luteum degenerates about 4 to 5 days prior to menses by a process of cellular vascularization and hyalinization, forming a homogeneous mass, the corpus albicans. The surrounding ovarian stroma invades the corpus albicans, reducing it to a small scarlike area. If the ovum is fertilized and securely embedded, trophoblastic secretions maintain the corpus luteum for about 3 months as the corpus luteum of pregnancy. This important secretory body elaborates estrogen and progesterone.

Estrogen

The three major natural estrogens are estradiol-17β, estrone, and estriol (Fig. 20-1). Several pathways of steroidogenic biosynthesis have been traced in the ovary (Fig. 20-2). It has been shown that homogenates of follicular cells readily convert progesterone to estrone and estradiol-17β, but homogenates of luteal tissue manufacture androstenedione and no estrogen. Thecal cells in humans are capable of complete cycle to androgen and estrogen, whereas granulosa cells produce progesterone predominantly. If the biosynthetic pathway in the ovary is abnormal because of genetic or acquired abnormalities of the converting enzymes, estrogen synthesis may be impaired and diverted to the production of androgens, including testosterone.

Estrogen metabolism. During menstruation the total estrogen (estradiol-17β, estrone, and estriol) ranges from 4 to 22 μg./24 hr., gradually rises to a peak of 35 to 100 μg./24 hr. just prior to ovula-

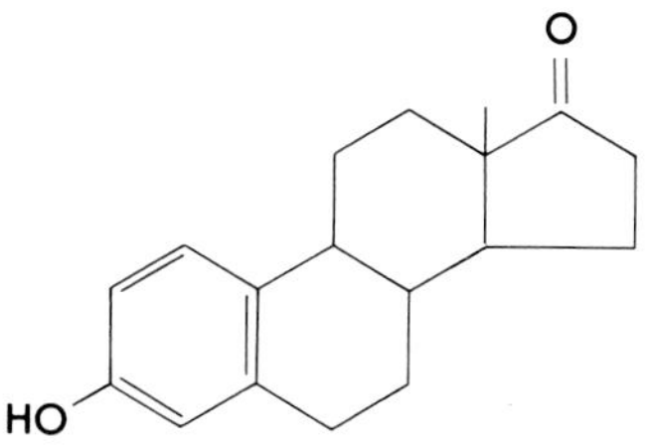

Estrone

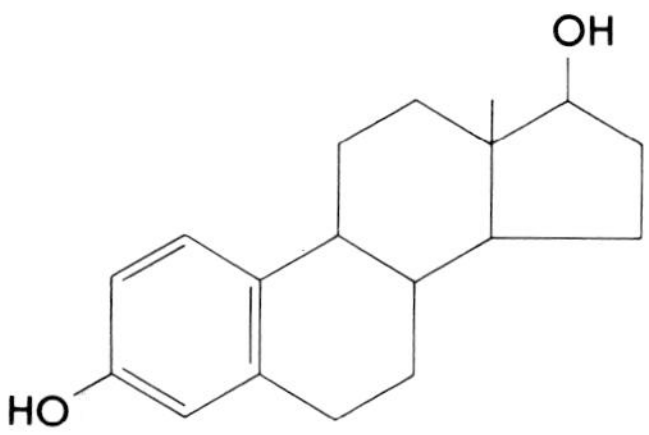

Estradiol-17β

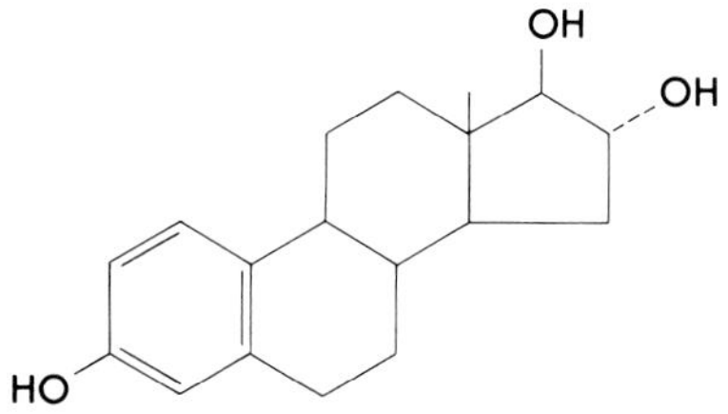

Estriol

Natural estrogens

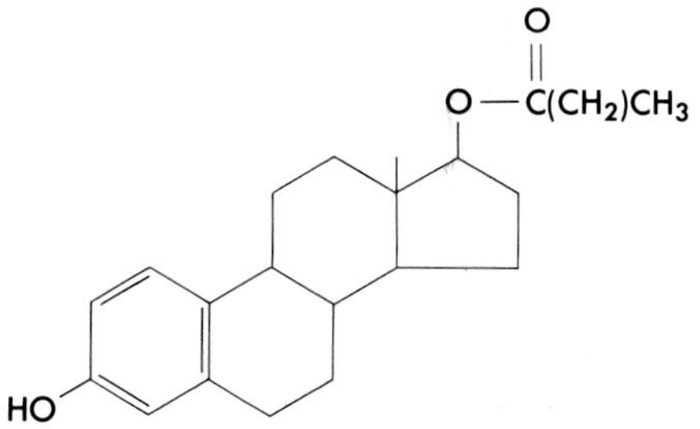

Estradiol valerate

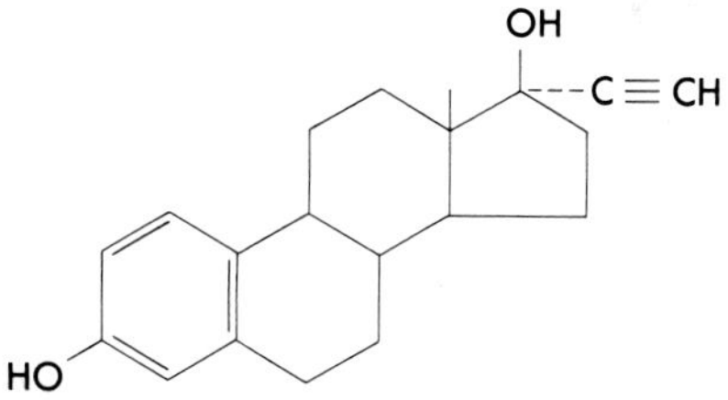

Ethinyl estradiol

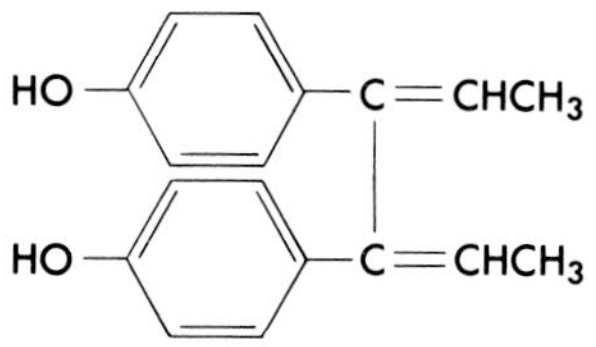

Dienestrol

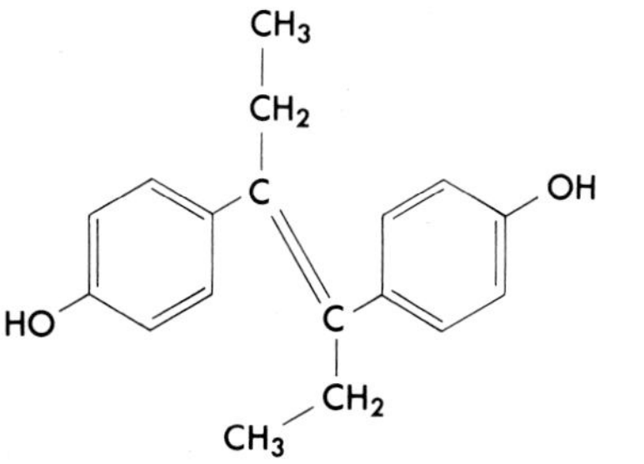

Diethylstilbestrol

Synthetic estrogens

Fig. 20-1. Some natural and synthetic estrogens.

tion, and falls again 24 to 48 hours prior to menstruation. The normal range varies widely both with each woman and with each month. During pregnancy, the concentration of estrogen in the blood and urine greatly increases. Estrogen in the blood is bound to a beta globulin. It is excreted by the kidneys as a water-soluble sulfate or glucuronide conjugate derived from the liver. The total quantity of estro-

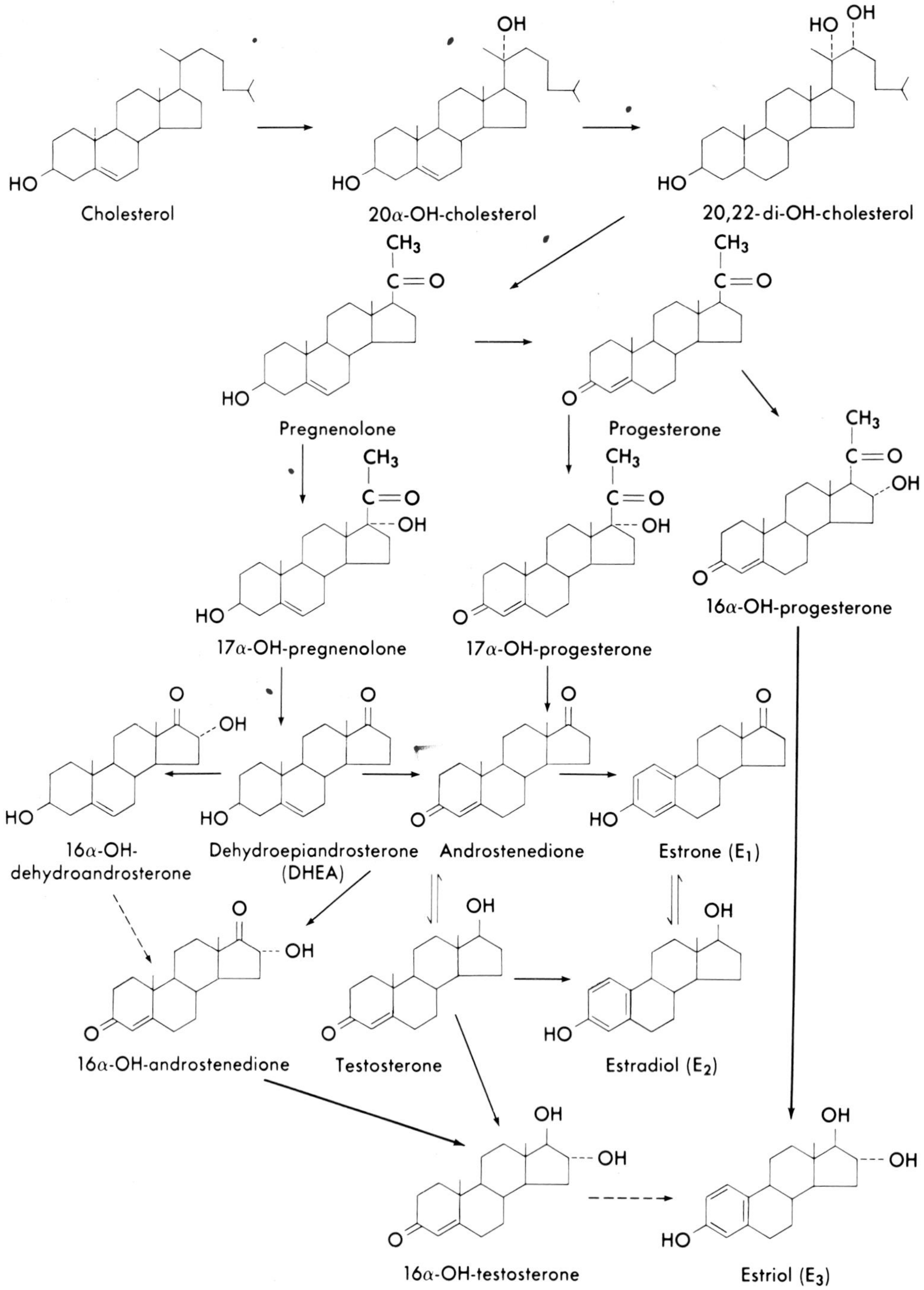

Fig. 20-2. Biosynthetic pathways in the ovary.

gen excreted following its oral or I.M. administration is not more than 50% and is highest in the first 24 hours. The release of estrogen from the enterohepatic circulation is slowed, causing a latent period of 2 to 4 days before excretion again occurs. The liver removes estrogen from the blood and conjugates approximately one half the total to favor renal excretion; the bound remainder circulates through the enterohepatic circulation. For a review of ovarian steroidogenesis see Savard et al., 1965. Ribonucleic acid (RNA) extracted from estrogen-stimulated cells is capable of initiating morphologic changes in the endometrium characteristic of estrogen itself. Hence, estrogens may activate the process of protein synthesis through RNA mechanisms, though the precise molecular mechanism is unknown.

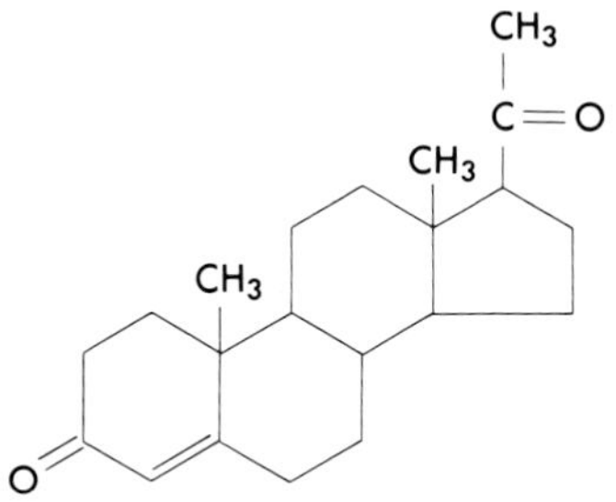

Progesterone

Progesterone derivatives

Medroxyprogesterone acetate (Provera)

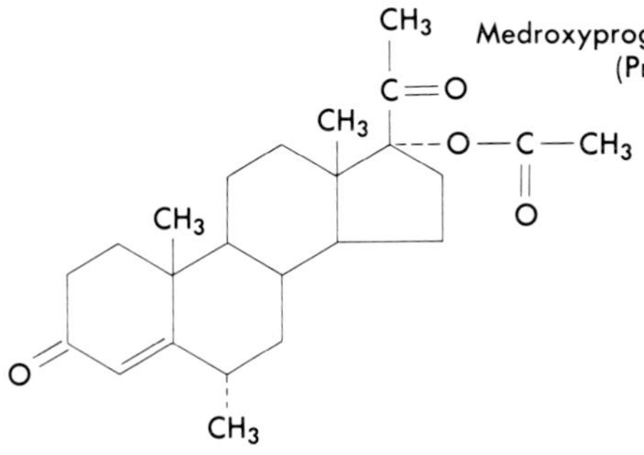

Hydroxyprogesterone (Delalutin)

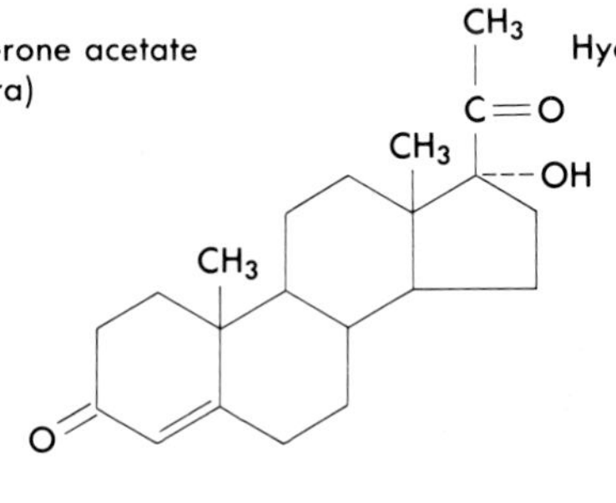

6α-Methyl-17α-acetoxyprogesterone

17α-Hydroxyprogesterone

19-Nortestosterone derivatives

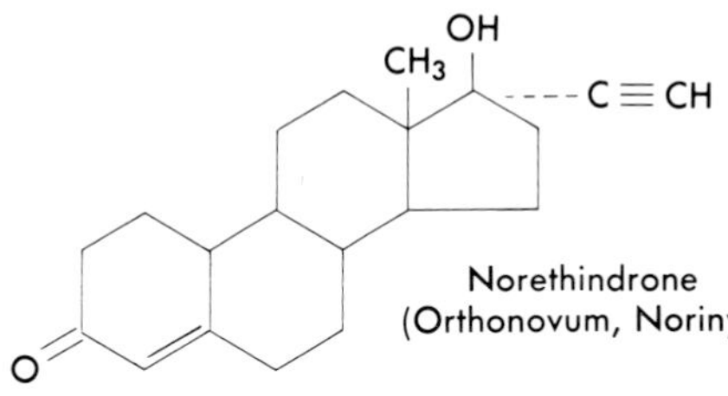

Norethindrone (Orthonovum, Norinyl)

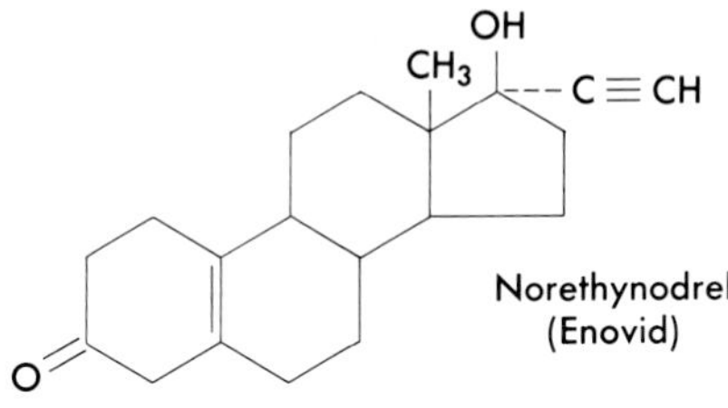

Norethynodrel (Enovid)

19-Nor-17α-ethynyltestosterone

17α-Ethynyl-17-hydroxy-5(10)-estren-3-one

Fig. 20-3. Progesterone and synthetic progestins.

Progesterone (Fig. 20-3)

The best index of progesterone production is the primary metabolite, pregnanediol. It appears in the urine 36 to 48 hours after ovulation, is excreted in a concentration of 5 to 10 mg./day, and disappears just before the onset of menstruation. This range continues through the first 2 months of pregnancy and then rises to a peak of 80 to 120 mg./24 hr. by the fifth month, a level it maintains until labor ensues. Plasma progesterone levels during the second half of the cycle are 2 to 5 μg./100 ml., 5 to 10 μg./100 ml. during the first trimester of pregnancy, and up to 40 μg./100 ml. as pregnancy advances. Progesterone has been found in the blood as early as 48 hours prior to ovulation. Exogenously administered progesterone is rapidly lost from the blood; body fat may store portions of the hormone (particularly where the molecule is both metabolized and conjugated). The enterohepatic circulation permits a large fecal loss of progesterone metabolites.

Progestogens. Compounds resembling crystallized progesterone, often of adrenocortical and androgenic origin, and possessing varying degrees of progestational activities have been isolated and synthesized. The assay of progesterone-like compounds depends on their effect upon the endometrium. Other changes, desired or undesired, include inhibition of pituitary gonadotrophin, alteration of cervical mucus, virilization action, myometrial blockage, and therapeutic efficacy in controlling or reducing uterine bleeding (Table 20-1). The general term *progestin* was employed to designate a substance capable of producing progestational changes in the estrogen-primed endometrium without reference to its state of chemical purity or source. The newer term *"progestogen"* has now come into general use to indicate a synthetic progestin, classification of which is shown in Fig. 20-3.

Ovarian-endometrial cycle

Normal menstrual cycles vary from 23 to 35 days, with a bleeding period of 3 to 7 days. Menstruation is defined as bleeding following an ovulation when fertilization does not occur. The endometrium, prepared for nidation, becomes necrotic and is discharged vaginally. The cycle is divisible into three phases—menstrual phase, proliferative or preovulatory phase, and secretory or postovulatory phase.

Menstrual phase

The endometrium of a menstruating woman consists of three layers, of which (1) the compacta and (2) the spongiosa are functional, and (3) the basal layer, next to the myometrium, is regenerative. Histologic sections of endometrium show only small, inactive glands in the probably functionless basal layer of stroma. The compacta and most of the spongiosa are shed at the time of menstruation. The total blood loss averages 60 ml. (range 25 to 180 ml.). Since neither menstrual blood nor blood from a cervical wound during menstruation clots, an unknown anticoagulant or a hemolytic agent probably origi-

Table 20-1. Clinical results with progestogens

	Progesterone	Progesterone derivatives	Nortestosterone derivatives
Ovulation inhibition	—	+4	+3
Dysmenorrhea	—	+3	+2
Endometriosis	—	+4	+3
Pregnancy maintenance	+4	+4	—
Endometrial hyperplasia	—	+2	+3
Basal body temperature elevation	+4	+3	—
Myometrium relaxation	+4	+4	+2

nates in the endometrial stroma. Menstrual discharge contains 75% blood, 10% cholesterol and lipids, approximately 15% estrogen, and small quantities of unknown protein substances. The cause of menstruation is unknown but has been variously explained as due to (1) estrogen deprivation, (2) progesterone deprivation, (3) menstrual toxins, (4) inadequate lymphatic drainage, and (5) unknown endometrial bleeding factors.

Proliferative or preovulatory phase

The endometrium proliferates after menstruation in response to ovarian secretion. It grows at first from the residual spongiosa and intact basal layers, with the appearance of rather narrow and widely scattered tubular endometrial glands in a dense stroma, lined by low columnar cells with irregularly placed nuclei exhibiting active mitosis. Small blood vessels run obliquely through the basal layers toward the surface in the stroma where they form a loose capillary network. Immediately before ovulation, the endometrium approximates a thickness of 3.5 mm. and the numerous glands are lined by centrally nucleated columnar cells.

Ovulation

Pituitary FSH, acting together with LH, ripens an ovarian follicle to a mature graafian follicle. Many believe that increasing quantities of LH cause a minute perifollicular hematoma that prepares the stigma, or point of rupture, for ovulation by increasing the interfollicular tension within a few hours. Some feel that the ovum release is mechanical and the abruptness of the escape of the ovum correlates with the degree of intrafollicular pressure. Human ovulation has been timed variously as 20 seconds to 15 minutes. Ovulation occurs in 85% of women about 14 days prior to onset of flow, regardless of the length of the menstrual cycle. Unlike humans, several species of animals ovulate in relationship to mating, sexual excitation, or other external stimuli.

Secretory or postovulatory phase

Ovarian-theca lutein cells continue to secrete estrogen while the granulosa lutein cells produce progesterone. Within 5 to 7 days following ovulation, the final endometrial phase occurs when the estrogen and progesterone ratio is optimal. The glands are hyperplastic, tortuous, and filled with secretions, and the compacta layer has enlarged surface cells. The secreting cells lining the glands increase in size, and intercellular vacuoles and basal nuclei appear. Engorged capillaries and large stromal cells containing abundant cytoplasm and large round nuclei can be seen between the secreting glands. The stroma becomes edematous, its cells closely resembling the decidual cells of pregnancy.

The spongiosa is composed of dilated tortuous glands, many arterioles, and narrow bridges of decidua-like stroma. The nonfunctional layer in the basalis contains inactive glands that remain almost unchanged throughout all phases. There is a progressive increase in vascularization in all layers, with wide areas in the stroma that are probably sinuslike end organs. Profound vasoconstriction of the spiral blood vessels leads to the limited bleeding seen with menses. If there is no fertilization, the corpus luteum disintegrates in 1 or 2 days with the withdrawal of these hormones. The menstrual flow again occurs

Cycle of ovarian—secondary sexual tissues
Estrogen

Secondary sexual tissues are controlled primarily by estrogen and progesterone. The mechanism is not fully understood, although there is evidence of an estrogen-sensitive, enzyme-substrate system. The general metabolism acts primarily by an effective transhydrogenation reaction, as coenzyme, in the transfer of hydrogen from TPN to DPN. This estrogen-sensitive enzyme exists in certain target end organs (endometrium, myometrium, placenta, mammary glands). Cyclic AMP also plays a regulatory role.

Fallopian tubes. Estrogen causes (1) cyclic changes in the tubal mucosa, (2) rhythmic contractions of the musculature that brings the fimbriated end of the fallopian tube into contact with the ovary during ovulation, and (3) motion of tubal cilia to help move follicular fluid and ovum through the tube.

Uterus. Estrogen causes myometrial hypertrophy as well as rhythmic contractions and increases uterine tonus, particularly during the follicular phase. There is stimulation of endometrial growth and marked changes in alkaline phosphatase, glycogen formation, and tissue fluid. It produces coiling of the spiral arterioles. A fall in the estrogen level of 45% to 55% is followed by a series of vascular changes that cause bleeding. This withdrawal of estrogen results in a nonovulatory type of dysfunctional bleeding.

Cervix. Estrogens cause elongation of the columnar cells lining the endocervical glands, with resulting increased secretory activity. An increase in the amount of cervical mucus with a lowered viscosity promotes migration, motility, and longevity of the spermatozoa.

Vagina. As estrogen increases, the superficial layer thickens; as estrogen activity wanes, the epithelium of the vagina becomes thinner and has a parabasal or basal type of structure. Estrogen causes the deposition of glycogen in human vaginal epithelial cells, which maintains the acidity of vaginal flora.

External genitalia. With approaching puberty, the size of the labia minora, labia majora, and the clitoris increase. In adults, estrogen increases vascularity and tissue edema.

Breasts. Estrogens stimulate the growth of the breast by inducing proliferation of the duct system and increasing pigmentation, growth, and development of the nipple.

Effects are also produced in the urinary tract, in genital skin, in the nasal and buccal mucosa, and in certain male reproductive glands. It has a direct effect on other endocrine glands, such as the pituitary, by means of feedback mechanisms; on the ovary itself by its apparent trophic effect, as well as on the coiled arterioles of the ovary; on the thyroid gland either directly or peripherally; and on the adrenal by its appreciable sex dimorphism with regard to adrenal weight.

Progesterone

Progesterone prepares the uterus for nidation of a fertilized ovum and aids in the maintenance of pregnancy. Its activities require the concomitant presence of estrogen with which it can act synergistically or antagonistically. Large amounts of progesterone exert an androgenic effect, possibly due to its conversion to androgenic metabolites.

Fallopian tubes. There is diminished fallopian-tube motility and decreased ciliation and activity within the lining of the tubes.

Uterus. It reduces the synchrony of uterine muscle fibers, thus reducing the force and frequency of contractions. In the estrogen-primed endometrium, it induces secretory changes and stimulates the growth of coiled spiral arterioles.

Cervix. Progesterone causes regression of the estrogen effect in stimulating the columnar epithelium. There is a decrease in the cell size, with diminished secretion and decreased viscosity of the mucus.

Vagina. There is marked desquamation of the superficial layer, diminution of the thickness of the epithelium, and infiltration by leukocytes. In vaginal smears, the desquamated cells are curled and folded and the cytoplasm loses some acidophilic staining that was present in the late follicular phase.

Breasts. Progesterone, in conjunction with estrogen, causes development of the alveolar system from the ducts. The combination produces a marked increase in breast parenchyma and prepares and sensitizes the breast for the action of lactogenic hormone for milk formation.

Lactogenic hormone—physiology of lactation

After pregnancy and immediately following placental separation, gonadotrophin releasing factors and prolactin-inhibiting factor are blocked, leading to diminished gonadotrophic secretion and a release of prolactin. The latter acts on the estrogen- and progesterone-primed breast to cause milk formation in the alveolar holocrine glands and generalized venous engorgement (Menczer and Eskin, 1969). Myoepithelial cell contractions, stimulated by oxytocin released from the posterior pituitary, cause the secretion of milk through the collection ducts.

LABORATORY STUDIES USEFUL IN GYNECOLOGIC ENDOCRINOLOGY

The presence or absence of ovulation indicates the state of the functional relationships between the trophic centers, endocrine organs, and final pathways. The cause of anovulation must be elucidated whenever possible. (See Fig. 20-4.)

Office studies

Vaginal smears. Specimens are obtained from the lateral vaginal wall by gentle removal of the epithelium without scraping, using a wooden spatula or nonabsorbent swab. This material is then rolled onto a slide that is preserved in an alcohol fixative,

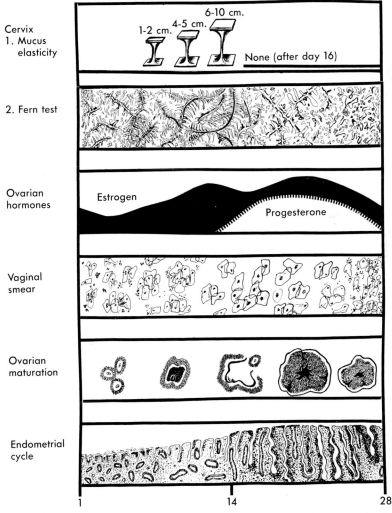

Fig. 20-4. Ovulation detection methods used in gynecologic-endocrine evaluations.

and stained by Papanicolaou, Rakoff, or quinaldine blue stain, or TMK-101 Shaeffer's ink. The percentage of cells with nuclear pyknosis is defined as the *karyopyknotic index* (KI). The percentage of cells showing cytoplasmic acidophilia is termed the *cornification index* (CI). The *maturation index* (MI) is a ratio of the three major types of cells shed from the stratified squamous epithelium. The MI expresses numerically the ratio of parabasal cells to intermediate cells to superficial cells, from a total of 100 counted cells. Examples are shown in Fig. 20-5.

Endometrial biopsy. An endometrial biopsy provides an index of ovarian hormonal secretions. It is most informative when performed just prior to menses; pregnancy must be ruled out prior to biopsy. If carcinoma is suspected, a complete dilatation and curettage (D&C) is necessary.

Chromatin smears. Genetic sex determination is described in Chapter 23.

Cervical mucus and fern tests. Cervical

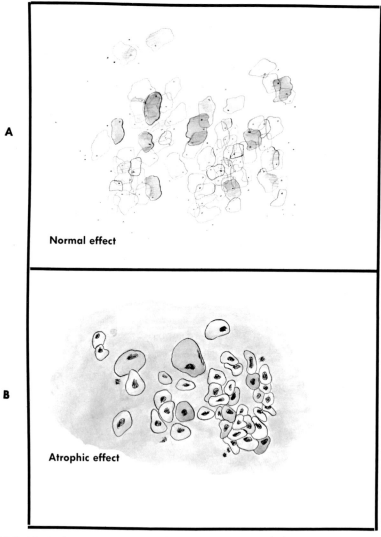

A

Normal effect

B

Atrophic effect

Fig. 20-5. Vaginal smears. **A,** Normal estrogen effect seen with superficial cornified cells with pyknotic nuclei predominating (MI 0:0:100). **B,** Atrophic effect showing parabasal cells of vagina with large vesicular nuclei (MI 100:0:0).

mucus characteristics are outlined in Table 20-2. The mucus is allowed to dry on a clean slide and examined under the microscope for crystallized fernlike patterns. One may make a quantitative evaluation of estrogen, since ferning, caused by the precipitation of NaCl in crystalline form, may be graded as 1+ to 4+. The fern test is negative when progesterone antagonizes estrogen.

Pregnancy tests. Besides the standard Friedman, A-Z, and amphibian tests, several immunologic tests (hemagglutination-inhibition, precipitin, latex-fixation) permit an office diagnosis of pregnancy in 20 seconds to 2 hours. All tests depend on high titers of chorionic gonadotrophins.

Basal body temperature (BBT) studies. The BBT, an index of ovulation, is measured with an oral clinical thermometer in the morning, before the patient arises. Estrogen alone lowers, whereas estrogen and progesterone together elevate, the temperature. It is believed that the thermogenic effect of progesterone acts via the hypothalamus. A normal BBT is shown in Fig. 20-6.

Surgical procedures

Culdoscopy. Culdoscopy utilizes an endoscope to visualize and often to biopsy the pelvic organs through the posterior vaginal vault. Tubal patency may also be studied after the insertion of dye through the cervix for direct observation of the dye traversing the tubes to the fimbriated ends.

Laparotomy. Laparotomy may be necessary to obtain tissue for diagnosis of ovarian or tubal disease, uterine abnormalities, or diseases of the nongenital pelvic organs. Ovarian section, wedge resection of polycystic ovaries, and uterine biopsies are sometimes required in gynecologic endocrine problems.

Endocrine laboratory procedures

Marked elevation of pituitary gonadotrophins suggests a nonfunctioning ovary from lack of feedback control, whereas a reduction points to insufficiency of the hypothalamic-pituitary axis. 17-KS and 17-OHCS are discussed in Chapter 12. Twenty-four–hour total estrogen values may be important in the study of hormone-secreting ovarian tumors (granulosa cell tumors or thecomas) or in hypo-ovarianism. Estriol determinations reflect fetal-placental vitality in the last 12 weeks of gestation. Urinary pregnanediol levels correlate with progesterone secretion and are evidence of ovulation. Serum or urinary testosterone may serve to diagnose polycystic ovarian disease under certain conditions. Thyroid tests (Chapter 6) are important when abnormal thyroid states affect the menstrual cycle or fertility. X-ray studies such as

Table 20-2. Ovulatory changes in cervical mucus

	Preovulatory	Ovulatory
Viscosity	High ("thick")	Low ("runny")
Daily quantity	Up to 60 mg.	200 to 700 mg.
Spinnbarkeit (ability to be drawn into threads)	1 cm.	10 to 13 cm.
Elastic recoil	8 to 10 mm.	30 mm. or more
Visible character	Opaque or translucent	Clear, glairy, or transparent
Fern formation	None or atypical	Typical
Water content	92% to 94%	97% to 98%
Leukocytes	Moderate to many	Few to none
Spermatozoal penetrability	0.2 to 0.5 mm./min.	1.7 to 2 mm./min.

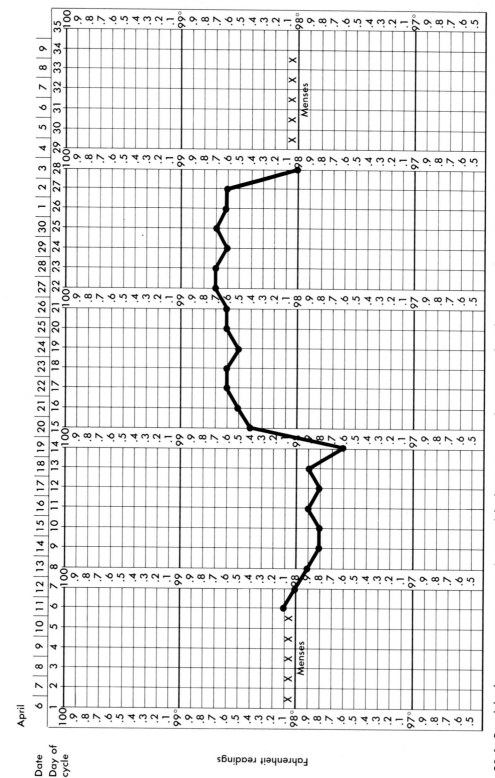

Fig. 20-6. Basal body temperature curve. A normal biphasic curve is demonstrated with a preovulatory dip and rise and rapid premenstrual drop.

skull x-ray examination for size of sella turcica, adrenal air studies, etc. are performed when indicated.

CLINICAL ASPECTS OF GYNECOLOGIC ENDOCRINOLOGY

Abnormalities of menstruation

Amenorrhea of endocrine origin

Amenorrhea is *primary* when menstruation has never begun, or *secondary* when menstruation has regularly occurred. *Oligomenorrhea* is amenorrhea of short duration, usually defined as 3 months; *hypomenorrhea* is the quantitative lessening of menstruation and implies scanty flow; *cryptomenorrhea* is occult menstruation caused by a mechanical barrier.

Central nervous system (hypothalamic)

The normal menstrual cycle depends on the harmonious relationship of the central nervous system through the hypothalamus to the anterior lobe of the pituitary, the ovaries, and the uterus. *Acute emotional disturbances,* particularly those associated with galactorrhea, pseudocyesis, and anorexia nervosa, have been implicated in amenorrhea. Anorexia nervosa is a psychogenic illness that causes amenorrhea through starvation producing functional hypogonadotrophism. Amenorrhea with obesity may have a hypothalamic origin. Sensory abnormalities, particularly of sight and smell, have often been implicated in changing menstrual behavior and infertility. *Pseudocyesis,* the yearning for a pregnancy, suppresses menstrual function and is an aggregate of the physical signs of a nonexisting gestation. *Secondary amenorrhea from acute psychosis* may be a result of interference with the release of LRF from the hypothalamus, leading to inadequate LH. Certain tranquilizers used in the treatment of psychoses, such as Mellaril and Trilafon, also cause menstrual problems, which sometimes are mistakenly considered to have been caused by the psychiatric illness.

Galactorrhea. *Chiari-Frommel syndrome* is characterized by amenorrhea, prolonged galactorrhea, and moderate obesity occurring post partum. It may be a hypothalamic abnormality inhibiting secretion of the gonadotrophin releasing factors and the prolactin-inhibiting factor thus producing excessive quantities of the lactogenic hormone from the anterior pituitary. *Ahumada–del Castillo syndrome* is similar but is a nonpuerperal disease for which treatment is more difficult. Both of these syndromes have been successfully treated by clomiphene citrate or high-dosage progestogen therapy. *Forbes-Albright syndrome,* a nonpuerperal galactorrhea, is associated with a chromophobe adenoma of the pituitary. Differentiation of these three entities is often difficult (Table 20-3). Certain phenothiazide derivatives can cause both galactorrhea and amenorrhea.

Pituitary insufficiency

The amenorrhea is the result of gonadotrophic insufficiency (p. 57). When pregnancy is desired, the use of available gonadotrophic hormones in proper sequence

Table 20-3. Differentiation of the types of galactorrhea

	Sella enlargement	Onset	Duration
Chiari-Frommel	—	Postpartum	Usually transient
del Castillo	—	Spontaneous	Usually permanent
Forbes-Albright	+	Either	Permanent

is utilized with some success. The recent separation of gonadotrophins from menopausal urine (HMG) has produced a more potent FSH product. When fertility is not important, the patient's psyche can be satisfied by steroid cyclic therapy, with withdrawal uterine bleeding.

Several forms of gonadotrophic hormones are in clinical use, although some of these are not commercially available. Patients are observed for evidence of ovarian overstimulation with these substances.

Ovarian hyperstimulation syndrome (Ferin and Renaer, 1968). The dosage of FSH is the principal factor in both the mild form of the ovarian hyperstimulation syndrome (lower abdominal pain, nausea, vomiting, abdominal distention, and cystic enlargement of the ovaries) and the severe form (risk of rupture of ovarian cysts and possible acute Meigs' syndrome). A safe dose of FSH is determined by measurement of total urinary estrogens or estriol, or by pelvic examination to palpate ovarian size.

Gonadotrophins. Therapies that may be used for replacement are grouped relative to their primary gonadotrophic activity.

PRIMARILY FSH ACTIVITY

1. Pregnant mare serum (PMS) has primarily a follicle-stimulating effect. (It is available as PMS.)

2. Human pituitary gonadotrophin (HPG), most of which is human pituitary follicle-stimulating hormone (HPFSH), stimulates the ovarian follicle, leading to ovarian estrogen secretion. (It is not available.)

3. Human menopausal gonadotrophin (HMG) consists of FSH extracted from menopausal urine. (It will be available soon as Pregova, or Pergonal.)

PRIMARILY LH ACTIVITY

1. Human chorionic gonadotrophin (HCG) is extracted from abundantly available pregnancy urine. (It is available as A.P.L. or Follutein.)

2. Luteinizing hormone (LH) is a purified form extracted from a urine source now in only small supply. (It is not available.)

Ovarian abnormalities

Gonadal dysgenesis (Turner's syndrome, Bonnevie-Ullrich syndrome, ovarian dysgenesis, ovarian dwarfism, and ovarian agenesis). There is primary amenorrhea, failure to develop secondary sexual characteristics, short stature (48 to 56 inches), rarely normal height, absence of breast tissue, immature nipples, scanty axillary hair, and usually fine sparse pubic hair. Multiple stigmas often seen are short-webbed neck, broad shieldlike chest, low hairline especially on the back of the neck, underdeveloped mandible, high-arched palate, reversed carrying angle of elbow (cubitus valgus), and moles on face and neck (Fig. 20-7). Webbing of fingers and toes because of impairment of lymphatic drainage has been described. One or several congenital anomalies may occur, such as coarctation of the aorta, cardiac septal defects, ocular nerve defects, nerve deafness, mental deficiency, osteoporosis, spina bifida, short metacarpals, pigmented nevi, renal anomalies, Madelung's deformity, abnormalities of fusion of the cervical vertebrae, cataract and corneal abnormalities, and multiple telangiectasia of the bowel. The external genitalia are immature, the vagina is narrow with a thin mucosal lining, the cervix is small, the uterus is hypoplastic, and occasionally the clitoris is enlarged.

Although clinical variations are legion, the etiology of the cases is similar. Gonadal dysgenesis results from embryonic defects due to errors in chromosomal transmission often giving rise to problems of intersexuality. Approximately 80% of patients have a chromatin-negative buccal smear and an XO karyotype.

An understanding of the variations seen in gonadal dysgenesis requires comprehension of present-day concepts of sexual organization. Presently it is considered that sexual characteristics, both primary and secondary, develop in the following three

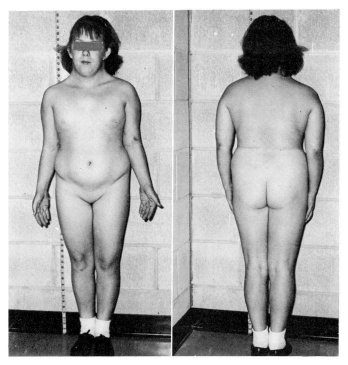

Fig. 20-7. Turner's syndrome. Patient, 19 years of age, shows short stature (56 inches), marked webbing of neck, shieldlike chest configuration, minimal breast development, generalized sexual infantilism, no pubic or axillary hair, increased carrying angle of elbow (cubitus valgus), lowered hairline in the back of neck, and receding chin (due to underdeveloped mandible). (Courtesy Dr. M. B. Dratman, Philadelphia, Pa.)

stages: (1) chromosomal determinants produce sex of developing gonads; (2) gonadal organizers program the formation of müllerian or wolffian systems; and (3) sex hormonal secretions decide the secondary sexual characteristics. Recent evidence suggests the presence of nonchromosomal determinants of sex, a fact that clarifies certain aspects of hermaphrodism. Since in many animals fetal castration produces female reproductive organs, the theory has also been advanced that only the male chromosome may cause organ differentiation.

In ovarian agenesis or total lack of the gonads, some hormonally functional tissue, androgenic or estrogenic, often remains. Androgenic manifestations are usually seen as clusters of hilus cells in the gonadal-streak area. The chromosomal pattern is discussed in Chapter 23.

The diagnosis of gonadal dysgenesis is made in a patient with primary amenorrhea, a chromatin-negative buccal or vaginal smear, and an elevated urinary gonadotrophin titer. The differentiation from a virilized female hermaphrodite with adrenal hyperplasia must be made.

TREATMENT. If the patient's karyotype is XO, estrogen treatment is started as soon as maximal growth is attained. If the pattern is XY or a mosaic containing the Y chromosome, an exploratory laparotomy with removal of the gonads associated with the dysgenetic Y chromosome is done before any steroid treatment is instituted. Estrogen alone or together with progesterone improves the development of the female secondary sex characteristics and, since the müllerian tract is usually well formed, cyclic uterine bleeding can be induced. The patient is permanently infertile. If some partially male or rather ambiguous external genitalia are present in the female, a reconstructive operation should be done.

Polycystic ovary disease (Stein-Leventhal syndrome)

PATHOLOGY. The ovaries are enlarged 3 to 5 times, with hyperthecosis just beneath a thick capsule. The general appearance of the enlarged ovary reflects a microcystic and thickened fibrotic surface. There is a scarcity of prominent granulosa cells and a singular absence of both graaf-

ian follicles and corpus luteum, which characterize the anovulation (Fig. 20-8). Since metabolic abnormalities have been determined, ovaries of polycystic ovary disease have been variously described as normal-sized or even small ovaries with the microcystic characteristics becoming the crucial diagnostic criteria. With culdoscopy, the ovary is a shiny, grayish white, firmly cystic, generally enlarged and elongated (two to three times) ovoid that, despite overall smoothness of contour, has

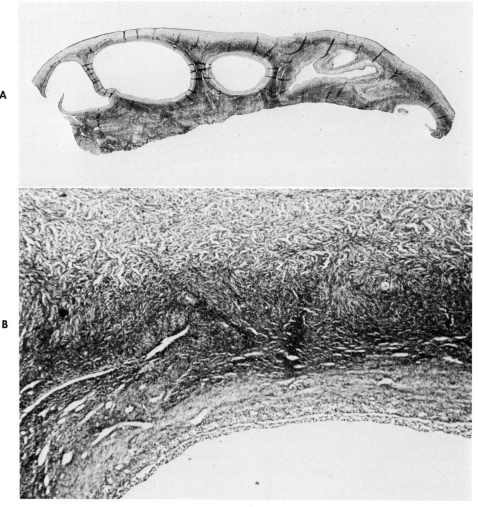

Fig. 20-8. Polycystic ovary disease. Sections through cortex of polycystic ovary. **A,** Ovarian cortex (X10). Multiple cystic follicles with thickened capsule. **B,** Section through wall of cyst (X24). Pathognomonic findings of fibrous thickening of the ovarian cortex and an increased thecal layer (hyperthecosis).

a moderately irregular surface because of the superficial cysts.

ETIOLOGY. Four theories that have evolved are adrenocortical abnormality, hypothyroidism, hypothalamic-pituitary effects, and ovarian biosynthetic abnormality.

Adrenal cortex. An adrenocortical abnormality has been described in 5% to 12% of patients. In some patients having hirsutism without virilization, there is high-normal or slightly elevated urinary 17-KS. These patients respond to corticosteroid suppressive therapy, at least initially, with ovulatory cycles and pregnancies. Ovarian wedge resections are usually unsuccessful. Several authors have indicated a specific biochemical adrenal-ovarian axis in which steroidogenic abnormalities in the ovary adversely affect the adrenal and vice versa, producing increasing amounts of androgens. Evidence of secretion of significant levels of pregnanetriolone in patients with adrenal hyperplasia favors the presence of an adrenal component. Some studies conclude that dysfunctional changes in adrenals are secondary to ovarian steroid biosynthetic modulations. Competitive inhibition of enzyme systems in the ovary could affect such cortisol systems as 11β-hydroxylation, with resulting adrenal abnormalities.

Hypothyroidism. Polycystic ovary disease can be produced in hypothyroid animals in the presence of adequate or elevated gonadotrophin and is found in some hypothyroid patients.

Hypothalamic-pituitary effects. There can be alterations in the secretion of FSH and LH (Singh, 1969). Whether the ovarian abnormality is primary, causing feedback at the hypothalamus or pituitary, or whether direct CNS affects on the hypothalamic-pituitary axis initiates this sequence, is not settled. Polycystic ovaries are an important source of elevated androgens in the female. This may not always be an enzymatic ovarian defect, since the androgen concentration in some polycystic ovaries can be reduced when the involved ovaries are stimulated with gonadotrophin.

Thus there may be a deficiency or imbalance of endogenous gonadotrophins, resulting in the disturbed steroid synthesis. Treatment of prepubertal rats with testosterone always produces polycystic ovary disease. The resulting "masculinization of the hypothalamus" is apparently refractory to everything except median eminence stimulus after progesterone is given, showing evidence of feedback masculinization from the androgen (Barraclough and Gorski, 1961).

Therapy with gonadotrophins or clomiphene citrate produces ovulation in polycystic ovary disease only when FSH levels are low. Findings of persistently elevated urinary LH in patients with polycystic ovary disease has likened this problem to that of the male in whom a singular gonadotrophin, LH (ICSH), secretion exists. These patients show gonadal biosynthetic pathways that are similar to those seen in the male.

Ovarian biosynthetic abnormality. There may be (1) an enzymatic defect preventing aromatization of ring A, causing excessive secretion of androstenedione, (2) a defect in the 3β-ol-dehydrogenase enzyme, causing heightened secretion of dehydroepiandrosterone (DHEA), and (3) an augmentation of testosterone produced by a direct pathway from progesterone. Although some estrogen is produced, the androgen-estrogen ratio is increased, resulting in hirsuitism, slightly elevated 17-KS, and elevated plasma and urinary testosterone. The last two cause pathologic changes in the ovary with disturbed ovulation, with or without amenorrhea.

CLINICAL FEATURES. The principal clinical features are secondary amenorrhea, sterility, and hirsutism. The finding of demonstrable microcystic changes in both ovaries is pathognomonic (Fig. 20-8). Secondary amenorrhea can occur presumably when the condition develops slowly over a period of years. Usually mild, infrequent, irregular, anovular uterine bleeding accompanies sterility. Some patients have normal menarche with irregularity occurring after adolescence, characterized by lengthening intervals with scanty flow. In 50% of such patients there is a male escutcheon, excessive facial hair (notably on the chin and the sideburn areas), and long hairs around the mammary areolae.

Polycystic ovary disease accounts for approximately 18% of patients with irregular menstrual problems in the 17- to 25-year-age group. Basal temperature curves are monophasic, vaginal smears are mildly estrogenic, and endometrial biopsies show early proliferative patterns. Body contour and breast development are normal; occasionally there is obesity (15% to 20%).

DIAGNOSIS. Pelvic examination reveals bilateral ovarian enlargement, but proof may require culdoscopy, gynecography, culpotomy, or laparotomy. Urinary estrogen and FSH levels are usually normal, LH is generally increased, and urinary 17-KS may be normal or elevated. Increased plasma testosterone in patients with polycystic ovaries following the administration of HCG may be useful as a diagnostic test in differentiating the cause as pituitary rather than ovarian. The endometrium is atrophic, proliferative, or hyperplastic, but consistently anovular.

Differential diagnosis of polycystic ovary disease should include (1) masculinizing ovarian tumor, (2) adrenocortical hyperfunction (Chapter 15), (3) hypopituitarism (Chapter 5), and (4) idiopathic hirsutism. Masculinizing tumors exhibit elevated urinary 17-KS and marked virilization. Polycystic ovary disease usually has only heterosexual hirsutism. In idiopathic hirsutism there is normal-appearing ovarian tissue by culdoscopy and normal adrenocortical function tests.

TREATMENT. Medical treatment should be employed before surgical intervention is contemplated. When increased urinary 17-KS and hirsutism occur, the adrenal cortex is suppressed with prednisone in doses up to 10 mg. daily (2.5 mg. four times daily). The urinary 17-KS should be reduced to less than 8 mg. and should be maintained for at least 6 months unless complications ensue. When there appears to be a pituitary or ovarian etiology, human pituitary gonadotrophin (HPG) or human menopausal gonadotrophin (HMG) (see p. 372) as well as clomiphene citrate may be efficacious. Low doses of HPG are first employed for 5 to 7 days, with ovulation usually occurring 2 to 4 days later. Enlarged ovarian cysts with occasional rupture can occur. HMG followed by HCG in sequence can stimulate ovulation. The dosage schedule has not been established yet; follicular cysts are common. Clomiphene citrate (Clomid) may be employed in sequence with HMG, or alone. Clomid is generally the first compound used in a daily dosage of 50 mg. for 5 days; ovulation occurs 3 to 8 days later. Hypothyroidism is treated as described in Chapter 9. Bilateral ovarian wedge resection is successful in 80% of primarily ovarian cases. It is employed only when medical therapy has failed or was not indicated, or when pregnancy is desired immediately. Therefore, surgical treatment should not be recommended in unmarried women or teenagers, inasmuch as polycystic ovaries do not progress without therapy. Severe hirsutism constitutes an exception; however, adrenal suppression therapy should be employed first. Wedge resection is believed effective because the removal of malfunctioning ovarian tissue eliminates the feedback inhibition of the hypothalamic-pituitary axis.

Testicular feminization (or androgen insensitivity) syndrome. See p. 398.

Primary hypogonadism and premature menopause

PRIMARY HYPOGONADISM. Primary ovarian failure is genetic or acquired. Prepubertally acquired conditions that may lead to primary amenorrhea include severe childhood infections (viral or bacterial), oophorectomy, and radiation therapy. Eunuchoid hypogonadism is characterized by abnormally long bones of extremities, underdeveloped breasts, scantiness of pubic hair, undersized genitalia, and late menarche. It has been classified by some authors as tall ovarian-dysgenesis patients with rudimentary ovaries and 46 XO karyotype.

PREMATURE MENOPAUSE. Spontaneous menopause before the age of 40 years occurs in about 8% of women. The deficiency is created by a lack of germinal ova at birth or, less likely, reduced pituitary gonadotrophin. The diagnosis depends on finding either an elevation of urinary FSH or gonadotrophins (greater than 70 mU./24 hr.) and hypoestrinism, indicating ovarian failure or a markedly reduced gonadotrophin level from pituitary insufficiency. Therapy is individualized to the diagnosed endocrine defect.

Ovarian endocrine tumors

FEMINIZING TUMORS

Granulosa cell tumor. In children the tumor gives rise to precocious puberty, hypertrophy of the uterus, and, in many cases, precocious anovulatory vaginal bleeding. During the reproductive years, amenorrhea or oligomenorrhea is followed by periods of excessive or irregular bleeding. Usually, ovarian function is inhibited by continuous estrogen production, but rarely there is fertility. The principle clinical features are pain, abdominal enlargement, and the findings of a pelvic mass. Postmenopausal women, who constitute a large proportion of cases, experience uterine bleeding at regular intervals, enlarged breasts that may be restored to their premenopausal fullness and firmness, disappearance of vasomotor menopausal symptoms if present, and local signs due to the pelvic mass. Carcinoma of the endometrium is present in approximately 20% of postmenopausal cases. The treatment is resection, being relatively conservative in childhood and radical in the reproductive and postmenopausal years.

Thecoma. Thecomas constitute 1% to 3% of solid ovarian tumors and are often confused with ovarian fibromas. More than 65% occur after the menopause. The clinical findings of the hormonally active thecoma are the same as in granulosa cell tumors.

Feminizing luteomas. Feminizing luteomas consist predominantly of cells resembling the corpus luteum and produce estrogen and/or progesterone. They probably result from lutein transformation of theca and granulosa cells.

MASCULINIZING TUMORS

Arrhenoblastoma. Arrhenoblastomas, rare unilateral tumors, are thought to arise from tubular structures in the ovarian hilus interpreted as remnants of early phases of fetal gonadogenesis when both ovary and testis arise from undifferentiated tissue. Although considered potentially malignant, extension beyond the capsule or metastasis is unusual. Clinical manifestations vary from marked virilization to absence of endocrine stigmas with only the mechanical effects of the tumor. Urinary 17-KS are normal or slightly elevated; urine and plasma testosterone is high. Treatment is surgical resection.

Adrenal-like ovarian tumor. The rare, potentially malignant, masculinizing tumors called adrenal-like ovarian tumors have lipid-containing cells resembling those of the adrenal cortex or corpus luteum and occur during the reproductive years. The diagnosis is made by the presence of an enlarging ovary in a patient with manifestations of an adrenogenital or Cushing's syndrome and moderately elevated urinary 17-KS. Treatment is simple oophorectomy when the tumor is benign and in the young patient, and radical extirpation in malignant cases and in older patients. Those exhibiting cushingoid features require similar preoperative and postoperative treatment as in adrenal surgery, since postoperative collapse and death can occur.

Hilar cell tumors. Hilar cell tumors arise from sympathicotropic hilar cells in the hilus of the ovary and resemble testicular Leydig cells. They produce varying degrees of masculinization; 17-KS may be normal or moderately elevated. Surgical extirpation is the treatment of choice.

CHORIOEPITHELIOMA OF THE OVARY. Although chorioepithelioma exists in rare cases as a primary ovarian neoplasm, it usually occurs secondarily to chorioepithelioma of the uterus. They secrete chorionic gonadotrophin. The clinical features include a rapidly growing ovarian mass and systemic manifestations from an excessive production of estrogen and progesterone. In children, there are evidences of precocious pseudopuberty; in adults, there is excessive or irregular bleeding or amenorrhea, and occasional secretion from the breasts. The diagnosis is made by finding elevated urinary chorionic gonadotrophin with an associated adnexal mass. Radical pelvic surgery is mandatory because the lesion is highly malignant. Methotrexate and Viablastine have been beneficial.

Other endocrine tumors related to pregnancy and the source of large quantities of chorionic gonadotrophins are hydatidiform mole and chorioadenoma destruens. Commonly producing amenorrhea, they often manifest some mild vaginal bleeding, which, with an increasing uterine size simulating pregnancy, is diagnostic.

Endocrine-metabolic disorders

Disorders of the menstrual cycle are common accompaniments of thyroid and adrenocortical diseases. Well-controlled diabetes mellitus is compatible with regular ovulatory menstruation. Malnutrition and cachectic states, anorexia nervosa, and severe chronic infections result in functional hypopituitarism with oligomenorrhea or amenorrhea. In liver cirrhosis estrogen degradation is impaired, circulatory estrogens increase, and there is endometrial hyperplasia with irregular shedding and bleeding or amenorrhea. Amenorrhea in obesity may be the result of hypothalamic dysfunction.

Hormone suppression and contraception

Menstrual abnormalities following the use of contraceptive estrogen-progestin hormones have ranged from prolonged amenorrhea to hypopituitarism. The amenorrhea is self-limiting and lasts maximally from 6 to 9 months. Withdrawal bleeding may be effected by the cyclic utilization of estrogen and progesterone; however, such hormonal therapy generally does not assist in the return of ovulatory cycles since it maintains suppression of the hypophysiotrophic hormones. Clomid therapy in daily doses of 50 mg. for 5 days has met with some success. Using contraceptive pills to improve fertility by potentiating rebound gonadotrophins after they are withdrawn would seem unwarranted in light of the abnormal amenorrhea seen.

Dysfunctional uterine bleeding (DUB)

Dysfunctional uterine bleeding (DUB) is defined as vaginal bleeding that occurs at unexpected times and/or in excess of normal expectations in the absence of any systemic or local organic abnormality. Since DUB may be symptomatic of many endocrinopathies, an endocrine evaluation is mandatory after the exclusion of organic causes. Vaginal bleeding is classified according to quantity and type as follows: (1) *menorrhagia*—either excessive daily uterine bleeding or a prolonged flow (hypermenorrhea) occurring at the time of anticipated menses, and (2) *metrorrhagia*—prolonged excessive uterine bleeding following amenorrhea or as premenstrual or intermenstrual staining. The quantity of blood loss ranges from scant to profuse. Although DUB occurs at any age from puberty to menopause, it is usually found during the rise and decline of menstrual activity when luteinization is defective or absent. Though DUB is rare in women with regular menstrual cycles, those who have irregular patterns, particularly with infrequent menses, are prone to abnormal bleeding.

The endometrium may bleed irrespective of its histologic condition. DUB occurs when ovarian steroid effects on the endometrium are abnormal qualitatively or quantitatively. Two types of uterine bleeding are due to endocrine factors: (1) estrogen withdrawal bleeding, which occurs by lysis of basal endometrial blood vessels and is, hence, both irregular and unpredictable, and (2) progesterone arteriolar bleeding activated from spiral arterioles that break down, causing menstrual-like bleeding.

Pathophysiology

ANOVULATORY DUB. Anovulatory irregularities are more common in adolescent and menopausal individuals than in the mid years of menstruating women. The endometrium is usually hyperplastic and the menstrual pattern shows marked irregularities with variable intermenstrual bleeding. The following are the major abnormalities:

1. *Estrogen excess* is found with persistent follicular cysts, hormonal ovarian tumors, and liver cirrhosis. This excess promotes endometrial hyperplasia with irregular cyclic bleeding.

2. *Inadequate estrogen* is a common cause of DUB. The quantity of estrogen that produces endometrial hyperplasia is seldom in excess of the normal titers. Hence, the duration of endometrial exposure rather than the quantity of estrogen is the determining factor.

3. *Ovarian response failure* to pituitary stimulation results in failure of the maturing follicle to complete its cycle of ovulation and luteinization, particularly in the premenopausal or pubertal ovary. Follicles remain unruptured or merge into a functionally defective corpus luteum after rupture. On the other hand, when the ovaries are in a responsive state, inadequate pituitary stimulation may cause either failure of ovulation or defective luteinization.

4. *Other endocrine abnormalities* causing menstrual irregularities are described in the section on amenorrhea. The ovarian abnormality may be primary, secondary to improper performance of another endocrine gland, or the result of improper ovarian steroidogenesis. End-organ variations may be critical, such as unresponsiveness of the ovary to trophic stimulation or of the endometrial lining to ovarian hormone stimulation. This speculation is supported by recent studies on the lack of predictability of endometrial response to hormonal dosages of contraceptive preparations. DUB is frequent in *hypothyroidism* and sometimes is associated with disorders of the *adrenal cortex.*

5. *Central factors* or *psychogenic factors* acting through the hypothalamus have been considered. Evidence of external stimuli on the hypothalamus has been seen in cases of both psychiatric and neurologic abnormalities. Irregularities in menses have been studied in female students in emotional crises with no other cause present.

OVULATORY DUB. When DUB occurs during ovulatory cycles, progesterone secretion qualitatively or quantitatively must be abnormal. Ovulatory DUB is more prevalent in the midyears of childbearing. The endometrium is secretory and heavy bleeding occurs at or immediately preceding menses.

Inadequate progesterone. Inadequate progesterone may promote DUB, since this hormone plays an important role in the utilization and metabolism of estrogen and in maintaining an intact endometrium. Following the withdrawal of estrogen and progesterone, the inability of the endometrium to disintegrate completely within the usual time also causes bleeding abnormalities. There is irregular shedding, the diagnosis of which is made by endometrial biopsy during menses.

Prolonged corpus luteum activity. Corpus luteum retention cysts of the ovary maintain progesterone secretion and produce a thickened, highly vascular endometrium. The waxing and waning of the progesterone titer causes irregular bleeding episodes that are often difficult to control. The relaxing effect of progesterone on uterine muscle also poses a problem of hemostasis.

Midcycle hormone deprivation. The problem of acute midcycle hormone deprivation at the time of ovum release affects the level of estrogen and more prominently the progesterone titer. The bleeding that follows is usually minimal and self-limited as the developing corpus luteum begins secreting within 24 to 48 hours.

Diagnosis. One must rule out systemic,

local, or other endocrine-metabolic diseases. If hemostasis is a problem and the patient is bleeding heavily, the parenteral use of progesterone or estrogen or, if necessary, an emergency dilatation and curettage (D&C) is indicated. The knowledge that the patient is ovulatory or anovulatory is essential for diagnosis and therapy. Anovulatory DUB is characterized by persistent estrogen titers without progesterone. The retention follicular cyst is usually easily diagnosed by finding a large ovarian cyst on pelvic examination or by Doppler x-ray methods. Ovulatory DUB is manifested by an endometrium showing irregular shedding or a mixed type (secretory and proliferative cells). Since these patients have unusually prolonged or heavy bleeding, abortion must be differentiated. The diagnosis is made by curettage on the fourth or fifth day of bleeding. A persistent secreting corpus luteum is responsible and an enlarging ovarian cyst is found by pelvic examination. In addition, there is elevated urinary pregnanediol or serum progesterone.

Treatment. Heavy bleeding can be controlled in 36 to 48 hours using 20 mg. conjugated estrogens I.V. slowly, 100 mg. progesterone U.S.P. I.M., 50 or 100 mg. medroxyprogesterone acetate I.M., or 250 mg. hydroxyprogesterone caproate I.M. Progesterone dampens further proliferation of the endometrium, induces secretory changes, and, when withdrawn, promotes desquamation and shedding of the endometrium. Estrogen-testosterone combinations are no more effective. A D&C may be necessary and in rare cases hysterectomy or hypogastric artery ligation may be required for hemostasis. After the diagnosis is made, therapy is given on the basis of the etiology.

ANOVULATORY DUB

Estrogen excess

1. *Progesterone therapy.* Progesterone U.S.P., 100 mg., I.M. once or medroxyprogesterone acetate, 2.5 mg. orally is given daily for 5 days. Reevaluation of a retention cyst should be made at monthly intervals.

2. *Suppressive therapy.* Cyclic therapy with 1.25 mg. conjugated estrogens daily for 24 days and either 125 mg. hydroxyprogesterone caproate I.M. or 50 mg. medroxyprogesterone acetate I.M. on day 14 of the cycle, or 2.5 mg. medroxyprogesterone acetate orally and daily, from day 15 through day 24, may be given. Sequential contraceptives, such as Oracon and C-Quens, have also been used.

3. *Surgical treatment.* If there is a retention follicular cyst less than 5 cm. in size, progesterone and suppressive methods may be tried; however, an enlarging cyst should be removed. Hormonal ovarian tumors require surgical intervention.

Inadequate estrogen

1. *Estrogen replacement.* Small doses of estrogen stimulate ovulation on rare occasions (0.05 mg. stilbestrol, 0.65 mg. conjugated estrogens, or 0.02 mg. ethinylestradiol daily).

2. *Ovulation stimulation.* Clomiphene citrate, 50 mg., is given daily for 5 days, from day 6 through day 10. HMG and HPFSH have been used experimentally. The cyclic use of gonadotrophins has been described.

3. *Cyclic therapy.* In those cases in which ovulation is not desired, estrogen and progesterone in sequence can be given. Although there are occasional patients in whom cyclic therapy may regulate the cycle, usually, when therapy is discontinued, the dysfunctional problem recurs. Since the time of onset of regular menses is unknown in many adolescent girls, cyclic therapy may tide the patient over until normal regulation and maturity occur. Conversely, the premenopausal woman will hopefully go into her menopause.

Ovarian response failure

When the ovary is not responsive to pituitary stimulation, the prognosis is poor. Differentiation from polycystic ovary disease or premature menopause must be made. Therapy consists of combinations of gonadotrophin and clomiphene citrate as described in polycystic ovary disease.

OVULATORY DUB

Inadequate progesterone

Progesterone levels can be enhanced

with dydrogesterone orally 5 or 10 mg. daily, from day 15 through day 25; medroxyprogesterone acetate orally, 2.5 mg. daily, from day 15 through day 25; hydroxyprogesterone caproate I.M., 125 mg., day 15 (Table 20-4).

Prolonged corpus luteum activity

1. *Suppressive therapy.* Therapy is described under the discussion on estrogen excess on p. 380.

2. *Surgical treatment.* Since corpus luteum cysts are less likely to respond to hormone therapy than are follicular cysts, follow-up is mandatory. Although the condition may be corrected by a simple curettage or cyclic therapy, surgical removal may be required.

Dysmenorrhea

Primary dysmenorrhea (essential dysmenorrhea) is menstrual pain in the absence of an organic pelvic lesion. It has been attributed to ovulation, estrogen-progesterone imbalance, and/or psychologic factors. *Secondary dysmenorrhea* is of organic origin and includes constitutional changes, cervical stenosis, nonpatent hymen, hypoplasia of the uterus, or endometriosis. The incidence of the incommoding type of primary dysmenorrhea is approximately 10%. Typically, the pain begins with the onset of menstruation and lasts a few hours, only occasionally continuing for several days. It is most frequently of a colicky, laborlike nature and, if severe, may be accompanied by diarrhea, nausea, and vomiting.

Treatment

SYMPTOMATIC. Often analgesics, tranquilizers, and sedation suffice. A prescription containing aspirin in combination with an antispasmodic, such as Pavatrine or Vasodilan or with a sympathomimetic, such as amphetamine sulfate, is efficacious. Bed rest is helpful, and symptomatic relief can be obtained by medication when there is nausea, vomiting, or diarrhea.

ENDOCRINE. Endocrine treatment aims at

Table 20-4. Estrogen and progesterone for clinical use

Generic name	Doses	Trade name	Mode of administration
Estrogen effects			
Conjugated estrogens	0.65, 1.25, and 2.5 mg. tablets	Premarin	P.O.
		Amnestrogen	P.O.
		Conjutabs	P.O.
		Estratab	P.O.
		Ogen	P.O.
	20 mg. ampule	Premarin IV	I.V.
Diethylstilbestrol or stilbestrol	0.05, 0.1, 1, and 5 mg. tablets	Stilbetin	P.O.
Ethinylestradiol	0.02, 0.05, and 0.5 mg. tablets	Estinyl	P.O.
Progesterone effects			
Progesterone U.S.P.	50 and 100 mg./ml.	Progesterone in oil	I.M.
Dydrogesterone	5 and 10 mg. tablets	Duphaston	P.O.
		Gynorest	P.O.
Medroxyprogesterone acetate	2.5 and 5 mg. tablets	Provera	P.O.
	50 and 100 mg./ml.	Depo-Provera	I.M.
Hydroxyprogesterone caproate	125 and 250 mg./ml.	Delalutin	I.M.
Others			
Clomiphene citrate	50 mg. tablets	Clomid	P.O.

abolishing ovulation and consists of estrogen, progesterone, or the combination given cyclically. Oral contraceptive compounds can be used to inhibit ovulation. This method affords an inexpensive therapy, but the related side effects and contraindications must be considered. Endocrine therapy is not curative, for the pain usually returns after medication is discontinued.

SURGICAL. Presacral neurectomy or sympathectomy may be necessary in the unusual case of intractable dysmenorrhea.

PSYCHOGENIC THERAPY. Acquisition of insight, stemming from the physician's explanation of the innocuous nature of the pain and its probable self-limited existence, is salutary.

EXERCISES. Postural treatment is based on the assumption that the severe spasmodic pain is peripheral and not visceral.

Endometriosis, a cause of secondary dysmenorrhea, is treated with progesterone-estrogen combinations in large doses over 6- to 9-month periods. Enovid (norethynodrel plus mestranol), 10 to 30 mg., orally every day, and Depo-Provera, 50 or 100 mg. I.M. every 2 to 3 weeks, is used. The dosage employed is that amount providing relief from symptoms without vaginal bleeding. Surgery is used only if the medical regimen is not effective. Testosterone may be of some value in endometriosis but has no place in dysmenorrhea.

Climacteric and menopause

Climacteric describes the manifold changes resulting from the decline in ovarian function over a span of several years. *Menopause* refers to the physiologic cessation of menstruation. The climacteric covers approximately the 15 years that constitute the involutional phase of life between 45 and 60 years of age. Loss of menstrual cyclicity in women creates a temporary imbalance in the endocrine system, with subsequent manifestations that are severe in 15% of women and moderate in an additional 25%. Surgical or x-ray castration during childbearing years causes more severe climacteric symptoms, probably due to the acuteness of the deactivating process. Climacteric occurs primarily between the ages of 45 and 50 years. In most women, menstruation disappears gradually; however, in a small minority the period abruptly ceases.

Pathophysiology. Sclerosis of the ovaries and their unresponsiveness to pituitary stimulation causes cessation of menstruation. Glandular hyperplasia occurs in the endometrium, and there is a thin atrophic mucosa with no active proliferation in the vagina. Atrophy of the vagina and vulva are quite apparent. This aging of the ovary, occasionally accompanied by benign hyperplasia of the stroma, follows a progressive pattern. When ovulation and luteinization disappear, the anovulatory state itself creates no symptoms. The absence of progesterone results in endometrial changes and the disappearance of pregnanediol. The growth of follicles continues for some time, a process that promotes estrogen production and occasional irregular episodes of bleeding. Gradual loss of all phases of follicular activity, accompanied by progressive shrinking of the ovarian cortex and diminution of estrogen production, eventually occurs. There is a high state of activity in the pituitary basophilic cells, with an increase in both the rate of elaboration and release of FSH.

The genital organs and the uterus atrophy. The endometrium, ovulatory or nonovulatory in the terminal cycles, usually shows a thin proliferative type of endometrium. The vaginal mucosa gradually loses its cornified epithelium, decreases its glycogen content, and alters its protective vaginal flora. Cytologic smears at this time show more and more parabasal cells. If an estrogenic effect does occur, it is due to the activity of the remaining ovarian follicles and the accepted fact that the vaginal mucosa is remarkably sensitive to estrogen (Fig. 20-4). Genital-muscle tone and fascial strength decrease and atrophic skin changes occur about the vulvar area.

Clinical features. The type and severity of symptoms vary and may commence before complete cessation of menstruation.

Specific hormonal mechanisms of the menopausal syndrome are unknown, but they may be (1) estrogen deprivation, (2) high levels of pituitary gonadotrophins, or (3) hyperfunction of the anterior hypophysis. The last embraces not only the gonadotrophic-producing cells but also those elaborating ACTH and TSH that may result in an upheaval of the closely linked autonomic nervous system. The usual diagnostic evidence is (1) lengthening interval, (2) missed menses, (3) episodes of profuse or prolonged bleeding, and (4) periods of scant flow. Gynecologic diagnostic problems that occur at the premenopausal-menopausal interval must be ruled out, as they are often confused with the irregular onset of this syndrome. Symptoms include (1) vasomotor lability with hot flushes, sweating, and chills; (2) nervousness, headache, insomnia, and vertigo; and (3) mental and emotional instability, depression, weeping, fatigue, self-deprecation, and morbid worrying. There is usually a reduction of blood estrogen and urine and an increase in urinary FSH.

Treatment

TRANQUILIZERS AND SEDATIVES. Tranquilizers and sedatives may be of some value but the effects are not specific and not consistent.

ESTROGEN THERAPY. In recent years there has been much discussion concerning the use of estrogen for menopausal women. Utilization of 0.1 mg. of diethylstilbestrol, 0.625 mg. of conjugated estrogens, or 0.02 mg. of ethinylestradiol, daily, seems quite adequate (Table 20-4). Some authorities prefer cyclic administration for 24- to 30-day intervals. The question of cyclic therapy with estrogen and progesterone has also been raised, but the increase in breakthrough bleeding creates a problem. The smallest effective dose of hormone should be employed. Estrogens should be continued for at least 6 months, after which they may be withdrawn. If symptoms recur, continuation of estrogen for the duration of life, if necessary, would not seem unwarranted. Since many elusive feminine traits, such as skin texture, hair, breast form, and female contours, may be maintained by the continual use of estrogens, treatment for life has been advocated by many. When estrogen is employed, occasional bleeding or spotting may occur; however, if it persists, a diagnostic D&C is required.

Approximately 25% of postmenopausal women develop skeletal osteoporosis and estrogen arrests this demineralization by decreasing bone resorption (Chapter 17). Cardiovascular disease is more prevalent after surgical menopause. The ability of estrogen to lower elevated serum lipids favors its use in the prevention and therapy of coronary atherosclerosis in postmenopausal women.

Contraindications to the use of estrogens in menopausal women are (1) breast or genital carcinoma, (2) myomata uteri, and (3) endometriosis. Estrogen has not been shown to cause carcinoma of the breast or genitalia by itself. A sensitivity imposed by other factors may be modified and an existing cancer worsened by estrogen. Myomata uteri usually decrease in size with the menopause after estrogen secretion is reduced but can be stimulated to growth by estrogen therapy. Patient suffering with endometriosis, particularly of the ovaries, are usually cured by ovariectomy with resulting estrogen deprivation. The addition of estrogen too early in the menopause may cause a recurrence. However, after secondary atrophy of the pelvic region has begun, a reactivation of the endometriosis does not occur or at least has never been described.

REFERENCES

Barraclough, C. A., and Gorski, R. A.: Endocrinology **68**:68, 1961.

Ferin, J., and Renaer, M.: Amer. J. Obstet. Gynec. **101**:439, 1968.

Menczer, J., and Eskin, B. A.: Obstet. Gynec. **33**:260, 1969.

*Savard, K., et al.: Recent Progr. Hormone Res. **21**:285, 1965.

Singh, K. B.: Obstet. Gynec. Survey **24**:2, 1969.

─────────

*Significant review.

Chapter 21

The testes*

Emil Steinberger, M.D.

STRUCTURAL AND PHYSIOLOGIC CONSIDERATIONS

The testes are composed of seminiferous tubules in which spermatogenesis takes place and through which the formed spermatozoa are transported to the excretory duct system. The interstitial cells of Leydig, concerned with elaboration of hormones, are interspersed between the seminiferous tubules. The testis is surrounded by a connective tissue layer, the tunica albuginea, which is covered by a membrane derived from the peritoneum, the tunica vaginalis. In some species, including the human, connective tissue septa extend from the tunica albuginea into the substances of the testes, forming compartments or lobules. The septa converge toward the posterior aspect of the testis, where they merge to form the mediastinum of the testis, through which some of the blood vessels, lymph channels, and nerves enter the organ.

Development of the testes

In the 27 mm. fetus the gonads first acquire the histologic characteristics of the testes. The interstitial cells acquire the characteristic specialization in the 31 mm. fetus. At birth the testicular tissue is composed of solid cords that contain supporting cells (precursors of Sertoli cells), and interspersed among the cords are gonocytes (precursors of the germ cell line of adult testes). The interstitial area is packed with easily recognizable large Leydig cells. A few weeks after birth the Leydig cells atrophy, and the testes appear to remain quiescent until puberty. (For reviews see Charny et al., 1952, and Albert, 1961). However, a process of differentiation during this time cannot be ruled out. Studies in lower species show definite changes in the pattern of the steroid biosynthetic capacity of developing testes (Steinberger and Ficher, 1969). The possibility of important changes occurring during this so-called "period of quiescence" should be entertained, since this is frequently the time when therapeutic intervention is contemplated.

With the onset of puberty, a rapid increase in size of the testes, sex accessories, and the phallus occurs concomitant with the appearance of gonadotrophins and steroid sex hormones (Figs. 21-1 and 21-2). This change is associated with an increase in size and tortuosity of the seminiferous tubules, differentiation of Leydig cells and Sertoli cells, and formation of adult seminiferous epithelium (Fig. 21-3).

Blood supply

The human testicular artery passes through the plexus pampiniformis, thus permitting precooling by the venous blood (Harrison and Barclay, 1948). During its

*This work has been supported by grants from the National Institutes of Health, No. AM 05449, and from The Ford Foundation.

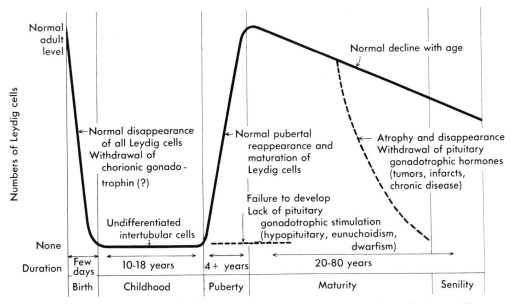

Fig. 21-1. Schematic summary of the life history of the human Leydig cell. (From Albert, A.: The mammalian testis. In Young, W. C., ed.: Sex and internal secretion, ed. 3, Baltimore, 1961, The Williams & Wilkins Co., vol. 1.)

intra-abdominal course the artery gives off branches to the cord and epididymis. Upon reaching the posterior border of the testis, the testicular artery forms two branches that pass under the tunica albuginea and further ramify to form the tunica vasculosa over the medial and lateral aspects of the testes, respectively. From this superficial vascular network, numerous terminal branches that enter the testicular parenchyma are given off. This anatomic arrangement of testicular vasculature has to be considered when surgical procedures are undertaken, since a ligature placed over an end artery may block the blood supply to a large segment of the testicular parenchyma.

Kinetics of the spermatogenic process

Subsequent to clarification of the kinetics of spermatogenesis in the rat, a tentative model for the human spermatogenic process had been proposed (Clermont, 1963). Clermont described six stages of the "cycle of seminiferous epithelium" in the human testis (Fig. 21-4). However, in contrast to rodents, areas in the seminiferous tubules occupied by any one of the stages of the cycle are very small. Thus several different "stages" or cellular associations are manifest in each cross section of a seminiferous tubule, and disruption of the pattern of the cellular associations may occur in any given area of the seminiferous tubule (Fig. 21-3). The irregularities preclude the use of the kinetics of spermatogenesis for quantitation of spermatogenesis, analogous to that achieved in the rodents. Nevertheless, this concept permitted morphologic definition of the various cell types and development of methods for quantitative analysis of seminiferous epithelium, which may lead to better understanding of the pathophysiology of testicular disorders (Steinberger and Tjioe, 1968).

Leydig cells. Recent biochemical studies, particularly in patients with Klinefelter's syndrome, called attention to the discrepancy between morphologic characteristics of the Leydig cells and plasma levels or production rates of testosterone. On the other hand, physiologic studies involving experimental stimulation of the testes with HCG or suppression of pituitary gonadotrophins with synthetic andro-

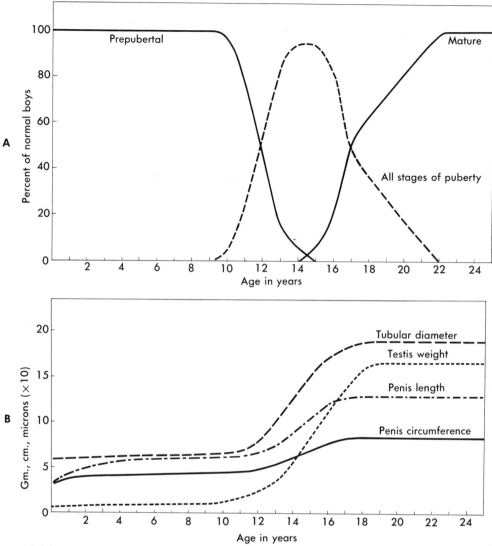

Fig. 21-2. A, Frequency of puberty. **B,** Measurements of testis and penis. **C,** Excretion of hormones during puberty in man (From Albert, A., et al.: Proc. Mayo Clin. **28:**409, 1953.)

gens or estrogens showed good correlation between the gonadotrophins and plasma levels or production rates of testosterone. These findings stress the value of testing procedures based on physiologic parameters and call for caution in interpretation of purely morphologic characteristics of the Leydig cells for diagnostic purposes.

Testosterone

Testosterone produced by the Leydig cells is the major testicular androgen. The biosynthetic pathways are outlined in Fig. 21-5. Testosterone blood levels show no diurnal variation and remain relatively constant during the adult life of the male. With advancing age, the production rate, as well as the metabolic clearance rate, declines, suggesting that in the older male the unchanged plasma levels in the face of reduced production rates could be related to diminished metabolic clearance rates. This possibility is supported by findings of a progressive drop in urinary

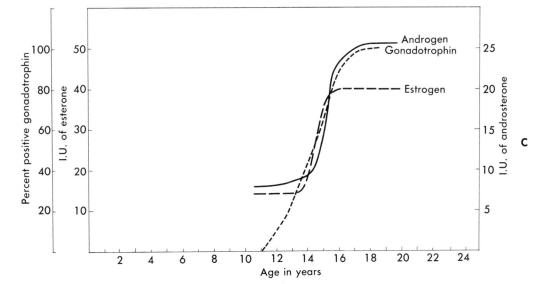

Fig. 21-2, cont'd. For legend see opposite page.

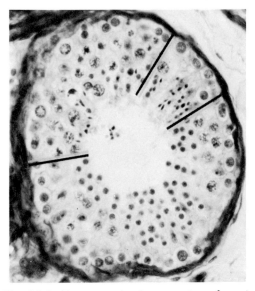

Fig. 21-3. Human testis. Cross section of seminiferous tubule showing several different cellular associations (lines drawn to illustrate the natural boundaries between the associations).

excretion of testosterone in males after the age of 40.

Most of the circulating testosterone is bound reversibly to proteins and is physiologically inactive. This mechanism provides for transport of testosterone and for rapidly available biologically active testosterone. The main site for testosterone metabolism is the liver, where it is converted to ketosteroids, conjugated with glucuronic and sulfuric acids, and excreted in the urine (Fig. 21-6). Recent studies focused attention on the importance of extragonadal sites of androgen metabolism. Not only is it clear that levels of urinary 17-KS do not reflect testicular androgen production, since at least 70% is derived from the adrenal cortex, but the extragonadal interconversion of various metabolites (17-hydroxyprogesterone, androstenedione, etc.) to testosterone has to be interpreted with great care to obtain a clear picture of testicular secretory function.

Testosterone is responsible for the development and maintenance of male sex characteristics (Schonfeld, 1943) (Chapter 24). The anabolic effects of testosterone are manifested by increased protein synthesis and retention of nitrogen, calcium, and phosphorus, together with a decrease of amino acid catabolism. The mechanism of this effect has not been entirely elucidated, but recent studies have implicated the DNA-dependent RNA synthesis mechanism.

Pathologic cessation of Leydig cell func-

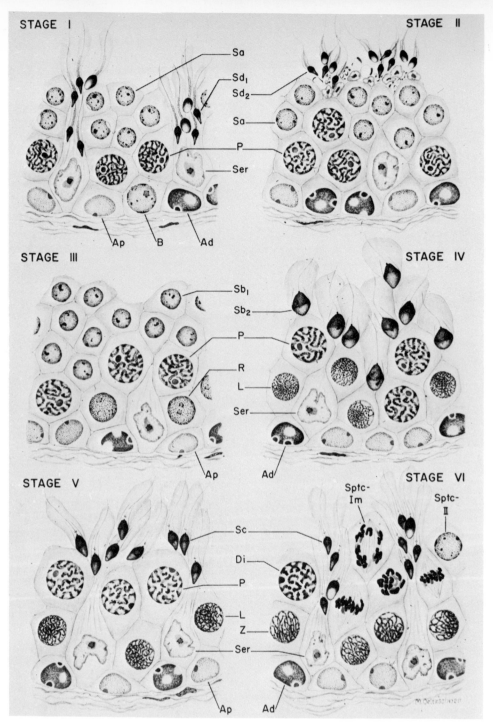

Fig. 21-4. Cycle of the seminiferous epithelium. Drawings diagrammatically representing the cellular composition and topography of the six typical cellular associations found repeatedly in human seminiferous tubules. These cell associations (stages I to VI) correspond to the stages of the cycle of the seminiferous epithelium. **Ap** and **Ad,** Pale and dark, type A spermatogonia; **B,** type B spermatogonia; **Di,** diplotene primary spermatocytes; **L,** leptotene primary spermatocytes; **P,** pachytene primary spermatocytes; **R,** resting primary spermatocytes; **RB,** residual bodies; **Sa, Sb, Sc,** and **Sd,** spermatids at various steps of spermiogenesis; **Ser,** Sertoli nuclei; **Sptc-Im,** primary spermatocytes in division; **Sptc-II,** secondary spermatocytes in interphase; **Z,** zygotene primary spermatocytes. (Courtesy Dr. Y. Clermont, Montreal.)

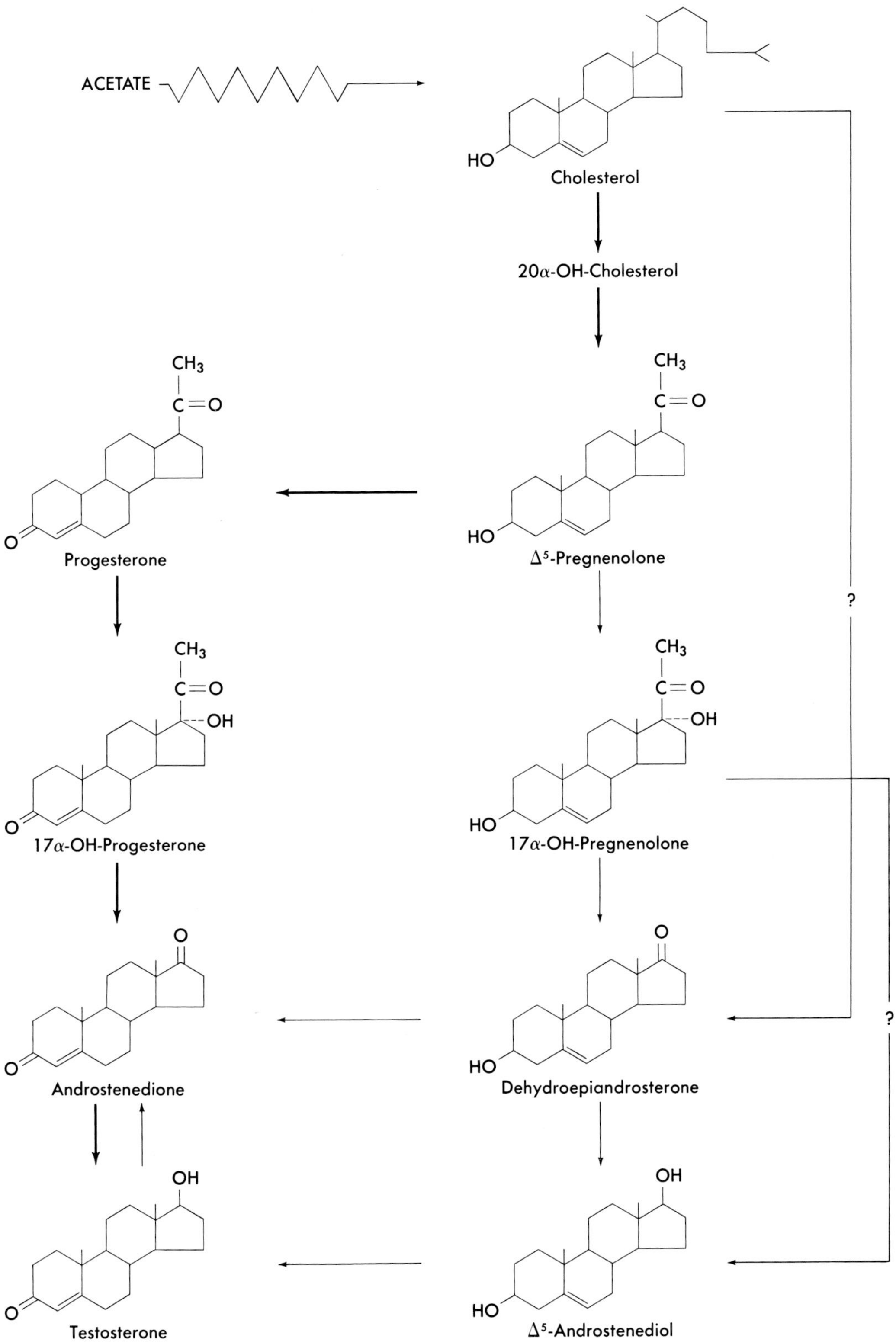

Fig. 21-5. Biogenesis of testosterone in the human testis.

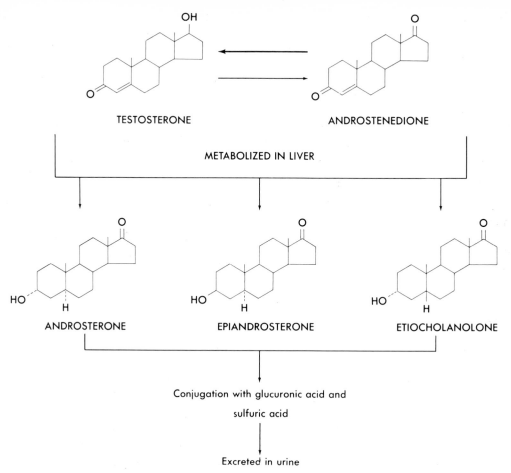

Fig. 21-6. Major pathways of testosterone metabolism.

tion in postpuberal individuals is not associated with rapid regression of secondary sexual characteristics. However, ultimately androgen withdrawal will result in not only somatic changes but also loss of potentia, and in some instances loss of libido; emotional instability characterized by irritability, depression, and lack of the capacity for concentration; and in some cases hot flushes and formication. All of these symptoms can be ameliorated by the administration of testosterone.

Hormonal control of testicular function

Pituitary ablation produces testicular atrophy. In the human, both interstitial cell–stimulating hormone (ICSH) and follicle-stimulating hormone (FSH) are essential for normal testicular function; testosterone administration to normal or oligospermic individuals produces atrophy of seminiferous epithelium. It has been demonstrated that human chorionic gonadotrophin (HCG) (predominantly ICSH activity) stimulates Leydig cells in normal men, thus inducing increased testosterone production and atrophy of seminiferous tubules (Maddock and Nelson, 1952). However, in individuals with deficient pituitary gonadotrophic function (hypogonadotrophic hypogonadism), HCG not only stimulates Leydig cells but may also induce a certain degree, though not complete, of maturation of seminiferous epithelium (Heller and Nelson, 1948). Recently, with the availability of gonadotrophins of human origin, further investigations into their role in maintaining spermatogenesis became possible. Gemzell and Kjessler, 1964, suggested that gonadotrophins are essential for the "maturation process of transforming spermatid to mature spermatozoa." MacLeod et al., 1966, and other investigators concluded that gonadotrophins are essential for the spermatogenic process commencing with spermatogonia.

DISORDERS OF TESTICULAR FUNCTION

Since testes are concerned with the production of sex hormones and of spermatozoa, testicular disorders may involve deficiency in either one or both of these functions. Since normal levels of testicular hormones in the male are essential for proper somatic growth and sexual maturation, the age at which the testicular abnormality first becomes manifest will determine the clinical appearance of the patient. Disturbances of testicular function can be due either to pituitary deficiency or to primary failure of the testis.

Testicular disorders associated with low urinary gonadotrophin levels

In patients with deficient gonadotrophic function of the pituitary gland, both the hormonal and spermatogenic activities of the testes are affected. An exception is the "fertile" eunuch (see below). The condition can occur in prepuberal or postpuberal individuals. It can be associated with selective failure of gonadotrophin secretion, a failure of gonadotrophic and one or more of the other pituitary trophic hormones, or a complete pituitary failure (panhypopituitarism). Furthermore, the gonadotrophic failure can be partial or complete.

Complete selective gonadotrophic failure occurring prior to puberty (hypogonadotrophic eunuchoidism)

Gonadotrophic failure occurring prior to puberty is difficult to recognize with presently available laboratory techniques, since normally the prepuberal state is charac-

terized by absent or low levels of gonadotrophins. However, after the age of expected puberty these individuals assume the characteristic clinical features of classical eunuchoidism and a presumptive diagnosis can be made on a clinical basis (Table 21-1). A number of reports of familial occurrence of this disorder have been made, and X-linked inheritance has been suggested. Association with other congenital anomalies like anosmia, cerebellar ataxia, ichythyosis, harelip, and cleft palate has also been reported. Pathologic studies of the brains of patients with anosmia and eunuchoidism revealed hypoplasia of the hypothalamus, mammillary bodies, and anterior portions of the white commissure and strongly suggested congenital involvement of the hypothalamus as the etiologic factor.

Since, in some instances, gonadotrophic function may commence spontaneously in late adolescence, therapy should be withheld until about the age of 17. The only commercially available gonadotrophin of human origin is human chorionic gonadotrophin (HCG), which evokes mainly Leydig cell response. HCG is administered intramuscularly, 3,000 I.U. three times weekly for 6 to 12 months. The duration of treatment will depend on the rapidity and completeness of response, as evinced by the development of the secondary sex characteristics. Once this stage is achieved, the dosage of HCG can be decreased to 2,000 I.U. three times weekly for an additional 4 months, followed by an interruption of several months. It is hoped that the patient's own gonadotrophin function becomes established and completion of testicular development occurs. If regression of stimulatory effects occurs, therapy should be restarted, since otherwise permanent damage to the seminiferous epithelium may occur. In some patients two or three courses of therapy may result in stimulation of normal gonadotrophic function.

In patients with permanent gonadotrophic failure, HCG alone may not stimu-

Table 21-1. Clinical and laboratory features of hypogonadotrophic hypogonadism

	Selective gonadotrophin failure		Panhypopituitarism	
	Prepuberal onset	Postpuberal onset	Prepuberal onset	Postpuberal onset
Clinical features	Eunuchoidal skeleton Span > height Pubis to floor × 2 > height	Normal skeletal development	Dwarfism (normal dimensions)	Noneunuchoid skeleton Decreased libido and impotency
	High-pitched voice	Normal voice	High-pitched voice	Normal voice
	No gynecomastia	Gynecomastia may be present	No gynecomastia	No gynecomastia
	Testes small (1 × 2 cm.) normal consistency	Testes soft, smaller than normal, but larger than prepuberal	Testes normal prepuberal consistency	Testes atrophic and soft
	Sparse or absent body and pubic hair	Body and pubic hair normal or diminished		Facial, body, and pubic hair decrease
	Lack of bitemporal scalp recession	Bitemporal scalp recession may be present		
			Symptoms of hypoadrenal corticism may be present Usually no clinical signs of hypothyroidism Hypoglycemic episodes may occur	Symptoms of hypoadrenal and hypothyroidism
				No congenital anomalies
Pituitary	No lesion	No lesions or early stages of lesions producing panhypopituitarism	Craniopharyngioma Histiocytosis (Hand-Schüller-Christian disease) Pituitary or hypothalamic cyst Tumor Post infection Post trauma	Idiopathic necrosis Tumor Post infection Post trauma
Testes	Normal prepuberal histology	Hyalinization of seminiferous tubules with destruction of germinal cells and atrophy of Leydig cells	Normal prepuberal histology	Various degrees of spermatogenic arrest, peritubular fibrosis, atrophic Leydig cells

Table 21-1. Clinical and laboratory features of hypogonadotrophic hypogonadism—cont'd

	Selective gonadotrophin failure		*Panhypopituitarism*	
	Prepuberal onset	*Postpuberal onset*	*Prepuberal onset*	*Postpuberal onset*
Laboratory findings	Azoospermia	Azoospermia or oligospermia	Azoospermia	Same as prepuberal
	Low or absent gonadotrophins Normal growth hormone levels	Low or absent gonadotrophins	Low or absent gonadotrophin, growth hormone, ACTH and TSH functions	
	Normal thyroid and adrenal function	In early stages, normal thyroid and adrenal function		

late complete spermatogenesis. Addition of human FSH to the therapeutic regimen is necessary, but there is no commercially available FSH preparation. For the secondary sex characteristics, libido, normal bone structure, etc., to be maintained, the patient may have to be treated ultimately with testosterone rather than HCG because of financial and logistic considerations.

Prepuberal partial selective gonadotrophin failure

In prepuberal partial selective gonadotrophin failure, puberal development may commence at the expected age but will proceed slowly (Table 21-1) and complete sexual maturation may never be attained. The clinical picture varies, depending on the age at which the individual is first seen. Usually some degree of puberal development is present, as well as puberal gynecomastia. The testes are larger than in prepuberal individuals and are of normal consistency. Testicular histology reveals early stages of spermatogenesis, but the Leydig cells are usually undifferentiated. The total urinary gonadotrophin levels are in the low-normal range. One course of therapy with chorionic go-

nadotrophin (3,000 I.U. three times weekly for 8 weeks) usually induces the patient's own pituitary to assume its normal function and to stimulate complete sexual development.

Complete selective gonadotrophic failure occurring after sexual maturation (hypogonadotrophic hypogonadism)

Complete selective gonadotrophic failure after sexual maturation is a rare condition. The classical picture of eunuchoidism is absent (Table 21-1) since skeletal, muscular, and sexual development was completed prior to the onset of the gonadotrophin insufficiency. The condition is idiopathic and may not be associated with any demonstrable organic disorder to the pituitary gland or the hypothalamus (tumors or cysts). Replacement therapy with gonadotrophins (if fertility is a factor) or with androgens is indicated. Several long-acting preparations of androgens for I.M. use are available: testosterone phenylacetate, testosterone cyclopentylpropionate, and testosterone enanthate. The usual dose is 200 mg. every 3 weeks. Oral preparations like methyl testosterone or fluoxymesterone usually do not elicit full clinical response/ and may produce alterations in liver function.

Testicular dysfunction associated with high urinary gonadotrophin levels
Adult seminiferous tubule failure

Idiopathic adult seminiferous tubule failure. Oligospermia is most commonly associated with abnormalities of the seminiferous epithelium and normal or relatively normal Leydig cell function. The etiology is unknown and the pathophysiology unclear. The condition is apparently progressive. In most but not all cases, urinary gonadotrophins are elevated. Since Leydig cell function is not compromised, secondary sex characteristics, libido, and potency are not affected. The testes may vary in size from perfectly normal to markedly atrophic. No therapy is available.

Postorchitis adult seminiferous tubule failure. Mumps orchitis is the most common infectious process that can produce irreversible damage to the seminiferous tubules. It apparently does not damage the prepuberal testes. Since it is ordinarily unilateral, azoospermia is rare. The onset is rapid; testicular atrophy can occur within a few weeks. Tubular damage is usually patchy, with some areas showing complete atrophy, hyalinization, and fibrosis, whereas other areas exhibit normal spermatogenesis. Leydig cell function is usually not affected. Following severe bilateral involvement, however, there can be complete loss of testicular function. Urinary gonadotrophins are usually elevated. Treatment during the acute stage is supportive and consists of bed rest, cool compresses, analgesics, and antipyretics. Administration of estrogen during the acute phase of the process has been advocated by some to "put the germinal epithelium at rest," but supporting evidence is lacking.

Varicocele. Tulloch, 1952, first gave serious consideration to varicocele as an important factor in oligospermia. Subsequently this factor was confirmed by others.

In 98% of cases, the varicocele is on the left side. Recent venographic studies have shown that a varicocele is an abnormal dilatation of the entire venous system of the testis. It is of interest to note that in cases of unilateral varicocele the contralateral testis may also be affected. Considerable success in the treatment of "male infertility" by means of varicocelectomy has been reported (Charny, 1962; MacLeod, 1965).

Ionizing radiation. Men accidentally exposed to high levels of ionizing radiation sustained deleterious effects on spermatogenesis (MacLeod et al., 1964). The maximum single dose of X irradiation that permits recovery lies probably between 400 and 600 R. The changes in germinal epithelium occur rapidly, but the Leydig cells appear to be quite resistant (Paulsen, 1967).

Heat. The deleterious effect of heat on the germinal epithelium has been studied in detail in lower species. Tokuyama, 1963, demonstrated untoward effects of locally elevated temperature on the human testes. It has been suggested that tight-fitting underwear (jockey shorts) may be harmful to the spermatogenic process.

Klinefelter's syndrome

In 1942, Klinefelter et al. described nine males with azoospermia, hyalinization of the seminiferous tubules, normal Leydig cells, elevated urinary gonadotrophins, and gynecomastia. Heller and Nelson, 1945, later described the lack of constancy of certain clinical features, especially gynecomastia, high-pitched voice, eunuchoidism, female distribution of body hair, and light facial hair growth. Furthermore, the apparent eunuchoid build frequently seen in individuals with Klinefelter's syndrome has been shown to have a different etiology from the classic eunuchoidism of hypogonadotrophic eunuchs. It is not due to delay of epiphysial closure secondary to low androgen levels, but to increased rate of linear growth of long bones in the lower extremities commencing before puberty.

The sex-chromosome complex usually consists of XXY; thus the total number of chromosomes is 47 rather than the normal 46. Subsequently, a number of variants were described (XXXY, XXYY, etc.) and mosaics were reported (Chapter 23). Surveys of newborn, phenotypically male infants for the presence of sex chromatin in buccal smears revealed an incidence of 0.2%; a similar incidence was observed in surveys of adult populations (Paulsen et al., 1964).

Although a genetic etiology is implicated, the pathophysiology remains unclear. Since the normal female requires two X chromosomes, and since one Y chromosome is sufficient for normal male development, the presence of XXY suggests intersexuality. Patients, however, appear somatotypically to be normal males at birth and not until the prepuberal period do changes occur in the testes.

Although the histologic appearance of the Leydig cells suggests unimpaired androgenic function and urinary levels of 17-KS are normal or low normal, the clinical picture strongly suggests a hypoandrogenic state. Testosterone production rates and plasma levels are either subnormal or low normal, and stimulation with HCG usually fails to increase the production rate. The hypogonadal state is progressive and more readily observed in older patients, who may develop frank symptoms of androgenic deficiency.

The incidence of Klinefelter's syndrome in mentally retarded individuals is higher than in the normal population. Psychologic testing of a series of Klinefelter's syndrome patients revealed a tendency toward serious emotional disorders, psychopathic personalities, with difficulties concerning aggressive impulses, and defensive and inferiority feelings in the sexual spheres. In patients with poly-X disorders (XXXXY and XXXY), severe mental retardation is common. An increased incidence of obesity, psychiatric disorders, diabetes mellitus, emphysema, and autoimmune diseases has been suggested.

Studies of serial sections of testes from chromatin-positive adults have revealed small areas of spermatogenesis (Bunge and Bradbury, 1956). Studies of prepuberal boys with positive sex chromatin revealed the presence of gonocytes. The number of gonocytes diminishes with increase in age (Ferguson-Smith, 1959). Recently, individuals with positive sex chromatin, classic 47,XXY karyotypes and areas of spermatogenesis in the testes were reported (Steinberger et al., 1965). Steinberger et al. suggest that the abnormality of spermatogenesis in Klinefelter's syndrome is not the result of congenital absence of germinal cells in the gonads, but inability of the primitive germinal cells (gonocytes) to enter the spermatogenic process; instead, they usually degenerate.

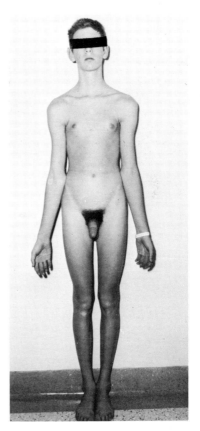

Fig. 21-7. A 16-year-old male with gynecomastia, small firm testes, elevated levels of urinary gonadotrophins and karyotype 47, XXY.

Clinical features. It is difficult to diagnose Klinefelter's syndrome before puberty unless a chromosome analysis is done. The prepuberal testes are of relatively normal size and consistency. The only clue may be the excessive growth of the long bones of the lower extremities. In adults, the characteristic clinical features of diminished androgenicity, as scant beard and body hair, characteristic female pubic hair distribution, poor muscular development, gynecomastia, excessive length of lower extremities, and small (1.5 to 2.5 cm.), very firm testes, call attention to the diagnosis (Fig. 21-7). Useful laboratory tests are determination of urinary gonadotrophin levels (usually elevated in Klinefelter's syndrome), chromosomal analysis (Chapter 23), semen analysis (usually azoospermic), and testicular biopsy. The latter shows hyalinized seminiferous tubules or an occasional tubule lined with Sertoli cells; in some instances there are small patches of spermatogenesis. The Leydig cells are hypertrophic and arranged in large clumps, at times suggestive of small adenomas (Fig. 21-8).

Treatment. Some individuals with Klinefelter's syndrome may undergo apparently normal puberty and experience no difficulty until later in life, when there is infertility or impotency. Various degrees of involvement may be exhibited and the condition may progress at different rates in different individuals. Ultimately a deficiency of androgens will develop and require therapy. Testosterone replacement, as outlined above, is mandatory in cases showing a hypoandrogenic state. The azoospermia is not amenable to treatment. If gynecomastia is a problem, surgical intervention is indicated.

Ullrich-Turner syndrome (male Turner's syndrome)

A syndrome of diminished testicular function and phenotypic characteristics of Turner's syndrome has been described (Chaves-Carballo and Hayles, 1966). The chromosal studies usually have revealed normal 46,XY karyotypes and in others various chromosomal abnormalities (XO, XXY, XO/XY, XO/XY/XYY, etc.). The characteristic clinical findings are short stature, webbed neck, low-set ears, ocular anomalies, "shield" chest, cubitus valgus, cardiovascular anomalies, cryptorchidism, and signs of diminished androgenic function. In some cases gynecomastia, lymphedema of the dorsum of feet and hands, and mental retardation may be present. The histologic picture of the testes is highly variable, ranging from complete fibrosis of seminiferous tubules to various degrees of spermatogenic activity. In postpuberal individuals the urinary gonadotrophin levels are usually elevated. Therapy is directed toward correction of the hypoandrogenic state.

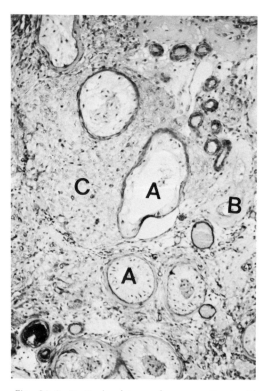

Fig. 21-8. Testicular biopsy from a patient with Klinefelter's syndrome. Note the characteristic features: **A,** seminiferous tubules lined with Sertoli cells only; **B,** completely hyalinized seminiferous tubules; **C,** masses of Leydig cells.

Reifenstein's syndrome

Reifenstein's syndrome resembles Klinefelter's and is characterized by a eunuchoid body build, testicular atrophy, hypospadias, azoospermia, and gynecomastia (Bowen et al., 1965). However, the karyotype is that of a normal male (46,XY). Histologic studies of the testes reveal varying amounts of spermatogenic activity and the presence of elastic fibers in the wall of the seminiferous tubules, indicating that the testes have undergone puberal changes. Treatment consists of surgical correction of gynecomastia and hypospadias and replacement therapy with testosterone.

Sertoli cell syndrome

The syndrome whereby only Sertoli cells are found includes azoospermia or extremely severe oligospermia, elevated gonadotrophin levels, and intact androgenic function. The testes are of normal size and consistency, there are no associated congenital abnormalities, and the skeletal and muscular development is normal. The karyotype is 46,XY. Microscopic examination of the testes reveals seminiferous tubules lacking germinal elements but lined with Sertoli cells. There is no peritubular fibrosis or hyalinization, and the Leydig cells appear normal. Congenital absence of germinal cells has been considered as the etiologic factor in this condition. However, in some instances, particularly in young individuals, areas of spermatogenesis have been observed, arguing against this concept. Since these individuals do not exhibit any androgenic deficiency, replacement therapy with androgens is not indicated.

Cryptorchidism

At birth the incidence is 10%, whereas in adults it is 0.3% to 0.4%, indicating that most cryptorchid testes descend spontaneously. Multiple factors may be responsible—hormonal, anatomic, and even genetic. As associated testicular disorder must be suspected (Klinefelter's, etc.), an endocrinologic evaluation and biopsy of the testes at the time of orchiopexy are essential.

Therapy is hormonal and/or surgical. There is controversy concerning the age at which treatment should be started. Most authors favor treatment before the tenth year, and Nelson et al., 1951, suggested 6 to 7 years of age as the optimal time. The critical issue concerns the interval when irreversible damage to the germinal epithelium can occur by exposure to an intra-abdominal environment and later to the effects of elevated pituitary gonadotrophins, with the onset of puberty. Fertility following orchiopexy is the ultimate criterion of successful therapy. Opinions vary from the pessimism of Charny, 1960, to the reported high incidence of success by Hortling et al., 1967. Surgical damage to the blood supply is an ever-present threat, particularly in young children. Surgery should always be preceded by hormonal therapy. Testicular descent is often accomplished and, if not, gonadal and vasculature structures enlarge, making surgery less difficult. Human chorionic gonadotrophin (HCG) is given in a dosage of 2,000 I.U. thrice weekly for 4 to 5 weeks. If excessive androgenic stimulation occurs (penile growth and erections, pubic hair, etc.), treatment is stopped. A second course can be instituted after a rest period of 2 months if descent fails with the first attempt.

The reported increased incidence of neoplasm in cryptorchid testes provides a further rationale for therapy. Placing the testes into the scrotum, however, does not protect against the possibility of malignant transformation. Because of the extremely low incidence of testicular carcinoma (0.002%) orchiectomy hardly seems justified.

Functional prepuberal castrate syndrome

Functional prepuberal castrate syndrome is characterized by anorchia of unknown etiology. Disturbances in embryologic development of the genital tract have been implicated but not proved. There is no evidence for a genetic disturbance. The testicular destruction, however, must occur after the seventh to fourteenth week of fetal life, since absence of the gonad in earlier stages of development would result in a female phenotype. Definite diagnosis prior to puberty is difficult, since absence of testes from the scrotum can be due to cryptorchidism. At or after puberty the diagnosis still requires exploratory surgery for confirmation but can be made on the basis of clinical and laboratory findings. Since there are no functional Leydig cells, puberal changes fail to occur and the scrotum is empty. A classical picture of sexual infantilism is present. The urinary gonadotrophins are extremely high. Also, in contradistinction to hypogonadotrophic eunuchoidism, in which the patients are tall, these individuals are short. Usually no other congenital anomalies or cytogenetic abnormalities are present. The treatment is androgenic replacement and has to be continued for life.

Testicular feminization

In 1953, Morris coined the term "testicular feminization syndrome" to describe individuals with a female phenotype and testes instead of ovaries.

Clinical features. There is primary amenorrhea, infertility, or dyspareunia. The classic history is that of a normal "female" who experienced somatic development at puberty but failed to properly develop axillary and pubic hair and menstrual cycles. Occasionally there is a history of tender inguinal swellings. A family history of a similar disorder in a sister or maternal aunt is not uncommon. On physical examination the body habitus is feminine, with well-developed breasts and rounded hips. Pelvic examination reveals a vagina with normal mucosa ending in a blind pouch. No cervix or uterus is palpable, and there is no clitoral hypertrophy. Not uncommonly, the testes are palpable in the inguinal canals as tender lumps resembling hernias. Chromosomal analysis reveals a male karyotype (46,XY). Other laboratory studies, and particularly endocrine studies, are usually normal. The findings of normal male levels of testosterone and estrogen, feminine habitus of the patient, and failure to demonstrate any androgenic effect after administration of massive doses of androgen, suggest that there is genetic insensitivity of body tissues to androgen. A recent report implicates the absence of 5α-reduction of testosterone in peripheral tissues.

Treatment consists of castration followed by replacement estrogen therapy. Castration is indicated because of increased incidence of malignancy in the ectopic testes. In a prepuberal patient, it may be wise to delay castration until after puberty and thus obtain as normal a puberal development as possible.

REFERENCES

Albert, A.: The mammalian testis. In Young, W. C., and Corner, G. W., editors: Sex and Internal Secretions, Baltimore, 1961, The Williams & Wilkins Co., p. 305.

Bowen, P., et al.: Ann. Intern. Med. **62**:252, 1965.

Bunge, R. G., and Bradbury, J. T.: J. Urol. **76**:758, 1956.

Charny, C. W.: J. Urol. **83**:697, 1960.

Charny, C. W.: Fertil. Steril. **13**:47, 1962.

Charny, C. W., et al.: Ann. N. Y. Acad. Sci. **55**:597, 1952.

Chaves-Carballo, E., and Hayles, A. B.: Mayo Clin. Proc. **41**:843, 1966.

Clermont, Y.: Amer. J. Anat. **112**:35, 1963.

Ferguson-Smith, M. A.: Lancet **1**:219 (1959).

Gemzell, C. A., and Kjessler, B.: Lancet **1**:644, 1964.

Harrison, R. G., and Barclay, A. E.: Brit. J. Urol. **20**:57, 1948.

Heller, C. G., and Nelson, W. O.: J. Clin. Endocr. **5**:1, 1945.

Heller, C. G., and Nelson, W. O.: J. Clin. Endocr. **8**:345, 1948.

Hortling, H., et al.: J. Clin. Endocr. **27**:120, 1967.

Klinefelter, H. F., et al.: J. Clin. Endocr. **2**:615, 1942.

MacLeod, J.: Fertil. Steril. **16**:735, 1965.

MacLeod, J., et al.: J.A.M.A. **187**:637, 1964.

MacLeod, J., et al.: Fertil. Steril. **17**:7, 1966.

Maddock, W. O., and Nelson, W. O.: J. Clin. Endocr. **12**:985, 1952.

Morris, M. J.: Amer. J. Obstet. Gynec. **65**:1192, 1953.

Nelson, W. O.: Recent Progr. Hormone Res. 6:29, 1951.

Paulsen, C. A.: Nuclear Science Abstr. **21**:abst. 408, 1967.

Paulsen, C. A., et al.: J. Clin. Endocr. **24**:1182, 1964.

Schonfeld, W. A.: Amer. J. Dis. Child. **65**:535, 1943.

Steinberger, E., et al.: J. Clin. Endocr. **25**:1340, 1965.

Steinberger, E., and Tjioe, D. Y.: Fertil. Steril. **19**:960, 1968.

Steinberger, E., and Ficher, M.: Biol. Reprod. **1**:119, 1969.

Tokuyama, I.: Quoted by Leblond, C. P., et al. In Hartman, C. G., editor: Mechanisms concerned with conception, New York, 1963, The Macmillan Co. p. 38.

Tulloch, W. S.: Trans. Edinburgh Obstet. Soc., p. 29, 1952; in Edinburgh Med. J. March, 1952.

Chapter 22

Hermaphroditism and abnormalities of sexual development

Emil Steinberger, M.D.
Keith D. Smith, M.D.

The gender of an individual is distinguished by specific combinations of a number of morphologic, physiologic, and psychologic characteristics. During embryonal and postnatal developmental stages, these characteristics become established in the proper sequence, and their expression results in normal sexual development. Any departure, be it congenital or acquired, can be considered a sexual abnormality.

Although no classification of sexual abnormalities satisfies all criteria, it is advantageous to group these disorders into several categories for discussion. Since the clinical manifestations of a number of these abnormalities are presented in other chapters, we will appropriately limit our discussion of these categories and emphasize the clinical approach to differential diagnosis.

CONGENITAL ABNORMALITIES
Chromosomal abnormalities

Individuals with Klinefelter's syndrome or Turner's syndrome are examples of chromosomal abnormalities, expressed developmentally by deficient differentiation of the gonads. Since the external genitalia of these individuals are usually normal at birth and not inconsistent with their gonadal sex, no problems arise in assignment to the proper sex on the basis of the phenotypic characteristics. Later in life gyne-

comastia is often seen in patients with Klinefelter's syndrome, and immaturity of genitalia in those with Turner's syndrome. Nevertheless, these individuals do not present sexual ambiguity and should not be considered as examples of intersex. The clinical and cytogenetic aspects of these disorders are discussed in Chapters 20 and 21.

Endocrine abnormalities

Male pseudohermaphroditism. Individuals having male pseudohermaphroditism are genetic males with testes yet demonstrate a female phenotype that results from an inappropriate response of peripheral tissue to androgens or a congenital adrenal disorder of steroid synthesis.

TESTICULAR FEMINIZATION. Patients with testicular feminization are reared as females and develop a relatively normal female habitus. Clinical manifestations and pathophysiology are discussed in Chapter 21.

VARIANTS OF CONGENITAL ADRENAL HYPERPLASIA. The severity of the adrenal lesion precludes survival in these extremely rare conditions. The pathophysiology consists of blockage in both adrenal and testicular steroid biogenesis, secondary to absence or deficiency of enzymes necessary for conversion of cholesterol to pregnenolone (congenital lipoid hyperplasia) or pregnenolone to progesterone (deficiency of Δ^5-3β-hydroxysteroid dehydrogenase). This blockage results not only in adrenal insufficiency but also in failure of testosterone production by the fetal testis, yielding incomplete masculinization of the external genitalia (see Chapter 15).

Female pseudohermaphroditism. This condition of female pseudohermaphroditism is characterized by the presence of ovaries and female karyotypes in individuals with frank virilization, secondary to congenital adrenal disease or administration of androgens to the mother during pregnancy.

CONGENITAL VIRILIZING ADRENAL HYPERPLASIA. In this disorder a biochemical lesion of the adrenal gland results in excessive production of androgens in the female fetus, which induces masculinization of its external genitalia. Details are discussed in Chapter 15.

IATROGENIC CONDITION. Administration of steroids with androgenic activity to pregnant females may result in virilization of a female fetus. The type and degree of virilization depend on the stage of gestation at which the fetus is exposed to the offending agent. In addition to androgens (methyl testosterone), a number of synthetic progestins (Norlutin, Progestoral, Pranone) have been implicated. It is of interest that Bongiovanni et al., 1959, have reported masculinization in 4 infants whose mothers received stilbestrol during pregnancy.

True hermaphroditism

The diagnosis of true hermaphroditism requires histologic demonstration of both ovarian and testicular elements. Although this condition is relatively rare, Overzier, 1963, was able to collect 171 cases from the literature between 1900 and 1962.

Clinical findings. In newborns the external genitalia usually reveal some ambiguity such as an enlarged phallus in a female infant, or cryptorchidism and/or hypospadias in a male. In puberal individuals one may find gynecomastia, cryptor-chidism, hypospadias, and probably every gradation between normal male and female external genitalia. Most patients have a uterus that is well developed, whereas a prostate is less common. Testis, ovary, or an ovotestis may be found in the scrotum or in the inguinal canal, and inguinal hernias are common. The presence of seminal vesicles, epididymides, vasa deferentia, fallopian tubes, and a vagina is variable. The urethra may vary from fully penile to typically female. Other than having symptoms associated with ambiguity of the external genitalia, patients may occasionally complain of cyclic hematuria, which, of course, is menstruation. Although no patients have been found to be fertile, the presence of spermatozoa in the seminal fluid has been reported.

The karyotype is usually 46,XX, but 46,XY or mosaics occur. Determination of pituitary and gonadal hormones is also of no diagnostic value.

Therapy is dependent on the patient's age at diagnosis, specific physical characteristics, and gonadal type. In general, one tries to assign a sex consistent with prior rearing and desire, or consistent with anticipated future development. If necessary, one or both gonads may be removed and appropriate replacement therapy instituted.

Isolated genital duct abnormalities

Although genital duct abnormalities may be associated with any congenital disorder, they may also occur independently.

Male

HYPOSPADIAS. Various degrees of hypospadias in the male are relatively common and occasionally familial. Deficient function of fetal Leydig cells resulting in inadequate virilization during embryonal development has been postulated as the mechanism of this disorder. It should be emphasized that in most instances no abnormality of gonadal function develops postnatally.

HERNIAE UTERI INGUINALES. Failure of fetal testes to elaborate duct-organizing substance or failure of the müllerian duct to respond to this substance may result in the presence of derivatives of this structure in otherwise normal males. In most instances a uterus, fallopian tubes, and at least one ectopic testis are found at abdominal surgery or herniorrhaphy in otherwise normal males. Instances of fertility in some patients have been recorded. Treatment is hysterosalpingectomy.

Female

UTERINE, TUBAL, AND VAGINAL ANOMALIES. Various forms of anomalies from reduplication to absence have been reported. They are commonly associated with congenital abnormalities of the urinary tract. Since hormonal etiology is unlikely, the abnormal differentiation of these müllerian duct derivatives is, most likely, a result of defective embryogenesis of the urogenital ridge in early fetal life.

URETHRAL ANOMALIES. The presence of an accessory urethra traversing the clitoris and producing an apparent clitoral hypertrophy may cause a diagnostic problem. Other abnormalities, such as urogenital sinus (common orifice of urethra and vagina) in otherwise normal females, have been reported.

ACQUIRED ABNORMALITIES

If it is accepted that an individual's gender is determined by certain morphologic, physiologic, and psychologic characteristics, acquired changes in any one of these characteristics could then, by definition, be considered as an abnormality in sexual development, even though it may occur after full development has taken place.

Psychologic abnormality

Serious disturbances in psychosexual development may result in homosexuality or transvestism. In these individuals the morphologic and genetic sex characteristics are in conflict with the psychologic expression of sexuality. Numerous studies have shown no evidence of endocrine disturbances. The discussion of the pathophysiology of these conditions is beyond the scope of this chapter.

Endocrine abnormality

Feminization in males. Acquired feminization in males can be expressed by development of gynecomastia, change in body contours, changes in facial and body hair, and testicular atrophy.

TUMORS. Estrogen-producing tumors of the adrenals (Chapter 15) and interstitial cell tumors or choriocarcinoma of the testes have been reported to produce feminization. When the tumor occurs in prepuberal individuals, the development of gynecomastia may be the only sign of feminization; in an adult, one of the first symptoms may be decline in potency and libido. Subsequently, changes in body and facial hair, gynecomastia, and testicular atrophy (except for the affected testis in case of testicular tumor) appear. In most instances, elevated urinary estrogen levels can be demonstrated.

METABOLIC AND IDIOPATHIC ABNORMALITY. Gynecomastia is the most obvious sign of a feminizing disorder in a male. The association of liver cirrhosis with gynecomastia and testicular atrophy has been considered to be due to defective estrogen conjugation resulting in elevated levels of free, thus biologically active, estrogens. Recently, utilizing sophisticated techniques, Korenman et al., 1969, demonstrated definite elevation of plasma estradiol levels in patients with liver cirrhosis. Testosterone is also capable of inducing transient gynecomastia when administered to hypogonadal males. The pathophysiology of this process is poorly understood, but it should be noted that testosterone is convertible in vivo to estrogens. A similar mechanism may be operative in the induction of puberal gynecomastia, a relatively common condition that is usually transitory and leaves no residual breast enlargement. When the breast enlargement persists until adulthood, surgical excision is the only form of therapy.

Painful gynecomastia was noted after

refeeding in malnourished prisoners of war, concentration camp inmates, and individuals with malnutrition caused by other factors ("refeeding gynecomastia"). The pathophysiology is unclear. Gynecomastia has also been described in association with hyperthyroidism, hypothyroidism, multiple myeloma, ulcerative colitis, pituitary tumors, bronchogenic carcinoma, and pulmonary osteoarthropathy. Drugs such as digitalis, phenothiazines, reserpine, and spironolactone can induce gynecomastia.

Masculinization in females. Acquired changes in sexual characteristics are a relatively common finding in the female. The major difficulty in discerning these disturbances lies in the approach one takes toward defining which abnormality constitutes masculinization. All authors accept the diagnosis of virilization when the full-blown picture of clitoral hypertrophy, severe hirsutism, skeletal muscle changes, bitemporal balding, change in voice, and breast atrophy is present. Although some authors will limit the diagnosis to only those patients showing all of the above changes, others will consider it also when minor changes of hirsutism or clitoral hypertrophy are present. If we accept the concept that any change in the morphologic, physiologic, or psychologic determinants disturbs the normal expression of sexual development, then the latter view would be acceptable.

The symptomatology leading to masculinization is usually caused by neoplastic or metabolic disorders of the adrenal and/or the ovary. The details of these conditions are discussed in the chapters on the adrenal and the ovary. The occurrence of iatrogenic masculinization has been declining in recent years, particularly because of diminished use of androgens in the treatment of the menopause. However, iatrogenic etiologies should be considered, since androgens are still being used in a variety of metabolic and neoplastic conditions.

REFERENCES

Bongiovanni, A. M., et al.: J. Clin. Endocr. **19:** 1004, 1959.

Korenman, S. G., et al.,: American Society for Clinical Investigation, 61st annual meeting, abst. 144, 1969.

Overzier, C.: Intersexuality, New York, 1963, Academic Press, Inc., p. 182.

Chapter 23

Cytogenetics in endocrinology*

Emil Steinberger, M.D.
Anna Steinberger, Ph.D.

SEX CHROMATIN

Moore and Barr, 1954, first described a characteristic chromatin mass in cell nuclei of the human female. This elliptical or planoconvex "Barr body" measures approximately 1 μ in its largest diameter. It usually appears close to or is attached to the membrane of an interphase nucleus (Fig. 23-1). It has an affinity for basic dyes and gives reactions specific for deoxyribonucleic acid (DNA). On the basis of its staining properties, it can thus be easily distinguished from nucleoli of similar size and shape that exhibit staining characteristics of ribonucleic acid (RNA). Barr bodies are found in 20% to 80% of cells in the female and in zero to several percent of cells in the male. Another form of sex chromatin is a nuclear appendage called a "drumstick" found in circulating polymorphonucleated luekocytes. The drumstick consists of a small nuclear lobe 1.5 μ in diameter attached to the rest of the nucleus by a thin chromatin thread (Fig. 23-2), and is found in 2% to 5% of cells in females and is absent in males.

It was originally thought that the Barr body was formed by fusion of the heterochromatic portions of two X chromosomes. This suggested that "chromatin-positive" patients with Klinefelter's syndrome were chromosomal females (XX), and "chromatin-negative" individuals, as in Turner's syndrome, were chromosomal males. Thus the expressions "male chromatin pattern" and "female chromatin pattern" evolved. However, studies dealing with the dynamics of chromosome duplication and cell division provided evidence for a single X chromosome origin of the Barr body. It is now accepted that the Barr body represents the "heteropyknotic" X chromosome. In view of these findings, the terms "male chromatin pattern" and "female chromatin pattern" are misleading.

Lyon, 1962, advanced the hypothesis that the heteropyknotic X chromosome is genetically inactive. She postulated that in the female the genes located on one X chromosome are inactivated early in embryonic life. Recent studies in animals have demonstrated that the selection of the inactive X chromosome is random in each cell. Therefore, in the female the active X chromosome is approximately equally representative of paternal and maternal origins. In the normal male it is, of course, always of maternal origin. Thus both sexes have a single set of X chromosome–linked genes.

Except for polyploid cells, the number

*This work has been supported by U. S. Public Health Grants, numbers HD-00399 and AM-05449, and also by a grant from The Ford Foundation.

Grateful acknowledgment is made to Mrs. A. Sweiman and Mrs. M. Hollander for their editorial assistance.

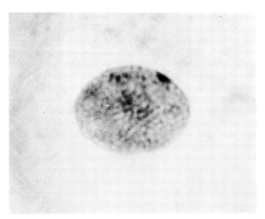

Fig. 23-1. Sex chromatin in nucleus of a buccal epithelium cell.

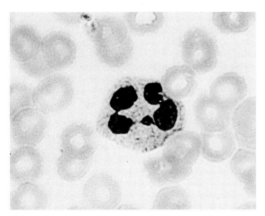

Fig. 23-2. Drumstick in a circulating polymorphonuclear leukocyte.

of Barr bodies per nucleus is equal to the number of X chromosomes minus one. Consequently, in cells containing only one X chromosome, no Barr bodies are found (normal male, XY; ovarian dysgenesis, XO). In cells with two X chromosomes (normal female, XX; Klinefelter's syndrome, XXY) there is one Barr body; in cells with three X chromosomes ("superfemale," XXX) there are two Barr bodies, etc.

The techniques for detection of sex chromatin can be used for screening a large number of individuals, as well as in the initial diagnostic investigation of patients with suspected sex chromosome abnormalities. The determination is not helpful in the diagnosis of genetic dis-

turbances that are not related to sex chromosomes, nor does it provide information concerning the Y chromosome. Absence of sex chromatin can be observed in individuals with markedly diverse sex chromosome complements. Similarly, study of sex chromatin may not reveal the presence of some forms of mosaics. For example, absence of Barr bodies in a male would suggest normality, whereas a detailed chromosomal analysis may reveal a mosaic of XO/XY. Furthermore, in patients with mosaicism, the number of sex chromosomes may vary, depending on the source of tissue being examined.

Technique for sex chromatin study

1. The inside of the cheek is scraped with a spatula, some pressure being exerted to obtain cells from the deeper epithelial layers.

2. The material is spread thinly on a slide that is placed immediately into freshly prepared chilled ether and absolute ethanol (equal parts).

3. The preparation is fixed for a minimum of 15 minutes (up to 24 hours) at 4° C.; then it is hydrated in 50% ethanol and two changes of water, 5 minutes each.

4. The cell nuclei are stained with 0.5% solution of cresyl fast violet for 5 minutes; the slide is rinsed in water to remove excess dye, then dehydrated and differentiated in ethanol.

5. For permanent storage the preparation can be mounted under a coverslip. The percentage of nuclei containing the Barr body is ascertained by microscopic examination.

CHROMOSOMAL ABNORMALITIES

Abnormalities in a karyotype can be expressed by changes in the number of chromosomes or changes in their morphologic appearance (deletions, translocations, ring chromosome, or isochromosome formation). It is certain that gross morphologic abnormalities observed in the chromosomes must involve a large number of genes.

Somatic cells, which are normally dip-

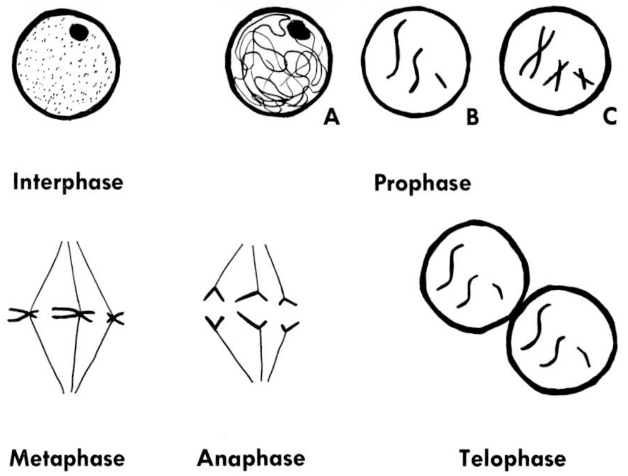

Interphase · Prophase

Metaphase · Anaphase · Telophase

Fig. 23-3. Diagram of nuclear changes during mitosis. For simplicity only three chromosomes are shown. *Prophase:* **A,** Chromatin forms a continuous thread; **B,** nucleolus disappears, and individual chromosomes become visible; **C,** synthesis of DNA takes place so that each chromosome becomes duplicated but is held together by the centromere. *Metaphase:* Nuclear membrane disappears; chromosomes arrange themselves in the equatorial plate and become attached to the mitotic spindle by the centromeres. In this stage the chromosomes are most suitable for cytogenetic analysis. *Anaphase:* Duplicated chromosomes move toward opposite poles of the cell. *Telophase:* Nuclear membrane reappears, enclosing a diploid number of chromosomes in each newly formed cell.

loid, divide by a process of mitosis and yield two daughter cells, which contain chromosomal complements identical to those of the original cell (Fig. 23-3). The formation of a gamete requires the occurrence of a miotic division, during which the number of chromosomes is reduced to half (Fig. 23-4). An abnormal number of chromosomes can be produced as a result of nondisjunction or anaphase lagging taking place during mitosis (Fig. 23-5) or miosis (Fig. 23-6). The term denoting a normal number of chromosomes is *euploid*; the gametes have a *haploid* (one-half) number of chromosomes in comparison with the diploid number of somatic cells. Cells containing a number of chromosomes other than the normal are called *heteroploid*. If the number of chromosomes is greater than normal, it is *hyperploid*; if lesser, *hypoploid*. A chromosome number that is an exact multiple of the normal haploid complement is called *polyploid*, whereas a number deviating from the exact multiple is *aneuploid*.

Structural chromosomal abnormalities usually result from breaks. A piece of a chromosome after breaking off may become lost, a process called *deletion*. If the detached fragment unites with another chromosome, the process is called *translocation*. When there is an exchange of genetic material between two chromosomes, the process is called *reciprocal translocation*.

CHROMOSOMAL ANALYSIS

Refinements of the original technique of Tjio and Levan, 1956, particularly by methods that permit chromosomal analysis on a drop or two of whole blood (Steinberger et al., 1964), brought chromosomal analysis from the realm of the research laboratory to the patient's bedside. Advantage is taken of the fact that chromosomes become morphologically best defined during the metaphase in cell division. Theoretically any tissue in which cell multiplication takes place can be utilized. In several instances like bone marrow or testes, the rate of cell divisions is naturally high and the chromosomal analysis can be performed on the original tissues. How-

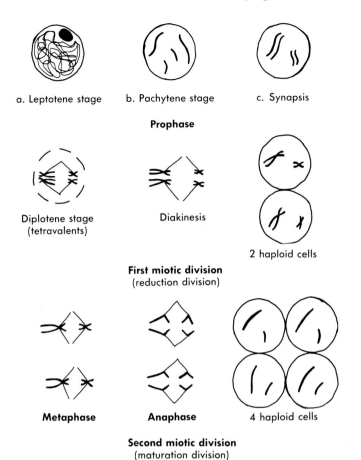

a. Leptotene stage   b. Pachytene stage   c. Synapsis

Prophase

Diplotene stage (tetravalents)   Diakinesis   2 haploid cells

First miotic division (reduction division)

Metaphase   Anaphase   4 haploid cells

Second miotic division (maturation division)

Fig. 23-4. Diagram of nuclear changes during miosis. For simplicity only four chromosomes (two homologous pairs) are shown. *Prophase:* **a,** Leptotene stage; **b,** pachytene stage—individual chromosomes become discernible; **c,** synapsis—homologous chromosomes pair up. *First miotic division:* Diplotene stage—duplicated chromosomes appear as tetravalents in the equatorial plate. Diakinesis—nuclear membrane disappears. Members of homologous pairs begin to separate toward opposite poles of the cell forming two cells with haploid number of duplicated chromosomes. *Second miotic division:* Chromosomes separate to form four haploid cells.

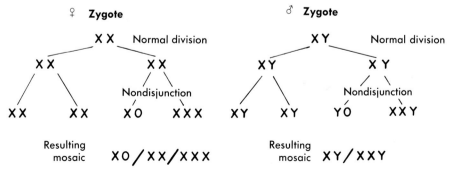

Fig. 23-5. Mitotic nondisjunction of sex chromosomes giving rise to cell stem lines with different karyotypes.

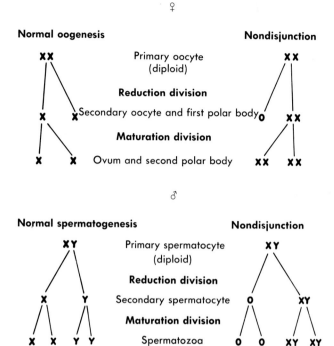

Fig. 23-6. Miotic nondisjunction of sex chromosomes. An ovum containing XX or O chromosomes fertilized by normal X or Y sperm may give rise to XO (Turner); XXX (superfemale); YO (probably nonviable); or XXY (Klinefelter) sex chromosomes; spermatozoon containing XY or O sex chromosomes fertilizing a normal ovum may give rise to a zygote with XO (Turner) or XXY (Klinefelter) sex chromosomes.

ever, in most other cases the tissue has to be cultured in order to obtain a sufficiently high rate of cell divisions. Since the discovery that leukocytes from peripheral blood can be induced to divide in culture by phytohemagglutinin, blood has been most frequently used for karyotyping. It is readily available and requires only 3 days of culture, compared to several weeks required for skin.

The techniques for obtaining slide preparations suitable for karyotyping, using various tissue sources, have been reviewed by Moorehead and Nowell (1964). Well-spread metaphases (Fig. 23-7, A) are examined microscopically and the chromosomes are analyzed for numerical or gross morphologic abnormalities. The metaphase is photographed and enlarged in printing, and the individual chromosomes are arranged into appropriate pairs and groups,

according to the Denver system of classification (see p. 410). Artifacts during preparation must be recognized. For example, a chromosome may become dislodged from one metaphase and become associated with another, resulting in two abnormal counts, one higher and one lower than the modal number. In case of numerical abnormality, it becomes important to establish which chromosome is involved. A true abnormality will consistently involve a specific chromosome, whereas deviations resulting from technique artifacts will usually involve different chromosomes. Analysis of distribution of chromosome counts in a large number of cells in individuals with normal modal number of 46 showed that the count distribution is not symmetrical but negatively skewed; approximately 12.1% of cells have counts lower than 46, and only 2.9% have

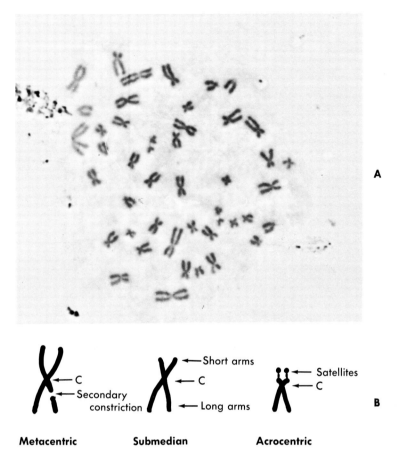

Metacentric   **Submedian**   **Acrocentric**

Fig. 23-7. A, Well-spread metaphase prepared according to the standard cytogenetic techniques. **B,** Diagram of basic shapes of chromosomes during metaphase (**C,** centromere).

counts in excess of 46 (Court-Brown et al., 1960).

Morphology of chromosomes during metaphase

The microscopic appearance of chromosomes during metaphase is shown in Fig. 23-7, *A,* and diagrammatically represented in Fig. 23-7, *B.* A chromosome has two sets of arms, short and long, separated by the primary constriction called *centromere.* Some chromosomes also have bits of chromatin material connected to the rest of the chromosome by thin chromatin strands, called *satellites.* Based on the position of the centromere, chromosomes are classified into several morphologic types. They are *median* or *metacentric* when the short-

arm long-arm ratio is close to 1; *submedian* or *submetacentric* when this ratio is slightly less than 1; and *subterminal* or *acrocentric* when one set of arms is extremely short. Recently it has been demonstrated that with proper staining techniques achromatic regions (secondary constrictions) can be observed in certain chromosomes—a fact which may be used for their identification.

Karyotype

The normal karyotype in the human consists of 44 autosomes (22 pairs) and two sex chromosomes—X and Y in the male, and two X chromosomes in the female for a total of 46. Half of the diploid number (23) is called haploid and is characteristic

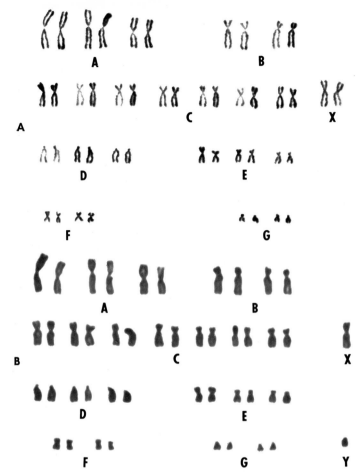

Fig. 23-8. A, Karyotype of a normal female. **B,** Karyotype of a normal male.

for the sperm and for the ovum. These cells have 22 autosomes and a single sex chromosome. The spermatozoon contains either an X or a Y chromosome, whereas an ovum always contains one X chromosome.

The first classification of chromosomes was adopted in 1960 (Denver Conference, 1960) and is referred to as the Denver classification. The chromosomal pairs are matched and arranged in a descending order of size (Fig. 23-8). On the basis of the size and position of the centromere, they form seven groups. The X chromosome is grouped together with pairs 6 to 12, since morphologically it often cannot be distinguished from them. The Y chromosome is acrocentric and simi-

lar in size to chromosomes in pairs 19 and 20. During the second conference on chromosomal classification (The London Conference on the Normal Human Karyotype, 1963), further refinements in defining specific chromosomes were made and the seven groups were designated by letters of the alphabet, A to G. Recently a third conference was held, called Standardization in Human Cytogenetics (Chicago Conference, 1966), in which further changes and additions in nomenclature were adopted. Since this nomenclature is presently in use, it will be described in greater detail.

Karyotypes are described by recording the total number of chromosomes, followed by a comma, followed by the sex chromosome complement. For example, Klinefelter's syndrome, with a total of 47 chromosomes and XXY sex chromosome complement, is recorded as *47,XXY*. A normal male karyotoype with 46 chromosomes and XY sex chromosome complement is recorded as *46,XY*.

Numerical alterations

In cases with a numerical abnormality of autosomes, the group in which this abnormality is observed is indicated and followed by a *minus* sign when a chromosome is missing and a *plus* sign when an extra chromosome is present. For example, when a chromosome is missing in group C in an otherwise normal female karyotype, it will be recorded as *45,XX,C–*. When an extra chromosome is found in group C, the karyotype is recorded as *47,XX,C+*. When the missing chromosome has been identified with certainty, the chromosome number may be used instead of the group designation as *45,XX,16–*. If a karyotype contains 46 chromosomes with XX sex chromosomes, an extra number 16 chromosome, and a missing number 21 chromosome, it would be written as *46,XX,16+,21–*. A polyploidy or heteroploidy is evident from the chromosomal number. Presence of endoreduplication is indicated by the abbreviation *END* as *END 46,XX*. Chromosomal mosaics are recorded by separating the various karyotype designations by a diagonal line as *47,XXY/46,XY*.

Structural alterations

An increase in length of the short arm is indicated by *p+* and of the long arm by *q+*, a decrease in their length by *p–* or *q–*, respectively. For example, a deletion of a short arm in the number 4 chromosome in an otherwise normal karyotype of a male is recorded as *46,XY,4p–*. A translocation is indicated by the letter *t* preceding the parenthesis in which the involved chromosomes are indicated. For example, translocation between the short arm of a chromosome from group A and the long arm of a chromosome from group B is indicated as *46,XY,t(Ap–;Bq+)*. Isochromosome is indicated by the letter *i* placed after the arm designation for the involved chromosome. For example, an isochromosome that originated from the long arm of the X chromosome in a male is indicated as *46,XqiY*. Ring chromosomes are indicated by the letter *r* placed after the involved chromosome. Therefore, a ring formation involving chromosome 19 is indicated as *46,XY,19r*. Satellites are designated by the letter *s*, secondary constriction by the letter *h*; the centromere is abbreviated *cen*. For additional details see the Chicago Conference (1966).

CHROMOSOMAL ABNORMALITIES IN CLINICAL ENDOCRINOLOGY

Following the description by Lejeune et al., 1959 of a specific chromosomal abnormality in mongolism, there were reports on the abnormalities in Turner's and in Klinefelter's syndromes. In the ensuing years there were innumerable reports of a wide variety of sex chromosomal abnormalities. However, only a small number of abnormalities of the autosomal chromosomes were observed, suggesting that such abnormalities have a more deleterious effect on the development of an organism than do abnormalities of sex chromosomes. Grumbach et al., 1963, and the studies by Lyon, 1962, which indicated that viability of zygote depends, most likely, on the presence of only one X chromosome, support this hypothesis. Consequently, abnormalities in the number of X chromosomes are compatible with life.

When the characteristic abnormalities of Klinefelter's and Turner's syndromes were described, it was hoped that sex chromosomal abnormalities would clearly define certain disease entities. However, in addition to the lack of a definite chromosomal pattern in hermaphrodites, a great array of chromosomal abnormalities that do not correspond to specific clinical phenotypes have been reported. Conversely, it has been shown that often the degree of observed phenotypic abnormality is not related to the degree of chromosomal derangement.

Klinefelter's syndrome

The clinical features of Klinefelter's syndrome are discussed in Chapter 21. Sex chromatin is found in a large proportion of nuclei in buccal smears from these patients, and the karyotype is 47,XXY (Fig. 23-9). It has been suggested that a chromosome complement of XXY is related to absence of germinal epithelium in the testes. However, recent reports provided evidence of spermatogenesis in patients with Klinefelter's syndrome and a 47,XXY karyotype, based on study of the peripheral blood (Steinberger et al., 1965).

XXY sex chromosomes. The XXY pattern is probably the most common sex chromosome abnormality. It is encountered in 0.2% to 0.3% of all live births among Caucasians (Marden et al., 1964). The pathophysiology in most cases is maternal meiotic nondisjunction.

Supernumerary X chromosomes. Numerous cases of Klinefelter's syndrome with a complement of more than two X chromosomes have been reported. These patients show mental retardation and increased severity of testicular lesions, but no additional specific physical changes have been detected. However, in patients with XXXY there is a severe degree of mental retarda-

tion, together with the classic testicular picture and hypoplasia of the genitals, and various skeletal anomalies, the most constant being proximal radial-ulnar synostosis, hypertelorism, strabismus, epicanthic folds, and mongoloid slanting of the palpebral tissues (Scherz and Roeckel, 1963). The mechanism of XXXXY or XXXY formation is, most likely, double nondisjunction occurring during the first and second meiotic division in oogenesis. Under these circumstances, depending on whether three or four chromosomes segregate together, an ovum with XXXX or XXX sex chromosome complement will be formed. Fertilization of such an ovum with a normal sperm carrying a Y chromosome will produce a zygote with XXXXY or XXXY sex chromosomes.

Chromosomal mosaicism. Numerous reports of chromosomal mosaics in Klinefelter's syndrome have been reported. The number of cell lines may vary and may contain any one of the abnormal sex chromosome complements such as an XY/XXY mosaic, XX/XXY or a triple line XY/XXY/XXYY. It is difficult to predict the degree of gonadal damage in mosaicism, because it depends on whether the abnormal cell line involves the germinal cells. This difficulty is illustrated by a report of a patient with an XY/XXXY mosaic who was mentally deficient but had perfectly normal testes and secondary sex

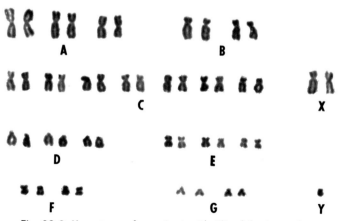

Fig. 23-9. Karyotype of a patient with Klinefelter's syndrome.

characteristics (Barr et al., 1962). Possibly the XY cell line was responsible for the normal differentiation of gonads, while the XXXY cells in some way affected the development of the nervous system. It would seem that a chromosomal analysis performed directly on the germ cells could yield more reliable information on the relationship between the chromosomal abnormalities and the extent of testicular damage.

Turner's syndrome

Numerous cases of Turner's syndrome have been reported with various clinical manifestations. Different terms like ovarian aplasia, ovarian hypoplasia, and ovarian dysplasia, as well as gonadal dysgenesis and gonadal agenesis, have been used, sometimes interchangeably, not only for the classic Turner's syndrome but also for similar syndromes. The authors prefer to reserve the term ovarian dysgenesis for the classic Turner's syndrome, which may correspond to Wilkins' ovarian aplasia. In these cases there is no evidence of a mosaic and the sex chromosomal complement is consistently XO (Fig. 23-10). There is a "streak" gonad, absence of nuclear sex chromatin, female external and internal genitalia and poor secondary sex development. Besides this "pure" syndrome, a variety of gradations exist with streak gonads and positive nuclear sex chromatin associated with a chromosomal mosaic like XX/XO. Other combinations associated with a variety of mosaics, deletion of a part of or the whole X chromosome, translocations, etc., may be clinically labeled as ovarian hypoplasias or dysplasias. The clinical diagnosis of Turner's syndrome may not become evident until puberty, except when webbing of the neck, short stature, or congenital lymphedema exists. Turner's syndrome represents a rare chromosomal abnormality occurring about once in 2,000 female births.

XO. In XO there is neck webbing, epicanthic folds, congenital lymphedema, and coarctation of the aorta. The mechanism of formation of the XO complex is not as clearly defined as that of the XXY, but in most cases it is probably nondisjunction of maternal origin.

XO/XX mosaicism. Cases vary from typical Turner's syndrome, with the many associated anomalies, to those with normal gonadal and somatic development. Patients reported as having a typical XX pattern with characteristic clinical signs and symptoms may represent undetected XO/XX mosaics. Mosaicism should be suspected whenever there is a discrepancy between nuclear sex chromatin and the karyotype or when an unusually low percentage of chromatin-positive nuclei is found in a

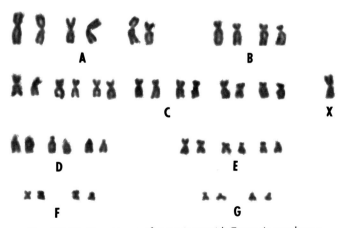

Fig. 23-10. Karyotype of a patient with Turner's syndrome.

phenotypic female. The detection of mosaicism is difficult even with extensive study of several tissues.

Isochromosome X. Lindsten, 1963, in his report of 56 cases of Turner's syndrome, includes 2 patients having 46 chromosomes, one of whom had a large metacentric chromosome resembling an extra chromosome number 3. He asumed that this was an isochromosome for the long arm of one X chromosome, that is, 46,XqiX. In the same report he mentions 9 patients with 46,XqiX/45,XO mosaic.

Partial loss of an X chromosome. Deletion of the short arm or the long arm of X chromosome has been reported. However, the evidence for it was only presumptive, since it was based solely on morphology. Recently more definitive evidence for partial loss of an X chromosome was presented by Atkins et al., 1965, and Steinberger et al., 1966. The latter case involved a 9-year-old female whose only clinical symptom was loss of eyebrows. Chromosomal analysis revealed 46 chromosomes, with apparently one normal and one deleted X chromosome. Radioautographic studies showed the deleted chromosome being late labeling, thus confirming its X chromosome origin (Fig. 23-11).

Ring X chromosome. Lindsten, 1963, suggested the association between a ring X chromosome and ovarian dysgenesis. The ring chromosome appears to be formed by deletion of parts of both the short and the long arms of an X chromosome, with a subsequent fusion of the broken ends.

XO/XY mosaicism

The mosaic of XO/XY is associated with the greatest variation in phenotypic and clinical manifestations, possibly because the XO pattern leads to undifferentiated gonads and female sexual characteristics, whereas the XY complement leads to the formation of male gonads and wolffian ducts. Thus, in combination, a variety of phenotypic effects can be expected, depending on the degree of involvement of these two cell lines. Such mosaicism has been described in phentoypic males and in individuals with ambiguous external genitalia.

True hermaphroditism

Although the majority of true hermaphrodites are sex chromatin–positive, they may exhibit a variety of sex chromosome complements. A number of individuals were reported to have 46 chromosomes with XX chromosome complement or various mosaics such as XX/XY, XX/XXY, XX/XXY/XXYYY.

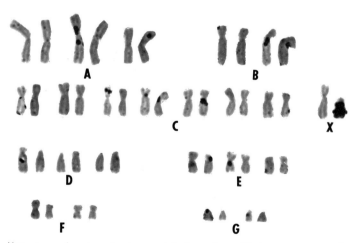

Fig. 23-11. Karyotype showing short-arm deletion of one X chromosome; radioautography shows late labeling of the partially deleted chromosome.

Trisomy, tetrasomy, and pentasomy of X

The presence of extra X chromosomes is compatible with life and produces relatively mild phenotypic changes when compared with autosomal polysomics. Jacobs et al., 1959, described an XXX female who experienced premature menopause. Rather ironically, such subjects were labeled "superfemales." In an XXX chromosomal anomaly, the phenotype varies greatly and the clinical picture ranges from amenorrhea to various menstrual disorders. A number of these patients have relatively normal ovarian function and may bear children without chromosomal abnormalities. Individuals with tetrasomy and pentasomy of X chromosome are characterized mainly by mental retardation.

Y chromosome abnormalities

It has been assumed that the Y chromosome bears a masculinizing factor and that it is necessary for development of the testis. This may hold true, except for the fact that male gonads were found in patients who were true hermaphrodites with XX chromosome complement. However, as emphasized above, possible existence of mosaicism cannot be ruled out and may have played a role in these cases. The Y chromosome behaves to a great extent like the heterochromatic X chromosome.

Numerical aberrations. Sandberg et al.,

1961, described a fertile and phenotypically normal male with 47 chromosomes and an extra Y chromosome. On the other hand, an extra Y chromosome can be found in association with Klinefelter's syndrome. A variety of other numerical abnormalities involving Y chromosomes have been reported such as XXXYY, XX/XYY, and XX/XXY/XXYYY. More recently, accumulated evidence indicates a correlation of XYY sex chromosomal complement with unusual tallness, mental deficiency, and aggressive behavior.

Structural abnormalities. It is difficult to assign any phenotypic abnormality to abnormal Y chromosome morphology, since the Y chromosome classically exhibits a great degree of polymorphism. A small familial Y chromosome was described by Yunis, 1965. An abnormally long Y chromosome (Fig. 23-12) has been observed in individuals with oligospermia and azoospermia (van Wijck et al., 1962; Makino and Muramoto, 1964), as well as in phenotypically normal individuals (Smith and Steinberger, 1963; de la Chapelle et al., 1963). The length of the Y chromosome has been found to be variable among cells from different individuals, as well as among cells within the same individuals. There is, however, some evidence for the existence of heritable large Y chromosome.

Extra chromosomal fragments. The ab-

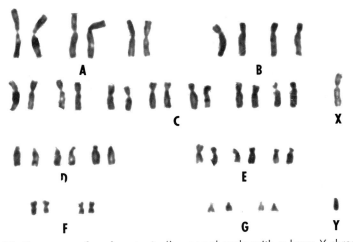

Fig. 23-12. Karyotype of a phenotypically normal male with a large Y chromosome.

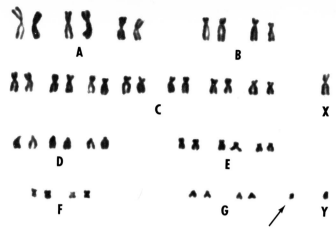

Fig. 23-13. Karyotype of an oligospermic male with an extra centric chromosomal fragment.

normality of extra chromosomal fragments is rare. An acentric chromosomal fragment was reported by Haylock, 1962, in a male infant with multiple congenital anomalies. Vaharu et al., 1961, reported a 4½-year-old female with gonadal dysplasia, 45,XO karyotype, plus a small fragment. Smith et al., 1965, reported a small centric chromosomal fragment (Fig. 23-13) in a male with oligospermia and an otherwise normal karyotype (46,XY). A similar chromosomal fragment was present in the karyotype of this patient's mother.

REFERENCES

Atkins, L., et al.: Ann. Hum. Genet. **29**:89, 1965.

Barr, M. L., et al.: J. Ment. Defic. Res. **6**:65, 1962.

Chicago Conference: Standardization in human cytogenetics; birth defects; original article series vol. II, no. 2, New York, 1966, The National Foundation, March of Dimes.

Court-Brown, W. M., et al.: Lancet **1**:160, 1960.

de la Chapelle, A.: Acta Endocr. Suppl. **65**:9, 1962.

de la Chapelle, A., et al.: Hereditas **50**:351, 1963.

Denver Conference: Ann. Hum. Genet. **24**:319, 1960.

Grumbach, M. M., et al.: Proc. Nat. Acad. Sci. U.S.A. **49**:581, 1963.

Haylock, J.: Conference on Genetics and Mental Retardation, Department of Public Health, New South Wales, Sydney, Australia, 1962, p. 63.

Jacobs, P. A., et al.: Lancet **2**:423, 1959.

Lejeune, J., et al.: C. R. Acad. Sci. (Paris) **248**:1721, 1959.

*Lindsten, J.: The nature and origin of X chromosome aberrations in Turner's syndrome, Uppsala, 1963, Almqvist & Wiksell.

The London Conference on the Normal Human Karyotype: Cytogenetics **2**:264, 1963.

Lyon, M. F.: Amer. J. Hum. Genet. **14**:135, 1962.

Makino, S., and Muramoto, J.: Proc. Japan Acad. **40**:757, 1964.

Marden, P. M., et al.: J. Pediat. **64**:357, 1964.

Moore, K. L., and Barr, M. L.: Acta Anat. **21**:197, 1954.

*Moorehead, P. S., and Nowell, P. C.: Meth. Med. Res. **10**:310, 1964.

Sandberg, A. A., et al.: Lancet **2**:488, 1961.

Scherz, R. G., and Roeckel, J. E.: J. Pediat. **63**:1093, 1963.

Smith, K. D., and Steinberger, E.: J. Einstein Med. Cent. **11**:134, 1963.

Smith, K. D., et al.: Cytogenetics **4**:219, 1965.

Steinberger, A., et al.: J. Einstein Med. Cent. **12**:5, 1964.

Steinberger, E., et al.: J. Clin. Endocr. **25**:1325, 1965.

Steinberger, E., et al.: J. Med. Genet. **3**:226, 1966.

Tjio, J. H., and Levan, A.: Hereditas **42**:1, 1956.

Vaharu, T., et al.: Lancet **1**:1351, 1961.

van Wijck, J. A. M., et al.: Lancet **1**:218, 1962.

Yunis, J. J., editor: Human chromosome methodology, New York, 1965, Academic Press, Inc.

*Significant reviews.

Chapter 24

Endocrine problems of puberty and adolescence

Puberty and adolescence, the transition stages from childhood to adulthood, are characterized by a profound somatic, mental, and emotional metamorphosis. The endocrinologist is primarily concerned with the changes relating to growth and sexual maturation.

GROWTH

The hormonal stimuli to growth have been discussed in previous chapters. Adult stature is the resultant of the rate of growth, the length of growing time, and the genetic background. Growth commences after fertilization of the ovum and ceases when the skeletal epiphyses fuse. The rate of statural increase continously diminishes from birth to sexual maturity, except for a brief spurt that commences with the onset of puberty. In Simmons' study (1944) puberal growth acceleration was observed in girls from age 9 to 12 years and in boys from 11 to 14 years. Maximum growth occurred in the twelfth year in girls and the fourteenth year in boys. The total duration of the puberal growth spurt averages 2 years. The mean yearly growth rate during childhood is approximately 2 inches, but during the growth spurt the rate is 3 inches. Final epiphysial fusion and cessation of linear growth is accomplished from 1 to 3 years after the menarche. During this statural spurt there are anthropometric changes that broaden the hips of girls from about 10 years onward, whereas in boys the hips remain narrow, but the shoulder breadth increases. A number of publications list the changes in anthropometric measurements for each year throughout childhood and adolescence (Stuart, 1946). The time of onset and the magnitude of the adolescent growth spurt vary widely among individual children, but the sequence of events, once initiated, exhibits considerable uniformity. Children with an early growth spurt may complete this phase in approximately 1 year and tend to show a more feminine habitus with broad hips and short legs.

SKELETAL DEVELOPMENT

Roentgenograms of the epiphyses provide an objective marker of the stage of osseous development by comparing the presence of epiphysial centers and the characteristics of the epiphysial lines to the chronologic age of the individual. They are of predictive value in determining the probable growth potential of an adolescent. Bayley et al., 1952, found a high correlation between the skeletal age as read from hand x-ray films and the proportion of adult stature achieved by children 9 or more years of age, and prepared tables for predicting adult height from skeletal age. The radiologist obtains films from several epiphysial centers, since variation from one to the other is characteristic, and by consulting suitable tables (Todd, 1937; Greulich and Pyle, 1959), arrives at an estimate of the *bone age*.

417

Skeletal proportions of particular importance in endocrinology are the height, the upper measurement (crown to symphysis pubis), the lower measurement (symphysis pubis to floor), and the span (distance between fingertips of outstretched hands and arms). In sexually mature adults the span and height are equal (±2 inches) and the upper and lower measurements are approximately equal. In eunuchoid subjects the extremities are long, rendering the span disproportionately greater than the height and the lower segment greater than the upper.

SEXUAL DEVELOPMENT

The mechanism that triggers the onset of hypothalamic-pituitary-gonadal activity is unknown. It is apparently stimulated by central nervous system influences modified by the genetic background of the individual. The removal of a hypothalamic inhibitor to gonadotrophin release has been proposed. A number of investigators have found evidences of gonadotrophic activity in the pituitary glands of immature animals, but there are few quantitative data available for humans through childhood or at the beginning of puberty. Despite the lack of sensitivity of assays for urinary gonadotrophins, there are a few reports of positive assays in prepuberal children. Substantial quantities usually appear in the urine only at the time of puberty. Odell et al., 1966, studied sera by radioimmunassay for LH, with the following average results: 25 eugonadal males, 1.5 mμg./ml.; 12 postmenopausal females, 7.8 mμg./ml.; and 9 prepubertal children, 0.88 mμg./ml. Gonadotrophic hormones are secreted in increasing quantities and stimulate the growth and function of the immature gonad, whose responsiveness to the pituitary hormone may be enhanced.

Male sexual development (Schonfeld, 1943)

The sequence of appearance of the primary and secondary sexual characters is shown in Table 24-1 and Fig. 24-1. Each of these phenomena is initiated at

Table 24-1. Chronologic appearance of primary and secondary sex characters in the male*

Characteristic	Average age in years
Enlargement of testes	
Growth of penis	10½-12½
Growth of prostate, with secretion	
Pubic hair	11-12
Axillary hair, sweat, odor	12-13
Breast and nipple enlargement, subareolar nodule	13-14
Rapid growth of testes and penis	14-17
Downy hair on upper lip	14-15
Voice deepens / Acne	15
Motile, mature sperm	15-16
Beard, full pubic, axillary, and body hair	16-18

*Adapted from data in Schonfeld, W. A.: Amer. J. Dis. Child. **65**:535, 1943; Stuart, H. C.: New Eng. J. Med. **234**:666, 1946; and Wilkins, L.: The diagnosis and treatment of endocrine disorders in childhood and adolescence, ed. 3, Springfield, Ill., 1965, Charles C Thomas, Publisher, p. 201.

the approximate age listed and proceeds in concert with the others at varying rates to full maturity. The beginning of puberty is marked at about age 11½ years (±1 year) by enlargement of the testes, the almost coincidental growth of the penis and prostate, and the appearance of downy pubic hair; and the end is marked by the presence of a deep voice and full growth of axillary, facial, and pubic hair and finally by completion of linear growth.

The stages of sexual development and maturation are shown in Fig. 24-1 and the age distribution of the various stages

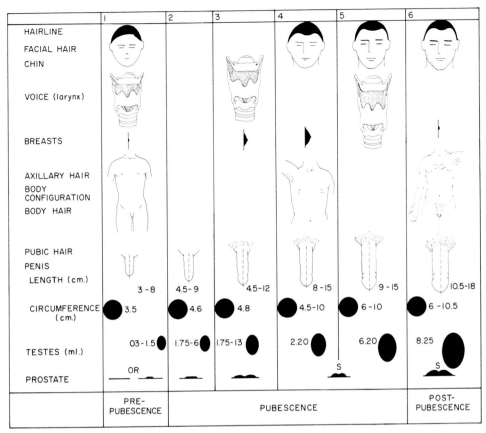

Fig. 24-1. Stages of sexual development and maturation. (From Schonfeld, W. A.: Amer. J. Dis. Child. **65:**535, 1943.)

is shown in Table 24-2 from Schonfeld's study (1943). At puberty the scrotal sac enlarges and becomes more vascular, pigmented, wrinkled, and corrugated, and the distal portion begins to distend to contain the enlarging testes and epididymis. The prostate becomes palpable early in puberty, and a median raphe and palpable lateral lobes become apparent somewhat later. At varying times in early puberty, secretion can be massaged from the prostate, and seminal fluid appears as a nocturnal emission or by masturbation. Pubic hair first appears as a downy growth of villous hair at the base of the penis and suprapubic mound. Later the hair becomes more profuse and curly and extends laterally toward the inguinal region. In the final stage the hair grows over the lower midabdomen and extends to the umbilicus,

forming the typical male escutcheon. Axillary hair begins to grow about 1 year after the first appearance of pubic hair and is shortly accompanied by the secretion of adult axillary sweat and sebaceous secretion. The axilla of the prepubertal male is dry and odorless, whereas that of the adult male is slightly moist, oily, and odoriferous.

Coincidental with the first appearance of axillary hair, fine downy hair grows just inside the corners of the mouth and coarsens as it gradually spreads toward the midline. The sideburns and chin hairs begin to grow shortly thereafter and gradually form a full beard in late adolescence. Temporal recession of scalp hair is a late development, usually beginning at age 16 to 18 years in some boys, later in others. A subareolar firm, often tender plaquelike

Table 24-2. Age distribution, in percent, of the stages of sexual maturation in males*†

Years	Pre-pubescent	2	3	4	5	Fully matured
1-9	100	—	—	—	—	—
10	96	4	—	—	—	—
11	76	12	12	—	—	—
12	44	14	32	10	—	—
13	15	18	38	21	8	—
14	6	15	26	26	27	—
15	—	2	16	22	53	7
16	—	1	9	11	59	20
17	—	—	3	7	39	51
18	—	—	—	7	30	63
19	—	—	—	—	26	74
20-21	—	—	—	—	17	83
22-25	—	—	—	—	—	100

*From Schonfeld, W. A.: Amer. J. Dis. Child. **65**:535, 1943.
†Classes 2 to 5 correspond with Fig. 24-1.

Table 24-3. Chronologic appearance of female sex characteristics

Characteristic	Average age in years
Elevation of breast areolae	
Budding of breasts	10-12
Growth and remodeling of pelvis	
Pubic hair (unpigmented, downy)	10½-12½
Vaginal growth, rugation, cornification	11-12
Axillary hair	12-13
Pubic hair (dense, mature)	12-14
Leukorrhea	12½-13
Menarche	13½

nodule frequently emerges in one or both breasts at 13 to 14 years and usually regresses within 6 to 12 months. Occasionally it persists as "puberal gynecomastia." The voice begins to crack and break at midpuberty and gradually or rapidly drops about one octave in pitch.

Female sexual development

Table 24-3 outlines chronologic female sexual development; more information is given by Stuart, 1946. Before pubarche (appearance of pubic hair) and at a mean age of 10½ years (±1¼ years), the breast areolae become elevated, producing a small conical protuberance on the chest, the "bud stage." Thereafter fat becomes deposited, some glandular tissue may or may not become palpable, and the areolae and nipples become enlarged and pigmented. Normally the menarche follows breast budding by 1 to 3 years. The early appearance of secondary sexual characteristics, however, does not always lead to a precocious menarche but may slowly mature, with menarche occurring at the usual age. Broadening and molding of the pelvic bones and the deposition of subcutaneous fat produce rounding of the hips. Pubic hair develops much as in the male but does not extend to the umbilicus, so that the typical female escutcheon is a triangle with the base at the suprapubic area and the apex toward the perineum. The secretion of a mucoid leukorrhea, the first evidence of mucus-producing cervical glands, usually precedes the menarche by about 6 months (Israel, 1967). The average age of menarche is 13½ years; the range is 11 to 15 years with about 3% above and 3% below these limits. The average age has tended to become younger in succeeding generations probably because of improved nutrition. Menstrual irregularity is common until about 2 years after the menarche, when regular cycles are usually established.

The range of normality is wide, and the differences in the state of maturity of children of the same age are frequently striking. A boy of 14 years may have attained almost full adult stature and sexual development, whereas his companion of the same age may fail to exhibit any sign of puberty; yet both boys are normal. Thus using chronologic age as the sole index of normality during the adolescent years is often misleading. If chronologic age is ignored and the age of either the growth spurt or of the onset of sexual development is substituted, there is considerable uniformity in the sequence of events. The bone age may be a more suitable landmark of the stage of adolescent development.

DELAYED PUBERTY

Normal children occasionally do not exhibit puberal changes until 16 or 17 years of age. When a male fails to initiate sexual development by age 14 or 15 years, or the female by age 13 or 14 years, one must distinguish sexual infantilism from delayed puberty. Many of the boys, and less frequently the girls, have been small throughout childhood and then become short, though not dwarfed, adults. There is often a family history of short stature and perhaps of delay in puberal onset. The differential diagnosis of dwarfism has been discussed on p. 65. Delayed sexual maturation is commonly an associated problem. Some of the clinical and laboratory criteria that may be of help are listed in Table 24-4.

Primordial dwarfs. Although primordial dwarfs (p. 65), who are miniature adults, usually manifest puberal changes at the normal age, there is occasionally some delay that may closely resemble delayed puberty in children of short stature.

Parenchymatous pineal tumor. A parenchymatous pineal tumor exerts an inhibitory effect on the secretion of gonadotrophin-releasing factors and results in sexual infantilism (p. 14).

Hypothalamic lesions. Space-taking or infiltrative lesions interfere with the elaboration of various releasing factors that are necessary for the production of ante-rior pituitary trophic hormones. The resulting clinical picture resembles hypopituitarism. The most common tumor is a craniopharyngioma. Added to sexual infantilism there may be other aspects of hypopituitarism plus signs of hypothalamic disease (p. 78). Sexual infantilism with obesity is called "Fröhlich's syndrome," an extraordinarily rare disorder that is commonly misdiagnosed in obese boys with delayed puberty. The *Laurence-Moon-Biedl* syndrome is discussed on p. 433.

Hypopituitarism. The differential diagnosis from delayed puberty may be difficult and, at times, must await future events before a decision is possible. In hypopituitarism there is permanent sexual infantilism. Usually the patient with pituitary insufficiency is short in stature, physically weak, and lacking in vigor. Some of the differential features are listed in Table 24-4. Martin et al., 1968, described several sexually immature males, age 15 to 18, who failed to demonstrate a normal HGH response to insulin hypoglycemia or arginine but, after androgenic stimulation, responded normally. Thus the growth-promoting effects of androgens may be mediated through enhanced GH release by the pituitary. Observing the effects of administered androgen may prove to be a good test to differentiate hypopituitarism from delayed puberty. Particular difficulty may be encountered in the recognition of isolated loss of gonadotrophins. The patient may appear healthy and attains normal stature but either fails to mature sexually or exhibits some degree of hypogonadism. An organic lesion or various nutritional or emotional factors may lead to failure to secrete gonadotrophins, the most vulnerable type of anterior pituitary hormones. Anorexia nervosa, for example, is often associated with a functional reduction or loss of gonadotrophins. Diseases in which anoxia is a prominent feature, such as chronic anemia and congenital heart or pulmonary disease, can result in various degrees of sexual infantilism or,

Table 24-4. Differential diagnosis of delayed puberty versus various causes of hypogonadism (sexual infantilism)*

	Stature	Other signs of hypopituitarism (Chapter 5)	Urinary gonado-trophin	Plasma HGH	Metyrapone test	Thyroid tests	Adrenocortical tests
Delayed puberty	N or ↓	0	N	N	N	N	N
Primordial dwarfs	↓	0	N	N	N	N	N
Pineal (parenchymatous)	N	0	0	N	N	N	N
Hypothalamic	N or ↓	0 or +	0	N or ↓	↓	N or ↓	N or ↓
Hypopituitary							
Isolated { Deficient GH	↓	0	N	0	N	N	N
Deficient gonadotrophins	N	0	0	N	N	N	N
Panhypopituitarism	↓	+	0	0	↓	↓	↓
Hypothyroid	↓	0	N or 0	N?	N or ↓	↓	N or slightly ↓
Primary testicular failure	N	0	↑	N	N	N	N

*N = normal, ↓ = lower than normal or decreased, ↑ = elevated, + = positive, 0 = none.

at the least, in a markedly delayed onset of puberty.

Hypothyroidism. Juvenile hypothyroidism can impede the onset of puberty and may lead to various degrees of hypogonadal function, depending on the severity of the thyroid deficiency.

Primary testicular disease. The most common cause of male hypogonadism is Klinefelter's syndrome (p. 394). It should be suspected in mentally defective boys with apparent delayed puberty, exceptionally long legs, and small very firm testes and can be proved by finding an XXY karyotype or a mosaic variation.

Treatment

The keystone of therapy is reassurance of both the patient and the parents that, given time, there will be both normal growth and sexual maturity. The lack of any therapeutic agent to date that can augment the stature that the patient will ultimately and spontaneously attain must be discussed. Human growth hormone (HGH) is not available for general use, nor is there evidence to suggest that an endocrinologically normal adolescent can acquire greater stature with HGH injections than nature intended. Thyroid therapy, with or without androgens, has been suggested, but it is doubtful that it exerts any effect if the patient is euthyroid. Androgen therapy or chorionic gonadotrophin in males can usually trigger the initiation of puberty, but careful supervision is necessary to ensure that bone age does not advance disproportionately to height age. A number of synthetic steroids have been designed to dissociate growth-promoting and androgenic effects, but the evidence to substantiate this dichotomy of action has not been established. Where emotional maladjustment is an important consideration in a male who has passed his fifteenth birthday without signs of puberty, cautious therapy is justified. Therapy is not indicated if there is any sign of beginning puberty (pubic down, forehead acne, etc.). Human chorionic gonadotrophin (HCG) is usually favored over testosterone, though it must be given by injection. The dosage is approximately 2,000 units I.M. thrice weekly for not more than 3 months. Prolonged use of HCG may cause testicular degeneration. If the testicle is responsive, it will increase in size and secrete testosterone, resulting in other manifestations of sexual maturation. If there is no response, a second therapeutic trial is justified after a 4-month interval. If again there is no response, a primary testicular defect is probable. If a response that was established is not maintained after injections are completed, a gonadotrophin deficiency is likely. In normal adolescents, once puberal changes are instituted, therapy is omitted and sexual development usually proceeds normally. In lieu of HCG, a testosterone preparation can be used by injection (200 mg. testosterone enanthate every 3 to 4 weeks for 4 months), by buccal tablet (10 mg. methyltestosterone once or twice daily), or orally (2 mg. fluoxymesterone daily). Again the first sign of puberal onset constitutes a signal to stop treatment.

In girls, androgens may cause hirsutism, enlargement of the clitoris, or deepening of the voice, and should be avoided. Estrogen serves as both a growth stimulant and a trigger of the secretion of pituitary gonadotrophins. The daily dosage is 1 mg. of stilbestrol or its equivalent for 3 months, followed by cyclic therapy to induce withdrawal bleeding for another 3 to 6 months. If this trial is unsuccessful, the dosage is doubled in a second trial. If menses are not thereafter established, a gynecologic and endocrine study is mandatory. HCG is not effective, and a potent FSH is not available; human menopausal gonadotrophin (HMG) is rich in FSH but

has not been released for general use.

PRECOCIOUS PUBERTY

Precocious puberty is an uncommon condition defined as the onset of puberty prior to 8 years of age in girls and 10 years of age in boys. Striking examples have been recorded, such as menarche occurring in a 9½-month-old child who had a secretory endometrium at 11½ months of age (Marten et al., 1965) and the famous Lina Medina of Peru, whose menarche was at the age of 8 months and who was delivered by cesarean section of a live infant at the age of 5 years 8 months (Escomel, 1939). In Wilkins' series (1965b), of a total of 893 cases, there were 601 females (67%) and 292 males (33%).

Idiopathic sexual precocity ("constitutional," "cryptogenic"). Idiopathic sexual precocity is the most common form (64% of Wilkins' 893 cases), and accounts for 80% to 90% of cases in girls. Females outnumber males 4 to 1. In a few reported instances, particularly in males, more than one member of a family was affected. The diagnosis is applied to children with premature activation of the hypothalamic–anterior pituitary–gonad pathway in whom no organic lesion can be found. There is, of course, no assurance that a small organic lesion in the region of the hypothalamus that cannot be demonstrated may not masquerade as idiopathic precocity. Liu et al., 1965, described abnormal EEG patterns in 87% of 42 children in whom a diagnosis of idiopathic precocity had been made and suggested that an underlying dysfunction of the central nervous system might prematurely trigger the onset of puberty. It has been demonstrated experimentally that the immature pituitary and the gonad are capable of responding to neural stimuli, so that the onset of puberty is possible at any age.

In this variety of premature sexual maturation, the sequential appearance of sex characters may follow the normal or exhibit unusual patterns and may or may not be greatly accelerated. The females show regular menses, eventually ovulate, and are fertile, and the males produce mature sperm. In both sexes statural growth is accelerated, and the bone age is advanced. Rarely dwarfism occurs.

Neurogenic precocity. Intracranial pathology causing precocity is more common in males than in females (2:1). Lesions are located principally in the posterior hypothalamus, particularly involving the mamillary bodies and tuber cinereum. Gliomas and astrocytomas that invade the third ventricle may cause hydrocephalus and compress the hypothalamus. Craniopharyngiomas most often cause sexual infantilism but may occasionally induce precocity. Hamartomas, localized pea-sized collections of normal nerve tissue, are found in the tuber cinereum. Precocity may occur following various forms of encephalitis and from any variety of infiltrative, invasive, or destructive lesion. The opinion has been held for a number of years that pineal tumors induce precocity only when they impinge on the posterior hypothalamus. However, the recent descriptions (p. 14) of a pineal secretion, melatonin, which inhibits ovarian maturation, may require modification of this hypothesis, though at present the physiologic role of the pineal gland is unknown. Neurogenic precocity follows the same pattern as the idiopathic constitutional variety. There is normal gonadotrophin-induced maturation of the testes, with spermatogenesis, and of the ovaries, with ovulatory menstruation. Positive neurologic findings may be present or absent, depending on the size and location of the lesion. Involvement of the hypothalamus can, in addition, induce a variety of hypothalamic symptoms (p. 12). The prognosis is usually poor because of the nature of the underlying lesion, but there have been long survivals. An example of a subject with hydrocephalus is shown in Fig. 24-2.

Premature thelarche, pubarche, or adrenarche. When bilateral breast hypertrophy occurs unaccompanied by other signs of precocity in the first 2 years of life *(premature thelarche)*, it usually lasts for 12 to 36 months but may occasionally persist until the onset of normal puberty. Nipples and areolae remain small and immature, and there are no other signs of estrogenic stimulation, though examination of desquamated cells in the urinary sediment may show an estrin effect. The cause is unknown, but a transient slight increase of estrogen production together with enhanced breast sensitivity has been suggested. Treatment is unnecessary, but the child should be kept under observation to rule out an organic lesion. Exposure

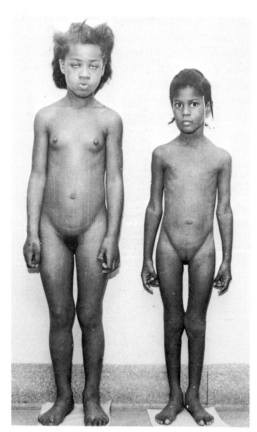

Fig. 24-2. A 7½-year-old female with hydrocephalus and precocious puberty on the left compared to a normal 7-year-old female on the right. Pubic hair was present at birth, menarche occurred at 2 years of age. Weight 61 lb., height 130 cm. Urinary gonadotrophins 6 to 48 mU./24 hr., 17-KS 2.3 mg./24 hr. Vaginal smear showed moderate estrogen effect.

to an estrogenic medication must be ruled out. The premature appearance of pubic and sometimes axillary hair without other manifestations of sexual development has been called "premature pubarche," or "premature adrenarche" when the growth of axillary hair predominates. It is rare in boys. Approximately 2 to 7 years elapse between pubarche and the beginning of breast development. Though the disorder is benign, organic brain lesions and mental retardation may be associated.

Treatment

There is no reliable therapeutic method for retarding the appearance of the manifestations of precocity. Various hormonal agents, particularly the synthetic progestins such as 17α-hydroxy-6α-methylprogesterone acetate (medroxyprogesterone acetate, Depo-Provera), have been ineffective in the hands of most investigators, though thera-

peutic trials are continuing. The parents and the child should be given, when feasible, a simple physiologic explanation of the condition. Menstruation should be explained to sexually precocious girls, preferably before the onset of menarche. Psychologic maladjustment is unusual (Money and Hampson, 1955).

Albright's syndrome. In 1937 Albright et al., and McCune and Bruch, independently described a syndrome that combined a triad of bone lesions, cutaneous pigmentation, and, in the female, precocious puberty. The last has been reported in only 4 males (Benedict, 1962). The bones show painless discrete, spotty, or disseminated replacement of the medullary structure with fibrous tissue producing areas of patchy pseudocystic rarefactions called "polyostotic fibrous dysplasia." Pathologic fractures can occur particularly in the femur. Lesions in the skull differ from the

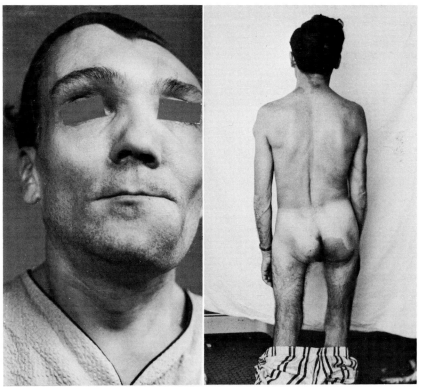

Fig. 24-3. Albright's syndrome in a 47-year-old male. Note skull deformity, asymmetry of face, swelling of left lower jaw from a mandibular tumor (fibrous dysplasia), characteristic pigmentation of back of neck and buttock, and short stature.

other skeletal lesions, in that osteosclerosis with increased density involving the base is characteristic. The thickened bone may cause deformity of the skull (Fig. 24-3), orbit, paranasal sinuses, and nasal passages and may impinge on cranial nerves. Areas of normal bone are found adjacent to areas of pathology, in contrast to the diffuse demineralization of hyperparathyroidism. The pigmentation occurs in the form of isolated dark brown or café-au-lait macules with a jagged, irregular ("coast-of-Maine") border. The macules are usually confined to one side of the midline, may be isolated or arranged in a linear or segmental pattern, and tend to occur most often over one buttock, the sacrum, one thigh, or the back of the neck (Fig. 24-3). Hair on the scalp overlying a lesion shows deeper pigmentation (Benedict et al., 1968). Benedict and his co-workers found that the only certain method of differentiating the skin lesions of Albright's syndrome from those of neurofibromatosis was by finding giant pigment granules in malpighian cells or melanocytes in the latter, whereas they were absent in 9 of 10 cases of Albright's syndrome. The mechanism of the precocious puberty is as unknown as is the etiology of the syndrome. It may well be a genetic disorder, but no hereditary tendency has been found. Only a few cases have been studied at autopsy, and the findings have shed little light on possible causes, though pathology of the hypothalamus has been suspected. Albright and Reifenstein, 1948, found one very small mamillary body and an extra nucleus in the adjacent tissue. Sternberg and Joseph, 1942, described an enlarged pituitary with a basophil adenoma, a parathyroid adenoma, an enlarged thyroid, and slight dilatation of the third ventricle of the brain. Benedict, 1962, studied 20 patients and found 7 cases of hyperthyroidism, 4 nontoxic goiters, and 2 hyperplastic parathyroids (of 4 patients examined).

Gonadal causes of precocious puberty. Granulosa cell tumors of the ovary, discussed on p. 377, are a rare cause of precocity in females. Although they were reported in 65 of 601 females in Wilkins' review, they probably comprise only 1% to 2% of the total. Other ovarian neoplasms are rare causes of precocity, such as teratomas, thecomas, luteomas, and chorionepitheliomas. Pseudopuberty produced precociously in girls by the ingestion of estrogens, particularly stilbestrol, has been reported. Intense dark brown areolar pigmentation of the breasts is a characteristic finding. Since the effect of estrogen on the vaginal epithelium subsides within 14 to 30 days after withdrawal of the hormone, a waiting period of at least 4 weeks is suggested before any definitive diagnostic procedures are pursued. In boys gynecomastia and areolar pigmentation result from exposure to estrogens. *Leydig cell (interstitial cell) tumors of the testes,* discussed on p. 257, were found in 33 of 292 males in Wilkins' review. They inhibit pituitary gonadotrophins, so that the nontumorous testis atrophies and there is no stimulus to spermatogenesis.

Adrenocortical causes of precocity (Chapter 15). Tumors or bilateral adrenal hyperplasia induces "macrogenitosomia praecox" in the male with virilization but suppresses testicular function. In females postnatal virilization occurs rather than premature female precocity.

Hepatomas causing precocity. Hepatomas, being extremely rare, highly malignant tumors of the liver, have been found only in males and induce rapid sexual development. It has been suggested that the tumor generates a chorionic-gonadotrophin–like protein that stimulates Leydig cell function (Wilkins, 1965).

Precocity with hypothyroidism. Hypothyroidism usually retards puberal onset, but sexual precocity has been reported. Replacement thyroid therapy causes regression of sexual development. The finding of an enlarged sella turcica in 10 patients and of enlarged ovaries and galactorrhea in others suggested to Van Wyk and Grumbach, 1960, that excessive gonadotrophin secretion and perhaps mammotrophin were an inappropriate response to thyroid failure.

Diagnostic studies in sexual precocity

Listed are diagnostic studies in sexual precocity:

Female
  History
    Age of onset, speed of development, familial factors, source of exogenous estrogens
  Physical examination
    Especially palpation of breasts for glandular elements, galactorrhea, nipple and areolar development and pigment
    Rectoabdominal exam for palpable tumor, vaginal exam with speculum (anesthesia if necessary)
    Culdoscopy if ovarian tumor is strongly suspected
  Neurologic exam
    Physical, fundoscopy, visual fields; if required, EEG, brain scan, pneumoencephalography, cerebral angiography
  Hormone studies
    Urinary gonadotrophins, estrogens, 17-KS (with suppression test if elevated), plasma and/or urinary testosterone, pregnanediol; vaginal smear and/or urinary sediment exam for estrin effect
Male
  History
    Same as that for female plus history of exogenous androgen, injections of chorionic gonadotrophin
  Physical examination
    Careful palpation of testes for tumor; biopsy if warranted; semen exam if possible
  Neurologic exam
    Same as for female
  Hormone Studies
    Urinary gonadotrophins, estrogens, 17-KS (with suppression if elevated), plasma and/or urinary testosterone

The diagnosis of precocious puberty is confirmed by the finding of gonadotrophins, estrogens, and 17-KS in the urine in keeping with the degree of sexual maturation, but the laboratory's chief value is to exclude other causes of precocity. Sigurjonsdottir and Hayles, 1968, in a large series, often could not detect urinary gonadotrophins when the patient was first seen, though urinary estrogens were positive in the majority of girls and the 17-KS were within the expected normal range.

Potentially dangerous and drastic procedures or exploratory laparotomy should not be employed without significant indications, particularly in females, in whom approximately 90% are of the idiopathic constitutional variety. A waiting period of at least a month should be observed if there is any likelihood of exogenous estrogens causing the precocity. In males there is a strong preponderance of neurogenic lesions.

In females with precocity due to premature gonadotrophin secretion, regular and often ovulatory menstruation occurs, whereas with ovarian and adrenal lesions, the bleeding is anovulatory and irregular. In males with premature gonadotrophin secretion, the testes enlarge and eventually produce mature sperm, whereas in testicular and adrenocortical precocity the testes remain small and produce neither testosterone nor spermatozoa.

For a review of sexual precocity see Jolly, 1955.

REFERENCES

Albright, F., et al.: New Eng. J. Med. **216:**727, 1937.

Albright, F., and Reifenstein, E. C., Jr.: The parathyroid glands and metabolic bone disease, Baltimore, 1948, The Williams & Wilkins Co., p. 269.

Bayley, N.: J. Pediat. **40:**423, 1952.

Benedict, P. H.: Metabolism **11:**30, 1962.

Benedict, P. H., et al.: J.A.M.A. **205:**618, 1968.

Escomel, E.: Presse Med. **47:**1648, 1939.

Greulich, W. W., and Pyle, S. I.: Radiographic atlas of skeletal development of the hand and wrist, ed. 2, Stanford, Calif., 1959, Stanford University Press.

Israel, S. L.: Diagnosis and treatment of menstrual disorders and sterility, ed. 5, New York, 1967, Paul B. Hoeber, Inc., Medical Book Dept. of Harper & Row, Publishers, pp. 66-68.

*Jolly, H.: Sexual precocity, Springfield, Ill., 1955, Charles C Thomas, Publisher.

Liu, N., et al.: J. Clin. Endocr. **25:**1296, 1965.

Marten, D. J., et al.: Amer. J. Obstet. Gynec. **91:**457, 1965.

Martin, L. G., et al.: J. Clin. Endocr. **28:**425, 1968.

McCune, D. J., and Bruch, H.: Amer. J. Dis. Child. **54:**806, 1937.

*Significant reviews.

Money, J., and Hampson, J. G.: Psychosom. Med. **17**:1, 1955.

Odell, W. D., et al.: Metabolism **15**:287, 1966.

Schonfeld, W. A.: Amer. J. Dis. Child. **65**:535, 1943.

Sigurjonsdottir, T. J., and Hayles, A. B.: Amer. J. Dis. Child. **115**:309, 1968.

*Simmons, K.: The Brush Foundation study of child growth and development. II. Physical growth and development. Monogr. Soc. Res. Child. Develop. **9**:1, 1944.

Sternberg, W. H., and Joseph, V.: Amer. J. Dis. Child. **63**:748, 1942.

*Stuart, H. C.: New Eng. J. Med. **234**:666, 693, 732, 1946.

Todd, T. W.: Atlas of skeletal maturation, St. Louis, 1937, The C. V. Mosby Co.

Van Wyk, J. J., and Grumbach, M. M.: J. Pediat. **57**:416, 1960.

Wilkins, L.: The diagnosis and treatment of endocrine disorders in childhood and adolescence, ed. 3, Springfield, Ill., 1965, Charles C Thomas, Publisher, (a) p. 201, (b) p. 226, (c) p. 235.

Chapter 25

Disorders, probably not of endocrine origin, of interest to the endocrinologist

Norman G. Schneeberg, M.D.
Sukhamoy Paul, M.D.

OBESITY

Because obesity almost defies definition, the designation "pathologic overweight" as a description of the excessive accumulation of adipose tissue that characterizes this disorder can be accepted.

Etiology

Obesity results from a positive caloric balance, but other factors appear to play a role.

Genetic-familial factors. Danforth, 1927, described a hereditary tendency to obesity in a strain of yellow mice that was transmitted as a dominant gene, and Ingalls et al., 1950, described a hereditary obese hyperglycemic syndrome in mice that was carried by a recessive gene. Gurney, 1936, found that when both parents were obese, 73% of the offspring were affected, whereas the incidence was 9% when neither parent was obese. If one parent was affected, 41% of the children became obese. The contribution of environmental factors is difficult to negate in familial groups, though studies of twins may be more informative. Newman et al., 1927, found a high correlation of the weight of identical twins, whereas there were significant differences between fraternal twins. Withers, 1964, found less correlation between the weights of adopted children and their foster parents than between the weights of natural offspring and their parents. The dietary habits of certain ethnic groups must undoubtedly contribute to the increased prevalence of obesity of their members.

Central nervous system. Obesity can be produced in animals from bilateral destruction of the ventromedial nuclei (satiety center) of the hypothalamus, or by lesions near the mammillary bodies or tuber cinereum, suprachiasmatic and tuberal lesions, and lesions caudal to the paraventricular nuclei (Fertman, 1955). The human counterpart is rare. Suprasellar lesions such as craniopharyngioma, as well as frontal lobectomy and damage to the frontal cortex, may be associated with obesity. Hyperphagia is a necessary accompaniment of all CNS lesions for weight gain to occur. Han, 1967, observed hypothalamus-damaged rats that did not outgain controls but did accumulate more than twice the amount of body fat. In hypothalamic obesity the mechanism of satiety is impaired.

Emotional and psychologic factors. Food can be used to ameliorate anxiety and tension. Emotional instability is prevalent in obese individuals. Schachter, 1967, Nisbett, 1968, and Stunkard, 1968, have performed ingenious experiments to elucidate the mechanisms that regulate food intake in man. In general, they discovered that obese subjects are governed by different biologic-psychologic drives to food-taking from those of individuals of normal weight. The obese subject rarely experiences hunger, and his desire to eat is governed to a large extent by external circumstances (availability of food, taste, smell, privacy). Impediments to eating result in reduced intake and weight loss. The individual of normal weight is guided by internal factors, eats when he is hungry, and is less affected by external factors.

Socioeconomic factors. An inverse relationship between socioeconomic status and obesity was found in the Midtown Manhattan Study (Srole et al., 1962). The prevalence of obesity in women was 5% in the upper class, 16% in women of "middle status" and 30% in those of the lower socioeconomic level.

Physical activity. A number of studies have shown that obese subjects are considerably less physically active than are lean subjects. In one prolonged observation of adolescent girls (Bullen et al., 1964), it was found that the obese consumed fewer calories than their lean peers, but their physical lethargy accounted for their positive caloric balance. Enforced or voluntary inactivity from illness or aging, unless accompanied by a reduction of caloric intake, results in weight gain.

Endocrine factors. Despite attempts to discover an endocrine cause, none has been forthcoming. Mayer, 1955, proposed a "glucostatic theory" of appetite regulation. The feeding center is stimulated and the satiety mechanism is inhibited by a reduction of glucose utilization by the hypothalamus. Glucose utilization can be reduced by both an increased blood sugar as in diabetes mellitus, or by a reduced blood sugar as in hypoglycemia. Thus various endocrine-metabolic changes can influence appetite and food consumption. A number of endocrine-metabolic aberrations have been discovered but are more likely effect than cause. Obese subjects show an excessive response of immunoreactive insulin and growth hormone (GH) from glucose or glucagon infusions, and the GH response to hypoglycemia, 2-deoxy-D-glucose, exercise, or arginine infusion is blunted (Copinschi et al., 1967). Vallance-Owen, 1965, found an increase of synalbumin antagonism in obesity, resulting in hyperinsulinism. There is insulin insensitivity in obesity, so that hyperinsulinism may be a compensatory metabolic adjustment that favors lipogenesis, reduces lipolysis, and promotes the deposition of fat.

Glucocorticoids can induce truncal obesity; patients with Cushing's syndrome usually gain weight and exhibit a characteristic redistribution of adipose tissue. Nevertheless, there is no evidence that hyperadrenocorticism plays a role in obesity. The weight gain of the hypothyroid subject is due more to deposition of myxedema tissue than of fat. Studies have failed to demonstrate any hypothyroid tendency in obese subjects. The weight gain that accompanies middle age and the menopause is probably more a consequence of physical inactivity combined with the retention of the eating habits of youth than of any hormonal influence. Nevertheless, castration of experimental animals, male eunuchoidism, and the Stein-Leventhal syndrome are often accompanied by obesity that may have a metabolic origin. The ratio of fat to protein is reversed in male hypogonadism, causing a preponderance of fat.

Anthropomorphic and anatomic factors. Seltzer and Mayer, 1964, found that although obese adolescent girls were not somatotypically homogeneous there was a distinct preponderance of endomorphism (abdominal mass overshadows thoracic bulk, all regions are notable for softness and roundness, hands and feet are relatively small) and mesomorphism (massive muscular chest, strong muscular relief, prominent body joints), and considerably less ectomorphism (slender, lanky, thin, delicate bone structure and stringy muscular development). They suggested that a prime requisite for the development of obesity was at least a moderate amount of endomorphy that predisposes to the accumulation of fat. Hirsch et al., 1966, found that obese subjects had double the number of adipocytes compared to subjects of normal weight despite the fact that their number is constant in human adults.

Diagnosis

The height-weight tables devised according to sex, age, and body build have certain limitations. The mesomorph (often a wrestler or football player) may be mistakenly labeled overweight because of a large skeletal and muscle mass. As individuals age, their weight may not change, though muscle is gradually replaced by fat. A number of methods such as densitometry, whole body ^{40}K, or determination of specific gravity by underwater weighing have been devised to gauge the ratio of fat to protein tissue. A practical method is the use of skin-fold calipers usually applied to the triceps region and comparison of the results with standard tables such as those of Tanner and Whitehouse, 1962. According to Mayer, 1959, obesity is a valid diagnosis when a male's fat content exceeds 25% to 30% or a female's 30% to 35% of body weight.

Differential diagnosis. In the majority of patients, obesity is a "simple" uncomplicated disorder. One must be on the alert to recognize certain specific categories, however:

1. Cushing's syndrome. The differential has been discussed in Chapter 14.

2. Myxedema. See Chapter 9.

3. Hyperinsulinism. Occasionally a functioning pancreatic adenoma may provoke weight gain because of the lipogenic action of insulin and because the patient learns that frequent eating averts symptoms.

4. Hypothalamic lesion. A suprasellar lesion can provoke hyperphagia.

5. Stein-Leventhal syndrome. The Stein-Leventhal syndrome should be suspected when obesity is associated with anovulatory oligomenorrhea or amenorrhea and mild hirsutism.

Complications. Life insurance statistics have documented the increased mortality rate of the obese, an increase that is positively correlated with the severity of the disorder. Obesity is associated with an increased mortality from cardiovascular-renal disease, diabetes mellitus, infections, cancer, and accidents. Atherosclerosis is twice as common among autopsied obese subjects as compared to the poorly nourished. The prevalence, mortality, and morbidity of coronary heart disease is greater in obese-hypertensive subjects than in non–obese-hypertensive patients. (Kannel et al., 1967). Obesity exerts an adverse effect upon almost every category of human pathology; increases the risk associated with anesthesia, surgery, and obstetrical delivery; promotes the onset of degenerative arthritis of spine, hips, and knees and of varicosities; and contributes to the onset of various gastrointestinal disorders, particularly of the biliary tract, and the onset of hiatal hernia. The most serious consequence is the *Pickwickian syndrome,* characterized by somnolence, alveolar hypoventilation, CO_2 retention, hypoxia, secondary polycythemia, pulmonary hypertension, and heart failure. There is limited diaphragmatic excursion and conversion of the normally resilient thoracic cage into a more rigid, immobile structure.

Treatment

The goal is to effect a negative caloric balance by reducing intake and increasing expenditure. Because obesity often commences in childhood and adolescence, vigorous treatment of the young to prevent chronicity is important. The obese customarily omit breakfast, eat little or no lunch, and become interested in food late in the day and in the evening. They therefore tend to ingest their total daily caloric intake in a short span of time. Cohn, 1961, demonstrated experimentally that consumption of full spaced meals, as contrasted to equicaloric nibbling of frequent small meals, results in increased body fat, decreased body protein and water, altered thyroid and tissue enzymatic activities, increased atherosclerosis, and increased severity of diabetes.

Diet therapy. Reproductions of low calorie diets are ubiquitous and will not be included in this discussion. They must provide adequate protein (0.75 to 1 gram/kg.) but will usually be deficient in certain vitamins, so that supplements are necessary for long-continued dieting. The total calorie content is the critical factor; there is no evidence to sustain the notion that diets of a certain specific composition of fat, protein, or carbohydrate are determining factors of success. The speed of weight loss is conditioned by the size of the deficit, provided that calorie expenditure remains relatively constant. The predictability of weight loss may be used to foster the patient's cooperation. Weight loss does not follow a smooth downward curve with equal daily decrements but is characterized by short bursts of fluid loss, especially in the first or second week, interspersed with plateaus of a few days up to 2 weeks, during which fluid is retained and there is little or no weight change. Several approaches have been advocated:

1. *Moderate restriction* is the provision of 1,000 to 1,500 calories daily or a deficit of 500 to 1,000 calories. By using the caloric requirement of the average subject, usually about 35 cal./kg. for a sedentary worker, one can calculate a diet with the desired deficit.

2. *Semistarvation* diets provide 300 to 600 cal./day and should contain 50 grams of protein. They result in more rapid weight loss with little hunger. In the first few days a marked water and solute (Na, K) diuresis occurs, with a fall of plasma volume and blood pressure. Orthostatic hypotension may result and constitutes a hazard to patients with coronary heart disease or cerebral vascular insufficiency. Ketonemia, a not uncommon occurrence, suppresses hunger.

3. *Total fasting* (Bloom, 1959; Duncan, 1965) may be a necessary measure in subjects refractory to more conventional

regimens. The fast is continued for 7 to 14 days preferably in the hospital. Noncaloric fluids (artificially sweetened drinks, water, tea, coffee, carbonated water) are permitted ad lib. Supplementary vitamins are given and sedation is prescribed when necesary. Anorexia is fostered by the accompanying ketonemia. Hyperuricemia can provoke gout in susceptible patients; probenecid is prescribed as a prophylactic. When the fast is terminated, a low calorie diet is prescribed together with one fast day per week.

4. *Formula diets* can be devised as liquid or solid nutrient mixtures and may be useful in the initial stage of treatment.

5. *Psychologic assistance* and even psychotherapy may be helpful or necessary in emotionally disturbed subjects. Stuart, 1967, has manipulated the environmental situation of eating and has reported excellent results. Group therapy provides a sympathetic setting for discussion of problems of weight reduction and introduces an element of competition.

6. *Small-intestine bypass operations* have been employed in seriously obese subjects to reduce the absorption of foodstuffs. The method is experimental.

Drug therapy. Most patients insist on receiving anorexigenic compounds. Many admit that this was the principal reason for consulting a physician. These compounds, mainly amphetamines, supposedly act on the hypothalamus and cerebral cortex to reduce appetite, speed up the experience of satiety, and induce euphoria. They are not universally effective; the anorectic effect, when experienced, is usually transient. Discontinuance may cause a psychologic letdown, fatigue, and occasionally depression. Diuretics tend to eliminate plateaus in the weight reduction curve by promoting water excretion but do not affect the ultimate result. They are useful in patients who suffer from "idiopathic edema" and obesity. Thyroid therapy is effective only if it produces substantial hypermetabolism (iatrogenic) and may therefore be dangerous.

Exercise. The value of increased physical

activity has only recently been emphasized. It is especially important to engender habits of regular exercise in the young.

Contraindications to weight reduction

There are scarcely any absolute contra-indications. Tuberculosis, Addison's disease, ulcerative colitis, active peptic ulcer, and malignancy are usually cited but are rarely encountered in obese individuals. Moderate weight reduction is a safe procedure during pregnancy, childhood, and adolescence if carefully supervised. Starvation diets are best avoided in gout because of hyperuricemia and in cardio- and cerebrovascular disorders because of orthostatic hypotension. Rarely depression or psychosis is precipitated.

Prognosis

The outlook for permanent weight reduction is poor. Stunkard and McLaren-Hume, 1959, reviewed eight published reports comprising 1,368 obese subjects. Forty-five percent of subjects lost less than 10 lb., 27% lost 10 to 20 lb., 28% lost more than 20 lb., and only 8% lost more than 40 lb. The best results were obtained by Feinstein et al., 1958; 31% lost more than 40 lb. using a 900-calorie formula diet. In Stunkard and McLaren-Hume's study of 100 of their own patients, only 2 maintained their weight loss after 2 years.

LAURENCE-MOON-BIEDL SYNDROME

In the Laurence-Moon-Biedl syndrome there is mental retardation, obesity, retinitis pigmentosa, polydactyly, and hypogonadism. The mode of inheritance is autosomal recessive. The hypogonadism may be due to pituitary or primary gonadal deficiency and several patients have shown sex-chromosome abnormalities. No consistent anatomic lesion has been found at autopsy.

MARFAN'S SYNDROME
(ARACHNODACTYLY)

Marfan's syndrome, presumed to be a genetic deficiency of mesodermal tissue, is characterized by excessively long, slender extremities, spiderlike fingers, poor muscular development, cardiovascular lesions (usually cardiac septal defects or dissecting aneurysm), pulmonary anomalies, and subluxation of the ocular lens. Various endocrine abnormalities have been described, but they probably play no causative role.

PROGERIA
(HUTCHINSON-GILFORD SYNDROME)

Progeria, a bizarre disorder of unknown etiology, is characterized by the rapid onset of senility in an individual with a life-span of 10 to 15 years, ending in coronary occlusion or hemiplegia. There is failure to gain weight, loss of hair by 2 years of age, and dwarfism. All subjects show a striking resemblance, with a small face, hydrocephalic look, prominent eyes, absence of eyebrows and lashes, atrophic inelastic skin, absent subcutaneous fat, thin limbs, poorly developed muscles, arthritic changes, and an I.Q. that is normal or above normal.

WERNER'S SYNDROME

Werner's syndrome, inherited as an autosomal recessive, is characterized by growth retardation, absence of the adolescent growth spurt, premature graying of the hair, premature baldness, alterations of the voice, cataracts, atrophy and hyperkeratosis of the skin, ulcerations of the skin of the feet, hypogonadism, vascular calcification, osteoporosis, a tendency to diabetes mellitus, and hypogonadism.

REFERENCES

Bloom, W. L.: Metabolism 8:214, 1959.
Brozek, J.: Body measurements, including skinfold thickness as indicators of body composition, techniques for measuring body composition, 1961, National Academy of Science—National Research Council.
Bullen, G. A., et al.: Amer. J. Clin. Nutr. **14:** 211, 1964.
Cohn, C.: J. Amer. Diet. Ass. 38:433, 1961.
Copinschi, G., et al.: Metabolism 16:485, 1967.
Danforth, C. H.: J. Hered. **18:**153, 1927.

*Significant reviews.

Duncan, G. G., et al.: Postgrad. Med. **38**:523, 1965.

Feinstein, A. R., et al.: Ann. Intern. Med. **48**: 330, 1958.

*Fertman, M. B.: Arch. Intern. Med. **95**:794, 1955.

Gurney, R.: Arch. Intern. Med. **57**:577, 1936.

Han, P. W.: Trans. N. Y. Acad. Sci. **30**:229, 1967.

Hirsch, J., et al.: J. Clin. Invest. **45**:1023, 1966.

Ingalls, A. M., et al.: J. Hered. **41**:317, 1950.

Kannel, W. B., et al.: Circulation **35**:734, 1967.

Mayer, J.: Ann. N. Y. Acad. Sci. **63**:68, 1955.

Mayer, J.: Postgrad. Med. **25**:469, 1959.

Newman, H. H., et al.: Twins, a study of heredity and environment, Chicago, 1937, University of Chicago Press.

Nisbett, R. E.: Science **159**:1254, 1968.

*Schachter, S.: Biology and behavior: neurophysiology and emotion—cognitive effects on bodily functioning. In Glass, D. C., editor: studies of obesity and eating; New York, 1967, The Rockefeller University Press p. 117.

Seltzer, C. C., and Mayer, J.: J.A.M.A. **189**:677, 1964.

Srole, L., et al.: Mental health in the metropolis: midtown Manhattan study, vol. 1, New York, 1962, McGraw-Hill Book Co.

Stuart, R. B.: Behavior Res. Ther. **5**:357, 1967.

Stunkard, A., and McLaren-Hume, M.: Arch. Intern. Med. **103**:79, 1959.

*Stunkard, A. J.: Fed. Proc. **27**:1367, 1968.

Tanner, J. M., and Whitehouse, R. H.: Brit. Med. J. **155**:446, 1962.

Vallance-Owen, J.: Ann. N. Y. Acad. Sci. **131**: 315, 1965.

Withers, R. F. J.: Eugen. Rev. **56**:81, 1964.

Appendix

ABBREVIATIONS

ACI adrenocortical insufficiency.
ACTH adrenocorticotrophic hormone, cortico-trophin.
ADH antidiuretic hormone, vasopressin.
AIU absolute iodine uptake.
AMP, see **C-AMP.**
ASR aldosterone secretion rate.
ATP adenosine triphosphate.
B, see Compound B.
BEI butanol-extractable iodine.
BMR basal metabolic rate.
B.P. blood pressure.
BUN blood urea nitrogen.
Ca calcium.
Ca⁺⁺ calcium ion.
CAH congenital adrenal hyperplasia.
C-AMP cyclic adenosine-3′,5′-monophosphate, cyclic 3′,5′-AMP.
CBG cortisol-binding globulin.
C.F.T. complement-fixing thyroid antibody.
CGTT corticosteroid glucose tolerance test.
Cl chloride.
CNS central nervous system.
Compound B corticosterone.
Compound E cortisone.
Compound F cortisol, hydrocortisone, Kendall's compound F.
Compound S deoxycortisol, desoxycortisol, 11-deoxycortisol, Compound S of Reichstein.
C$_p$ phosphate clearance.
CRF corticotrophin releasing factor.
CSF cerebrospinal fluid.
CSR cortisol secretion rate.
C-TBP cellular thyroxine-binding protein.
D&C dilatation and curettage.
DCA desoxycorticosterone acetate.
DFP diisopropyl fluorophosphate.
DHEA dehydroepiandrosterone.
D.I. diabetes insipidus.
DIT diiodotyrosine.

DNA deoxyribonucleic acid.
DOC desoxycorticosterone.
DOPA 3,4-dihydroxyphenylalanine.
DUB disfunctional uterine bleeding.
E epinephrine.
E, see Compound E.
ECF extracellular fluids.
ECG electrocardiogram.
EDTA ethylenediaminetetraacetic acid sodium salt, edetic acid, Versene, Disodium Edetate Injection U.S.P.
EEG electroencephalogram.
EKG, see **ECG.**
EPF exophthalmos-producing factor.
EPS exophthalmos-producing substance.
ET₃ T₃ red cell (erythrocyte) test.
FBG fasting blood glucose.
F, see Compound F.
FFA free fatty acids.
5-HIAA 5-hydroxyindole acetic acid.
5-HT serotonin, 5-hydroxytryptamine.
5-HTP 5-hydroxytryptophan.
FRF follicle-stimulating hormone releasing factor.
FSH follicle-stimulating hormone.
GFR glomerular filtration rate.
GH growth hormone, somatotrophin.
G1P glucose-1-phosphate.
GRF growth hormone releasing factor.
G6P glucose-6-phosphate.
GTT glucose tolerance test.
H⁺ hydrogen ion.
HCG human chorionic gonadotrophin.
HGH human growth hormone.
HMG human menopausal gonadotrophin.
HPFSH human pituitary follicle-stimulating hormone.
HPG human pituitary gonadotrophin.
HypoP hypoparathyroidism.
ICD isocitric dehydrogenase.
ICSH interstitial cell–stimulating hormone.
IdHypoP idiopathic hypoparathyroidism.

435

I.M. intramuscular.
IP inorganic phosphate.
I.U. international unit.
I.V. intravenous.
K potassium.
LATS long-acting thyroid stimulator.
LDH lactic acid dehydrogenase.
LH luteinizing hormone.
LRF luteinizing hormone releasing factor.
LTH luteotrophic hormone, luteotrophin, prolactin, lactogenic hormone, mammatrophic hormone.
MAO monamine oxidase.
μCi, μc. microcurie.
mCi, mc. millicurie.
MEAS multiple endocrine adenoma syndrome.
mEq. milliequivalent.
Mg magnesium.
μg. microgram.
MHPG methoxyhydroxyphenyl glycol.
MI maturation index.
MIF MSH-inhibiting factor.
MIT monoiodotyrosine.
mμg. millimicrogram, nanogram.
MN metanephrine.
mOsm milliosmole.
mRNA messenger ribonucleic acid.
msec. millisecond.
MSH-RF, MRF melanocyte-stimulating hormone releasing factor.
MSH melanocyte-stimulating hormone, melanotrophin, intermedin.
mU. milliunit.
M.U. Mouse unit.
mv. millivolt.
Na sodium.
NAD nicotinamide adenine dinucleotide.
NADP nicotinamide adenine dinucleotide phosphate.
NE norepinephrine.
ng. nanogram, millimicrogram.
NMN normetanephrine.
NPH neutral protamine Hagedorn.
O oxytocin.
OGTT oral glucose tolerance test.
PA primary aldosteronism.
PAH para-aminohippurate.
PAS periodic acid–Schiff stain.
PBI, PB^{131}I protein-bound iodine (or with radioactive iodine).
PEI phosphate excretion index.
PHP primary hyperparathyroidism.
PIF prolactin inhibiting factor.
PII plasma inorganic iodide.
PMS, PMSG pregnant mare serum gonadotrophin.
P.O. orally (per os).
PO$_4$ phosphate.
PPBG postprandial blood glucose.
PRA plasma renin activity.
PS Porter-Silber reaction.

Pseudo-HP pseudohyperparathyroidism.
PTE parathyroid extract.
PTH parathyroid hormone.
PTU propylthiouracil.
PTX parathyroidectomy.
P.V. paraventricular.
q.s. sufficient quantity
R roentgen.
RAI radioactive iodine.
RAIU radioactive iodine uptake.
RBC red blood cell (count).
RF releasing factor.
RNA ribonucleic acid.
S, *see* Compound S.
SA secondary aldosteronism.
S.D. standard deviation.
S.E. standard error.
17-KGS 17-ketogenic steroids.
17-KS 17-ketosteroids, 17-oxosteroids.
17-OHCS 17-hydroxycorticosteroids, 17-hydroxycorticoids.
SGOT serum glutamic oxaloacetic transaminase.
SH pseudohypoparathyroidism.
SHP secondary hyperparathyroidism.
SIP serum inorganic phosphate.
S.O. supraoptic.
SRF somatotrophin-releasing factor, GRF.
SSH pseudo-pseudohypoparathyroidism.
Stat. immediately.
STH growth hormone, somatotrophic hormone, somatotrophin.
T$_4$, L-T$_4$ thyroxine, levo-thyroxine.
T$_3$, L-T$_3$ triiodothyronine, levo-triiodothyronine, liothyronine.
T$_3$-RBC (ET$_3$) triiodothyronine erythrocyte test.
T$_3$-resin triiodothyronine resin test.
T$_2$ diiodothyronine.
TBG thyroxine-binding globulin.
TBP thyroxine-binding protein.
TBPA thyroxine-binding prealbumin.
TCT thyrocalcitonin, calcitonin.
Tetrac tetraiodothyroacetic acid.
TH thyroid hormones.
THS tetrahydrodeoxycortisol.
Tm tubular maximum reabsorption or maximum tubular reabsorption.
TmP, TmPO$_4$ Tm of phosphate.
TPN triphosphopyridine nucleotide.
TPNH reduced triphosphopyridine nucleotide.
TPTX thyroparathyroidectomy.
TRC tanned red blood cell agglutination.
TRF thyrotrophin-releasing factor.
Triac triiodothyroacetic acid.
Triprop triiodothyropropionic acid.
TRP tubular reabsorption of phosphate.
TSH thyroid-stimulating hormone, thyrotrophin.
U. unit.
UDPG uridine diphosphoglucose.
VMA vanillylmandelic acid.
WBC white blood cell (count).

Index